Equitable and Inclusive Care in Pediatrics

A Compendium of AAP Clinical Practice Guidelines and Policies

With a Foreword by Joseph L. Wright, MD, MPH, FAAP

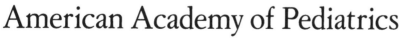

American Academy of Pediatrics

DEDICATED TO THE HEALTH OF ALL CHILDREN®

American Academy of Pediatrics Publishing Staff

Mary Lou White, *Chief Product and Services Officer/SVP, Membership, Marketing, and Publishing*

Mark Grimes, *Vice President, Publishing*

Carrie Peters, *Editor, Professional/Clinical Publishing*

Leesa Levin-Doroba, *Production Manager, Practice Management*

Soraya Alem, *Digital Production Specialist*

Sara Hoerdeman, *Marketing and Acquisitions Manager, Consumer Products*

Published by the American Academy of Pediatrics

345 Park Blvd

Itasca, IL 60143

Telephone: 630/626-6000

Facsimile: 847/434-8000

www.aap.org

The American Academy of Pediatrics is an organization of 67,000 primary care pediatricians, pediatric medical subspecialists, and pediatric surgical specialists dedicated to the health, safety, and well-being of all infants, children, adolescents, and young adults.

The recommendations in this publication do not indicate an exclusive course of treatment or serve as a standard of medical care. Variations, taking into account individual circumstances, may be appropriate.

Any websites, brand names, products, or manufacturers are mentioned for informational and identification purposes only and do not imply an endorsement by the American Academy of Pediatrics (AAP). The AAP is not responsible for the content of external resources. Information was current at the time of publication.

This publication has been developed by the American Academy of Pediatrics. The contributors are expert authorities in the field of pediatrics. No commercial involvement of any kind has been solicited or accepted in the development of the content of this publication.

Every effort has been made to ensure that the drug selection and dosages set forth in this publication are in accordance with the current recommendations and practice at the time of publication. It is the responsibility of the health care professional to check the package insert of each drug for any change in indications or dosage and for added warnings and precautions.

Every effort is made to keep *Equitable and Inclusive Care in Pediatrics: A Compendium of AAP Clinical Practice Guidelines and Policies* consistent with the most recent advice and information available from the American Academy of Pediatrics.

Please visit www.aap.org/errata for an up-to-date list of any applicable errata for this publication.

Special discounts are available for bulk purchases of this publication. Email Special Sales at nationalaccounts@aap.org for more information.

Printed in the United States of America

9-510/0624   1 2 3 4 5 6 7 8 9 10

MA1143

ISBN: 978-1-61002-747-2

eBook: 978-1-61002-748-9

Cover and publication design by LSD DESIGN LLC

Library of Congress Control Number: 2023951230

Clinical practice guidelines have long provided physicians with evidence-based decision-making tools for managing common pediatric conditions. Policy statements issued by the American Academy of Pediatrics (AAP) are developed to provide physicians with a quick reference guide to the AAP position on child health care issues. We have combined these 2 authoritative resources into 1 comprehensive manual to provide easy access to important clinical and policy information.

This manual contains an AAP clinical practice guideline, as well as AAP policy statements and clinical reports. Abstracts are included for online clinical practice guidelines, policy statements, and clinical reports and are linked by a QR code or URL.

Additional information about AAP policy can be found in a variety of professional publications such as *Pediatric Clinical Practice Guidelines & Policies,* 24th Edition; *Red Book®,* 33rd Edition; and *Red Book® Online* (http://redbook.solutions.aap.org).

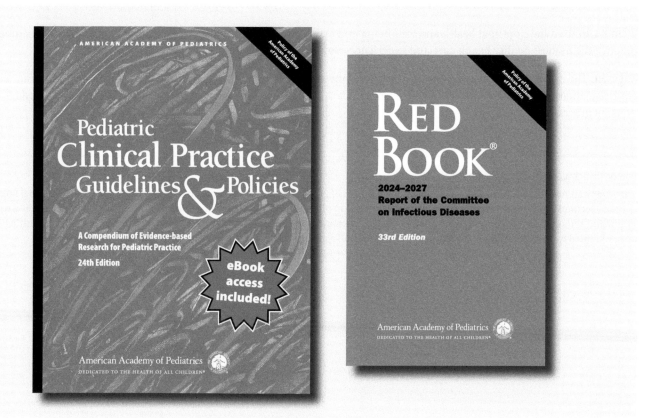

The American Academy of Pediatrics (AAP) and its member pediatricians dedicate their efforts and resources to the health, safety, and well-being of infants, children, adolescents, and young adults. The AAP has approximately 67,000 members in the United States, Canada, and Latin America. Members include pediatricians, pediatric medical subspecialists, and pediatric surgical specialists.

Core Values. We believe

- In the inherent worth of all children; they are our most enduring and vulnerable legacy.
- Children deserve optimal health and the highest quality health care.
- Pediatricians, pediatric medical subspecialists, and pediatric surgical specialists are the best qualified to provide child health care.
- Multidisciplinary teams including patients and families are integral to delivering the highest quality health care.
- The AAP is the organization to advance child health and well-being and the profession of pediatrics.

Vision. Children have optimal health and well-being and are valued by society. American Academy of Pediatrics members practice the highest quality health care and experience professional satisfaction and personal well-being.

Mission. The mission of the AAP is to attain optimal physical, mental, and social health and well-being for all infants, children, adolescents, and young adults. To accomplish this mission, the AAP shall support the professional needs of its members.

Equity, Diversity, and Inclusion Statement

The American Academy of Pediatrics is committed to principles of equity, diversity, and inclusion in its publishing program. Editorial boards, author selections, and author transitions (publication succession plans) are designed to include diverse voices that reflect society as a whole. Editor and author teams are encouraged to actively seek out diverse authors and reviewers at all stages of the editorial process. Publishing staff are committed to promoting equity, diversity, and inclusion in all aspects of publication writing, review, and production.

CONTENTS

SECTION 9
Obesity and Overweight

SECTION 10
Pediatric Workforce

SECTION 11
Socioeconomic Factors

SECTION 12
Substance Use Disorders and Substance Use Prevention

SECTION 13
Trauma-Informed Care and the Effects of Armed Conflict on Children

SECTION 14
Vulnerable and Exploited Youth

The American Academy of Pediatrics (AAP) has long addressed care delivery in its clinical practice guidelines and policy statements directed at populations of children and adolescents who may be uniquely marginalized or historically minoritized based on particular diagnoses or conditions, socioeconomic circumstances, sexual orientation, and/or racial or ethnic identity. A significant proportion of contemporary pediatric practice involves navigating systems of care on behalf of children and their families that may reside outside of the immediate longitudinal trajectory of the primary care or office-based setting. In fact, more than 40 years ago, former AAP President Dr Robert Haggerty coined the phrase "the new morbidities" to capture the profound effect that the increasing emergence of chronic health conditions, intellectual differences, physical disabilities, substance use disorders, vulnerable and exploited youth, and other of the myriad social drivers of health were specifically having on the practice of pediatrics and on the state of child health in general. Further, with the ever-increasing racial and ethnic diversification of the population of children younger than 18 years in the United States (ie, less than 50% white non-Hispanic), focus on the health and well-being of Black, Indigenous, and People of Color is paramount. This compendium takes a broad swath of content related to the delivery of equitable and inclusive care as chronicled in more than 50 clinical practice guidelines and policies and coalesces them across 14 topically related sections. The comprehensive nature of the material that comprises this compendium renders it valuable both as an encyclopedic reference as well as a modular education resource based on how the array of statements are organized into focused topics.

All the included statements represent active peer-reviewed and evidence-informed AAP clinical guidance or policy. Notably, several of the sections contain newly authored or recently revised statements that have been published within the last few years. Similarly, several of the statements have been recently reaffirmed, along with their original recommendations, within that same time frame.

Beginning with the "AAP Diversity and Inclusion Statement," the principles that link all the content in this publication together are part of the unwavering and mission-driven AAP commitment to equity, diversity, and inclusion. While, indeed, each of the different sections brings together distinct statements that share topically related content, identifying inequities in care delivery and the potential for resultant health disparities is a unifying theme that undergirds all the compendium's contributions. Further, acknowledgment and respect for the effect of differential lived experiences, especially as it relates to bias, discrimination, or racism, also grounds the content.

Lastly, this collection emphasizes meeting children and their families where they are regardless of circumstance, identity, historical disposition, condition, or diagnosis. Providing equitable and inclusive care certainly depends on working knowledge of what it means, for example, to be trauma informed or race conscious in approaches to care delivery. This compendium successfully places access to the latest science and thought leadership on content that is vital to pediatric care all in one place. By doing so, this collection also establishes an appreciation for the potential effect on health status of intersecting circumstances, identities, and/or social drivers on clinical outcomes for all children.

Joseph L. Wright, MD, MPH
Chief Health Equity Officer/SVP, Equity Initiatives
American Academy of Pediatrics

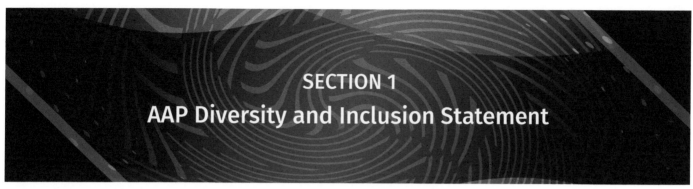

SECTION 1
AAP Diversity and Inclusion Statement

Some articles are available online only; scan the QR code to access online content.

POLICY STATEMENT Organizational Principles to Guide and Define the Child Health Care System and/or Improve the Health of all Children

American Academy
of Pediatrics

DEDICATED TO THE HEALTH OF ALL CHILDREN™

AAP Diversity and Inclusion Statement

The vision of the American Academy of Pediatrics (AAP) is that all children have optimal health and well-being and are valued by society and that AAP members practice the highest quality health care and experience professional satisfaction and personal well-being. From the founding of the AAP, pursuing this vision has included treasuring the uniqueness of each child and fostering a profession, health care system, and communities that celebrate all aspects of the diversity of each child and family.

The AAP appreciates that children are increasingly diverse, with differences that may include race, ethnicity, language spoken at home, religion, disability and special health care need, socioeconomic status, sexual orientation, gender identity, and other attributes.

The AAP, as an organization of pediatricians, pediatric medical subspecialists, and pediatric surgical specialists, recognizes that our membership is composed of a broad and diverse community. The AAP is strengthened by our diversity. The variety of skills, characteristics, and attributes offered by our members creates the vitality and success of the Academy and improves the care of all children and youth. Maximizing the diversity of our members and leaders allows the AAP to benefit from the rich talents and different perspectives of these individuals.

The AAP, as a national nonprofit organization, fervently respects, values, and promotes diversity and inclusiveness among all the individuals, groups, and vendors with whom we interact, collaborate, and partner.

The AAP is committed to being a learning organization that recruits, supports, and promotes talented, diverse individuals as employees and to fostering a work environment that embraces and celebrates diversity, promotes inclusiveness, and treats all employees with dignity and respect.

Celebrating the diversity of children and families and promoting nurturing, inclusive environments means actively opposing intolerance, bigotry, bias, and discrimination. The AAP is committed to using policy, advocacy, and education to encourage inclusivity and cultural effectiveness for all.

Policy statements from the American Academy of Pediatrics benefit from expertise and resources of liaisons and internal (AAP) and external reviewers. However, policy statements from the American Academy of Pediatrics may not reflect the views of the liaisons or the organizations or government agencies that they represent.

The guidance in this statement does not indicate an exclusive course of treatment or serve as a standard of medical care. Variations, taking into account individual circumstances, may be appropriate.

All policy statements from the American Academy of Pediatrics automatically expire 5 years after publication unless reaffirmed, revised, or retired at or before that time.

DOI: https://doi.org/10.1542/peds.2018-0193

PEDIATRICS (ISSN Numbers: Print, 0031-4005; Online, 1098-4275).

COMPANION PAPER: A companion to this article can be found online at www.pediatrics.org/cgi/doi/10.1542/peds.2018-0177.

ABBREVIATION

AAP: American Academy of
    Pediatrics

To cite: AAP Diversity and Inclusion Statement. *Pediatrics.* 2018;141(4):e20180193

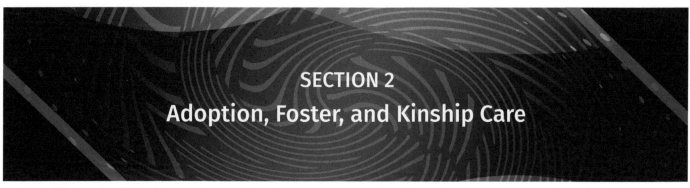

SECTION 2
Adoption, Foster, and Kinship Care

Some articles are available online only; scan the QR code to access online content.

CLINICAL REPORT Guidance for the Clinician in Rendering Pediatric Care

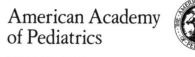

American Academy
of Pediatrics

DEDICATED TO THE HEALTH OF ALL CHILDREN®

Pediatrician Guidance in Supporting Families of Children Who Are Adopted, Fostered, or in Kinship Care

Veronnie F. Jones, MD, MSPH, FAAP,[a] Elaine E. Schulte, MD, MPH, FAAP,[b] Douglas Waite, MD, FAAP,[c] COUNCIL ON FOSTER CARE, ADOPTION, AND KINSHIP CARE

abstract

The child welfare system strives to provide children and adolescents in foster care with a safe, nurturing environment through kinship and nonkinship foster care placement with the goal of either reunification with birth parents or adoption. Pediatricians can support families who care for children and adolescents who are fostered and adopted while attending to children's medical needs and helping each child attain their developmental potential. Although this report primarily focuses on children in the US child welfare system, private and internationally adopted children often have similar needs.

THE FACES OF CHILD WELFARE IN THE UNITED STATES

The child welfare system strives to protect the safety of children while supporting families whose children are placed in foster care. In this document, the term "child" includes infants, children, adolescents, and young adults. The child welfare system also serves as a bridge to the primary goal of permanency through reunification or adoption. On September 30, 2018, the Adoption and Foster Care Analysis and Reporting System reported that 437 283 children and adolescents were in foster care.[1] Of these children, 262 956 entered foster care during the fiscal year of 2018, with 250 103 exiting foster care. The number of children served in the foster care system during 2018 was 687 345. There were 125 422 children waiting to be adopted, with 71 254 having parental rights terminated and 63 123 subsequently being adopted from care. Primary reasons for entering foster care include neglect (62%), parental substance use (36%), poor coping skills of the caregiver (14%), physical abuse (13%), and inadequate housing (10%). Other reasons that account for less than 10% in each category include child behavior problems, parental incarceration, parental alcoholism, abandonment, sexual abuse, child disability, relinquishment, parental death, and child alcohol and other substance use.[1] A growing number of children, estimated to be 5% to 10%

[a]Department of Pediatrics, School of Medicine, University of Louisville, Louisville, Kentucky; [b]The Children's Hospital at Montefiore, Bronx, New York; and [c]Department of Pediatrics, Icahn School of Medicine at Mount Sinai, New York, New York

Clinical reports from the American Academy of Pediatrics benefit from expertise and resources of liaisons and internal (AAP) and external reviewers. However, clinical reports from the American Academy of Pediatrics may not reflect the views of the liaisons or the organizations or government agencies that they represent.

All authors participated in the concept and design, analysis and interpretation of data, and drafting or revising of the manuscript; and all authors approved the final manuscript as submitted.

The guidance in this report does not indicate an exclusive course of treatment or serve as a standard of medical care. Variations, taking into account individual circumstances, may be appropriate.

All clinical reports from the American Academy of Pediatrics automatically expire 5 years after publication unless reaffirmed, revised, or retired at or before that time.

This document is copyrighted and is property of the American Academy of Pediatrics and its Board of Directors. All authors have filed conflict of interest statements with the American Academy of Pediatrics. Any conflicts have been resolved through a process approved by the Board of Directors. The American Academy of Pediatrics has neither solicited nor accepted any commercial involvement in the development of the content of this publication.

DOI: https://doi.org/10.1542/peds.2020-034629

Address correspondence to V. Faye Jones, MD, PhD. E-mail: vfjone01@louisville.edu

To cite: Jones VF, Waite D, AAP COUNCIL ON FOSTER CARE, ADOPTION, AND KINSHIP CARE. Pediatrician Guidance in Supporting Families of Children Who Are Adopted, Fostered, or in Kinship Care. *Pediatrics.* 2020; 146(6):e2020034629

of the total foster care population, are specifically placed because of complex medical needs.[2] In many cases, a combination of these factors leads to foster care placement.

The 2018 Adoption and Foster Care Analysis and Reporting System reports the mean age of children in foster care is 8.3 years of age, with 42% of children 5 years or younger. Of note, adolescents 13 to 20 years of age account for 21% of the population in foster care.[1] Black or African American children account for 23% of the foster care population, and Hispanic and Latino children make up 21%. Children who identify as ≥2 races account for 8% of the foster care population, and children of American Indian or Alaskan native, Asian American, and Native Hawaiian or other Pacific or unknown ethnicity represent 4% of the population.[1] Forty-six percent of children are placed in nonrelative foster care, with another 32% placed in a relative or kinship foster home. Other placement categories include institutional (6%), group home (4%), trial home discharge (5%), preadoptive home placement (4%), supervised independent living (2%), and runaways (1%). Fifty-nine percent of children exiting foster care in 2018 returned to a parent or primary caregiver, and 25% were adopted, 7% were emancipated, 7% were living with other relatives, 11% were placed in guardianship care, and 1% transferred to another agency.[1] In 2017, a report by the National Council of Juvenile and Family Court Judges revealed Black and African American and American Indian and Alaska Native children constitute 27.5% and 2% of the population in care, respectively, although African American and American Indian and Alaska Native children represent approximately 14% and 1%, respectively, of the general population.[3] Although the data during the time period did not reveal overrepresentation for Hispanic and

Latino children nationally, they did reveal disproportionate representations in several states.[3] These disproportionate rates of children in the child welfare system may result from social factors related to poverty, race, and class bias in initial reporting and subsequent processing of children in the child welfare system.[3-6] The effects of structural racism in the child welfare system also should be acknowledged and addressed in the disproportionate rates of minority children in the system.[7,8]

LEGISLATION SUPPORTING THE CARE OF CHILDREN IN FOSTER CARE AND ADOPTION

In 2018, the Family First Prevention Services Act was signed into law.[9-11] This law evolved in response to an increase in child welfare placements as a result of the opioid epidemic. The current increase in placements is similar to increases observed in 1999 at the height of the crack cocaine epidemic, when 567 000 children were in foster care.[12] The Family First Act allows reallocation of annual foster care funding to states, territories, and tribes to be redirected toward evidence-based preventive programs for mental health services, substance use treatment, and in-home parenting skill training with the goal of keeping children with their families, focusing especially on families affected by substance use and psychiatric illness.[9-11] The Family First Act also seeks to improve the well-being of children in foster care by placing children in the least restrictive environment within the child welfare system while setting standards of care for children with special needs placed in residential treatment programs, including timely assessments and periodic reviews to ensure continued need for a high level of care.[9-11,13] Summaries of the Family First Prevention Services Act and other significant federal legislation passed to protect children

in foster care are highlighted in Table 1.[13-15]

KINSHIP CARE

Approximately 4% of all children in the general population are cared for by extended family members. Although the vast majority of these more than 2.7 million children in the United States live in extended family homes without involvement of the child welfare system, approximately 104 000 of these children have been formally placed in kinship care as part of the state-supervised foster care system.[23] One-quarter of all children who have been removed from their homes by the child welfare system are subsequently placed in a kinship home. Over the past decade, the number of children in kinship care has grown 6 times faster than the number of children in the general population (18% vs 3%, respectively). It is estimated that 1 in 11 children live in kinship care for at least 3 consecutive months at some point before the age of 18 years. The likelihood that African American children will experience kinship care is more than double that of the overall population, with 1 in 5 African American children spending time in kinship care at some point during their childhood.[23] The passage of the Adoption and Safe Families Act in 1997 promoted placement in kinship care as a means of shortening length of child placement in foster care while continuing a child's relationship with his or her birth parent.[20] Kinship care is relatively cost-effective and may keep children more connected with their families, communities, and cultures compared with nonkinship care.[24,25]

Multiple studies suggest specific advantages when children are placed with members of their birth family.[26-32] In a systematic review, authors found that children placed in kinship foster care experienced fewer behavioral problems, mental health

TABLE 1 Federal Mandates for Adopted and Foster Children

	Description
Family First Prevention Services Act of 2018 (Pub L No. 115-123)[13]	This act reforms the federal child welfare financing streams Title IV-E and Title IV-B of the Social Security Act to provide prevention services, including mental health services, substance use treatment, and in-home parenting training.
	Allows IV-E funds to support inpatient substance use disorder treatment settings that allow the placement of children with their parents when those settings can treat the needs of both the parent and child.
	Reauthorizes the Regional Partnership Grant program, which supports multidisciplinary approaches to addressing the effects of parental substance use on child welfare.
	Mandates that services be trauma informed and evidence based.
	Seeks to improve the well-being of children already in foster care by incentivizing states to reduce placement of children in congregate care while raising standards for residential treatment programs.
Fostering Connections to Success and Increasing Adoptions Act of 2008 (Pub L No. 110-351)[16–18]	States must make reasonable efforts to place siblings in the same foster home unless doing so would be contrary to the safety or well-being of any of the siblings.
	If siblings are not placed together, the state must make reasonable efforts to provide frequent visitation or other ongoing interaction between siblings unless this interaction would be contrary to a sibling's safety or well-being.
	Ensure that children have permanency goals to improve the well-being of children served by public child welfare agencies.
	Child welfare agencies are required to notify relatives of the child's removal from the custody of the parent.
	Promote permanent placement with relatives.
	Maintain connections with siblings and family.
	Increase the number of adoptions for waiting children.
	Improve outcomes and transition for older youth.
	Improve outcomes for American Indian and Alaska Native children.
	Improve competencies of individuals working with children involved in the child welfare system.
	Improve education stability and coordination of medical needs.
Child and Family Services Improvement and Innovation Act of 2011 (Pub L No. 112-34)[19]	Requires states to monitor children removed from the home for emotional trauma
	States must track and enact protocols for appropriate use of psychotropic medications
	States must report on steps taken to ensure developmental health for young children in state care
Adoption and Safe Families Act of 1997 (Pub L No. 105-89)[20]	Provides a fundamental change in child welfare philosophy from a primary focus of reunification with the biological parents as the principal goal without regard to parental history, to a process of considering child well-being related to the child's health and safety in permanency planning.
	Improves the safety and promotes permanency for fostered children through adoption or the establishment of other permanent homes.
	Gives preference to the placement of abused and neglected children with relatives.
	Provides provisions to ensure family support.
	Places an emphasis on timeliness to permanency.
Indian Child Welfare Act of 1978 (Pub L No. 95–608).[21,22]	Enacted "to protect the best interests of Indian children and to promote the stability and security of Indian tribes and families by the establishment of minimum federal standards for the removal of Indian children from their families and the placement of such children in foster or adoptive homes which will reflect the unique values of Indian culture, and by providing for assistance to Indian tribes in the operation of child and family service programs."
	Gives greater authority to tribal governments to collaborate in decision-making in child custody proceedings.
	When a child lives on a reservation or is a ward of the tribe, tribal leadership can assert exclusive decision-making power.

disorders, and placement disruptions compared with their counterparts in nonkinship care.[26] Thirty-two percent of children placed in early kinship care showed behavioral problems 36 months after placement, compared with 46% of children placed in nonkinship homes when controlling for baseline behavior before placement.[27] Children also experienced less stigma and trauma from the separation from parents and were more likely to remain connected to siblings and maintain family cultural traditions.[28–32] Researchers have consistently shown that relative caregivers are more likely to be single, poorer, and older; to have less formal education than nonkin foster parents; to care for large sibling groups; and to have chronic health conditions or disabilities because of their age.[33,34] Children who come to the attention of child protection and are placed with a relative but are not taken into state custody (voluntary kinship care) are more likely to be cared for by a grandparent (87%) than children placed in kinship foster care after being taken into state custody (43%). Conversely, children in kinship foster care are more likely to be in the care of an aunt or uncle (37%) than those in voluntary kinship care (10%).[33] Children in kinship care are more likely to be removed from the birth parent's home because of parental substance use and neglect than children in nonkinship care.[34] For kinship families, unexpected placement of children with relatives may exacerbate financial and daily life stress. A report by the Annie E. Casey Foundation revealed 38% of children living in kinship care live below the federal poverty threshold, and 63% live below 200% of the poverty level.[23] A recent report by Generations United revealed that of the 2 572 146 grandparents responsible for their grandchildren, 57% were in the workforce, with 20% living below the poverty line.[35]

Despite these challenges, voluntary and kinship foster caregivers are less likely to be aware of financial benefits and other support services available to children in nonkinship foster care.[23,36,37] The Annie E. Casey Foundation reports that fewer than 12% of kin caregivers receive help from Temporary Assistance for Needy Families program, although the majority of families are eligible to receive benefits.[23,37] Fifty-eight percent of low-income kinship families do not receive Supplemental Nutritional Assistance Program benefits (food stamps) or Medicaid health coverage.[23,37] Only 17% of families receive child care assistance, with a mere 15% seeking housing cost support.[23] These statistics highlight how little our current child welfare system and communities support kinship families, especially those outside of the child welfare

system, and why pediatricians, through referral to benefit resources and simple acknowledgment of the dedication of kinship parents, can be an important part of a support network to kinship families who care for children who would otherwise be placed in a nonkinship home.

The Families First Act has several provisions to support kinship families by extending Title IV-E eligibility requirements at the end of 12 months while ensuring that programs provided to children are not counted against a kinship caregiver's eligibility for other programs.[9-11,13] The Family First Act funds the development of an electronic interstate database to help facilitate placement of children with relatives who live in states other than the child's state of origin. Additionally, the Family First Act allows states to receive funding for up to 50% of the state's expenditures on kinship navigator programs that work to help locate potential kinship placements for children in the child welfare system.[9-11,13]

In addition to placement in kinship care, placement of siblings in the same foster home helps maintain ties to a child's family of origin. Approximately two-thirds of children in the child welfare system have a sibling in care.[38,39] The Fostering Connections to Success and Increasing Adoptions Act of 2008 was the first federal law to address the placement and welfare of siblings and promote ongoing relationships with siblings, requiring:

[S]tates to make reasonable efforts to place siblings in the same foster care, kinship guardianship, or adoptive placement, unless doing so would be contrary to the safety or well-being of any of the siblings. If siblings are not placed together, the state must make reasonable efforts to provide frequent visitation or other ongoing interaction between the siblings, unless this interaction would be contrary to a sibling's safety or well-being.[16-18]

Efforts to maintain sibling placement can be complicated because of inaccurate contact information after sibling separation.[40] Furthermore, specialized medical and psychiatric needs of a child may require an exceptional foster home placement, which further complicates attempts to keep siblings together.[41] Maintaining contact with siblings and other members of a kinship family in such cases helps ameliorate the strains such separations put on ties to a child's birth family.

An often-forgotten venue of kinship care and placement of siblings is the adult sibling caregiver, which is the third largest relative caregiver group behind grandparents and aunts and uncles.[42] In their study, Denby and Ayala[42] reported adult sibling caregivers have the same unmet service needs as other kinship caregivers, and the emotional toll may be even greater because of their unique sibling relationship to the child's birth parents. Although sibling caregivers who express a relatively high degree of parenting ability report strong support systems, others with low levels of family involvement and social support report a dissatisfaction with available services.[42] Additionally, when younger siblings have special health care needs, the adult sibling caregiver is more likely to commit to adopt their siblings.[42] Pediatricians can help adult sibling caregivers connect with peer-aged parents and caregivers to support parenting skills. By educating sibling caregivers on the developmental abilities of their younger siblings, pediatricians can ease unrealistic caregiver expectations while encouraging activities to promote child development.[42]

Kinship caregivers report significantly fewer support services than other foster caregivers, such as parent training, peer support, and respite care.[43] Grandparents who become adoptive parents may have the additional burden of grieving lost expectations of their own children becoming parents while coping with the stresses of raising another generation of children and managing the ongoing challenges that led to their grandchild's placement in care.[35] In some cases, the stress of taking in a grandchild may cause problems within a marriage, exacerbate preexisting health issues, and increase financial strain within the family. Kinship parents may experience guilt or resentment over the birth parents' inability to be primary caregivers for their children.[35] At the same time, kinship parents may face challenges from birth parents who may express anger over the circumstances that led to their children being placed in foster care and feel the kinship parent conspired against them to obtain custody.[35,44] In addition, children may not understand or may resent the kinship parent, blaming them for their inability to live with their birth parents.[28] Boundaries must be set regarding the type of contact, timing, and granting of parental responsibility to the birth parents. All family members may need to be reminded that the guardian or adoptive parent is the responsible parent.

ADOPTION AND PERMANENCY

Approximately 2.4% of the child population in the United States is adopted, accounting for 2.1 million children.[45] In 2014, there were a total of 110 373 adoptions, with 41 023 (37%) adoptions with at least 1 adoptive parent related to the child by blood or marriage, and 69 350 (63%) family-unrelated adoptions.[46] The number of children who are adopted in the United States has steadily declined, primarily because of a decrease in international adoptions. In 2004, 22 989 children were adopted internationally. In 2013, 7092 international adoptions occurred, dropping to 4714 in

2017.[47] Although this clinical report is focused on children who are served through the child welfare system, awareness of other venues for adoption is important, because many of the same issues exist for both groups.

Additional demographic data collected by the Children's Bureau at the Department of Health and Human Services Administration for Children and Families provide a broader picture of adoptive families.[48] Data reveal that the predominant family structures are married couples (68.8%) and female-headed households (26.5%). Previous families of fostered youth account for almost half of adoptions, with relatives making up 31% of adoptive families. Eighty-one percent of children adopted from the foster care system are classified as having special needs. Ninety-one percent of families receive an adoption subsidy. White children account for most adoptees (49%), whereas African American and Hispanic children represent 19% and 22%, respectively.[48] Younger children are more likely to be adopted than teenagers. According to a report from the Children's Bureau through a partnership with the Ad Council, AdoptUSKids, youth in the foster care system between the ages of 15 and 18 years represent 43% of all children with active photograph listings on AdoptUSKids.org, but only 5% of all children adopted in 2015 were in that age range.[49]

Two different forms of adoption influence a child's subsequent relationship to his or her family of origin. Closed adoption allows no sharing of identifying parental information with the adoptive parent, leaving large amounts of information and details of an adopted child's family of origin and birth unknown to the adoptive parent. In contrast to closed adoptions, open adoption allows a continuum of communication between birth families, adoptive parents, and the

adopted child.[50] Open adoption may be restricted to birth parents' participation in the selection of the adoptive parents or may extend to regular communication between, or face-to-face meetings with, the adoptive parents, adopted child, or both.[51,52] Open adoption is a dynamic and fluid process with the goal of child-centered integration of a child's family of origin with the adoptive family that ensures the child's awareness of his or her origins and culture. Open adoption may be particularly important to an older child or adolescent with long-standing bonds to members of his or her birth family. Postadoption contact between families is typically unregulated; in rare cases, a judge may order postadoption contact with birth family relatives, even over the adoptive parents' objection. Although these statutes are present in most states, their implementation is varied.[53]

As children age into adolescence and adulthood, they often wish to seek out more information about their biological families.[54] In attempting to gain information about their birth parents, adopted individuals who joined their families through intercountry adoption may choose to make a trip to their country of birth. Others seek information about their birth parents through commercially available DNA testing that matches an individual with those who share a similar DNA inheritance.[55] Advancements through social media have also made it much easier to locate relatives of their family of origin.[56] Other available routes include exploration of reunion registries, reestablishment of ties in a lapsed open adoption, or restoration of other ties that have connections to the child's family.

Although some adoptive parents may view their child's searching for his or her birth family as a sign of rejection, this transition is a normal sign of healthy emotional growth and establishment of identity. The experience of a reunion with the biological family may be rewarding but may also cause the child to re-experience his or her loss. In preparing for contact and reunion, those who have been adopted or experienced foster care may need to anticipate a whole range of realities, including rejection by the birth parent(s) and family members.[57,58] Pediatricians need to be aware of the feelings children may have after meeting a sibling, either one who is older or who remained with the birth parent(s) or one who was born after the child was placed. Adoptive parents may fear birth parents will interfere in the adoptive family's life or affect the child's bond with the adoptive family. All members of this triad may need the help of mental health professionals to work through these situations. An adoption-competent social worker and/or counselor can discuss the extent of communication between the adoptive family and birth family and provide needed support by identifying benefits and drawbacks to the relationship. Pediatricians are encouraged to become aware of local community resources, support groups, conferences, services, and mental health professionals to which families confronting these difficult issues can be referred. Some available resources are included later in the article.

MEDICAL ISSUES

Children, adolescents, and young adults involved in the child welfare system often have multiple health care needs.[59–66] Because children who have been in foster care may move through multiple placements, the resulting fracture of medical care places children at risk for having medical, developmental, and psychiatric needs that remain either unaddressed and/or untreated. In addition to developmental delays and behavioral issues that can occur

because of neglect and early environmental deprivation, physical and sexual abuse can lead to marked behavioral challenges at any age. The effects of toxic stress in early childhood on the neuroendocrine–immune system not only leads to psychological and psychiatric morbidity but also can result in higher risks for later medical morbidity. Additional information on the effects of early life adversity on brain development and both physical and mental health can be found in the 2012 American Academy of Pediatrics (AAP) policy statement and technical report on early childhood adversity and toxic stress in addition to the AAP Trauma Toolkit (https://www.aap.org/en-us/advocacy-and-policy/aap-health-initiatives/resilience/Pages/Training-Toolkit.aspx).[67,68]

Among the multiple factors associated with removal of a child from a parent's home, parental substance use is one of the most common. Although 36% of children in the child welfare system are referred because of documented parental substance use, children referred for neglect (62% of child welfare referrals) often have parental substance use that has not been documented at the time of intake.[1] Although parental substance use is often reported on foster care intake, the co-occurrence of alcohol use by the parents is often overlooked. This is especially important in caring for children born with neonatal abstinence syndrome. The prevalence of fetal alcohol spectrum disorders (FASDs) among children in foster care has been estimated to be 16.9%.[63] A recent study of children in foster care referred for developmental evaluation provides further evidence of the prevalence of FASD in foster care and lack of diagnosis of this disorder. Eighty percent of children subsequently diagnosed with an FASD had not been previously diagnosed with this disorder.[64] Given this prevalence, all children entering

foster care should be screened for prenatal alcohol exposure. The AAP has created an implementation guide for pediatric primary care providers to increase screening for prenatal alcohol exposure (https://www.aap.org/en-us/Documents/FASD_PAE_Implementation_Guide_FINAL.pdf). In addition, a comprehensive medical evaluation, including behavioral health assessment by using validated tools to identify needs, is most effective when completed soon after placement.[61,62,66] An early evaluation allows the pediatrician to identify and address existing medical diagnoses, uncover issues unaddressed before placement, discuss developmental and behavioral concerns with parents, and make appropriate referrals when appropriate.[61,62,66] Other issues for exploration, particularly in the adolescent and young adult population, include a history of their own substance use, mental health history, and the potential of the adolescent or young adult to be involved in sex trafficking.

Review of past medical records allows successful coordination of the child's medical, developmental, and mental health needs. Children in foster care may arrive at the office or hospital with little or no documented medical history. Despite reasonable efforts to obtain past records, information may be incomplete or uncomprehensive in scope. Barriers to obtaining consent from birth parents can make these efforts frustrating. Determining who has legal authority to give consent to care and allow access to past medical records is critical. Access to a child's medical history is particularly important for children with complex health care needs. At the time of admission to the child welfare system, the person with legal custody of the child signs consent for general and emergency medical care. Consent for further medical intervention beyond routine care must be obtained from the legal guardian. Foster parents may not be authorized to sign consent for medical care. Many states have passed medical consent laws that allow kinship caregivers to make health decisions on the child's behalf with parental consent and without having to obtain legal custody.[69] In cases in which, despite diligent efforts, obtaining consent is not possible or in cases of parent refusal to sign consent, local child welfare authorities or the family court system can override custody rights in acting toward the best interests of the child.[70] Such situations may include the need for surgery, medical tests, psychotropic medication, and developmental evaluation and intervention. These legal issues often require pediatricians to act as advocates for the child while working with the foster care agency and family court system. After adoption, adoptive parents gain the right to be legal guardians and make decisions separate from the birth parent. The AAP Council on Foster Care, Adoption, and Kinship Care has provided further guidance related to consent in "Health Care Issues for Children and Adolescents in Foster Care and Kinship Care"[61] and at the AAP Fostering Health Web site: https://www.aap.org/en-us/advocacy-and-policy/aap-health-initiatives/healthy-foster-care-america/Pages/Fostering-Health.aspx.

Particularly relevant parts of the health care record include past medical history; complications of pregnancy; late recognition of pregnancy; lack of prenatal care; prenatal exposures to maternal alcohol, substances, and/or tobacco; poor maternal nutrition; preterm birth; maternal and paternal psychiatric illness; and genetic diseases within the family. Important history also includes the number of previous placements, significant past relationships, developmental delays, abnormalities in growth, behavioral challenges, mental health history,

substance abuse, and any traumatic events such as physical and sexual abuse, including sex trafficking.[61,62,65,66] Pediatricians can use the time a child is in foster care to integrate the medical, developmental, and psychiatric history within an electronic health record that can be easily forwarded to new placements while working with their state child welfare system to advocate for centralized or portable records that can travel with the child across foster care placements. Examples of categories within such records may include birth and developmental history, prenatal drug and/or alcohol exposure risk factors, immunization records, past psychiatric treatment, and ongoing diseases and medications. When reviewing medical records, informed interpretation of the Health Insurance Portability and Accountability Act allows proper sharing of information to improve continuity and coordination of medical care. The Health Insurance Portability and Accountability Act contains several provisions that encourage information sharing regarding children in foster care.[71]

In collaboration with members of child welfare services, pediatricians can develop treatment recommendations that support caregivers in planning to best meet their child's physical and mental health needs while anticipating future challenges. Pediatricians without expertise in this area may seek resources through the AAP Council on Foster Care, Adoption, and Kinship Care to assist in this effort.[72] For internationally adopted children, this evaluation includes, but is not limited to, infectious disease and developmental screening tests and assessment of immunization status, as recommended in the AAP *Red Book*[73] and the Centers for Disease Control and Prevention *Yellow Book*.[74] The following AAP resources are also available to guide pediatricians: *Addressing Mental*

Health Concerns in Primary Care: A Clinician's Toolkit,[75] *Developmental and Behavioral Pediatrics*,[76] and *Adoption Medicine: Caring for Children and Families*.[77]

Finally, identification and documentation of a child's medical diagnoses may be necessary in establishing eligibility for financial subsidies to support the child's needs. Although the type and amount of assistance vary by state and typically are negotiated before the adoption is finalized, financial subsidy may specifically support medical and/or psychiatric care, counseling or therapy, special equipment, tutoring programs, or other support services that may help children who have special needs.[78-80] Community services, such as early child intervention programs, quality early childhood learning centers, parent support groups, financial assistance, respite care, trauma-informed care, and community organizations, including local child welfare agencies, can also help support families. Organizations such as the Child Welfare League of America[81] and Generations United[82] may be valuable resources for pediatricians and families.

COMMUNICATING WITH CHILDREN AND ADOLESCENTS ABOUT PLACEMENT AND PERMANENCY

Even before a child understands the words "adoption," "adopted," "foster care," "kinship care," "guardianship," and "biological family" or "birth family," these words should become a part of a family's natural conversation, whether the adoption is open or confidential, kinship, or foster-adoptive placement.[83,84] Positive language lays a foundation for a child's later understanding of the abstract concepts of foster care, adoption, and separation from birth parents. It is generally not advisable for families to wait until "just the right minute" to talk to children about their permanency status, because this may leave children feeling betrayed and wondering what else their parents may have hidden from them. Early communication that shares these sensitive histories, starting with placement or early childhood, helps maintain trust between the parent and child. Encouraging an honest, nonjudgmental discussion of a child's birth family and the placement or permanency process will give a child permission to ask questions and express thoughts and feelings that not only serve to develop trust and a feeling of security but also help ameliorate the shame and the stigma associated with being in the child welfare system.[85–87]

Some information in a child's past may be difficult to discuss, such as previous sexual or physical abuse or having been conceived in the context of rape or incest, and should be discussed on the basis of the child's questions and developmental ability to understand these difficult thoughts, feelings, and memories. Furthermore, for older youth and adolescents, discussion of parental psychiatric history, substance use disorder, and life challenges that might have hindered a parent from being a greater part of the child's life can help open future questions and dialogue. Pediatricians, potentially with the collaboration of a mental health specialist, may help the family decide how and when to disclose this information. Open discussion with a child is essential in building bridges of trust and security within a family, but it is also important that the discussion be framed with developmentally appropriate language.[87] Effective communication nurtures a child's self-esteem as he or she grows in the understanding of what it means to join a family and integrate disparate parts of their lives. A child's understanding of the meaning of permanency changes with his or her cognitive development. The pediatrician can counsel parents about the need to understand the

child's specific questions surrounding placement and permanency in the context of the child's current development and answer questions in a way that supports a child's sense of self and self-efficacy (Table 2).

Children placed in families at a young age may not understand that they have another family besides the family with whom they live. For many children and adolescents, separation anxiety and other internalizing and externalizing disorders may be pronounced, especially with children who remember the loss of birth or foster parents, siblings, or other relatives. Children may fear that their current family will abandon them in the same way once their "hidden flaws" are discovered. Some children may express yearnings to have been "in the belly" of their mother with whom they are presently living.[86] By kindergarten, many children realize that most of their peers are not in foster care, kinship care, or adopted, which may lead children to feel responsible for their birth parents' inability to raise them as well as for the repeated losses through moves in and out of foster care. This feeling of responsibility is especially true when a foster placement does not advance to adoption of the child.[89–93]

Pediatricians are encouraged to model positive adoption language for all families. Adoptive, foster care, and kinship care families are "real" families; siblings who joined a family through any of these channels are "real siblings." Birth parents do not "give up a child for adoption," which might imply to the child that he or she was of less worth and was given away. Rather, they "make an adoption plan for a child." Furthermore, in modeling positive language, pediatricians can use vocabulary that reflects respect and permanency about children and their families.[84] A "life book," that compiles both happy and difficult periods of a child's life experiences can be an effective tool

for parents in helping a child process their thoughts and feelings.[94] Some families choose to develop rituals with their child to honor the child's birth parents on birthdays or holidays or as a special prayer to commemorate the birth family. Rituals like these allow children to acknowledge and remember their past but also to honor their present status.[84]

LOSS, GRIEF, AND TRAUMA ASSOCIATED WITH FOSTER CARE PLACEMENT

Although birth parents may anticipate the loss of their parental rights or loss of their child through adoption, the surrendering of their child often precipitates grief and a sense of loss manifested as denial, sorrow, depression, anger, and guilt. Birth parents may grieve the loss of their role as a parent and of playing a significant part in their child's life. The later birth of other children may be a reminder of the loss of the child that they did not raise.[95] In cases in which change of custody is kept secret, friends and family may not even be aware of this loss or not understand the extent of the birth parent's loss.

Foster parents can experience loss and grief with each child for whom they care. In many instances, foster parents interact with birth families to support reunification of the family. Although reunification may be the mutually desired goal, the resulting separation can be traumatic to both the foster parent and child.[96] Moreover, other children in the home may experience loss and undergo their own grieving process. Birth children of foster parents report feelings of guilt, sadness, and blame at the departure of a child who had been fostered in their childhood home.[97] Anniversary reactions often occur for children with each passing year. Anniversaries may trigger thoughts of the birth family, and children may wonder whether their birth parents still love them or even

TABLE 2 Developmental Tasks and Issues Specific to Adopted and Foster Children

Age and Developmental Stage	Erikson's Psychosocial Stages of Development[88]	Issues That May Be Intensified for Adopted and Foster Children	Strategies for Families and Pediatricians
Birth to 16 mo	Trust versus mistrust	Difficulty or failure to develop a trusting, reliable attachment to caregivers Children may present with feeding problems, anxiety, depression, aggression, sleep disorders, and lack of trust[56]	Educate caregivers of the need to provide a consistent, sensitive, and responsive environment Caregivers should be vigilant for behavioral dysregulation that can be a sign of previous trauma and toxic stress[36]
18 mo to 3 y	Autonomy versus shame and doubt	A child's emerging self-centered perception of the world can become fragmented from experiences of multiple caregivers, previous neglect, and physical or sexual abuse	Caregivers should be aware of the manifestations of early childhood adversity and toxic stress[56,57] Create a highly structured, calm environment that provides a feeling of safety and security Address a child's questions and fears with acknowledgment tempered with reassurance of the child's current safety Be vigilant for developmental delays and behavioral problems, especially in cases of known or suspected prenatal alcohol or drug exposure and in such cases facilitate referral for evaluation for fetal alcohol spectrum disorders Refer to early intervention for developmental delays and behavioral concerns
3–5 y	Initiative versus guilt Problem-solving; attempts to understand permanency and past and current living arrangements	Children who have experienced trauma or been placed with multiple caregivers may exhibit anger, withdrawal, aggression, or sadness because of feelings of insecurity about their environment or caregivers Children who come into families by foster care or adoption experience loss in multiple areas of their life; loss should be viewed as a form of trauma and may manifest in variety of ways depending on the child's developmental level, the type of placement (temporary versus permanent), familiarity of surroundings and support systems[82–85]	Keep a daily, consistent routine Understand a child's current concerns and behaviors in the context of their past experiences and meet these challenges with acknowledgment and reassurance Validate a child's feelings while setting limits on problematic behavior Refer to mental health services when appropriate Refer for speech and other developmental or behavioral problems Consider referral to developmental-behavioral pediatrician and/or referral for evaluation for fetal alcohol spectrum disorders in cases of developmental or behavioral challenges Provide opportunities to nurture intellectual curiosity by allowing preschoolers to explore their environment through imaginative play and social engagement Encourage preschoolers to plan and participate in new activities of their own choosing within the bounds of a safe environment
Middle childhood	Industry versus inferiority Peer groups have increased influence over a child's self-esteem	Fostered or adopted children may experience low self-esteem and feelings of inferiority or rejection as they become aware of their differences from their peers. Such issues may be especially difficult for children placed in homes of a different racial or cultural background In addition to loss of their family of origin, fostered children may experience the loss of friends, surroundings, culture, and disruption of past routines	Caregivers can help their child integrate past experiences into their current life Caregivers can help a child begin to understand how current feelings and thoughts may be related to past experiences while grounding the child to their present life circumstances Refer to mental health services when appropriate Refer for educational support services if indicated Consider referral to developmental-behavioral pediatrician and/or referral for evaluation

TABLE 2 Continued

Age and Developmental Stage	Erikson's Psychosocial Stages of Development[88]	Issues That May Be Intensified for Adopted and Foster Children	Strategies for Families and Pediatricians
			for fetal alcohol spectrum disorders in cases of learning and/or behavioral challenges
			Caregivers can be encouraged to educate their child about their cultural history while being sensitive to nonverbal clues that they communicate about race and cultural differences
Adolescence	Identity versus role confusion Autonomy Abstract thought; concepts like adoption and permanency may be internalized and adolescents might go through an intense period of self-reflection in an attempt to define their identities. As adolescents develop and begin the task of separation and individuation, permanency issues commonly become important, changing relationships between the adolescent and family	Early life trauma and toxic stress can worsen as a child moves from childhood to adolescence, especially when compared with peers who have had more stable childhoods Adopted adolescents or adolescents in foster care often struggle to integrate their past life into their current life and their future Adolescents may challenge authority within and outside the family, which may result in conflict; Youth may "test" caregivers by challenging their commitment to their relationship Risk-taking or unhealthy peer relationships can place adolescents at high risk for substance use, chronic truancy, and/or involvement in the juvenile justice system; such behaviors are sometimes precipitated by contact with or identification with birth parents who may have had similar difficulties	Caregivers should be aware of the manifestations of past traumatic events and losses and meet challenging behaviors with understanding but age-appropriate limit setting Encourage diary and creative writing or other art forms as a path for integrating past and present experiences into a life story Ensure appropriate support services are provided in school Refer for mental health or substance use treatment services when indicated Consider referral for evaluation for fetal alcohol spectrum disorders Pediatricians can screen for and directly address risks for substance use, depression, suicidality, and criminal behavior in one-on-one conversations with the adolescent In cases in which adolescent risk-taking behavior becomes a risk to an adolescent's future or placement stability, caregivers can consider pursuing a person-in-need-of-supervision petition in family court
Young adulthood[86]	Experiment and exploration: love, work, and worldviews	Housing instability Educational dropout Unemployment Lack of trust, expectation of failure in life trials, and social acceptance Engagement in criminal activities	Support transition with extension of foster care to age 21 y Supportive housing Job placement Funding for college opportunities Social networks and mentoring

think about them. The Child Welfare Information Gateway provides useful resources for families on separation and grief.

FAMILY DIFFERENCES

Although all children, especially in adolescence, face the normal developmental task of clarifying their identity, adopted children and children living in foster care with parents of a different race, ethnicity, or cultural background face the additional challenges of assimilating disparate parts of their lives. Children as young as 3 or 4 years are aware of differences between themselves and members of other racial groups.[98-102] When children live in communities where they are members of an ethnic minority, the differences in racial identity will be easily apparent to classmates, other parents, and strangers. These differences may provoke a child's sense of confusion about their racial, ethnic, or cultural origins.[102]

Children may encounter racist remarks for the first time, particularly in situations in which they are not physically or emotionally safeguarded by their parents. Role-playing with children with respect to stereotypes and racist statements may help them to feel in control when they encounter comments from strangers, friends, or extended family members.[103,104] Parents who have not experienced racism personally may need to pay extra attention to teaching their children effective ways to respond to racism. Families should openly acknowledge racial differences while providing the child with relationships with others of the same race or ethnic group, including adults and children.[104] The child should also be given the opportunity to learn more about the heritage of his or her racial and ethnic group and country of origin.

An estimated 220 000 children are being raised by more than 111 000 same-sex couples, with approximately 12% of children identified as adopted or in the foster care system.[105,106] Gates et al[107] reported that same-sex couples are 4 times more likely to adopt and are 6 times more likely to foster children than their different-sex counterparts. Additionally, approximately 25% of same-sex couples raising children are involved in kinship care arrangements. In the past, same-sex couples raising adopted children were typically older, more educated, and had more economic resources compared with other adoptive parents.[107] More recently, however, this trend may be changing secondary to the evolving societal acceptance and legal climate within the United States.[108,109] Between 2014 and 2016, 16.2% of all same-sex couples were raising children.[109] The majority (68%) of the couples were raising biological children; however, same-sex couples were more likely to have a child who was adopted (21% vs 3.0%) and/or a child in foster care (2.9% vs 0.4%) compared with male-female couples.[109]

In 2002, the AAP published a policy statement and technical report supporting coparent or second-parent adoption and reaffirmed the policy statement in May 2009.[110,111] Regardless of the sexual identity of the parent, children thrive best when raised in a home that provides a caring, supportive, and secure home environment. Children who grow up with gay or lesbian parents show the same emotional, cognitive, social, and sexual development as children who grow up with heterosexual parents.[112] Authors of a recent study exploring the perspectives of youth who were adopted by gay and lesbian parents reported that although many children experienced more bullying and teasing than their counterparts,

children of gay or lesbian parents were more accepting, had greater understanding, and were more compassionate toward people and individual differences than their counterparts raised by heterosexual parents.[113] This growing literature supports pediatricians in their advocacy for all capable individuals to have the opportunity to become foster and adoptive parents.

EDUCATIONAL CHALLENGES

Information from a 2018 multistate study reveals that 65% of foster youth had had more than 1 foster care placement, 34% had experienced 5 or more school placements; up to 47% had been placed in special education, and 65% completed high school by age 21.[114] Additionally, 17- to 18-year-old youth in the child welfare system are 2 times more likely to be suspended and 3 times more likely to be expelled from school.[114] Researchers in the 2005 Midwest study of 736 foster care alumni found that although 57.8% of former foster youth earned a high school diploma and 5% completed a general equivalency diploma (GED), 37% had attained neither a high school diploma nor GED.[115] Youth who earn a high school diploma are 1.7 times more likely to complete an associate's degree and 3.9 times more likely to complete a bachelor's degree and have higher incomes than those with a GED credential.[115] A 2018 multistate study found that although 70% to 84% of high school graduates wished to pursue further college education, only 32% to 45% actually enrolled in college, and only 3% to 11% attained a bachelor's degree.[114]

Researchers have shown that a higher incidence of exposure to one or more traumatic adverse childhood experiences affects educational achievement.[116–118] Maltreatment experienced before kindergarten was associated with negative academic and behavioral outcomes by second

grade.[117,118] Kovan et al[119] report children involved with the child welfare system had poorer outcomes than their peers with no involvement with the child welfare system on measures of receptive vocabulary, math reasoning, and teacher ratings of anger or aggression and anxiety or withdrawal. These findings support previous studies with similar conclusions of poor outcomes of children who have experienced neglect in early childhood.[117] Similarly, poor science outcomes have also been reported for children who experience neglect before kindergarten compared with their peers.[117] Thus, disproportionate representation of children from minority populations in the child welfare system helps maintain disparities in academic outcomes.[3–6] Quality early child care and early education programs, such as Head Start and prekindergarten programs, can partially mitigate the effects of maltreatment on school readiness and child development.[118–121] For children younger than 3 years, referral to a federally funded early intervention program may be warranted. For children older than 3 years, Individualized Education Program and 504 plans under the Individual with Disabilities Act can be mechanisms to obtain services and resources to help meet the special needs of children in foster care or those who have been adopted.[122] In addition, the Uninterrupted Scholars Act (Pub L No. 112-278), passed in 2013, allows information sharing between schools, child welfare agencies, and tribal organizations without parental consent.[123]

TRANSITION CARE TO ADULTHOOD: BARRIERS AND OPPORTUNITIES

Most young adults not in foster care continue to receive ongoing financial and social support from their parents beyond age 18.[124] In 2018, approximately 19 000 young adults aged out of foster care, potentially losing the financial, educational, and social support services of state foster care overnight when they turned 18 to 21 years old, depending on the state in which they resided.[1,125] Adolescents in foster care enter the world of adulthood all too often ill prepared, their prospects compounded by mental health problems, substance use, and underemployment.[126,127] The Midwest outcome study revealed that fewer than half of young adults leaving foster care were currently employed at age 26, approximately half of the young adults who had worked during the past year reported annual earnings of $9000 or less, and more than one-quarter had no earnings at all.[127] Researchers in a study of aged-out youth found that 20% were chronically homeless, with housing instability associated with emotional and behavioral problems, physical and sexual victimization, criminal conviction, and high school dropout.[128]

Title IV-E of the Social Security Act was amended in 1986 to create the Independent Living Program, allowing states to receive funds to provide independent living services.[129] State child welfare agencies are required to develop a transition plan in collaboration with the youth aging out of foster care that includes housing, health insurance, education, local opportunities for mentors and continuing support services, workforce supports, and employment services.[16–18,129,130] The age limit for foster care varies by state, with some states extending care to 21 years of age. The Fostering Connections to Success and Increasing Adoptions Act of 2008 amended Title IV-E to extend the age of Title IV-E eligibility from 18 to 21 years.[16–18,129] In one study, youth living in a state that extended the age of foster care to 21 years were nearly twice as likely to complete at least 1 year of college education.[126] Awareness of state-specific age limits

on foster care placement allows early transition planning for all adolescents in the medical home.[131] Youth who remain in care past age 18 attain higher educational credentials, which translate into better employment outcomes.[126,127,132,133] Furthermore, even when the level of educational achievement is controlled for, the number of years in care after the age of 18 positively affects employment and higher wages of the youth.[134] This study suggests a window of opportunity within transition planning for obtaining employment before discharge from foster care. It also supports the extension of foster care from age 18 to age 21.[134]

Youth transitioning out of foster care report that the most important support for working toward their educational and employment goals are job preparation skills, transportation, child care, educational services, and overall life skills.[135] Yet, former fostered youth who currently live independently overwhelmingly describe a lack of resources in the areas of employment, education, finances, housing, access to independent living classes, personal care, and networking.[135] Although parents outside the foster care system often contribute to the development of young adult independence by advancing important skill-building activities early in life, empowering youth to make decisions for their own lives, and reinforcing the youth's ability to learn and cope with the consequences of those decisions in a supportive environment, this support often fails to be included in the transition care of children in foster care.[136]

Mental health challenges further complicate transition planning from foster care. More than half of young adults leaving care (54.4%) have current mental health problems, compared with less than one-quarter of the general population (22.1%).[137] The prevalence of posttraumatic

stress disorder within the previous 12 months is higher among young adults in foster care (25.2%) than among the general US population (4.0%) and nearly twice the rate of that experienced by American war veterans (Vietnam: 15%; Afghanistan: 6%; and Iraq: 12–13%).[137] The prevalence of major depression within the previous 12 months is significantly higher among foster alumni (20.1%) than among the general population (10.2%).[137] Although mental health challenges might be thought to be solely linked to foster care placement, researchers of studies among US adoptees suggest otherwise. Among 96% of the adopted children placed before 1 year of age and all children adopted before their second birthday, adoptees were 4 times more likely to attempt suicide than nonadoptees.[138] Potential contributing factors for the increased risk of suicide attempt include early trauma before adoption, prenatal substance and alcohol exposure, and genetic predisposition to psychiatric illness.[138]

In the face of these adversities lie barriers to medical and psychiatric care. In a study of foster care alumni, only 47% of young adults had health insurance as they prepared to leave foster care.[139] Young adults in foster care are more likely to have health conditions that limit their daily activities, report more emergency department visits and hospitalizations during the previous 5 years than their peers, and suffer medical problems that are left untreated because of lack of health insurance.[61,140] Pediatricians can help youth prepare to transition their health care needs by identifying medical issues that require regular follow-up and educating youth on how to use health insurance benefits and nonemergent medical care.[133] Information on billing for the delivery of health care transition services can be found in the 2017 Transition Coding and Reimbursement Tip

Sheet, as well as other resources, on the Got Transition Web site.[141]

Finally, children placed in foster care are at risk for "crossing over" to the juvenile justice system, and inversely, many juvenile justice–involved youth later become involved in the child welfare system. These youth are commonly referred to as crossover youth, whereas youth with concurrent involvement in both the child welfare and juvenile justice system are described as dually involved or dually adjudicated youth.[142,143] Children who have experienced maltreatment average a 47% greater risk for future delinquency relative to children who have not experienced abuse or neglect.[144] An estimated 56% of crossover youth have mental health problems. A growing body of research indicates that running away from foster care increases the probability of subsequent involvement in the juvenile and/or adult justice system, especially for male individuals, with 42% of youth with runaway histories in one study having at least 1 juvenile and/or adult conviction.[145] Approximately 16% of children placed into foster care experience at least 1 delinquency court involvement compared with 7% of all maltreatment victims who are not removed from their family.[144] Other characteristics related to delinquency include age at first child welfare placement, years in placement, number of placements, total length of time in residential care, and sex, race, and recurrence of maltreatment.[144,146] African American youth involved in the child welfare system are up to 13 times more likely than white fostered youth to become involved in the juvenile justice system.[147] Reasons for this disparity are complex; however, structural racism should be considered.[7,8,147] Structural racism refers to the policies and practices that reinforce racial group inequity by allowing privilege associated with

race, in this case white-colored skin, while withholding those same privileges from communities of color. Structural racism is insidious and embedded within historical, cultural, and ideological norms of organizations and systems.[8] Norms around language, behavior, and practices, such as policing and court judgments, are typically based on white middle class expectations and contribute to the disproportionate involvement of youth of color in both the child welfare and juvenile justice systems.[147] Recognition of structural racism in current systems allows for education and interventions to be put in place to mitigate its effects.

One of several promising approaches to juvenile court involvement is multisystemic therapy.[148] Multisystemic therapy interventions target problems identified by the child, family, and worker within and between the multiple systems of the home, school, and neighborhood to problem-solve challenges and support success.[146,148] Pediatricians can affect the outcomes of these youth by participating in a multidisciplinary team that includes members from the juvenile justice system, child welfare organizations, and the family. This coordinated approach provides opportunities to change the trajectory of children with judicial involvement and affect the long-term outcome of their lives.[149]

THE LAST WORD: RESILIENCE

Resilience is the developmental process by which an individual can use internal and external resources to negotiate and adapt to current challenges while developing skills to aid future challenges. Resilience implies the presence of adaptive capacities to negotiate life challenges effectively.[150] In a study of 164 young adults emancipated from foster care, nearly half (47%) managed challenges in education, employment, civic engagement, relationships, self-

esteem, and mental health, and 16.5% had low educational and low occupational competence, low civic engagement, problematic interpersonal relationships, low self-esteem, and high depressive symptoms. Yet among those youth having difficulties in their external life, 30% exhibited internal resilience, characterized by psychological well-being, despite having difficulties in external circumstances such as education, employment, homelessness, early parenthood, drug use, and criminal activity. In contrast, 6.5% of youth showed significant emotional difficulties despite the appearance of external competence.[151] Thus, young adults can demonstrate resilience in one area of their lives even as they struggle in others. The greatest association with improvement in resilience is having more than one strong network (biological family, peers, foster care), with multiple strong social networks ameliorating the psychological stress of life struggles.[152] In addition to biological family, foster parents, extended family, and peers, support can come from child welfare case workers, therapists, teachers, mentors, coaches, and pediatricians, many of whom often continue to be a resource after the formal placement has ended.[149] For this reason alone, pediatricians can never underestimate the effect of the day-to-day interactions they share with fostered youth. Conversations for even a simple medical concern can affect a child or foster parent in ways we can never foresee.

Further information on the care of children in foster care and children who have been adopted can be found on the AAP Council on Foster Care, Adoption, and Kinship Care Web site.

KEY POINTS AND RECOMMENDATIONS OF CLINICAL REPORT

- Children and adolescents involved in the child welfare system, whether formally or informally, often have multiple health care needs that require an interdisciplinary team to maximize their well-being. See the AAP Fostering Health Web site for further information: https://www.aap.org/en-us/advocacy-and-policy/aap-health-initiatives/healthy-foster-care-america/Pages/Fostering-Health.aspx.

- Children and adolescents in foster care and those who have been adopted are at far greater risk than the general population for neurodevelopmental disorders, such as fetal alcohol spectrum disorders. Pediatricians can provide surveillance and screening of socioemotional well-being using validated tools and being aware of developmental and mental health issues common among children and adolescents in foster care. See the AAP Fetal Alcohol Spectrum Disorders Toolkit for further information: https://www.aap.org/en-us/advocacy-and-policy/aap-health-initiatives/fetal-alcohol-spectrum-disorders-toolkit/.

- Many children and adolescents experience social and emotional issues during periods of transition. It is important for pediatricians to counsel and provide information to parents in the recognition and management of current and future medical, developmental, and behavioral problems.

- Pediatricians can advocate for the development of a standardized process for consent and transfer of health information with their local Department of Social Services.

- Pediatricians can address the effects of adverse childhood experiences, early childhood adversity, and trauma on early brain development and life course trajectory for both physical and mental health, as recommended by AAP policy.[39] See the AAP Trauma Toolkit for further information:

https://www.aap.org/en-us/advocacy-and-policy/aap-health-initiatives/resilience/Pages/Training-Toolkit.aspx.

- Pediatricians can encourage parents to have developmentally appropriate discussions using developmentally appropriate language with their child or adolescent. Words such as "adoption," "adopted," "foster care," "kinship care," "guardianship," and "biological family" or "birth family" should become a part of a family's natural conversation, whether the adoption is open or confidential, kinship, or foster-adoptive placement.[84,85] Positive language lays a foundation for a child's later understanding of the abstract concepts of foster care, adoption, and separation from birth parents and facilitates the formation of an integrated identity.

- Pediatricians can help parents acknowledge racial and cultural differences and support children and adolescents in coming to an understanding of these differences. See HealthyChildren.org for further information for pediatricians Talking to children about racial bias https://www.healthychildren.org/English/healthy-living/emotional-wellness/Building-Resilience/Pages/Talking-to-Children-About-Racial-Bias.aspx Teaching children cultural and racial pride https://www.healthychildren.org/English/family-life/family-dynamics/Pages/Teaching-Children-Cultural-and-Racial-Pride.aspx

- Pediatricians can be aware of the complexity of losses experienced by children and adolescents in foster care or kinship care or adopted, in addition to losses experienced by foster, adoptive, and birth parents, while facilitating mental health referral as needed.

- Pediatricians can advocate for young adults who are transitioning out of care and/or involved in the

juvenile justice system, because they are at risk for poor physical and mental health outcomes, low socioeconomic status, and lower educational attainment.

RESOURCES

Available resources include the following:

AAP, Council of Foster Care, Adoption, and Kinship Care (https://www.aap.org/en-us/about-the-aap/Committees-Councils-Sections/Council-on-Foster-Care-Adoption-Kinship/Pages/Foster-Care-Adoption-Kinship.aspx);

AAP, Healthy Children (https://www.healthychildren.org/English/Pages/default.aspx);

National Council for Adoption (http://www.adoptioncouncil.org/);

Child Welfare Information Gateway (https://www.childwelfare.gov/):

- Legal Issues in Adoption (https://www.childwelfare.gov/topics/systemwide/courts/processes/legal-issues-in-adoption/);

- Working With American Indian Children and Families in Adoption (https://www.childwelfare.gov/topics/systemwide/cultural/adoption/american-indian-families/);

- Helping Children and Families with Separation and Grief (https://www.childwelfare.gov/topics/outofhome/casework/helping/); and

- Helping Youth Transition to Adulthood: Guidance for Foster Parents (https://www.childwelfare.gov/pubPDFs/youth_transition.pdf);

Grandparents Raising Grandchildren (http://www.raisingyourgrandchildren.com/Index.htm);

AdoptUsKids: Families for Native American Children: Consideration When Fostering and Adopting (https://www.adoptuskids.org/adoption-and-foster-care/overview/who-can-adopt-foster/families-for-native-children);

Jones BJ, Tilden M, Gaines-Stoner K. *The Indian Child Welfare Act Handbook: A Legal Guide to the Custody and Adoption of Native American Children.* Chicago, IL: American Bar Association; 2008;

National Center for Mental Health and Juvenile Justice. Family Involvement in the Juvenile Justice System (https://www.ncmhjj.com/wp-content/uploads/2016/09/Family-Involvement-in-the-Juvenile-Justice-System-for-WEBSITE.pdf); and

Baker JL, Brown EJ, Schneiderman M, Sharma-Patel K, Berrill LM. Application of evidenced-based therapies to children in foster care: a survey of program developers.

APSAC Advisor. 2013;27(3):27–34 (http://www.apsacny.org/wp-content/uploads/2014/11/APSAC_Advisor_Vol_26_1-pp27-34.pdf).

LEAD AUTHORS

Veronnie F. Jones, MD, MSPH, FAAP
Elaine E. Schulte, MD, MPH, FAAP
Douglas Waite, MD, FAAP

COUNCIL ON FOSTER CARE, ADOPTION, AND KINSHIP CARE EXECUTIVE COMMITTEE, 2018–2020

Sarah Springer, MD, FAAP, Chairperson
Moira Ann Szilagyi, MD, PhD, FAAP, Immediate Past Chair
Heather Forkey, MD, FAAP
Kristine Fortin, MD, FAAP
Mary V. Greiner, MD, MS, FAAP
David Harmon, MD, FAAP
Veronnie Faye Jones, MD, MSPH, FAAP
Anu N. Partap, MD MPH, FAAP
Linda Davidson Sagor, MD, MPH, FAAP
Mary Allen Staat, MD MPH, FAAP
Jonathan D. Thackery, MD, FAAP

Douglas Waite, MD, FAAP
Lisa W. Zetley, MD, FAAP

LIAISONS

George Alex Fouras, MD – *American Academy of Child and Adolescent Psychiatry*
Jeremy Harvey – *Foster Care Alumni of America*
Camille Robinson, MD – *American Academy of Pediatrics Section on Pediatric Trainees*

STAFF

Mary Crane, PhD, LSW
Tammy Piazza Hurley, BS

ABBREVIATIONS

AAP: American Academy of Pediatrics
GED: general equivalency diploma
FASD: fetal alcohol spectrum disorder

PEDIATRICS (ISSN Numbers: Print, 0031-4005; Online, 1098-4275).

Copyright © 2020 by the American Academy of Pediatrics

FINANCIAL DISCLOSURE: The authors have indicated they have no financial relationships relevant to this article to disclose.

FUNDING: No external funding.

POTENTIAL CONFLICT OF INTEREST: The authors have indicated they have no potential conflicts of interest to disclose.

REFERENCES

1. US Department of Health and Human Services, Administration on Children, Youth and Families, Children's Bureau. *The AFCARS Report #26. Preliminary FY 2018 Estimates as of August 22, 2019 - No. 26.* Washington, DC: US Department of Health and Human Services; 2019. Available at: https://www.acf.hhs.gov/sites/default/files/cb/afcarsreport26.pdf. Accessed January 28, 2020

2. Seltzer RR, Henderson CM, Boss RD. Medical foster care: what happens when children with medical complexity cannot be cared for by their families? *Pediatr Res.* 2016; 79(1–2):191–196

3. National Council of Juvenile and Family Court Judges. Disproportionality rates for children of color in foster care 2015 Technical Assistance Bulletin. 2017. Available at: https://www.ncjfcj.org/wp-content/uploads/2017/09/NCJFCJ-Disproportionality-TAB-2015_0.pdf. Accessed May 10, 2019

4. National Indian Child Welfare Association. National Indian Child Welfare Association (NICWA) disproportionality statistics. 2014. Available at: https://www.nicwa.org/wp-content/uploads/2017/09/Disproportionality-Table.pdf. Accessed May 10, 2019

5. Child Welfare and Information Gateway. Racial disproportionality and disparity in the child welfare continuum. 2016. Available at: https://www.childwelfare.gov/pubPDFs/racial_disproportionality.pdf. Accessed May 10, 2019

6. Hines AM, Lemon K, Wyatt P, Merdinger J. Factors related to the disproportionate involvement of children of color in the child welfare system: a review and emerging themes. *Child Youth Serv Rev.* 2004; 26(6):507–527

7. Trent M, Dooley DG, Dougé J; Section on Adolescent Health; Council on Community Pediatrics; Committee on Adolescence. The impact of racism on child and adolescent health. *Pediatrics.* 2019;144(2): e20191765

8. Pryce J. Child welfare is not exempt from structural racism and implicit bias. The Imprint. 2019. Available at: https://chronicleofsocialchange.org/opinion/child-welfare-is-not-exempt-from-structural-racism-and-implicit-

bias/33315. Accessed November 10, 2019

9. Torres K, Mathur R. Family first prevention services act. Fact sheet. Available at: https://campaignforchildren.org/resources/fact-sheet/fact-sheet-family-first-prevention-services-act/. Assessed May 10, 2019

10. National Conference of State Legislatures. Family first prevention services act. Updates. Available at: www.ncsl.org/research/human-services/family-first-prevention-services-act-ffpsa.aspx. Accessed May 10, 2019

11. Children's Defense Fund. The Family First Prevention Services Act: historic reforms to the child welfare system will improve outcomes for vulnerable children. 2018. Available at: https://www.childrensdefense.org/wp-content/uploads/2018/08/family-first-detailed-summary.pdf. Accessed May 10, 2019

12. Trends Child. Key facts about foster care. 2018. Available at: https://www.childtrends.org/indicators/foster-care. Accessed September 26, 2018

13. Administration for Children and Families. Information memorandum. Subject: New Legislation – Public Law 115-123, the Family First Prevention Services Act within Division E, Title VII of the Bipartisan Budget Act of 2018. 2018. Available at: https://www.acf.hhs.gov/sites/default/files/cb/im1802.pdf. Accessed May 10, 2019

14. Child Welfare Information Gateway. Legal and court issues in permanency. Available at: https://www.childwelfare.gov/topics/permanency/legal-court/. Accessed May 10, 2019

15. Child Welfare Information Gateway. Federal laws related to permanency. Available at: https://www.childwelfare.gov/topics/permanency/legal-court/fedlaws/. Accessed May 10, 2019

16. Fostering Connections to Success and Increasing Adoptions Act of 2008, Pub L No. 110–351, 122 Stat 3949 (2008). Available at: https://www.congress.gov/110/plaws/publ351/PLAW-110publ351.pdf. Accessed October 7, 2018

17. Court Appointed Special Advocates for Children. Fostering connections to success act. Available at: https://www.

ncsc.org/services-and-experts/government-relations/child-welfare/fostering-connections-to-success-act. Accessed May 10, 2019

18. Children's Defense Fund. Fostering connections to success and increasing adoptions act summary. 2010. Available at: https://www.childrensdefense.org/wp-content/uploads/2018/08/FCSIAA-detailed-summary.pdf. Accessed May 10, 2019

19. The Child and Family Services Improvement and Innovation Act of 2011–2012, Pub L No. 112-34, 125 Stat 369 (2011). Available at: https://www.congress.gov/bill/112th-congress/house-bill/2883. Accessed May 10, 2019

20. Adoption and Safe Families Act of 1997, Pub L No. 105–89, 111 Stat 2115 (1997). Available at: https://www.gpo.gov/fdsys/pkg/PLAW-105publ89/pdf/PLAW-105publ89.pdf. Accessed May 10, 2019

21. Tribal Law and Policy Institute. The Indian child welfare act summary. Available at: http://nc.casaforchildren.org/files/public/community/programs/Tribal/indian-child-welfare-act-summary.pdf. Accessed May 10, 2019

22. Jones BJ. The Indian child welfare act. The need for a separate law. Available at: https://heinonline.org/HOL/LandingPage?handle=hein.journals/gpsolo12&div=46&id=&page=. Accessed May 28, 2019

23. Bissell M, Miller J. *Stepping Up for Kids: What Government and Communities Should Do to Support Kinship Families.* Baltimore, MD: The Annie E. Casey Foundation; 2012. Available at: https://www.aecf.org/resources/stepping-up-for-kids/. Accessed May 10, 2019

24. Jimenez J. The history of child protection in the African American community: implications for current child welfare policies. *Child Youth Serv Rev.* 2006;28(8):888–905

25. Xu Y, Bright CL. Children's mental health and its predictors in kinship and non-kinship foster care: a systematic review. *Child Youth Serv Rev.* 2018;89:243–262

26. Winokur M, Holtan A, Batchelder KE. Systemic review of kinship care effects on safety, permanency, and well-being outcomes. *Res Soc Work Pract.* 2018;28(1):19–32

27. Rubin DM, Downes KJ, O'Reilly ALR, Mekonnen R, Luan X, Localio R. Impact of kinship care on behavioral well-being for children in out-of-home care. *Arch Pediatr Adolesc Med.* 2008;162(6):550–556

28. Cywnar G. Kinship adoption: meeting the unique needs of a growing population. 2010. Available at: https://njarch.org/kinship-adoption-meeting-the-unique-needs-of-a-growing-population/. Accessed May 28, 2019

29. Cuddeback GS. Kinship family foster care: a methodological and substantive synthesis of research. *Child Youth Serv Rev.* 2004;26(7):623–639

30. Winokur M, Holtan A, Valentine D. Kinship care for the safety, permanency, and well-being of children removed from the home for maltreatment. *Cochrane Database Syst Rev.* 2009;(1):CD006546

31. Monahan DJ, Smith CJ, Greene VL. Kinship caregivers: health and burden. *J Fam Soc Work.* 2013;16(5):392–402

32. Peterson TL. Changes in health perceptions among older grandparents raising adolescent grandchildren. *Soc Work Public Health.* 2017;32(6):394–406

33. Ehrle J, Geen R. Kin and non-kin foster care—findings from a national survey. *Child Youth Serv Rev.* 2002;24(1–2):15–35

34. Rubin D, Springer SH, Zlotnik S, Kang-Yi CD; Council on Foster Care, Adoption, and Kinship Care. Needs of kinship care families and pediatric practice. *Pediatrics.* 2017;139(4):e20170099

35. Generations United. In loving arms: the protective role of grandparents and other relatives in raising children exposed to trauma. 2017. Available at: https://www.gu.org/app/uploads/2018/05/Grandfamilies-Report-SOGF-2017.pdf. Accessed November 11, 2019

36. Child Welfare and Information Gateway. Working with kinship caregivers. 2012. Available at: https://www.childwelfare.gov/pubPDFs/kinship.pdf. Accessed May 10, 2019

37. Annie E. Casey Foundation. What is kinship care? 2019. Available at: https://www.aecf.org/blog/what-is-kinship-care/. Accessed November 11, 2019

38. Webster D, Shlonsky A, Shaw T, Brookhart MA. The ties that bind II: reunification of siblings in out-of-home care using a statistical technique for examining non-independent observations. *Child Youth Serv Rev.* 2005;27(7):765–782

39. Wulczyn F, Zimmerman E. Sibling placements in longitudinal perspective. *Child Youth Serv Rev.* 2005;27(7): 741–763

40. Child Welfare Information Gateway. Sibling issues in foster care and adoption. 2014. Available at: https://www.childwelfare.gov/pubPDFs/siblingissues.pdf. Accessed May 10, 2019

41. Kernan E. Keeping siblings together: past, present, and future. 2006. Available at: https://youthlaw.org/publication/keeping-siblings-together-past-present-and-future/. Accessed May 10, 2019

42. Denby RW, Ayala J. Am I my brother's keeper: adult siblings raising younger siblings. *J Hum Behav Soc Environ.* 2013;23(2):192–210

43. Sakai C, Lin H, Flores G. Health outcomes and family services in kinship care: analysis of a national sample of children in the child welfare system. *Arch Pediatr Adolesc Med.* 2011;165(2):159–165

44. Lee E, Clarkson-Hendrix M, Lee Y. Parenting stress of grandparents and other kin as informal kinship caregivers: a mixed methods study. *Child Youth Serv Rev.* 2016;69:29–38

45. Lofquist D, Lugaila T, O'Connell M, Feli S. Households and families: 2010. 2012. Available at: https://www.census.gov/prod/cen2010/briefs/c2010br-14.pdf. Accessed May 10, 2019

46. Jones J, Placek P. *Adoption by the Numbers.* Alexandria, VA: National Council For Adoption; 2017. Available at: https://www.adoptioncouncil.org/publications/2017/02/adoption-by-the-numbers. Accessed May 10, 2019

47. Bureau of Consular Affairs, US Department of State. Intercountry adoption. 2016. Available at: https://travel.state.gov/content/travel/en/Intercountry-Adoption/adopt_ref/adoption-statistics.html. Accessed May 10, 2019

48. Children's Bureau. Adoption data 2014. Available at: https://www.acf.hhs.gov/cb/resource/adoption-data-2014. Accessed May 10, 2019

49. Children's Bureau, Department of Health and Human Services, Administration for Children and Families. New PSAs focus on the importance of adopting teenagers from foster care. 2017. Available at: https://www.acf.hhs.gov/media/press/2017/new-psas-focus-on-the-importance-of-adopting-teenagers-from-foster-care. Accessed May 10, 2019

50. Child Welfare Information Gateway. *Openness in Adoption: Building Relationships Between Adoptive and Birth Families.* Washington, DC: Department of Health and Human Services, Children's Bureau; 2013

51. Siegel DH. Open adoption of infants: adoptive parents' feelings seven years later. *Soc Work.* 2003;48(3): 409–419

52. Appell AR. The open adoption option. *Children's Rights Litigation.* 2010;13(1): 8–12

53. Child Welfare Information Gateway. Postadoption contact agreements between birth and adoptive families. Available at: https://www.childwelfare.gov/pubPDFs/cooperative.pdf. Accessed November 18, 2019

54. Muller U, Perry B. Adopted persons' search for and contact with their birth parents. I: who searches and why? *Adoption Q.* 2001;44(3):5–37

55. Kirkpatrick BE, Rashkin MD. Ancestry testing and the practice of genetic counseling. *J Genet Couns.* 2017;26(1): 6–20

56. Samuels J. Reframing adoptive family narratives through digital and social media technologies. *Interactions: Studies in Communication & Culture.* 2018;9(2):239–250

57. McWey LM, Acock A, Porter B. The impact of continued contact with biological parents upon the mental health of children in foster care. *Child Youth Serv Rev.* 2010;32(10): 1338–1345

58. Clapton G. Close relations? The long-term outcomes of adoption reunions. *Genealogy.* 2018;2(4):41

59. Schulte EE, Michaelson RL. *Caring for Your Adopted Child.* Elk Grove Village, IL: American Academy of Pediatrics; 2018

60. Child Welfare Information Gateway. *Access to Adoption Records.* Washington, DC: US Department of Health and Human Services, Administration for Children and Families, Children's Bureau; 2016

61. Szilagyi MA, Rosen DS, Rubin D, Zlotnik S; Council on Foster Care, Adoption, and Kinship Care; Committee on Adolescence; Council on Early Childhood. Health care issues for children and adolescents in foster care and kinship care. *Pediatrics.* 2015; 136(4). Available at: www.pediatrics.org/cgi/content/full/136/4/e1142

62. Jones VF, Schulte E; Committee On Early Childhood, Adoption, And Dependent Care. Comprehensive health evaluation of the newly adopted child. *Pediatrics.* 2012;129(1). Available at: www.pediatrics.org/cgi/content/full/129/1/e214

63. Lange S, Shield K, Rehm J, Popova S. Prevalence of fetal alcohol spectrum disorders in child care settings: a meta-analysis. *Pediatrics.* 2013;132(4). Available at: www.pediatrics.org/cgi/content/full/132/4/e980

64. Chasnoff IJ, Wells AM, King L. Misdiagnosis and missed diagnoses in foster and adopted children with prenatal alcohol exposure. *Pediatrics.* 2015;135(2):264–270

65. Beal SJ, Greiner MV. Children in nonparental care: health and social risks. *Pediatr Res.* 2016;79(1–2): 184–190

66. Pullmann MD, Jacobson J, Parker E, et al. Tracing the pathway from mental health screening to services for children and youth in foster care. *Child Youth Serv Rev.* 2018;89: 340–354

67. Shonkoff JP, Garner AS; Committee on Psychosocial Aspects of Child and Family Health; Committee on Early Childhood, Adoption, and Dependent Care; Section on Developmental and Behavioral Pediatrics. The lifelong effects of early childhood adversity and toxic stress. *Pediatrics.* 2012;129(1). Available at: www.pediatrics.org/cgi/content/full/129/1/e232

68. Garner AS, Shonkoff JP; Committee on Psychosocial Aspects of Child and Family Health; Committee on Early Childhood, Adoption, and Dependent Care; Section on Developmental and Behavioral Pediatrics. Early childhood adversity, toxic stress, and the role of the pediatrician: translating developmental science into lifelong health. *Pediatrics*. 2012;129(1). Available at: www.pediatrics.org/cgi/content/full/129/1/e224

69. National Conference of State Legislators. Education and medical consent laws. 2017. Available at: www.ncsl.org/research/human-services/educational-and-medical-consent-laws.aspx. Accessed May 10, 2019

70. Strassburger Z. Medical decision-making for youth in the foster care system. *John Marshall Law Rev.* 2016; 49(4):1103–1154

71. US Department of Health and Human Services, Administration on Children, Youth and Families, Children's Bureau. HIPAA for professionals. 2017. Available at: https://www.hhs.gov/hipaa/for-professionals/index.html. Accessed May 10, 2019

72. American Academy of Pediatrics. Council on Foster Care, Adoption, and Kinship Care Web site. Available at: https://www.aap.org/en-us/about-the-aap/Councils/Council-on-Foster-Care-Adoption-and-Kinship-Care/Pages/COFCAKC.aspx. Accessed January 28, 2020

73. American Academy of Pediatrics. Medical Evaluation of Internationally Adopted Children for Infectious Diseases. In: Kimberlin DW, Brady MT, Jackson MA, Long SS, eds. *Red Book: 2018 Report of the Committee on Infectious Diseases*, 31st ed. Elk Grove Village, IL: American Academy of Pediatrics; 2018:191–203

74. Centers for Disease Control and Prevention. *CDC Yellow Book 2020: Health Information for International Travel*. New York, NY: Oxford University Press; 2018

75. American Academy of Pediatrics, Task Force for Mental Health. *Addressing Mental Health Concerns in Primary Care: A Clinician's Toolkit*. Elk Grove Village, IL: American Academy of Pediatrics; 2010

76. American Academy of Pediatrics. *Section on Developmental and Behavioral Pediatrics*. Elk Grove, IL: American Academy of Pediatrics; 2010

77. American Academy of Pediatrics. *Adoption Medicine: Caring for Children and Families*. Elk Grove, IL: American Academy of Pediatrics; 2014

78. Child Welfare Information Gateway. Adoption assistance by state. Available at: https://www.childwelfare.gov/topics/adoption/adopt-assistance/?CWIGFunctionsaction=adoptionByState:main.getAnswersByQuestion&questionID=12. Accessed May 10, 2019

79. Child Welfare Information Gateway. Financial assistance for kinship caregivers: legal and financial information. Available at: https://www.childwelfare.gov/topics/outofhome/kinship/resourcesforcaregivers/legalinfo/. Accessed May 28, 2019

80. Child Welfare Information Gateway. Adoption assistance for children adopted from foster care. 2011. Available at: https://www.childwelfare.gov/pubpdfs/f_subsid.pdf. Accessed May 10, 2019

81. Child Welfare League of America. Social supports as (primary) maltreatment prevention. Available at: https://www.cwla.org/our-work/advocacy/family-community-support/social-supports-as-primary-maltreatment-prevention/. Accessed October 10, 2020

82. Generations United. Adoption and guardianship for children in kinship foster care. Available at: https://www.gu.org/resources/adoption-and-guardianship-for-children-in-kinship-foster-care/. Accessed October 10, 2020

83. American Academy of Pediatrics, Council on Foster Care, Adoption, and Kinship Care. Respectful ways to talk about adoption: a list of do's & dont's. 2015. Available at: https://www.healthychildren.org/English/family-life/family-dynamics/adoption-and-foster-care/Pages/Respectful-Ways-to-Talk-about-Adoption-A-List-of-Dos-Donts.aspx. Accessed May 10, 2019

84. AdoptiveFamlies. *Positive Adoption Conversations: The Complete Guide to Talking About Adoption*. New York, NY: Adoptive Families Magazine; 2015. Available at: https://www.adoptivefamilies.com/store/adoption-ebook/positive-adoption-conversations/. Accessed January 28, 2020

85. Keefer B, Schooler JE. *Telling the Truth to Your Adopted or Foster Child: Making Sense of the Past*. Westport, CT: Bergin & Garvey; 2000

86. Springer S; American Academy of Pediatrics, Council on Foster Care, Adoption, and Kinship Care. Anticipatory guidance for pediatricians on addressing difficult adoption, foster care, & kinship care topics. 2016. Available at: https://www.aap.org/en-us/Documents/cofcakc_anticipatory_guidance.pdf. Accessed January 28, 2020

87. Springer S; American Academy of Pediatrics, Council on Foster Care, Adoption, and Kinship Care. Talking with families about adoption, foster care & kinship care in the pediatrician's office. 2016. Available at: https://www.aap.org/en-us/advocacy-and-policy/aap-health-initiatives/healthy-foster-care-america/Documents/TalkingWithFamilies.pdf. Accessed January 28, 2020

88. Erikson EH. *Identity and the Life Cycle*. New York, NY: WW Norton & Company; 1994

89. Baxter C. Understanding adoption: a developmental approach. *Paediatr Child Health*. 2001;6(5):281–291

90. Singer E. *Children and Adoption The School Age Years (6-11)*. Burtonsville, MD: Center for Adoption Support and Education; 2016. Available at: https://adoptionsupport.org/wp-content/uploads/2015/12/02-The-School-Age-Years.pdf. Accessed January 28, 2020

91. Berrier S. The effects of grief and loss on children in foster care. *Fostering Perspectives*. 2001;6(1). Available at: https://fosteringperspectives.org/fp_vol6no1/effects_griefloss_children.htm. Accessed January 28, 2020

92. Forkey H, Garner A, Nalven L, Schilling S, Sterling J. *Helping Foster and Adoptive Families Cope With Trauma*. Elk Grove Village, IL: American Academy of Pediatrics and Dave Thomas Foundation for Adoption; 2015. Available at: https://www.aap.org/en-us/advocacy-and-policy/aap-health-initiatives/healthy-foster-care-america/Documents/Guide.pdf. Accessed January 28, 2020

93. Arnett JJ. Emerging adulthood. A theory of development from the late teens through the twenties. *Am Psychol.* 2000; 55(5):469–480

94. Child Welfare Information Gateway. Lifebooks. Available at: https://www.childwelfare.gov/topics/adoption/adopt-parenting/lifebooks/. Accessed November 20, 2019

95. Child Welfare Information Gateway. Impact of adoption on birth parents. 2013. Available at: https://www.childwelfare.gov/pubs/f_impact/index.cfm. Accessed May 10, 2019

96. Edelstein SB, Burge D, Waterman J. Helping foster parents cope with separation, loss, and grief. *Child Welfare.* 2001;80(1):5–25

97. Williams D. Grief, loss, and separation: experiences of birth children of foster careers. *Child Fam Soc Work.* 2017; 22(4):1448–1455

98. Clark KB, Clark MK. Segregation as a factor in the racial identification of Negro pre-school children: a preliminary report. *J Exp Educ.* 1939; 8(2):161–163

99. Clark KB, Clark MK. Skin color as a factor in racial identification of Negro preschool children. *J Soc Psychol.* 1940; 11(1):159–169

100. Quintana SM. Children's developmental understanding of ethnicity and race. *Appl Prev Psychol.* 1998;7:27–45

101. Singarajah A, Chanley J, Gutierrez Y, et al. Infant attention to same- and other-race faces. *Cognition.* 2017;159: 76–84

102. Brodzinsky DM. Adoptive Identity and Children's Understanding of Adoption: Implications for Pediatric Practice. In: Mason P, Johnson D, Albers Prock L, eds. *Adoption Medicine: Caring for Children and Families.* Elk Grove Village, IL: American Academy of Pediatrics; 2014

103. Ito-Gates J, Dariotos WM. Talking about race and racism. Available at: https://holtinternational.org/adoption/parent-training/wp-content/uploads/2018/08/Talking-About-Race-and-Racism-have-permission-to-reprint.pdf. Accessed November 20, 2019

104. Anderson A, Douge J. Talking to children about racial bias. Available at: https://www.healthychildren.org/English/healthy-living/emotional-wellness/Building-Resilience/Pages/Talking-to-Children-About-Racial-Bias.aspx. Accessed November 20, 2019

105. Gates GJ. LGBT parenting in the United States. 2013. Available at: http://williamsinstitute.law.ucla.edu/wp-content/uploads/LGBT-Parenting.pdf. Accessed May 10, 2019

106. Gates GJ. Marriage and family: LGBT individuals and same-sex couples. *Future Child.* 2015;25(2):67–87

107. Gates GJ, Lee Badgett MV, Macomber JE, Chambers K. *Adoption and Foster Care by Gay and Lesbian Parents in the United States.* Washington, DC: The Urban Institute and the Charles R. Williams Institute on Sexual Orientation and Policy; 2007. Available at: https://www.urban.org/sites/default/files/publication/46401/411437-Adoption-and-Foster-Care-by-Lesbian-and-Gay-Parents-in-the-United-States.PDF. Accessed January 28, 2020

108. Family Equity Council. LGBTQ family fact Sheet. 2017. Available at: https://www2.census.gov/cac/nac/meetings/2017-11/LGBTQ-families-factsheet.pdf. Accessed January 28, 2020

109. Goldberg SK, Conron KJ. How many same-sex couples in the U.S. are raising children? 2018. Available at: https://williamsinstitute.law.ucla.edu/wp-content/uploads/Parenting-Among-Same-Sex-Couples.pdf. Accessed November 11, 2019

110. Perrin EC; Committee on Psychosocial Aspects of Child and Family Health. Technical report: coparent or second-parent adoption by same-sex parents. *Pediatrics.* 2002;109(2): 341–344

111. Committee on Psychosocial Aspects of Child and Family Health. Coparent or second-parent adoption by same-sex parents. *Pediatrics.* 2002;109(2): 339–340

112. Perrin EC, Siegel BS; Committee on Psychosocial Aspects of Child and Family Health of the American Academy of Pediatrics. Promoting the well-being of children whose parents are gay or lesbian. *Pediatrics.* 2013;131(4). Available at: www.pediatrics.org/cgi/content/full/131/4/e1374

113. Cody PA, Farr RH, McRoy RG, Ayers-Lopez SJ, Lesdesma KJ. Youth perspectives on being adopted from foster care by lesbian and gay parents: implications for families and adoption professionals. *Adoption Q.* 2017;20(1): 98–118

114. National Working Group on Foster Care and Education. Fostering success in education: national factsheet on the educational outcomes of children in foster care. 2018. Available at: https://foster-ed.org/fostering-success-in-education-national-factsheet-on-the-educational-outcomes-of-children-in-foster-care/. Accessed January 28, 2020

115. Courtney ME, Dworsky A, Ruth G, Keller TE, Havlicek J, Bost N. Midwest evaluation of the adult functioning of former foster youths: outcomes at age 19. 2005. Available at: http://pdxscholar.library.pdx.edu/cgi/viewcontent.cgi?article=1015&context=socwork_fac. Accessed November 21, 2019

116. Metzler M, Merrick MT, Klevens J, Ports KA, Ford DC. Adverse childhood experiences and life opportunities: shifting the narrative. *Child Youth Serv Rev.* 2017;72:141–149

117. Fantuzzo JW, Perlman SM, Dobbins EK. Types and timing of child maltreatment and early school success: a population-based investigation. *Child Youth Serv Rev.* 2011;33:140–144

118. Klein S. *Benefits of Early Care and Education for Children in the Child Welfare System.* Washington, DC: Office of Planning, Research and Evaluation, Administration for Children and Families, US Department of Health and Human Services; 2016

119. Kovan N, Mishra S, Susman-Stillman A, Piescher KN, LaLiberte T. Differences in the early care and education needs of young children involved in child protection. *Child Youth Serv Rev.* 2014; 46:139–145

120. Lipscomb ST, Schmitt SA, Pratt M, Acock A, Pears KC. Living in non-parental care moderates effects of prekindergarten experiences on externalizing behavior problems in school. *Child Youth Serv Rev.* 2014;40:41–50

121. Merritt DH, Klein S. Do early care and education services improve language development for maltreated children? Evidence from a national child welfare

sample. *Child Abuse Negl.* 2015;39: 185–196

122. University of Washington. What is the difference between an IEP and a 504 plan? 2018. Available at: https://www.washington.edu/accesscomputing/what-difference-between-iep-and-504-plan. Accessed May 10, 2019

123. Styles KM, Yudin MK. Guidance on the amendments to the family educational rights and privacy act by the Uninterrupted Scholars Act. Available at: https://www2.ed.gov/policy/gen/guid/fpco/ferpa/uninterrupted-scholars-act-guidance.pdf. Accessed January 28, 2020

124. Barraso A, Parker K, Fry R. Majority of Americans say parents are doing too much for their young adult children. 2019. Available at: https://www.pewsocialtrends.org/2019/10/23/majority-of-americans-say-parents-are-doing-too-much-for-their-young-adult-children/. Accessed November 15, 2019

125. Fowler PJ, Marcal KE, Zhang J, Day O, Landsverk J. Homelessness and aging out of foster care: a national comparison of child welfare-involved adolescents. *Child Youth Serv Rev.* 2017; 77:27–33

126. Courtney ME, Dworsky A, Cusick GR, Havlicek J, Perez A, Keller T. Midwest evaluation of the adult functioning of former foster youth: outcomes at age 21. 2007. Available at: https://www.chapinhall.org/wp-content/uploads/Midwest-Eval-Outcomes-at-Age-21.pdf. Accessed May 10, 2019

127. Courtney M, Dworsky A, Brown A, Cary C, Love K, Vorhies V. *Midwest Evaluation of the Adult Functioning of Former Foster Youth: Outcomes at Age 26.* Chicago, IL: Chapin Hall at the University of Chicago; 2011. Available at https://www.researchgate.net/publication/264883847_Midwest_Evaluation_of_the_Adult_Functioning_of_Former_Foster_Youth_Outcomes_at_Age_26. Accessed May 10, 2019

128. Fowler PJ, Toro PA, Miles BW. Pathways to and from homelessness and associated psychosocial outcomes among adolescents leaving the foster care system. *Am J Public Health.* 2009; 99(8):1453–1458

129. US Department of Health and Human Services Administration for Children.

Youth and families. Independent living initiatives. Available at: https://www.acf.hhs.gov/sites/default/files/cb/pi8701.pdf. Accessed November 21, 2019

130. Fernandes-Alcantara AL. Youth transitioning from foster care: background and federal programs. 2016. Available at: https://fas.org/sgp/crs/misc/RL34499.pdf. Accessed May 10, 2019

131. US Department of Health and Human Services, Administration on Children, Youth and Families. Children's Bureau. Extension of foster care beyond age 18. 2017. Available at: https://www.childwelfare.gov/pubPDFs/extensionfc.pdf. Accessed October 11, 2020

132. Dworsky A, Courtney M. Does extending foster care beyond age 18 promote postsecondary educational attainment? 2010. Available at: https://www.chapinhall.org/wp-content/uploads/Midwest_IB1_Educational_Attainment.pdf. Accessed January 28, 2020

133. Courtney ME, Hook JL. The potential educational benefits of extending foster care to young adults: findings from a natural experiment. *Child Youth Serv Rev.* 2017;72:124–132

134. Hook JL, Courtney ME. Employment outcomes of former foster youth as young adults: the importance of human, personal, and social capital. *Child Youth Serv Rev.* 2011;3310:1855–1865

135. Thompson HM, Wojciak AS, Cooley ME. The experience with independent living services for youth in care and those formerly in care. *Child Youth Serv Rev.* 2018;84:17–25

136. Child Welfare Information Gateway. Helping youth transition to adulthood: guidance for foster parents. 2013. Available at: https://www.childwelfare.gov/pubPDFs/youth_transition.pdf. Accessed May 10, 2019

137. Pecora PJ, Kessler RC, Williams J, et al. *Improving Family Foster Care: Findings from the Northwest Foster Care Alumni Study. The Foster Care Alumni Studies.* Seattle, WA: Casey Family Programs; 2005. Available at: https://caseyfamilypro-wpengine.netdna-ssl.com/media/AlumniStudies_NW_Report_ES.pdf. Accessed May 10, 2019

138. Keyes MA, Malone SM, Sharma A, Iacono WG, McGue M. Risk of suicide attempt in

adopted and nonadopted offspring. *Pediatrics.* 2013;132(4):639–646

139. Jaudes P; Council on Foster Care, Adoption, and Kinship Care and Committee on Early Childhood. Health care of youth aging out of foster care. *Pediatrics.* 2012;130(6):1170–1173

140. Stolzfus E, Baumrucker EP, Fernandes-Alcantara AL, Fernandez B. Child welfare: Health care needs of children in foster care and related federal issues. Available at: https://www.everycrsreport.com/reports/R42378.html. Accessed January 28, 2020

141. McManus M, White P, Harwood C; National Alliance to Advance Adolescent Health. 2017 coding and reimbursement tip sheet for transition from pediatric to adult health care. Available at: www.gottransition.org/resourceGet.cfm?id=352. 2017. Accessed May 10, 2019

142. Herz D, Lee P, Lutz L, Stewart M, Tuell J, Wig J. *Addressing the Needs of Multi-System Youth: Strengthening the Connection Between Child Welfare and Juvenile Justice.* Washington, DC: Center for Juvenile Justice Reform-Georgetown University, Robert F. Kennedy Children's Action Corp; 2012

143. Herz DC, Ryan JP, Bilchik S. Challenges facing crossover youth: an examination of juvenile-justice decision-making and recidivism. *Fam Court Rev.* 2010;48(2): 305–321

144. Ryan JP, Testa MF. Child maltreatment and juvenile delinquency: investigating the role of placement and placement instability. *Child Youth Serv Rev.* 2005; 27(3):227–249

145. Sarri RC, Stoffregen E, Ryan JP. Running away from child welfare placements: justice system entry risk. *Child Youth Serv Rev.* 2016;67:191–197

146. Vidal S, Prince D, Connell CM, Caron CM, Kaufman JS, Tebes JK. Maltreatment, family environment, and social risk factors: Determinants of the child welfare to juvenile justice transition among maltreated children and adolescents. *Child Abuse Negl.* 2017;63: 7–18

147. Marshall JM, Haight WL. Understanding racial disproportionality affecting African American Youth who cross over from the child welfare to the juvenile justice system: communication, power,

race and social class. *Child Youth Serv Rev.* 2014;42:82–90

148. Borduin CM. Multisystemic treatment of criminality and violence in adolescents. *J Am Acad Child Adolesc Psychiatry.* 1999;38(3):242–249

149. Jones T, McMahon J. Tips for preventing delinquent behavior. *Fostering Perspectives.* 2014;18(2). Available at: http://fosteringperspectives.org/fpv18n2/tips.htm. Accessed January 28, 2020

150. Shpiegel S. Resilience among older adolescents in foster care: the impact of risk and protective factors. *Int J Ment Health Addict.* 2016;14:6–22

151. Yates TM, Grey IK. Adapting to aging out: profiles of risk and resilience among emancipated foster youth. *Dev Psychopathol.* 2012;24(2): 475–492

152. Collins ME, Spencer R, Ward R. Supporting youth in the transition from foster care: formal and informal connections. *Child Welfare.* 2010;89(1): 125–143

POLICY STATEMENT Organizational Principles to Guide and Define the Child Health Care System and/or Improve the Health of all Children

American Academy
of Pediatrics

DEDICATED TO THE HEALTH OF ALL CHILDREN™

This Policy Statement was reaffirmed June 2022.

Needs of Kinship Care Families and Pediatric Practice

David Rubin, MD, FAAP,[a,b] Sarah H. Springer, MD, FAAP,[c] Sarah Zlotnik, MSW, MSPH,[d] Christina D. Kang-Yi, PhD,[e] COUNCIL ON FOSTER CARE, ADOPTION, AND KINSHIP CARE

abstract

As many as 3% of children in the United States live in kinship care arrangements with caregivers who are relatives but not the biological parents of the child. A growing body of evidence suggests that children who cannot live with their biological parents fare better, overall, when living with extended family than with nonrelated foster parents. Acknowledging this, federal laws and public policies increasingly favor kinship care over nonrelative foster care when children are unable to live with their biological parents. Despite overall better outcomes, families providing kinship care experience many hardships, and the children experience many of the same adversities of children in traditional foster care. This policy statement reviews both the strengths and vulnerabilities of kinship families and suggests strategies for pediatricians to use to address the needs of individual patients and families. Strategies are also outlined for community, state, and federal advocacy on behalf of these children and their families.

[a]Policylab and Population Health, Children's Hospital of Philadelphia, Philadelphia, Pennsylvania; Departments of [b]Pediatrics and [e]Psychiatry, University of Pennsylvania, Perelman School of Medicine, Philadelphia, Pennsylvania; [c]Kids Plus Pediatrics, Pittsburgh, Pennsylvania; and [d]Stoneleigh Foundation, Philadelphia, Pennsylvania

Dr Kang-Yi conducted the literature review for the article and conceptualized and drafted the initial manuscript with Dr Rubin; Dr Springer and Ms Zlotnik reviewed the original draft as completed by Drs Rubin and Kang-Yi; they completed follow-up literature reviews, updated data and statistics, completed numerous draft updates and revisions, and addressed comments and concerns from American Academy of Pediatrics reviewers.

Policy statements from the American Academy of Pediatrics benefit from expertise and resources of liaisons and internal (AAP) and external reviewers. However, policy statements from the American Academy of Pediatrics may not reflect the views of the liaisons or the organizations or government agencies that they represent.

The guidance in this statement does not indicate an exclusive course of treatment or serve as a standard of medical care. Variations, taking into account individual circumstances, may be appropriate.

All policy statements from the American Academy of Pediatrics automatically expire 5 years after publication unless reaffirmed, revised, or retired at or before that time.

DOI: 10.1542/peds.2017-0099

INTRODUCTION

The number of children living with kin because of the absence of their parents is significant. In 2013, an estimated 2.5 million children in the United States, approximately 3% of the nation's children, lived in such kinship care arrangements.[1] Of the 427 910 children in foster care in 2015, 30%, or 127 821, are in the care of a relative[2] (Adoption and Foster Care Analysis and Reporting System AFCARS Report 23, accessed 2/18/17, available at: https://www.acf.hhs.gov/sites/default/files/cb/afcarsreport23.pdf). A child typically enters the custody of a kin caregiver when the child's biological parents are absent (including a parent[s] who is incarcerated, is receiving extended inpatient medical care, or is deployed or geographically separated while serving in the military). Most often, the kin caregiver is a grandparent but may be another relative or adult with whom the child has a long-standing, significant relationship. Kinship care arrangements may be temporary until the parent is again

To cite: Rubin D, Springer SH, Zlotnik S, et al. Needs of Kinship Care Families and Pediatric Practice. Pediatrics. 2017;139(4):e20170099

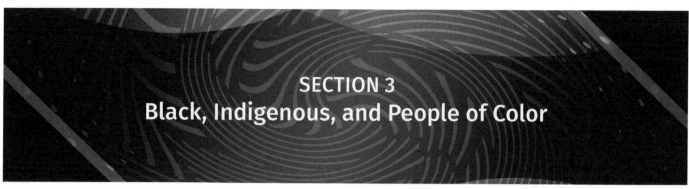

SECTION 3
Black, Indigenous, and People of Color

Some articles are available online only; scan the QR code to access online content.

Organizational Principles to Guide and Define the Child Health Care System and/or Improve the Health of all Children

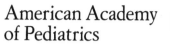

American Academy
of Pediatrics

DEDICATED TO THE HEALTH OF ALL CHILDREN™

Eliminating Race-Based Medicine

Joseph L. Wright, MD, MPH, FAAP,[a,b] Wendy S. Davis, MD, FAAP,[c] Madeline M. Joseph, MD, FAAP,[d] Angela M. Ellison, MD, MSc, FAAP,[e,f] Nia J. Heard-Garris, MD, MSc, FAAP,[f] Tiffani L. Johnson, MD, MSc, FAAP,[g] and the AAP Board Committee on Equity

Race-based medicine has been pervasively interwoven into the fabric of health care delivery in the United States for more than 400 years. Race is a historically derived social construct that has no place as a biologic proxy. In addition to valid measures of social determinants of health, the effects of racism require consideration in clinical decision-making tools in ways that are evidence informed and not inappropriately conflated with the limiting phenotype of race categorization. This policy statement addresses the elimination of race-based medicine as part of a broader commitment to dismantle the structural and systemic inequities that lead to racial health disparities.

In an address at the annual meeting of the Medical Committee for Human Rights in March of 1966, Dr Martin Luther King, Jr. said, "Of all the forms of inequality, injustice in health care is the most shocking and inhumane."[1] This oft cited quote presaged by nearly 4 decades the comprehensive and incontrovertible evidence documented in the Institute of Medicine's *Unequal Treatment* report that pervasive systemic inequities and historic structural barriers contribute directly to disparities disproportionately experienced by people of color in the health care system.[2] Race has been historically embedded into the foundations of health care in the United States for more than 400 years.[3] Race is a social, not a biologic, construct, and the use of race as a proxy for factors such as genetic ancestry is scientifically flawed.[4,5] Pediatricians may be unaware of this construct conflation. This policy statement specifically addresses race-based medicine, characterized as the misuse of race as a corrective or risk-adjusting variable in clinical algorithms or practice guidelines. The historic roots of race-based medicine and current reconsiderations are also discussed.

The role of race and racism in medicine has been vigorously debated.[6–11] Recognition of the determinative contribution of bias, whether implicit or explicit, to disparate and deleterious outcomes in a variety of settings, for a range of conditions, has been well chronicled.[12–20] Further, perceptions of physiologic differences based solely on racial phenotypes have long been intertwined and persist in the practice and teaching of medicine.[21,22] A 2016 study of White

[a]*Department of Pediatrics, University of Maryland School of Medicine, Baltimore, Maryland;* [b]*Department of Health Policy and Management, University of Maryland School of Public Health, College Park, Maryland;* [c]*Department of Pediatrics, Robert Larner, MD, College of Medicine, University of Vermont, Burlington, Vermont;* [d]*Departments of Emergency Medicine and Pediatrics, University of Florida College of Medicine – Jacksonville, Jacksonville, Florida;* [e]*Department of Pediatrics, Perelman School of Medicine, University of Pennsylvania, Philadelphia, Pennsylvania;* [f]*Department of Pediatrics, Northwestern University Feinberg School of Medicine, Chicago, Illinois;* [g]*Department of Emergency Medicine, University of California, Davis, Sacramento, California*

Dr Wright conceptualized the outline and content and drafted the initial manuscript; Drs Davis, Joseph, Ellison, Heard-Garris, and Johnson were each responsible for contributing to all aspects of reviewing and editing the document and responding to questions and comments from reviewers and the Board of Directors; and all authors approved the final manuscript as submitted and agree to be accountable for all aspects of the work.

DOI: https://doi.org/10.1542/peds.2022-057998

Address correspondence to: Joseph L. Wright, MD, MPH. E-mail: joseph.wright@umm.edu

PEDIATRICS (ISSN Numbers: Print, 0031-4005; Online, 1098-4275).

FUNDING: No external funding.

POTENTIAL CONFLICT OF INTEREST: Dr Heard-Garris has a financial relationship with XNY Genes, LLC. The other authors have indicated they have no potential conflicts of interest to disclose.

To cite: Wright JL, Davis WS, Joseph MM, et al. Eliminating Race-Based Medicine. *Pediatrics.* 2022;150(1):e2022057998

medical students and residents demonstrated that endorsement of false beliefs about the way in which Black people experience pain was associated with lower pain score assessments and inaccurate treatment recommendations for Black patients compared to White patients in mock clinical scenarios.[23,24]

Beginning in the late 16th and early 17th centuries, race and racism became the primary mechanism through which enslaved Africans, their descendants, and other people of color were systematically subjected to subordination and marginalization in the United States. The evolution of modern medicine, in this context, has not been immune from the historical influence of inequitable societal attitudes and an unjust belief in the validity of human hierarchy. Phenotypic difference was intentionally used by the colonists and their descendants to justify the institution of slavery, the seizure of native lands, and the establishment of political and economic advantage. Flawed science and unfounded evidence further fueled the codified existence of race-based medicine in many places across the health care landscape. Eliminating race-based medicine and moving toward race-conscious medicine[25] is an essential step on the journey to equitable health care and outcomes.

Background

In 2019, the American Academy of Pediatrics (AAP) policy statement "The Impact of Racism on Child and Adolescent Health" directly named racism as a social determinant of health and called out the fallacy of racial biology.[26] The statement definitively emphasized that race-based medicine serves to "solidify the permanence of race, reinforce the notions of racial superiority, and justify differential treatment on the

basis of phenotypic differences." In 2020, the AAP Annual Leadership Forum passed a resolution, "Prohibit the Use of Race-Based Medicine," through which "the Academy shall end the practice of using race as a proxy for biology or genetics in all their education events and literature, and … require [that] race be explicitly characterized as a social construct when describing risk factors for disease with all presentations at AAP-sponsored conferences."[27] In 2021, the AAP Board of Directors and Executive Committee published a perspective reiterating the organization's high prioritization of and focused intent to operationalize the elimination of race-based medicine.[28]

One of the steps that the AAP has already undertaken to address race-based medicine was retirement of "Urinary Tract Infection: Clinical Practice Guideline for the Diagnosis and Management of the Initial Urinary Tract Infection (UTI) in Febrile Infants and Children 2 to 24 Months."[29,30] The guideline came under scrutiny when Kowalsky et al questioned the systematic differential care recommended for Black or non-White children.[31] The inclusion of race as a decision-making factor in the clinical algorithm was based on a theoretical lower risk of UTI for children of color. Review of the guideline's cited references reveals that not only is the risk theoretical, but it is based on a blood group antigen-linked uroepithelial cell adherence hypothesis that the study authors state "requires additional study to substantiate or refute."[32,33] Further examination of the literature regarding the adherence hypothesis finds some evidence for blood group phenotyping as a potential biomarker for UTI risk but nothing specifically aligning this risk with subjective racial identification.[34] In this case, race was inappropriately

inserted as default biologic proxy in lieu of incompletely explained epidemiologic observation. The just approach is to confer equitable care to all young children regardless of race.

The Historic Roots of Race-Based Medicine

The origins of race-based medicine in the United States date back to the precolonial period and range from unproven hypothetical assumptions to outright cruel and inhumane practices. For example, Alabama physician J. Marion Sims, widely considered the father of modern gynecology, notoriously performed experimental vesico-vaginal fistula repair procedures on unanesthetized enslaved women.[35] He did so despite the availability and widespread use of ether, which he did employ with his White patients.[3] Sims' justification for this abusive practice was aligned with the broadly held belief in the medical community that, because of their thicker skin, Black people differentially experienced pain and were, therefore, more tolerant of surgical procedures, a concept espoused and published in 1851 by Sims' contemporary and fellow enslaver, Louisiana physician Samuel Cartwright.[36,37]

Another such example lies in the roots of race-based lung function assessment, which can be traced back to founding father Thomas Jefferson, considered an enlightened intellectual of the era. Jefferson wrote in his influential 1781 treatise "Notes on the State of Virginia" about differences in lung capacity between the enslaved and White colonists.[24,38] He remarked on the dysfunction of the pulmonary apparatus in Black individuals and that "among the real distinctions which nature has made is a lack of lung capacity."[24] Completely speculative, yet widely accepted, Jefferson's assertion remained empirically unchallenged until the second half of the 19th century when Cartwright, drawing directly from Jefferson's unfounded hypothesis, performed rudimentary experiments using the enslaved on his plantation as subjects.[39] Cartwright concluded and published that lung capacity in Black individuals was 20% deficient and went on to further theorize that, because small lungs prevent Blacks from inhaling enough air that "forced labor is a way to vitalize the blood and correct the problem."[36,40] This pseudoscience served to reinforce the practice of slavery and to perversely justify its necessity to help the enslaved.

False Equivalency and Flawed Science: The Case for Eliminating Race-Based Medicine

Although the blatant philosophical and cognitively dissonant justifications for slavery and the conditions of the enslaved are stunning, what is even more remarkable is how so much of this framework has persisted for hundreds of years in the form of race-based medicine. Despite growing acceptance of the false equivalency of race as a biologic proxy, there are numerous examples throughout the 21st century practice of medicine in which the attempted application of race correction or race adjustment factors have manifest in differential approaches to disease management and disparate outcomes.[41] Race assignment is not an independent proxy for genetic difference. However, there is recognition that differential lived experiences, particularly those that contribute to adversity, can impact physiologic and developmental mechanisms and, therefore, must be carefully accounted for in the transformative unwinding of race-based medicine.[42–45]

A unifying definition for epigenetic events is the structural adaptation

of chromosomal regions so as to register, signal, or perpetuate altered activity states.[46] Epigenetic induced changes of activity state can lead to combinations of genes that produce differential developmental outcomes.[46] Basic science work on the intergenerational elaboration of stress has elucidated that disruptive biological, physiologic, and neurodevelopmental mechanisms can manifest in utero and may persist in subsequent generational cohorts of the initially exposed.[47,48] The transmission of toxic stress across generations may sow the seeds of chronic disease development and contribute to the physiologic weathering described in some populations of color.[49,50,51] In other words, the impact of the trauma experienced by the enslaved and their descendants may be epigenetically embedded in ways yet to be completely understood.[52,53]

Further, transparency regarding the truth behind the intensity of ancestral admixture in the preemancipation United States is required. Recent analysis of genotype array data from more than 50 000 US research participants reveals an overrepresentation of women of African descent in the gene pool than would otherwise be expected based on the slave ship manifests that documented the forcible transatlantic exile of 12 million Africans known as the Middle Passage.[54] The biases in the gene pool toward enslaved African women and European men can, in part, be attributed to the well-documented sexual exploitation of enslaved women by their enslavers.[55–58] This overrepresentation, despite the relatively smaller proportion of women in the Middle Passage, points to this sordid practice as an accelerator of genetic admixture[53,59,60] and deflates any assertion that binary stratification based on the phenotypic presence of melanin, ie, the "one drop rule"[61,62] or "blood quantum rule,"[63] has any

legitimate scientific validity as an independent biologic proxy measure.[22] This history regarding admixing helps explain why social terms such as race are less precise and do not always reliably match with genetics.

Race, as a social construct, does not represent shared genetic ancestry. It is, instead, a way of categorizing people on the basis of physical characteristics and geographic ancestry. The United States Census identifies 5 racial categories: White, Black, Asian, American Indian and Alaska Native, and Native Hawaiian and Pacific Islander. These racial categories, however, are not universal, because they vary between societies and have changed over time. Therefore, careful consideration of anthropologic, ecologic, economic, historic, and social science contributions is necessary if we are to unravel the complex milieu that constitutes the socially determined factors that frame health status and their attendant outcomes. An interdisciplinary approach that rigorously acknowledges the longstanding effects of intergenerationally transmitted trauma and the role that structural racism and differential lived experiences play in conferring risk and resilience is a necessary framework for future exploration aimed at the promise of equitable care delivery.[64–67]

Race-Based Guidelines Across the Medical Landscape

In addition to the aforementioned and now retired UTI clinical practice guideline,[28–31] there are several examples of race-based clinical algorithms or practice guidelines currently undergoing reexamination and reconsideration that deserve mention.

Staging of Chronic Kidney Disease

The most mature efforts to reconsider race correction as part of clinical disease management have occurred in the calculation of estimated glomerular filtration rate (eGFR) in the assessment of renal function and the staging of chronic kidney disease (CKD).[68–71] Race as an independent variable was originally introduced into eGFR calculation on the basis of the unsubstantiated notion that the higher average serum creatinine concentrations seen in Black people is a result of more muscle mass.[72] The effective risk of this race adjustment is that Black patients with advanced clinical disease may experience delays in being referred to specialty care or transplantation on the basis of race assignment and eGFR calculation alone. Recent analysis of developmental data sets that have omitted race in eGFR calculation demonstrate that more accurate disease staging with smaller differences between Black and non-Black patients is possible.[73] Also, Black adults with CKD will be identified younger and at relatively earlier stages of disease.[74,75] A small but growing number of health systems across the country have already officially eliminated the race modifier from eGFR calculation.[76]

Lung Function Assessment

Racialization of the use of spirometry in the assessment of lung function has a long, tortuous history, as previously described.[23,36,38,39,40,77,78] The unsubstantiated assertions of deficient lung capacity in Black individuals by slave-holding medical professionals in the late 18th and early 19th centuries[36,37,40] persist today in the race norming that is programmed into spirometers.[79,80] In the United States, spirometers apply correction factors of 10% to 15% for individuals labeled Black and 4% to 6% for people labeled Asian.[76,81] Predictive reference equations have also been established for people from Hispanic backgrounds.[82] The ubiquitous application of pulmonary function

testing (PFT) for respiratory illnesses like asthma and chronic obstructive pulmonary disease, conditions in which populations of color are clinically disproportionately represented, provide ample opportunity for thoughtful exploration to examine the validity of race and ethnic correction in use of the spirometer.

There is recognition that race does not adequately capture the interplay of individual and population-based exposures rooted in the social determinants that may influence lung health, nor does it begin to approximate ancestral contributions in the context of genetic admixture. Investigators have posited that more granular incorporation of ancestry into normative PFT equations may improve lung function estimates.[83] A recent study found that explicit inclusion of measures of adverse exposure reduce the effect size of race categorization and blunt the potential for inaccuracy of pathology detection on the basis of race-specific prediction alone.[84] Omitting the use of race in PFT is motivating researchers to creatively search for a better understanding of the etiologies of lung health disparities.[85,86] The scientific community is now critically working to unwind the race-based evolution of lung function assessment.

Atherosclerotic Cardiovascular Disease Risk

In 2020, the American Heart Association (AHA) issued an organizational declaration that structural racism is a fundamental driver of health disparities.[87] In its call to action, the AHA went on to further state that the task of dismantling racism requires advocating for policies and practices that eliminate inequities in health care with a commitment to internally examine and correct its own shortcomings.[86] The role of race as part of the calculation of atherosclerotic cardiovascular disease

(ASCVD) risk has been identified as a reappraisal opportunity.

Based on practice guidelines developed and published by the American College of Cardiology and the AHA in 2013, the ASCVD Risk Estimator uses pooled race and sex-specific cohorts as the methodology through which to estimate 10-year susceptibility to the development of atherosclerosis.[88] The pooled cohort equation assigns race and uses an array of standard cardiovascular, behavioral, and lifestyle risk factors to estimate ASCVD risk. Critical analysis of estimator performance has revealed a 10-year increased risk differential as large as 22.8% for Black patients, the magnitude of which is described as "substantial and biologically implausible based on race alone."[89,90] The accuracy of the ASCVD Risk Estimator using the pooled cohort equation approach has been challenged on the basis of the statistical overfitting required because of the small sample size of Black patients in the original developmental cohorts. Investigators posit that this overestimation factor has ultimately led to a poorly calibrated tool for Black patients.[91,92]

One might argue that the ASCVD Risk Estimator may be protective in terms of potentially skewing early cardiovascular care toward Black patients. However, the inherent danger is directing differential treatment to Black versus White patients on the basis of a flawed phenotypic signal in the face of what might otherwise be identical underlying risk profiles. Incorporating race as proxy for the biological effects of differential lived experience is misplaced in this example. Moreover, the organized cardiovascular care community, having issued a clarion call to dismantle structural inequities, is well-positioned to consider removal of the race term in ASCVD risk assessment as an important step toward achieving equity.

Vaginal Birth After Cesarean Delivery

The vaginal birth after cesarean (VBAC) clinical algorithm was designed to predict risk associated with offering a trial of labor to someone who has undergone a previous cesarean delivery. The VBAC calculator, which has been endorsed as a predictive tool by the Eunice Kennedy Shriver National Institute of Child Health and Human Development, relies on specific factors such as age, BMI, and previous delivery history.[93] Race and ethnicity modifiers for women who identify as Black or Hispanic are also included, but they "correct" the calculation in a negative direction, signaling lower likelihood of successful VBAC. The evidence behind the inclusion of race or ethnicity in the VBAC calculator is rooted in thinly veiled racialized science. Late 19th-century medical descriptions of normative pelvic variation characterize the pelvic anatomy of non-White women with such terminology as "degraded or animalized arrangement seen in the lower races."[94] Even in 21st-century scientific literature, the residua of such characterization survives in the unsubstantiated hypothesis that race- and ethnicity-based variation in pelvic architecture is independently associated with lesser adequacy for successful vaginal delivery supporting a narrative of the white gynecoid pelvis as the standard.[95,96] This context influenced the inclusion of race and ethnicity as negative factors in the VBAC calculator, emphasizing the need for thorough reexamination. The National Institute of Child Health and Human Development Maternal-Fetal Medicine Units Network recently assessed the feasibility of using the VBAC calculator without race and ethnicity in the prediction model.[97] That study demonstrated that valid estimation is possible when race and ethnicity are eliminated and

that the probability of a successful VBAC can indeed be reliably predicted. Of note, the investigators added a variable for treatment of chronic hypertension before or during pregnancy to the revised equation, an excellent example of incorporation of an important evidence-informed measure. In recent practice advisories, the American College of Obstetricians and Gynecologists has stated that a VBAC calculator score should not be a barrier to the consideration of a trial of labor after cesarean delivery.[98] The American College of Obstetricians and Gynecologists Committee on Clinical Practice Guidelines justifies its position by noting the higher likelihood of inaccuracy exists in the lower probability range precisely where race and ethnicity modifiers skew the original model.[99]

Finally, disparities in maternal morbidity and mortality are an escalating problem. In the United States, the maternal mortality rate for non-Hispanic Black women is 44 deaths per 100 000, which is 2.5 times that for non-Hispanic White women.[100] Similarly, the maternal mortality rate for American Indian women is 2.3 times than for non-Hispanic White women.[101] Surgery is a recognized contributor to maternal morbidity and mortality, and non-White women in the United States have persistently higher rates of cesarean delivery than White women. Any opportunity to objectively and safely promote vaginal birth and avoid unnecessary repeat cesarean delivery would result in more equitable obstetric care.

Recommendations

The AAP has committed to laying the foundation for pediatricians to acknowledge and consider the social determinants of health in supporting every child to reach their fullest potential.[102] The integration of health equity principles into practice is vital to address the structural and

systemic inequities that drive disparities among children of color and minoritized populations in general. Race-based approaches to the delivery of clinical care are a tangible outgrowth of these long present inequities across the health care landscape. Whether at the professional society, institutional, or individual pediatrician level, the task at hand is dependent on transparent recognition, declared opposition, and active replacement of race-based medicine.[103] However, it is simply not enough to dismantle the processes through which race-based medicine has evolved. Balanced scientific discourse argues that, even in the face of insurmountable evidence that race is not a direct proxy for genetic difference, there is certainly a role for what race represents in terms of differential lived experiences and exposures.[42,104] Peeling back and rigorously sorting the social determinants of health, with integrity, is a core component of the necessary, transformative, and race-conscious discovery to which the scientific community must be accountable.[25,105] Now is the time to formally apply an equity lens to the development and reconsideration of all clinical decision-making tools, including clinical practice guidelines, clinical reports, policy statements, and technical reports.[106] Strategically, this is a mechanism through which organizations can tactically begin to incorporate antiracist principles into all of the work for which they are accountable and stimulate the creation of more equitable systems of care. It is through this lens that the following recommendations are framed:

American Academy of Pediatrics

- The AAP will critically examine all policies and practice guidelines for the presence of race-based approaches in their development and deconstruct, revise, and retire, if necessary, all policies and practice guidelines that include race assignment as a part of clinical decision-making.

- The AAP will critically examine all policies and guidelines currently under development as well as consideration of all such future documents to ensure the exclusion of race assignment as part of clinical decision-making.
- The AAP will leverage the "Words Matter" document to ensure that all authors, editors, presenters, media spokespersons, and other content contributors recognize race as a social construct only and desist from any use, or its reference, as a biological proxy.[107]

Professional Organizations and Medical Specialty Societies

- All professional organizations and medical specialty societies should implement a process to identify and critically examine all organizational policies and practice guidelines that may incorporate race or ethnicity as independent variables or modifying factors within a reasonable timeframe.
- All professional organizations and medical specialty societies should advocate for the elimination of race-based medicine in any form.

Institutions

- Institutions should collaborate with learner-facing organizations such as the Accreditation Council on Continuing Medical Education, the Accreditation Council on Graduate Medical Education, the Association of American Medical Colleges, the Association of Medical School Pediatric Department Chairs, the Association of Pediatric Program Directors, the Council on Medical Student Education in Pediatrics, the Latino Medical Student Association, and the Student National Medical Association to expose new and lifelong learners to health equity curricular content, including a specific focus on the elimination of race-based medicine.

- Institutions should collaborate with academic health systems, schools of medicine, and other higher education entities in support of the research and scholarship necessary to deconstruct race-based medicine and proactively reframe clinical decision-making tools using valid, evidence-informed measures that incorporate the social determinants of health.

Pediatricians

- Pediatricians should seek health equity continuing medical education programming and incorporate content on the elimination of raced-base medicine as a component of lifelong learning and maintenance of certification.
- Pediatricians should assess their practices and clinical environments for race-based care delivery and eliminate race-based medicine in any form from their practices.

Summary

Racism has infiltrated and impacted health care delivery and outcomes in this country for more than 400 years. The inclusion of race in algorithms and guidelines that direct clinical practice explicitly acknowledges this connection. Although it will continue to be important to collect clinical data disaggregated by race and ethnicity to help characterize the differential lived experiences of our patients, unwinding the roots of race-based medicine, debunking the fallacy of race as a biologic proxy, and replacing this flawed science with legitimate measures of the impact of racism and social determinants on health outcomes is necessary and long overdue.

LEAD AUTHORS

Joseph L. Wright, MD, MPH, FAAP
Wendy S. Davis, MD, FAAP
Madeline M. Joseph, MD, FAAP
Angela M. Ellison, MD, MSc, FAAP
Nia J. Heard-Garris, MD, MSc, FAAP
Tiffani L. Johnson, MD, MSc, FAAP

American Academy of Pediatrics, Board Committee on Equity, 2022

Joseph L. Wright, MD, MPH, FAAP (Chair)
Wendy S. Davis, MD, FAAP
Yasuko Fukuda, MD, FAAP
Madeline M. Joseph, MD, FAAP
Warren M. Seigel, MD, MBA, FAAP
Lee Savio Beers, MD, FAAP (Ex-officio)
Sandy L. Chung, MD, FAAP (Ex-officio)
Moira A. Szilagyi, MD, PhD, FAAP (Ex-officio)

STAFF

Madra Guinn-Jones, MPH
Kristin Ingstrup

ABBREVIATIONS

AAP: American Academy of Pediatrics
AHA: American Hospital Association
ASCVD: atherosclerotic cardiovascular disease
CKD: chronic kidney disease
eGFR: estimated glomerular filtration rate
PFT: pulmonary function testing
UTI: urinary tract infection
VBAC: vaginal birth after cesarean

REFERENCES

1. Dittmer J. The Medical Committee for Human Rights. *Virtual Mentor.* 2014; 16(9):745–748

2. Institute of Medicine, Board on Health Sciences Policy, Committee on Understanding and Eliminating Racial and Ethnic Disparities in Health Care. In: Smedley BD, Stith AY, Nelson AR, eds. *Unequal Treatment: Confronting Racial and Ethnic Disparities in Health Care.* Washington, DC: National Academies Press; 2002

3. Washington HA. *Medical Apartheid: The Dark History of Medical Experimentation on Black Americans from Colonial Times to the Present.* New York, NY: Doubleday; 2006

4. Smedley A, Smedley BD. Race as biology is fiction, racism as a social problem is real: Anthropological and historical perspectives on the social construction of race. *Am Psychol.* 2005;60(1):16–26

5. Mancilla VJ, Peeri NC, Silzer T, et al. Understanding the interplay between health disparities and epigenomics. *Front Genet.* 2020;11:903

6. Evans MK, Rosenbaum L, Malina D, Morrissey S, Rubin EJ. Diagnosing and treating systemic racism. *N Engl J Med.* 2020;383(3):274–276

7. Bailey ZD, Feldman JM, Bassett MT. How structural racism works - racist policies as a root cause of U.S. racial health inequities. *N Engl J Med.* 2021;384(8):768–773

8. Yearby R, Clark B, Figueroa JF. Structural racism in historical and modern US health care policy. *Health Aff (Millwood).* 2022;41(2):187–194

9. Snipes SA, Sellers SL, Tafawa AO, Cooper LA, Fields JC, Bonham VL. Is race medically relevant? A qualitative study of physicians' attitudes about the role of race in treatment decision-making. *BMC Health Serv Res.* 2011;11:183

10. Zambrana RE, Williams DR. The intellectual roots of current knowledge on racism and health: relevance to policy and the national equity discourse. *Health Aff (Millwood).* 2022;41(2):163–170

11. Braveman PA, Arkin E, Proctor D, Kauh T, Holm N. Systemic and structural racism: Definitions, examples, health damages, and approaches to dismantling. *Health Aff (Millwood).* 2022;41(2): 171–178

12. Goyal MK, Johnson TJ, Chamberlain JM, et al; Pediatric Care Applied Research Network (PECARN). Racial and ethnic differences in antibiotic use for viral illness in emergency departments. *Pediatrics.* 2017;140(4):e20170203

13. Nafiu OO, Mpody C, Kim SS, Uffman JC, Tobias JD. Race, postoperative complications, and death in apparently healthy children. *Pediatrics.* 2020;146(2):e20194113

14. Greenwood BN, Hardeman RR, Huang L, Sojourner A. Physician-patient racial concordance and disparities in birthing mortality for newborns. *Proc Natl Acad Sci USA.* 2020;117(35):21194–21200

15. Morden NE, Chyn D, Wood A, Meara E. Racial inequality in prescription opioid receipt—role of individual health systems. *N Engl J Med.* 2021;385(4):342–351

16. Johnson TJ. Intersection of bias, structural racism, and social determinants with health care inequities. *Pediatrics.* 2020;146(2):e2020003657

17. Sun M, Oliwa T, Peek ME, Tung EL. Negative patient descriptors: documenting racial bias in the electronic health record. *Health Aff (Millwood).* 2022;41(2):203–211

18. Goyal MK, Kuppermann N, Cleary SD, Teach SJ, Chamberlain JM. Racial disparities in pain management of children with appendicitis in emergency departments. *JAMA Pediatr.* 2015;169(11):996–1002

19. Goyal MK, Johnson TJ, Chamberlain JM, et al; Pediatric Emergency Care Applied Research Network (PECARN). Racial and ethnic differences in emergency department pain management of children with fractures. *Pediatrics.* 2020;145(5):e20193370

20. Goyal MK, Drendel AL, Chamberlain JM, et al; Pediatric Emergency Care Applied Research Network (PECARN) Registry Study Group. Racial/Ethnic differences in ED opioid prescriptions for long bone fractures: trends over time. *Pediatrics.* 2021;148(5):e2021052481

21. Amutah C, Greenidge K, Mante A, et al. Misrepresenting race—the role of medical schools in propagating physician bias. *N Engl J Med.* 2021;(9): 872–878

22. Lujan HL, DiCarlo SE. The racist "one drop rule" influencing science: it is time to stop teaching "race corrections" in medicine. *Adv Physiol Educ.* 2021;45(3):644–650

23. Hoffman KM, Trawalter S, Axt JR, Oliver MN. Racial bias in pain assessment and treatment recommendations, and false beliefs about biological differences between blacks and whites. *Proc Natl Acad Sci USA.* 2016;113(16):4296–4301

24. Villarosa L. Myths about physical racial dierences were used to justify slavery—and are still believed by doctors today. Available at: https://www. nytimes.com/interactive/2019/08/14/ magazine/racial-differences-doctors. html Published online August 14, 2019. Accessed January 30, 2022

25. Cerdeña JP, Plaisime MV, Tsai J. From race-based to race-conscious medicine: how anti-racist uprisings call us to act. *Lancet.* 2020;396(10257):1125–1128

26. Trent M, Dooley DG, Dougé J; Section on Adolescent Health; Council on Community Pediatrics; Committee on Adolescence. Committee on Adolescence. The impact of racism on child and adolescent health. *Pediatrics.* 2019;144(2):e20191765

27. Chomilo N. Prohibit the use of race-based medicine. Available at: https:// collaborate.aap.org/alf/Documents/ Prohibit%20the%20use%20of% 20Race-Based%20Medicine.pdf. Published 2019. Accessed January 29, 2022

28. American Academy of Pediatrics Board of Directors and Executive Committee. AAP Perspective: Race-based medicine. *Pediatrics.* 2021;148(4):e2021053829

29. Roberts KB; Subcommittee on Urinary Tract Infection, Steering Committee on Quality Improvement and Management. Urinary tract infection: clinical practice guideline for the diagnosis and management of the initial UTI in febrile infants and children 2 to 24 months. *Pediatrics.* 2011;128(3):595–610

30. American Academy of Pediatrics. AAP publications reaffirmed or retired. *Pediatrics.* 2021;148(2):e2021052583

31. Kowalsky RH, Rondini AC, Platt SL. The case for removing race from the American Academy of Pediatrics clinical

practice guideline for urinary tract infection in infants and young children with fever. *JAMA Pediatr.* 2020;174(3): 229–230

32. Shaw KN, Gorelick M, McGowan KL, Yakscoe NM, Schwartz JS. Prevalence of urinary tract infection in febrile young children in the emergency department. *Pediatrics.* 1998;102(2):e16

33. Hellerstein S. Recurrent urinary tract infections in children. *Pediatr Infect Dis.* 1982;1(4):271–281

34. Jantausch BA, Criss VR, O'Donnell R, et al. Association of Lewis blood group phenotypes with urinary tract infection in children. *J Pediatr.* 1994;124(6): 863–868

35. Sims JM. On the treatment of vesicovaginal fistula. *Am J Med Sci.* 1852; 45:226–246

36. Guillory JD. The pro-slavery arguments of Dr. Samuel A. Cartwright. *La Hist.* 1968;9(3):209–227

37. Haller JS Jr. The Negro and the Southern physician: a study of medical and racial attitudes 1800-1860. *Med Hist.* 1972;16(3):238–253

38. *Nineteenth-Century America.* New York, NY: Columbia University Press; 1985

39. Jefferson T. Notes on the State of Virginia. Boston, Lilly, and Wait, 1832. Available at: https://www.loc.gov/item/03004902/.pdf. Accessed January 30, 2022

40. Braun L. Race, ethnicity and lung function: A brief history. *Can J Respir Ther.* 2015;51(4):99–101

41. Cartwright SA. Report on the diseases and physical peculiarities of the negro race. *New Orleans Med Surg J.* 1851; VII:692–713

42. Vyas DA, Eisenstein LG, Jones DS. Hidden in plain sight – reconsidering the use of race correction in clinical algorithms. *N Engl J Med.* 2020;383(9): 874–882

43. Burchard EG, Ziv E, Coyle N, et al. The importance of race and ethnic background in biomedical research and clinical practice. *N Engl J Med.* 2003; 348(12):1170–1175

44. Cooper RS, Kaufman JS, Ward R. Race and genomics. *N Engl J Med.* 2003; 348(12):1166–1170

45. Phimister EG. Medicine and the racial divide. *N Engl J Med.* 2003;348 (12):1081–1082

46. Yearby R. Race based medicine, colorblind disease: how racism in medicine harms us all. *Am J Bioeth.* 2021;21(2): 19–27

47. Bird A. Perceptions of epigenetics. *Nature.* 2007;447(7143):396–398

48. Hong JY, Lim J, Carvalho F, et al. Long-term programming of CD8 T cell immunity by perinatal exposure to glucocorticoids. *Cell.* 2020;180(5):847–861.e15

49. Dias BG, Ressler KJ. Parental olfactory experience influences behavior and neural structure in subsequent generations. *Nat Neurosci.* 2014;17(1):89–96

50. Heard-Garris NJ, Cale M, Camaj L, Hamati MC, Dominguez TP. Transmitting trauma: A systematic review of vicarious racism and child health. *Soc Sci Med.* 2018;199:230–240

51. Simons RL, Lei MK, Klopack E, Zhang Y, Gibbons FX, Beach SRH. Racial discrimination, inflammation, and chronic illness among African American women at midlife: support for the weathering perspective. *J Racial Ethn Health Disparities.* 2021;8(2):339–349

52. Geronimus AT, Hicken M, Keene D, Bound J. "Weathering" and age patterns of allostatic load scores among blacks and whites in the United States. *Am J Public Health.* 2006;96(5):826–833

53. Johnstone SE, Baylin SB. Stress and the epigenetic landscape: a link to the pathobiology of human diseases? *Nat Rev Genet.* 2010;11(11):806–812

54. Wright JL, Jarvis JN, Pachter LM, Walker-Harding LR. "Racism as a public health issue" APS racism series: at the intersection of equity, science, and social justice. *Pediatr Res.* 2020;88(5): 696–698

55. Micheletti SJ, Bryc K, Ancona Esselmann SG, et al; 23andMe Research Team. 23andMe Research Team. Genetic consequences of the transatlantic slave trade in the Americas. *Am J Hum Genet.* 2020;107(2):265–277

56. Stevenson BE. What's love got to do with it?: Concubinage and enslaved women and girls in the antebellum south. In: Berry DR, Harris LM, eds. *Sexuality and Slavery: Reclaiming Intimate Histories in the Americas.* Athens, GA: University of Georgia Press; 2018:159–188

57. Chestnut MB. A Confederate woman's diary. Available at: https://wps.prenhall.com/wps/media/objects/172/176275/16_confe. HTM. Accessed February 1, 2022

58. Jennings T. "Us colored women had to go through a plenty": sexual exploitation of African-American slave women. *J Womens Hist.* 1990;1(3):45–74

59. Jacobs HA. In: Child LM, ed. *Incidents in the Life of a Slave Girl: Written by Herself.* London, England: Hodson and Son; 1862. Available at https://docsouth.unc.edu/fpn/jacobs/jacobs.html. Accessed February 23, 2022

60. Fortes-Lima C, Verdu P. Anthropological genetics perspectives on the transatlantic slave trade. *Hum Mol Genet.* 2021;30(R1):R79–R87

61. Bryc K, Durand EY, Macpherson JM, Reich D, Mountain JL. The genetic ancestry of African Americans, Latinos, and European Americans across the United States. *Am J Hum Genet.* 2015;96(1):37–53

62. Hollinger DA. The one drop rule and the one hate rule. *Daedalus.* 2005;134(1):18–28

63. Plecker WA. Virginia's attempt to adjust the color problem. *Am J Public Health (N Y).* 1925;15(2):111–115

64. Spruhan P. A legal history of blood quantum in federal Indian law to 1935. *S D Law Rev.* 2006;51(1):1–50

65. Heard-Garris N, Williams DR, Davis M. Structuring research to address discrimination as a factor in child and adolescent Health. *JAMA Pediatr.* 2018;172(10):910–912

66. Raphael JL, Oyeku SO. Implicit bias in pediatrics: an emerging focus in health equity research. *Pediatrics.* 2020;145(5):e20200512

67. Duffee J, Szilagyi M, Forkey H, Kelly ET; Council on Community Pediatrics, Council on Foster Care, Adoption and Kinship Care, Council on Child Abuse and Neglect, Committee on Psychosocial Aspects of the Child and Family Health. Committee on psychosocial aspects of child and family health. Trauma-informed care in child health systems. *Pediatrics.* 2021;148(2): e2021052579

68. Hardeman RR, Homan PA, Chantarat T, Davis BA, Brown TH. Improving the measurement of structural racism to achieve antiracist health policy. *Health Aff (Millwood)*. 2022;41(2): 179–186

69. Delgado C, Baweja M, Crews DC, et al. A unifying approach for GFR estimation: Recommendations of the NKF-ASN task force on reassessing the inclusion of race in diagnosing kidney disease. *Am J Kidney Dis*. 2022;79(2):268–288.e1

70. Delgado C, Baweja M, Burrows NR, et al. Reassessing the inclusion of race in diagnosing kidney diseases: An interim report from the NKF-ASN Task Force. *J Am Soc Nephrol*. 2021;32(6): 1305–1317

71. Feldman HI, Briggs JP. Race and the estimation of GFR: getting it right. *Am J Kidney Dis*. 2021;78(1):3–4

72. Diao JA, Inker LA, Levey AS, Tighiouart H, Powe NR, Manrai AK. In search of a better equation—performance and equity in estimates of kidney function. *N Engl J Med*. 2021;384(5):396–399

73. Eneanya ND, Yang W, Reese PP. Reconsidering the consequences of using race to estimate kidney function. *JAMA*. 2019;322(2):113–114

74. Inker LA, Eneanya ND, Coresh J, et al; Chronic Kidney Disease Epidemiology Collaboration. New creatinine- and cystatin C-based equations to estimate GFR without race. *N Engl J Med*. 2021; 385(19):1737–1749

75. Yan G, Nee R, Scialla JJ, et al. Estimation of black-white disparities in CKD outcomes: Comparison using the 2021 versus the 2009 CKD-EPI creatinine equations. *Am J Kidney Dis*. 2022:S0272-6386(21)01053-2

76. Meeusen JW, Kasozi RN, Larson TS, Lieske JC. Clinical impact of the refit CKD-EPI 2021 creatinine-based eGFR equation. *Clin Chem*. 2022;68(4):534–539

77. Wiggins O. University of Maryland Medical System drops race-based algorithm—officials say harms black patients. Available at: https://www.washingtonpost.com/local/md-politics/maryland-hospital-black-diagnostic-test-kidneys/2021/11/17/e69edcfc-4711-11ec-b05d-3cb9d96eb495_story.html. Published

online November 17, 2021. Accessed January 31, 2022

78. Lujan HL, DiCarlo SE. Science reflects history as society influences science: brief history of "race," "race correction," and the spirometer. *Adv Physiol Educ*. 2018;42(2):163–165

79. Braun L. *Breathing Race into the Machine: The Surprising Career of the Spirometer from Plantation to Genetics*. Minneapolis, MN: University of Minnesota Press; 2014

80. Braun L. Race correction and spirometry: why history matters. *Chest*. 2021;159(4):1670–1675

81. Braun L. Spirometry, measurement, and race in the nineteenth century. *J Hist Med Allied Sci*. 2005;60(2):135–169

82. Hankinson JL, Odencrantz JR, Fedan KB. Spirometric reference values from a sample of the general U.S. population. *Am J Respir Crit Care Med*. 1999;159(1):179–187

83. LaVange L, Davis SM, Hankinson J, et al. Spirometry reference equations from the HCHS/SOL (Hispanic Community Health Study/Study of Latinos). *Am J Respir Crit Care Med*. 2017;196(8): 993–1003

84. Kumar R, Seibold MA, Aldrich MC, et al. Genetic ancestry in lung-function predictions. *N Engl J Med*. 2010;363(4): 321–330

85. Baugh AD, Shiboski S, Hansel NN, et al. Reconsidering the utility of race-specific lung function prediction equations. *Am J Respir Crit Care Med*. 2022;205(7): 819–829

86. Bhakta NR, Kaminsky DA, Bime C, et al. Addressing race in pulmonary function testing by aligning intent and evidence with practice and perception. *Chest*. 2022;161(1):288–297

87. Anderson MA, Malhotra A, Non AL. Could routine race-adjustment of spirometers exacerbate racial disparities in COVID-19 recovery? *Lancet Respir Med*. 2021;9(2):124–125

88. Churchwell K, Elkind MSV, Benjamin RM, et al; American Heart Association. Call to action: Structural racism as a fundamental driver of health disparities: a presidential advisory from the American Heart Association. *Circulation*. 2020;142(24):e454–e468

89. Goff DC Jr, Lloyd-Jones DM, Bennett G, et al; American College of Cardiology/ American Heart Association Task Force on Practice Guidelines. 2013 ACC/AHA guideline on the assessment of cardiovascular risk: a report of the American College of Cardiology/American Heart Association Task Force on Practice Guidelines. *Circulation*. 2014;129(25 Suppl 2):S49–S73

90. Vyas DA, James A, Kormos W, Essien UR. Revising the atherosclerotic cardiovascular disease calculator without race. *Lancet Digit Health*. 2022;4(1):e4–e5

91. Vasan RS, van den Heuvel E. Differences in estimates for 10-year risk of cardiovascular disease in Black versus White individuals with identical risk factor profiles using pooled cohort equations: an in silico cohort study. *Lancet Digit Health*. 2022;4(1):e55–e63

92. Yadlowsky S, Hayward RA, Sussman JB, McClelland RL, Min YI, Basu S. Clinical implications of revised pooled cohort equations for estimating atherosclerotic cardiovascular disease risk. *Ann Intern Med*. 2018;169(1):20–29

93. National Heart, Lung and Blood Institute. Assessing cardiovascular risk: systematic evidence review from the Risk Assessment Work Group, 2013. Available at: https://www.nhlbi.nih.gov/sites/default/files/media/docs/risk-assessment.pdf Accessed February 1, 2022

94. National Institutes of Health, Consensus Development Conference Panel. National Institutes of Health Consensus Development conference statement: vaginal birth after cesarean: new insights March 8-10, 2010. *Obstet Gynecol*. 2010;115(6):1279–1295

95. Walrath D. Rethinking pelvic typologies and the human birth mechanism. *Curr Anthropol*. 2003;44(1):5–31

96. Vyas DA, Jones DS, Meadows AR, Diouf K, Nour NM, Schantz-Dunn J. Challenging the use of race in the vaginal birth after cesarean section calculator. *Womens Health Issues*. 2019;29(3):201–204

97. Hollard AL, Wing DA, Chung JH, et al. Ethnic disparity in the success of vaginal birth after cesarean delivery. *J Matern Fetal Neonatal Med*. 2006;19(8): 483–487

98. Grobman WA, Sandoval G, Rice MM, et al; Eunice Kennedy Shriver National Institute of Child Health and Human Development Maternal-Fetal Medicine Units Network. Prediction of vaginal birth after cesarean delivery in term gestations: a calculator without race and ethnicity. *Am J Obstet Gynecol.* 2021;225(6):664.e1–664.e7

99. American College of Obstetricians and Gynecologists. Vaginal birth after cesarean delivery. ACOG Practice Bulletin No. 205. *Obstet Gynecol.* 2019;133(2): e110–e127

100. American College of Obstetricians and Gynecologists. Practice advisory – counseling regarding approach to delivery after cesarean and the use of a vaginal birth after cesarean calculator. Available at: https://www.acog.org/clinical/clinical-guidance/practice-advisory/articles/2021/12/counseling-regarding-approach-to-delivery-after-cesarean-and-the-use-of-a-vaginal-birth-after-cesarean-calculator. Published online 2021. Accessed February 9, 2022

101. National Center for Health Statistics, Centers for Disease Control and Prevention. Maternal mortality rates in the United States, 2019. Available at: https://www.cdc.gov/nchs/data/hestat/maternal-mortality-2021/E-Stat-Maternal-Mortality-Rates-H.pdf. Accessed February 2, 2022

102. Petersen EE, Davis NL, Goodman D, et al. Racial/Ethnic disparities in pregnancy-related deaths—United States, 2007–2016. *MMWR Morb Mortal Wkly Rep.* 2019;68(35):762–765

103. Council on Community Pediatrics and Committee on Native American Child Health. Policy statement—health equity and children's rights. *Pediatrics.* 2010;125(4):838–849

104. Ward JV. *The Skin We're in: Teaching Our Teens to be Emotional Strong, Socially Smart, and Spiritually Connected.* New York, NY: Free Press; 2002

105. Borrell LN, Elhawary JR, Fuentes-Afflick E, et al. Race and genetic ancestry in medicine—a time for reckoning with racism. *N Engl J Med.* 2021;384(5): 474–480

106. Wright JL, Freed GL, Hendricks-Muñoz KD, et al; Committee on Diversity, Inclusion and Equity on behalf of the American Pediatric Society. Achieving equity through science and integrity: dismantling race-based medicine [published online ahead of print April 5, 2022]. *Pediatr Res.* 2022

107. Yaeger JP, Alio AP, Fiscella K. Addressing child health equity through clinical decision-making. *Pediatrics.* 2022;149(2): e2021053698

108. American Academy of Pediatrics. Words matter: AAP guidance on inclusive, anti-biased language. Itasca, IL: American Academy of Pediatrics; 2021. Available at: https://services.aap.org/en/about-the-aap/american-academy-of-pediatrics-equity-and-inclusion-efforts/words-matter-aap-guidance-on-inclusive-anti-biased-language. Accessed February 3, 2022

POLICY STATEMENT Organizational Principles to Guide and Define the Child Health Care System and/or Improve the Health of all Children

American Academy of Pediatrics

DEDICATED TO THE HEALTH OF ALL CHILDREN®

Early Childhood Caries in Indigenous Communities

Steve Holve, MD,[a] Patricia Braun, MD, MPH,[b,c] James D. Irvine, MD,[d] Kristen Nadeau, MD, MS,[e] Robert J. Schroth, DMD, MSc, PhD,[f,g,h] AMERICAN ACADEMY OF PEDIATRICS COMMITTEE ON NATIVE AMERICAN CHILD HEALTH AND SECTION ON ORAL HEALTH, CANADIAN PAEDIATRIC SOCIETY FIRST NATIONS, INUIT, AND MÉTIS HEALTH COMMITTEE

abstract

The oral health of Indigenous children of Canada (First Nations, Inuit, and Métis) and the United States (American Indian and Alaska native) is a major child health disparity when compared with the general population of both countries. Early childhood caries (ECC) occurs in Indigenous children at an earlier age, with a higher prevalence, and at much greater severity than in the general population. ECC results in adverse oral health, affecting childhood health and well-being, and may result in high rates of costly surgical treatment under general anesthesia. ECC is an infectious disease that is influenced by multiple factors, but the social determinants of health are particularly important. This policy statement includes recommendations for preventive and clinical oral health care for infants, toddlers, preschool-aged children, and pregnant women by primary health care providers. It also addresses community-based health-promotion initiatives and access to dental care for Indigenous children. This policy statement encourages oral health interventions at early ages in Indigenous children, including referral to dental care for the use of sealants, interim therapeutic restorations, and silver diamine fluoride. Further community-based research on the microbiology, epidemiology, prevention, and management of ECC in Indigenous communities is also needed to reduce the dismally high rate of caries in this population.

[a]Tuba City Regional Health Care Corporation, Tuba City, Arizona; [b]Denver Health and Hospital, Denver, Colorado; [c]Anschutz Medical Campus, University of Colorado, Aurora, Colorado [d]University of Saskatchewan, LaRonge, Saskatchewan, Canada; [e]Mentored Scholarly Activity Longitudinal Research Course and Colorado Clinical and Translational Sciences Institute Scientific Advisory and Review Committee, Anschutz Medical Campus, University of Colorado and Children's Hospital Colorado, Aurora, Colorado; [f]Departments of Preventive Dental Science, Pediatrics and Child Health, and Community Health Sciences, Rady Faculty of Health Sciences, University of Manitoba, Winnipeg, Manitoba, Canada; [g]Children's Hospital Research Institute of Manitoba, Winnipeg, Manitoba, Canada; and [h]Section of Pediatric Dentistry, Winnipeg Regional Health Authority, Winnipeg, Manitoba, Canada

Policy statements from the American Academy of Pediatrics benefit from expertise and resources of liaisons and internal (AAP) and external reviewers. However, policy statements from the American Academy of Pediatrics may not reflect the views of the liaisons or the organizations or government agencies that they represent.

Drs Holve and Schroth participated in the planning for this manuscript and writing and editing of the manuscript; Drs Braun, Irvine, and Nadeau participated in the writing and editing of the manuscript; and all authors approved the final manuscript as submitted.

The guidance in this statement does not indicate an exclusive course of treatment or serve as a standard of medical care. Variations, taking into account individual circumstances, may be appropriate.

All policy statements from the American Academy of Pediatrics automatically expire 5 years after publication unless reaffirmed, revised, or retired at or before that time.

To cite: Holve S, Braun P, Irvine JD, et al. AAP AMERICAN ACADEMY OF PEDIATRICS COMMITTEE ON NATIVE AMERICAN CHILD HEALTH AND SECTION ON ORAL HEALTH, CANADIAN PAEDIATRIC SOCIETY FIRST NATIONS, INUIT, AND MÉTIS HEALTH COMMITTEE. Early Childhood Caries in Indigenous Communities. Pediatrics. 2021;147(6):e2021051481

INTRODUCTION

Indigenous children of Canada (First Nations [FN], Inuit, and Métis) and the United States (American Indian and Alaska native [AI/AN]) face significant health disparities compared with non-Indigenous populations. The oral health disparities Indigenous children experience exemplify the inequities and major need for oral health promotion, caries prevention, and early, locally available dental care services for them. Although general guidelines on oral health promotion, caries prevention, and risk assessment exist, the severity of dental disease and the barriers to care in Indigenous communities require special consideration.

Early childhood caries (ECC) is defined as tooth decay in any primary tooth in a child younger than age 6 years.[1] Also referred to as early childhood tooth decay or baby-bottle tooth decay, the term ECC better characterizes the disease as complex and involving transmission of infectious bacteria, dietary habits, and oral hygiene. ECC is an infectious disease, with *Streptococcus mutans* being the most commonly recognized causative organism. The causative triad for caries includes cariogenic bacteria, fermentable carbohydrates, and host susceptibility (integrity of tooth enamel). Caries has been described as the most prevalent pediatric infectious disease and the most common chronic disease of children.[2]

Tooth loss as a result of ECC may result in malocclusion and low oral health–related quality of life.[3] Children with ECC are at increased risk of further caries throughout childhood and adolescence.[4,5] The effects of ECC go beyond the oral cavity and influence overall childhood health and well-being, which are already compromised for many Indigenous children.[3,6–8]

Severe early childhood caries (S-ECC) is an aggressive form of ECC and is classified by location of the caries, number of teeth affected, and age.[1] S-ECC commonly requires surgical treatment under general anesthesia (GA).[9] Children with S-ECC experience more nutritional problems, including iron-deficiency anemia, low vitamin D, and overweight or obesity. S-ECC that penetrates the tooth pulp can lead to painful dental infections or abscesses and, rarely, death.[6–8,10]

ORAL HEALTH STATUS IN INDIGENOUS CHILDREN

In 2011, the prevalence of ECC in 3- to 5-year-old FN and Inuit children was 85%, and the prevalence of S-ECC was as high as 25%.[11–13] Oral health surveys performed by the Indian Health Service (IHS) in 2014 revealed that 75% of AI/AN children between the ages of 3 and 5 years had ECC, and in many communities, the caries rate was >90% (5 times greater than that of the general US child population).[14,15] The true burden of ECC in Indigenous children is not only the disparate ECC prevalence but also the disease severity. The average number of decayed or filled teeth in AI/AN children 2 to 5 years old was 5.8, almost 5 times that of the general US preschool population.[15,16]

An important consequence of ECC severity is the need for dental surgery under GA.[9,13,17] Rehabilitative surgery is expensive and carries the potential risks of GA. Overall, the rate of dental surgery to treat ECC under GA in Canada was 7 times higher for children from communities with a high proportion of Indigenous peoples than communities with lower Indigenous populations.[9,17] In the more remote Indigenous regions of Canada, the rates of dental surgery under GA exceed 200 per 1000 children younger than 5 years each year, a rate 15 times higher than the overall annual Canadian rate.[9,17] Exact data on the overall number of AI/AN children undergoing dental surgery for caries are limited, but one study in the Yukon–Kuskokwim Delta of Alaska reported that by 6 years of age, 73% of Alaska native children had undergone dental surgery under GA, a rate at least 50 times that in the general US population.[18]

EPIDEMIOLOGY OF ECC

Indigenous children often develop ECC at earlier ages than other children. The 2014 IHS Oral Health Survey reported that 21% of AI/AN 1-year-olds and 40% of AI/AN 2-year-olds had caries, whereas most dental surveys suggest ECC is rare among US children before 12 months of age, and only 10% of US children younger than 2 years have ECC.[19] The etiology of ECC in Indigenous children is multifactorial. The typical "window of infectivity" for the acquisition of cariogenic microorganisms, including *S mutans*, is between 19 and 31 months. However, 2 recent studies reported that AI/AN children acquire *S mutans* at earlier ages: 37% of 12-month-olds and 60% of 16-month-olds had *S mutans* colonization.[20,21] Additionally, primary teeth erupt at an earlier age in AI/AN infants, which may result in earlier *S mutans* colonization and earlier progression to caries.[22] Authors of a recent review of caries reiterate that newly erupted teeth are much more prone to caries.[23] Additionally, a recent study of Canadian FN children revealed that children with S-ECC had a significantly different plaque microbiome than their caries-free counterparts, with the S-ECC group harboring higher levels of known cariogenic organisms, particularly *S mutans*.[24] The early acquisition of *S mutans* in Indigenous children is likely mediated by factors associated with poverty, including household crowding, family size, nutrition, and other health behaviors.[25] Unfortunately, Indigenous children in the United States and Canada experience poverty at rates 2 to 3 times greater than the general population. For children younger than 5 years, 52% of FN children live in poverty, as do 25% Inuit and 23% of Métis children, compared with 13% of nonracialized Canadian children.[26] More than 37% of AI/AN children in the United States live in poverty, compared with 10% of their white American counterparts.[27]

Other known ECC risk factors are commonly found in Indigenous children. Caries in parents is associated with increased risk in their infants.[28] ECC is also associated with prolonged bottle-feeding, consumption of sugar-containing drinks, high frequency of sugary snacks,[29–33] and exposure to tobacco smoke.[13,34] Breastfeeding for up to 12 months of age can reduce ECC risk by half, most likely via immune-modulating effects and promotion of a healthy microbiome. Furthermore, a recent study demonstrated that breastfeeding did not provoke a decrease in biofilm pH and, therefore, did not facilitate ECC.[35] If the infant breastfeeds to sleep, the gums and erupting teeth should be wiped to minimize the risk of caries.[36] However, breastfeeding beyond 12 months of age, especially with at-will nighttime feeding, is associated with increased risk of ECC.[37–39] Obesity has also been shown to be associated with ECC, although it is unclear whether this risk occurs independently from dietary factors.[3,10,40–42] In addition, gestational diabetes, which is prevalent in Indigenous populations, may have an effect on early childhood dental development and caries risk.[43–45]

PREVENTION STRATEGIES

Prenatal Oral Health Care

ECC prevention is optimal if initiated prenatally.[46] Given the evidence for transmission of cariogenic bacteria from mother to child, routine dental assessments and preventive dental care, oral hygiene education, optimal prenatal nutrition, and the use of fluoride toothpaste for pregnant women are strategies that may prevent or delay ECC in their children.[46] Recent guidelines conclude that dental care in pregnancy is safe.[47–49]

Fluoride

All major Canadian and American dental and pediatric societies endorse the use of fluorides as safe and effective for caries prevention.[50–54] All of the aforementioned organizations support the use of fluoridated toothpaste twice daily for all children. They recommend that children younger than 3 years have

their teeth brushed by an adult with a grain of rice–sized portion of fluoridated toothpaste and that children 3 to 6 years of age be assisted with brushing with a green pea–sized portion of fluoridated toothpaste.[51,52]

Community water fluoridation is safe, effective, and inexpensive and does not require daily adherence.[55,56] Community water fluoridation in AN communities has been associated with a 40% reduction in caries.[57] In North America, there is wide disparity in the access to community water fluoridation. In 2017, 38.7% of Canadians using community water supplies had access to fluoridated water, compared with only 2.3% of FN people.[58] Although 74.4% of US residents had access to fluoridated community water, only 50% of Alaskans received fluoridated community water, with only 5.3% receiving optimal fluoride levels.[18,59]

Topical fluorides have been shown to be effective in preventing caries.[18,59] Studies in Indigenous children in Canada and the United States have shown reduction in caries with fluoride varnish, although the results were not statistically significant.[60,61]

These modestly favorable results for fluoride varnish in AI/AN children are tempered by 2 larger studies with longer follow-up. First, a 5-year IHS program targeting AI/AN children initially resulted in a small decrease in ECC in children younger than 2 years, but these benefits were lost for children 2 to 5 years of age.[62] A second cluster-randomized controlled trial (RCT) testing 4 fluoride varnish applications (and oral health–promotion activities) by trained tribal health workers in Head Start classrooms did not yield a reduction in ECC.[63] These studies suggest that fluoride varnish should be initiated with the first tooth eruption in Indigenous children to achieve maximal benefit. Although the data on fluoride varnish are

mixed for Indigenous populations, fluoride varnish is still recommended because the potential benefits far outweigh any risks. Fluoride varnish applications help to enhance both the mineralization of healthy enamel (making it more resistant to caries) and the remineralization of early incipient caries lesions (ie, white spot lesions) in primary and permanent teeth that have not yet progressed to the cavitation (ie, cavity) stage. The American Dental Association still recommends fluoride varnish for all children. However, the challenge is that fluoride varnish is not effective in arresting and remineralizing more advanced lesions that have cavitated through the enamel (ie, cavities), which are known to be more prevalent in young Indigenous children. Therefore, early applications of fluoride varnish to newly erupted teeth, beginning at the eruption of the first primary tooth at the 6-month developmental age milestone, is paramount.

Oral Health Education

Evidence surrounding the effectiveness of conducting dental examinations and provision of parental counseling to prevent ECC in preschool-aged children is mixed.[60,61,64,65] Studies of oral health education in Indigenous families resulted in increased parental knowledge but rarely demonstrate reduction in caries.[63,66] One large RCT of motivational interviewing in parents of AI preschool-aged children reported increased parent and caregiver knowledge but no reduction in ECC.[63] A previous Canadian RCT reported that motivational interviewing was associated with a reduction in the degree of severe caries among Cree children in northern Quebec.[64] Other studies suggest that oral health education for pregnant women and mothers of infants can reduce S-ECC from 32% to 20%.[67–69] Like the early receipt of fluoride varnish, evidence suggests that receiving oral health education at the time of first tooth eruption is more beneficial.

Community-Based Strategies

Evidence is clear that caries were rare in Indigenous communities until the introduction to European settler diets, including refined sugar and other processed foods.[70-73] In Canada, there are several community-based efforts to reduce ECC, some of which promote traditional Indigenous diets.[74-77] One program in a Cree community encourages breastfeeding and promotes the introduction of traditional first foods instead of processed infant foods.[78] These efforts are promising, but there are no data regarding their effects on ECC.

ASSESSMENT AND TREATMENT STRATEGIES

Caries Risk Assessment

Timely caries risk assessment (CRA) is an important first step to reduce the risk for ECC. Several pediatric and dental organizations have developed easy-to-use CRA tools that can identify a child's risk of developing caries.[79] CRAs also assist nondental primary health care providers in assessing the need for anticipatory guidance, fluoride varnish, and referral for dental evaluation.

Sealants

Pit and fissure dental sealants have traditionally been used on occlusal tooth surfaces of permanent molars to reduce dental caries. Recent reviews concur that in populations at high risk of caries, such as Indigenous children, sealants can be placed on primary molars after eruption.[80,81] Studies suggest that 74% of sealed primary molars remain caries-free and that sealing primary molars is cost-effective in reducing caries progression and the need for operative repair.[82] The American Dental Association recommends sealants on primary molars and fluoride varnish every 3 to 6 months

to arrest or reverse noncavitated carious lesions on the occlusal surfaces of primary teeth.[83] However, dental sealants may be challenging to apply on the teeth of infants and toddlers.

Interim Therapeutic Restorations

Minimally invasive dental restorative techniques, such as glass ionomer products, provide a practical option for managing cavitated lesions in young children. Interim therapeutic restorations can be used to restore and prevent caries progression in young and uncooperative children, in children with special health care requirements, and in circumstances in which the placement of traditional restorations is not possible.[84] Interim therapeutic restorations can be provided by midlevel dental professionals, including dental therapists (DTs) and hygienists, in many locales.

Silver Diamine Fluoride

Silver diamine fluoride (SDF) has been used extensively outside North America for caries arrest, with good results.[85,86] SDF is indicated for the arrest of cavitated caries lesions in primary teeth as part of a comprehensive caries management program.[83] SDF will turn the carious lesion hard and black, but this side effect is generally well accepted by parents.[87] At present, the use of SDF in the United States and Canada is limited to the dental profession, because there are no formal guidelines for its use outside of dentistry.

Frank Mendoza, DDS, an IHS dentist, pioneered the use of silver ion products at a tribal health clinic for caries arrest and demonstrated that only 2% of treated patients needed eventual operative repair.[19] Several other IHS and tribal programs now use SDF, with positive results.[88] There is an emerging consensus that SDF may be an important treatment option for children at high risk for

progression to severe ECC.[89] If the use of SDF becomes more widespread, primary care health providers will play a critical role in identifying patients for referral and in promoting adherence to treatment. Evidence-based clinical guidelines from the American Dental Association and the American Academy of Pediatric Dentistry for nonrestorative treatment of caries recommend biannual applications of 38% SDF to arrest advanced cavitated lesions on primary teeth, with the recognition that additional applications may occasionally be necessary.[90]

Repair Under GA

Given the prevalence and severity of ECC in Indigenous children, operative repair is often required. However, because ECC is largely preventable, each child requiring operative repair is a costly failure of our preventive and treatment systems. Operative repair is expensive, and prevention is more cost-effective, less painful, and less time-consuming for the patient.[9,91] Furthermore, the acute risks associated with anesthesia and the evidence that GA in young children may have potential cognitive effects are additional reasons to avoid this consequence of ECC.[92,93]

Authors of a cost-effectiveness review of preventive interventions such as water fluoridation, fluoride varnish, tooth brushing with fluoride toothpaste, and use of sealants concluded that these interventions are collectively relatively inexpensive and cost-saving and, if fully used, could reduce S-ECC requiring operative repair.[18] The major benefit of increased use of SDF is the arrest of the progression of already established caries and a subsequent reduction in the need for operative repair with GA.

ACCESS TO EARLY ORAL HEALTH CARE

Severe dental workforce shortages in Indigenous communities contribute to the high rates of untreated caries in

Indigenous children. The 2014 Oral Health Survey reported the ratio of dentists per person was 1:2800 for AI/AN communities compared with the US average of 1:1500[16] and that 45% of 5-year-old AI/AN children had untreated caries compared with 19% of US children.[15]

All major Canadian and American dental and pediatric societies have called for comprehensive dental health care from dentists for children by 12 months of age: the "age-one dental visit."[94,95] The chronic shortage of dentists in Indigenous communities suggests we look to expanded roles of other dental providers (eg, DTs and hygienists) and other nondental providers to increase access to oral health care, with an emphasis on preventive services.

In the 1970s, Health Canada supported the use of DTs for FN communities, and many began practice in the northern communities of Canada.[96] DTs are midlevel dental providers who work under the supervision of a dentist. Reviews of DTs in more than 50 countries reported that DTs expand access to dental care in a safe and effective manner.[97] Unfortunately, over time, an increasing number of Canadian DTs chose to work in urban settings rather than rural communities. The urban migration of DTs and the ongoing opposition by professional dental societies led the Canadian federal government to discontinue funding DT training programs in 2011.[98]

As Canada was reducing its support for the training of DTs, the Alaska Native Tribal Health Consortium began a dental health aide therapist (DHAT) program. The Alaska DHAT program has been linked to better oral health access and outcomes in remote villages and has been well received by health care providers and community members.[99–101] DHAT programs also have been

implemented in tribal clinics in the states of Washington and Minnesota. The National Indian Health Board champions the use of DHATs as a strategy to increase access to oral health and a legitimate exercise of tribal sovereignty.[102] The Department of Indigenous Services Canada and the Canadian Dental Hygienists Association have recently proposed the reestablishment of a training program for dental therapy that would see dental hygienists complete an extra year of education to be able to provide expanded oral health services.[103]

Primary care providers (pediatricians, family physicians, nurse practitioners, community health nurses, physician assistants, and dietitians) in Indigenous communities in North America are in unique positions to complement the work of dental health professionals. These nondental providers provide early and frequent care to children before they see a dental provider. In many Indigenous communities, well-infant, infant health, and immunization clinics are provided on a regular basis through community health nurses and physicians. These nondental providers have an opportunity to assess children's risk for caries and promote oral health as part of their overall health-promotion activities. In addition, they can provide oral health screening for infants and young children, provide fluoride varnish, and coordinate referrals to dental health professionals. Moreover, because of the high rates of obesity and type 2 diabetes mellitus in Indigenous populations, Indigenous youth may undergo dietary assessments and may be seen by dietitians. These visits provide opportunities for collaboration between primary care and dentistry to encourage limited consumption of sugars, a shared risk factor for both obesity and caries.

ORAL HEALTH RECOMMENDATIONS FOR INDIGENOUS COMMUNITIES

Caries prevention interventions that have worked well in the general population have been less effective in Indigenous children; therefore, the prevention and treatment recommendations described here should be informed by what is known of ECC epidemiology in Indigenous children. Indigenous children acquire *S mutans* colonization at an earlier age, develop caries at an earlier age, and commonly experience severe ECC. The health care community needs to recognize that "two is too late" for preventive interventions in Indigenous children to be successful and that new strategies with earlier intervention are needed to reduce this health disparity.

Community-Based Promotion Initiatives

- Promote changes in Indigenous communities to reduce frequent consumption of sugar-containing drinks and sugary snacks through education and improved access to healthy foods in communities.

- Emphasize the importance of oral health for the pregnant woman and her infant(s) through community-based activities.

- Promote exclusive breastfeeding for the first 6 months and breastfeeding until 12 months of age.

- Ensure that Indigenous communities benefit from community water fluoridation and know the fluoridation level of their water supply.

- Promote collaboration between oral health and obesity and type 2 diabetes mellitus prevention efforts for Indigenous communities.

Clinical Care Recommendations

- Consider early childhood oral health as an integral part of overall childhood health and well-being.

- Ensure that Indigenous women receive preconception and prenatal screening for oral health, anticipatory guidance for oral health and hygiene, and referral for dental care.
- Discuss oral health during well-child care visits with a CRA and anticipatory guidance on oral hygiene and diet, starting with the first tooth eruption.
- Recommend the establishment of a dental home by 12 months of age.
- Promote supervised twice-daily use of fluoridated toothpaste for all Indigenous children beginning with the eruption of the first tooth (rice grain–sized portion of toothpaste for children <36 months of age and a green pea–sized portion for children ≥36 months of age).
- Provide fluoride varnish by either dental or nondental health care providers in primary care settings and by trained lay workers in other settings starting with the first tooth eruption (and then every 3–6 months thereafter).
- Promote the incorporation of SDF into caries management protocols for Indigenous children with ECC to decrease or arrest caries progression and reduce or avoid the reliance on GA to facilitate operative repair.
- Consider promoting the incorporation of interim therapeutic restoration into caries management protocols.
- Consider promoting the use of sealants on primary molars to prevent caries and the need for operative repair.

Workforce and Access

- Provide early access to dental health professionals by 12 months of age to establish a dental home with the full range of oral health–promotion and interceptive disease-prevention services.
- Consider roles that DTs, dental hygienists, and primary health care providers can assume in areas where it is difficult to recruit and retain a sufficient number of dentists to provide early oral health services.
- Ensure that dentists, dental hygienists, DTs, and assistants working in Indigenous communities receive education to practice in a culturally appropriate manner.

Advocacy

- Advocate for an adequate dental workforce that can include the training and use of midlevel professionals such as DTs.
- Advocate for increased representation of Indigenous people in oral health professions.
- Advocate for regular and sustained ambulatory dental care in or near Indigenous communities.

Research

- Support further community-based participatory research on the epidemiology, prevention, management, and microbiology of ECC and ECC-prevention projects in Indigenous communities.

RECOMMENDED RESOURCES

- American Academy of Pediatric Dentistry. *Best Practice on Fluoride Therapy*. Chicago, IL: American Academy of Pediatric Dentistry; 2018. Available at: http://www.aapd.org/media/Policies_Guidelines/BP_FluorideTherapy.pdf.
- American Academy of Pediatric Dentistry. *Clinical Practice Guideline on Use of Silver Diamine Fluoride for Dental Caries Management in Children and Adolescents, Including Those with Special Health Care Needs*. Chicago, IL: American Academy of Pediatric Dentistry; 2017. Available at: http://www.aapd.org/media/Policies_Guidelines/G_SDF.pdf.
- American Academy of Pediatric Dentistry. *Best Practice on Caries-Risk Assessment and Management for Infants, Children, and Adolescents*. Chicago, IL: American Academy of Pediatric Dentistry; 2014. Available at: http://www.aapd.org/media/Policies_Guidelines/BP_CariesRiskAssessment.pdf.
- American Academy of Pediatrics, Section on Oral Health. Protecting All Children's Teeth (PACT): a pediatric oral health training program. Available at: https://www.aap.org/en-us/advocacy-and-policy/aap-health-initiatives/Oral-Health/Pages/Protecting-All-Childrens-Teeth.aspx.
- American Academy of Pediatrics, Section on Oral Health. Maintaining and improving the oral health of young children. *Pediatrics*. 2014; 123(6):1224–1229. Available at: www.pediatrics.org/cgi/doi/10.1542/peds.2014-2984.
- American Academy of Pediatrics, Section on Oral Health. Oral Health Advocacy Toolkit. Available at: https://www.aap.org/en-us/advocacy-and-policy/aap-health-initiatives/Oral-Health/Pages/Oral-Health-Advocacy-Toolkit.aspx.
- American Academy of Pediatrics, Section on Oral Health. Campaign for Dental Health/Community Water Fluoridation Resource. Available at: https://ilikemyteeth.org/.
- American Academy of Pediatrics, Section on Oral Health. Fluoride use in caries prevention in the primary care setting. *Pediatrics*. 2014; 134(3):626–633. Available at: http://pediatrics.aappublications.org/content/134/3/626.
- American Academy of Pediatrics. Caries Risk Assessment Tool. Available at: https://www.aap.org/en-us/Documents/oralhealth_RiskAssessmentTool.pdf.
- Casamassimo P, Holt K, eds; National Maternal and Child Oral Health Resource Centre. *Bright Futures in Practice: Oral Health Pocket Guide*. 3rd ed. Washington, DC: Georgetown University; 2016. Available at: https://www.

mchoralhealth.org/PDFs/
BFOHPocketGuide-booklet.pdf.

- Indian Health Service. IHS Early Childhood Caries Collaborative. Available at: https://www.ihs.gov/doh/index.cfm?fuseaction=ecc.display.

- Oral Health and the Aboriginal Child. Knowledge transfer site. Available at: http://oralhealth.circumpolarhealth.org.

- Winnipeg Regional Health Authority. Early childhood tooth decay. Healthy Smile Happy Child pamphlets and other resources. Available at: https://wrha.mb.ca/oral-health/early-childhood-tooth-decay/.

- Smiles for Life: A National Oral Health Curriculum. Available at: https://www.smilesforlifeoralhealth.org/buildcontent.aspx?tut=555&pagekey=62948&cbreceipt=0.

- Canadian Caries Risk Assessment Tool (< 6 years). Available at: http://umanitoba.ca/CRA_Tool_ENG_Version.pdf.

LEAD AUTHORS

Steve Holve, MD
Patricia Braun, MD, MPH
James D. Irvine, MD
Kristen Nadeau, MD, MS
Robert J. Schroth, DMD, MSc, PhD

AMERICAN ACADEMY OF PEDIATRICS COMMITTEE ON NATIVE AMERICAN CHILD HEALTH, 2018–2019

Shaquita L. Bell, MD, Chairperson
Daniel J. Calac, MD
Allison Empey, MD
Kristen J. Nadeau, MD, MS
Jane A. Oski, MD, MPH
(Ret) CAPT Judith K. Thierry, DO, MPH
Ashley Weedn, MD

LIAISONS

Joseph T. Bell, MD – *Association of American Indian Physicians*

Angela Kueck, MD – *American College of Obstetricians and Gynecologists*
Rebecca S. Daily – *American Academy of Child and Adolescent Psychiatry*
Radha Jetty, MD – *Canadian Paediatric Society*
Melanie Mester, MD – *American Academy of Pediatrics Section on Pediatric Trainees*
Nelson Branco, MD – *American Academy of Pediatrics Indian Health Special Interest Group Chairperson*

CONSULTANTS

Diana Dunnigan, MD

STAFF

Madra Guinn Jones, MPH

AMERICAN ACADEMY OF PEDIATRICS SECTION ON ORAL HEALTH EXECUTIVE COMMITTEE, 2018–2019

Patricia Braun, MD, MPH, Chairperson
Susan Fisher-Owens, MD, MPH
Qadira Huff, MD, MPH
Jeffrey Karp, DMD, MS
Anupama Tate, DMD
John Unkel, MD, DDS, MS
David Krol, MD, MPH, Immediate Past Chairperson

STAFF

Ngozi Onyema-Melton, MPH

CANADIAN PAEDIATRIC SOCIETY, FIRST NATIONS, INUIT, AND MÉTIS COMMITTEE

Radha Jetty, MD, Chairperson
Roxanne Goldade, MD, Board Representative
Brett Schrewe, MD
Véronique Pelletier, MD
Ryan J.P. Giroux, MD
Margaret Berry, MD
Leigh Fraser-Roberts, MD

LIAISONS

Patricia Wiebe, MD, MPH – *Indigenous Services Canada, First Nations and Inuit Health Branch**

Laura Mitchell, BA, MA – *Indigenous Services Canada, First Nations and Inuit Health Branch**
Shaquita Bell, MD – *American Academy of Pediatrics Committee on Native American Child Health*
Melanie Morningstar – *Assembly of First Nations*
Karen Beddard – *Inuit Tapiriit Kanatami*
Marilee Nowgesic, RN – *Indigenous Nurses Association of Canada*
Vides Eduardo, MD – *Métis National Council*
Lisa Monkman, MD – *Indigenous Physicians Association of Canada*

CONSULTANTS

James Irvine, MD
Kent Saylor, MD

ACKNOWLEDGMENTS

This position statement has been reviewed by the Community Paediatrics, Drug Therapy and Hazardous Substances, Infectious Diseases and Immunization Committees, and the Paediatric Oral Health Section Executives of the Canadian Paediatric Society. This document has also been reviewed by representatives from the First Nations and Inuit Health Branch, Indigenous Services Canada* and the Canadian Dental Association.

ABBREVIATIONS

AI/AN: American Indian and Alaska native
CRA: caries risk assessment
DHAT: dental health aide therapist
DT: dental therapist
ECC: early childhood caries
FN: First Nations
GA: general anesthesia
IHS: Indian Health Service
RCT: randomized controlled trial
SDF: silver diamine fluoride
S-ECC: severe early childhood caries

---

* The views expressed in this article/publication or information resource do not necessarily represent the positions, decisions, or policies of the First Nations and Inuit Health Branch liaisons or their organization.

This policy statement was developed collaboratively between the American Academy of Pediatrics and the Canadian Pediatric Society and is published simultaneously in *Pediatrics* and *Pediatrics & Child Health*.

DOI: https://doi.org/10.1542/peds.2021-051481

Address correspondence to Steve Holve, MD. E-mail: sholve55@gmail.com

PEDIATRICS (ISSN Numbers: Print, 0031-4005; Online, 1098-4275).

FINANCIAL DISCLOSURE: Dr Schroth received compensation from the Canadian Dental Association for his role as Chair of the Committee on Clinical and Scientific Affairs; the other authors have indicated they have no financial relationships relevant to this article to disclose.

FUNDING: No external funding.

POTENTIAL CONFLICT OF INTEREST: Dr Schroth serves as the Chair of the Committee on Clinical and Scientific Affairs for the Canadian Dental Association and is Co-Chair of the Canada–US Chapter of the Alliance for a Cavity-Free Future; the other authors have indicated they have no potential conflicts of interest to disclose.

REFERENCES

1. American Academy of Pediatric Dentistry. Policy on early childhood caries (ECC): classifications, consequences, and preventive strategies. *Pediatr Dent.* 2017;39(6):59–61

2. US Department of Health and Human Services. *Oral Health in America: A Report of the Surgeon General.* Rockville, MD: US Department of Health and Human Services; 2000

3. Schroth RJ, Harrison RL, Moffatt ME. Oral health of indigenous children and the influence of early childhood caries on childhood health and well-being. *Pediatr Clin North Am.* 2009;56(6):1481–1499

4. Almeida AG, Roseman MM, Sheff M, Huntington N, Hughes CV. Future caries susceptibility in children with early childhood caries following treatment under general anesthesia. *Pediatr Dent.* 2000;22(4):302–306

5. Peretz B, Ram D, Azo E, Efrat Y. Preschool caries as an indicator of future caries: a longitudinal study. *Pediatr Dent.* 2003;25(2):114–118

6. Schroth RJ, Levi JA, Sellers EA, Friel J, Kliewer E, Moffatt ME. Vitamin D status of children with severe early childhood caries: a case-control study. *BMC Pediatr.* 2013;13:174

7. Schroth RJ, Levi J, Kliewer E, Friel J, Moffatt ME. Association between iron status, iron deficiency anaemia, and severe early childhood caries: a case-control study. *BMC Pediatr.* 2013;13(1):22

8. Deane S, Schroth RJ, Sharma A, Rodd C. Combined deficiencies of 25-hydroxyvitamin D and anemia in preschool children with severe early childhood caries: a case-control study. *Paediatr Child Health.* 2018;23(3):e40–e45

9. Schroth RJ, Quiñonez C, Shwart L, Wagar B. Treating early childhood caries under general anesthesia: a national review of Canadian data. *J Can Dent Assoc.* 2016;82:g20

10. Davidson K, Schroth RJ, Levi JA, Yaffe AB, Mittermuller BA, Sellers EAC. Higher body mass index associated with severe early childhood caries. *BMC Pediatr.* 2016;16:137

11. Health Canada. *Inuit Oral Health Survey Report 2008-2009.* Ottawa, Canada: Health Canada; 2011

12. The First Nations Information Governance C.. *Report on the Findings of the First Nations Oral Health Survey (FNOHS) 2009-10.* Ottawa, Canada: The First Nations Information Governance Centre; 2012

13. Schroth RJ, Halchuk S, Star L. Prevalence and risk factors of caregiver reported Severe Early Childhood Caries in Manitoba First Nations children: results from the RHS Phase 2 (2008-2010). *Int J Circumpolar Health.* 2013;72

14. Batliner T, Wilson AR, Tiwari T, et al. Oral health status in Navajo Nation Head Start children. *J Public Health Dent.* 2014;74(4):317–325

15. Phipps K, Ricks TL. *The Oral Health of American Indian and Alaska Native Children Aged 1-5 Years: Results of the 2014 IHS Oral Health Survey.* Rockville, MD: Indian Health Service; 2015

16. Indian Health Service. *An Oral Health Survey of American Indian and Alaska Native Dental Patients. Findings, Regional Differences and National Comparisons.* Rockville, MD: Indian Health Service; 1999

17. Canadian Institute for Health Information. *Treatment of Preventable Dental Cavities in Preschoolers: A Focus on Day Surgery Under General Anesthesia.* Ottawa, ON: Canadian Institute for Health Information; 2013

18. Thomas TK, Schroth RJ. Promising efforts to improve the oral health of indigenous children. In: 8th International Meeting on Indigenous Child Health; March 22–24, 2019; Calgary, Alberta

19. Robertson LD. The Warm Springs Model: a successful strategy for children at very high risk for dental caries. *CDA J.* 2018;46(2):8

20. Lynch DJ, Villhauer AL, Warren JJ, et al. Genotypic characterization of initial acquisition of Streptococcus mutans in American Indian children. *J Oral Microbiol.* 2015;7:27182

21. Warren JJ, Kramer KW, Phipps K, et al. Dental caries in a cohort of very young American Indian children. *J Public Health Dent.* 2012;72(4):265–268

22. Dawson DV, Blanchette DR, Douglass JM, et al. Evidence of early emergence of the primary dentition in a Northern Plains American Indian population. *JDR Clin Trans Res.* 2018;3(2):161–169

23. Pitts NB, Zero DT, Marsh PD, et al. Dental caries. *Nat Rev Dis Primers.* 2017;3: 17030

24. Agnello M, Marques J, Cen L, et al. Microbiome associated with severe caries in Canadian First Nations children. *J Dent Res.* 2017;96(12): 1378–1385

25. Gibson S, Williams S. Dental caries in pre-school children: associations with social class, toothbrushing habit and consumption of sugars and sugar-containing foods. Further analysis of data from the National Diet and Nutrition Survey of children aged 1.5-4.5 years. *Caries Res.* 1999;33(2):101–113

26. Macdonald D, Wilson D. *Shameful Neglect. Indigenous Child Poverty in Canada.* Ottawa, Canada: Canadian Centre for Policy Alternatives; 2016

27. US Census Bureau. American Community Survey, poverty status in past 12 months by sex and age. Available at: https://www.census.gov/a cs/www/data/data-tables-and-tools/a merican-factfinder/. Accessed April 15, 2021

28. Mattila ML, Rautava P, Sillanpää M, Paunio P. Caries in five-year-old children and associations with family-related factors. *J Dent Res.* 2000;79(3):875–881

29. Smith PJ, Moffatt ME. Baby-bottle tooth decay: are we on the right track? *Int J Circumpolar Health.* 1998;57(suppl 1): 155–162

30. Lawrence HP, Romanetz M, Rutherford I, Cappel L, Binguis D, Rodgers JB. Effects of a community-based prenatal nutrition program on the oral health of Aboriginal preschool children in northern Ontario. *Probe.* 2004;38(4): 172–190

31. Tsubouchi J, Tsubouchi M, Maynard RJ, Domoto PK, Weinstein P. A study of dental caries and risk factors among Native American infants. *ASDC J Dent Child.* 1995;62(4):283–287

32. Weinstein P, Troyer R, Jacobi D, Moccasin M. Dental experiences and parenting practices of Native American mothers and caretakers: what we can learn for the prevention of baby bottle tooth decay. *ASDC J Dent Child.* 1999; 66(2):120–126, 85

33. Schroth RJ, Smith PJ, Whalen JC, Lekic C, Moffatt ME. Prevalence of caries among preschool-aged children in a northern Manitoba community. *J Can Dent Assoc.* 2005;71(1):27

34. Aligne CA, Moss ME, Auinger P, Weitzman M. Association of pediatric dental caries with passive smoking. *JAMA.* 2003;289(10):1258–1264

35. Neves PA, Ribeiro CC, Tenuta LM, et al. Breastfeeding, dental biofilm acidogenicity, and early childhood caries. *Caries Res.* 2016;50(3):319–324

36. Wong JP, Venu I, Moodie RG, et al. Keeping caries at bay in breastfeeding babies. *J Fam Pract.* 2019;68(3):E1–E4

37. Tham R, Bowatte G, Dharmage SC, et al. Breastfeeding and the risk of dental caries: a systematic review and meta-analysis. *Acta Paediatr.* 2015;104(467): 62–84

38. American Dental Association. Statement on early childhood caries. 2000. Available at: https://www.ada.org/en/ about-the-ada/ada-positions-policies-and-statements/statement-on-early-childhood-caries. Accessed February 7, 2020

39. Wong PD, Birken CS, Parkin PC, et al.; TARGet Kids! Collaboration. Total breast-feeding duration and dental caries in healthy urban children. *Acad Pediatr.* 2017;17(3):310–315

40. Hooley M, Skouteris H, Boganin C, Satur J, Kilpatrick N. Body mass index and dental caries in children and adolescents: a systematic review of literature published 2004 to 2011. *Syst Rev.* 2012;1:57

41. Li LW, Wong HM, Peng SM, McGrath CP. Anthropometric measurements and dental caries in children: a systematic review of longitudinal studies. *Adv Nutr.* 2015;6(1):52–63

42. Vázquez-Nava F, Vázquez-Rodríguez EM, Saldívar-González AH, Lin-Ochoa D, Martinez-Perales GM, Joffre-Velázquez VM. Association between obesity and dental caries in a group of preschool children in Mexico. *J Public Health Dent.* 2010;70(2):124–130

43. Boone MR, Hartsfield JK, Avery DR, Dean JA, Sanders BJ, Ward RE. Maternal diabetes and its effect on dental development [abstract]. *Int J Paediatr Dent.* 2003;13(suppl 1):29

44. Grahnén H, Edlund K. Maternal diabetes and changes in the hard tissues of primary teeth. I. A clinical study. *Odontol Revy.* 1967;18(2):157–162

45. Grahnén H, Möller EB, Bergstrom AL. Maternal diabetes and changes in the hard tissues of primary teeth. 2. A further clinical study. *Caries Res.* 1968; 2(4):333–337

46. American Academy of Pediatric Dentistry. Perinatal and infant oral health care. 2016. Available at: www. aapd.org/media/Policies_Guidelines/ BP_PerinatalOralHealthCare.pdf. Accessed February 7, 2020

47. California Dental Association Foundation. *Oral Health During Pregnancy & Early Childhood. Evidence-Based Guidelines for Health Professionals.* Sacramento, CA: California Dental Association Foundation; 2010

48. Oral Health Care During Pregnancy Expert W.. *Oral Health Care During Pregnancy: A National Consensus Statement.* Washington, DC: National Maternal and Child Oral Health Resource Centre; 2012

49. New York State Department of Health. *Oral Health Care During Pregnancy and Early Childhood: Practice Guidelines.* Albany, NY: New York State Department of Health; 2006

50. American Dental Association. ADA fluoridation policy. American Dental Association supports fluoridation. 2018. Available at: https://www.ada.org/en/ public-programs/advocating-for-the-public/fluoride-and-fluoridation/ada-fluoridation-policy. Accessed February 7, 2020

51. American Academy of Pediatric Dentistry. Policy on use of fluoride. 2018. Available at: www.aapd.org/ media/Policies_Guidelines/P_ FluorideUse.pdf. Accessed February 7, 2020

52. Canadian Dental Association. CDA position fluoride. 2012. Available at:

www.cda-adc.ca/en/about/position_statements/fluoride/. Accessed February 7, 2020

53. Section on Pediatric Dentistry and Oral Health. Preventive oral health intervention for pediatricians. *Pediatrics.* 2008;122(6):1387–1394

54. Godel J. The use of fluoride in infants and children. *Paediatr Child Health.* 2002;7(8):569–582

55. Riley JC, Lennon MA, Ellwood RP. The effect of water fluoridation and social inequalities on dental caries in 5-year-old children. *Int J Epidemiol.* 1999;28(2):300–305

56. McLaren L, Emery JC. Drinking water fluoridation and oral health inequities in Canadian children. *Can J Public Health.* 2012;103(7, suppl 1):eS49-eS56

57. Centers for Disease Control and Prevention (CDC). Dental caries in rural Alaska Native children–Alaska, 2008. *MMWR Morb Mortal Wkly Rep.* 2011;60(37):1275–1278

58. Public Health Agency of Canada. *The State of Community Water Fluoridation Across Canada.* Ottawa, Canada: Public Health Agency of Canada; 2017

59. Alaska Department of Health and Social Services. *Complete Health Indicator Report of Water - Fluoridated Drinking Water (HA2020 Leading Health Indicator: 20).* Anchorage, AK: Alaska Department of Health and Social Services; 2018

60. Petti S. Why guidelines for early childhood caries prevention could be ineffective amongst children at high risk. *J Dent.* 2010;38(12):946–955

61. Garcia R, Borrelli B, Dhar V, et al. Progress in early childhood caries and opportunities in research, policy, and clinical management. *Pediatr Dent.* 2015;37(3):294–299

62. Ricks TL, Phipps KR, Bruerd B. The Indian Health Service Early Childhood Caries Collaborative: a five-year summary. *Pediatr Dent.* 2015;37(3):275–280

63. Braun PA, Quissell DO, Henderson WG, et al. A cluster-randomized, community-based, tribally delivered oral health promotion trial in Navajo Head Start children. *J Dent Res.* 2016;95(11):1237–1244

64. Harrison RL, Veronneau J, Leroux B. Effectiveness of maternal counseling in reducing caries in Cree children. *J Dent Res.* 2012;91(11):1032–1037

65. Ismail AI, Ondersma S, Jedele JM, Little RJ, Lepkowski JM. Evaluation of a brief tailored motivational intervention to prevent early childhood caries. *Community Dent Oral Epidemiol.* 2011;39(5):433–448

66. Naidu R, Nunn J, Irwin JD. The effect of motivational interviewing on oral healthcare knowledge, attitudes and behaviour of parents and caregivers of preschool children: an exploratory cluster randomised controlled study. *BMC Oral Health.* 2015;15:101

67. Feldens CA, Giugliani ER, Duncan BB, Drachler ML, Vítolo MR. Long-term effectiveness of a nutritional program in reducing early childhood caries: a randomized trial. *Community Dent Oral Epidemiol.* 2010;38(4):324–332

68. Kay E, Locker D. A systematic review of the effectiveness of health promotion aimed at improving oral health. *Community Dent Health.* 1998;15(3):132–144

69. Bader JD, Rozier RG, Lohr KN, Frame PS. Physicians' roles in preventing dental caries in preschool children: a summary of the evidence for the U.S. Preventive Services Task Force. *Am J Prev Med.* 2004;26(4):315–325

70. Steggerda MH, Hill TJ. Incidence of dental caries among Maya and Navajo Indians. *J Dent Res.* 1935;15(5):10

71. Collins H. Caries and crowding of teeth of the living Alaska Eskimo. *Am J Phys Anthropol.* 1932;16(4):12

72. Parfitt GJ. A survey of the oral health of Navajo Indian children. *Arch Oral Biol.* 1960;1:193–205

73. Levin A, Sokal-Gutierrez K, Hargrave A, Funsch E, Hoeft KS. Maintaining traditions: a qualitative study of early childhood caries risk and protective factors in an indigenous community. *Int J Environ Res Public Health.* 2017;14(8):e907

74. Harrison R, White L. A community-based approach to infant and child oral health promotion in a British Columbia First Nations community. *Can J Community Dent.* 1997;12:7–14

75. Harrison RL, MacNab AJ, Duffy DJ, Benton DH. Brighter Smiles: service learning, inter-professional collaboration and health promotion in a First Nations community. *Can J Public Health.* 2006;97(3):237–240

76. Schroth RJ, Edwards JM, Brothwell DJ, et al. Evaluating the impact of a community developed collaborative project for the prevention of early childhood caries: the Healthy Smile Happy Child project. *Rural Remote Health.* 2015;15(4):3566

77. Schroth RJ, Wilson A, Prowse S, et al. Looking back to move forward: understanding service provider, parent, and caregiver views on early childhood oral health promotion in Manitoba, Canada. *Can J Dent Hyg.* 2014;48(3):99–108

78. Cidro J, Zahayko L, Lawrence H, McGregor M, McKay K. Traditional and cultural approaches to childrearing: preventing early childhood caries in Norway House Cree Nation, Manitoba. *Rural Remote Health.* 2014;14(4):2968

79. American Academy of Pediatric Dentistry. Caries-Risk Assessment and Management for Infants, Children, and Adolescents. In: *The Reference Manual of Pediatric Dentistry.* Chicago, IL: American Academy of Pediatric Dentistry; 2020:243–247

80. Azarpazhooh A, Main PA. Pit and fissure sealants in the prevention of dental caries in children and adolescents: a systematic review. *J Can Dent Assoc.* 2008;74(2):171–177

81. Beauchamp J, Caufield PW, Crall JJ, et al.; American Dental Association Council on Scientific Affairs. Evidence-based clinical recommendations for the use of pit-and-fissure sealants: a report of the American Dental Association Council on Scientific Affairs. *J Am Dent Assoc.* 2008;139(3):257–268

82. Akinlotan M, Chen B, Fontanilla TM, Chen A, Fan VY. Economic evaluation of dental sealants: a systematic literature review. *Community Dent Oral Epidemiol.* 2018;46(1):38–46

83. Slayton RL, Urquhart O, Araujo MWB, et al. Evidence-based clinical practice guideline on nonrestorative treatments for carious lesions: a report from the American Dental Association. *J Am Dent Assoc.* 2018;149(10):837–849.e19

84. American Academy of Pediatric Dentistry. Policy on interim therapeutic restorations (ITR). *Pediatr Dent.* 2018; 40(6):58–59

85. Rosenblatt A, Stamford TC, Niederman R. Silver diamine fluoride: a caries "silver-fluoride bullet". *J Dent Res.* 2009; 88(2):116–125

86. Peng JJ, Botelho MG, Matinlinna JP. Silver compounds used in dentistry for caries management: a review. *J Dent.* 2012;40(7):531–541

87. Clemens J, Gold J, Chaffin J. Effect and acceptance of silver diamine fluoride treatment on dental caries in primary teeth. *J Public Health Dent.* 2018;78(1): 63–68

88. Robertson LD. *Early Childhood Caries in American Indian Children: Looking Beyond the Usual Causes.* Ottawa, Canada: Canadian Dental Association; 2018

89. Horst JA, Ellenikiotis H, Milgrom PL. UCSF protocol for caries arrest using silver diamine fluoride: rationale, indications and consent. *J Calif Dent Assoc.* 2016;44(1):16–28

90. Crystal YO, Marghalani AA, Ureles SD, et al. Use of silver diamine fluoride for dental caries management in children and adolescents, including those with special health care needs. *Pediatr Dent.* 2017;39(5):135–145

91. Schroth RJ, Morey B. Providing timely dental treatment for young children under general anesthesia is a government priority. *J Can Dent Assoc.* 2007;73(3):241–243

92. Casamassimo PS, Hammersmith K, Gross EL, Amini H. Infant oral health: an emerging dental public health measure. *Dent Clin North Am.* 2018;62(2):235–244

93. Lee H, Milgrom P, Huebner CE, et al. Ethics rounds: death after pediatric dental anesthesia: an avoidable tragedy? *Pediatrics.* 2017;140(6): e20172370

94. Canadian Dental Association. CDA position on first visit to the dentist. 2012. Available at: www.cda-adc.ca/_files/position_statements/firstVisit.pdf. Accessed January 7, 2020

95. Hale KJ; American Academy of Pediatrics Section on Pediatric Dentistry. Oral health risk assessment timing and establishment of the dental home. *Pediatrics.* 2003;111(5 pt 1): 1113–1116

96. Canada H. *First Nations and Inuit Health Program Compendium 2011/2012.* Ottawa, Canada: Health Canada; 2012

97. Nash DA, Friedman JW, Mathu-Muju KR, et al. A review of the global literature on dental therapists. *Community Dent Oral Epidemiol.* 2014;42(1):1–10

98. Leck V, Randall GE. The rise and fall of dental therapy in Canada: a policy analysis and assessment of equity of access to oral health care for Inuit and First Nations communities. *Int J Equity Health.* 2017;16(1):131

99. Chi DL, Lenaker D, Mancl L, Dunbar M, Babb M. *Dental Utilization for Communities Served by Dental Therapists in Alaska's Yukon Kuskokwim Delta: Finding from an Observational Quantitative Study.* Seattle, WA: University of Washington; 2017

100. Chi DL, Lenaker D, Mancl L, Dunbar M, Babb M. Dental therapists linked to improved dental outcomes for Alaska Native communities in the Yukon-Kuskokwim Delta. *J Public Health Dent.* 2018;78(2):175–182

101. Chi DL, Hopkins S, Zahlis E, et al. Provider and community perspectives of dental therapists in Alaska's Yukon-Kuskokwim Delta: a qualitative programme evaluation. *Community Dent Oral Epidemiol.* 2019;47(6):502–512

102. Cladoosby BS. Indian Country leads national movement to knock down barriers to oral health equity. *Am J Public Health.* 2017;107(S1):S81–S84

103. Canadian Dental Hygienists Association. *The Canadian Dental Hygienists Association 2017-2018 Annual Report.* Ottawa, Canada: Canadian Dental Hygienists Association; 2018

POLICY STATEMENT Organizational Principles to Guide and Define the Child Health
Care System and/or Improve the Health of all Children

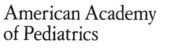

American Academy
of Pediatrics

DEDICATED TO THE HEALTH OF ALL CHILDREN®

Caring for American Indian and Alaska Native Children and Adolescents

Shaquita Bell, MD, FAAP,[a,*] Jason F. Deen, MD, FAAP,[a,*] Molly Fuentes, MD, MS,[b] Kelly Moore, MD, FAAP,[c] COMMITTEE ON NATIVE AMERICAN CHILD HEALTH

abstract

American Indian and Alaska Native (AI/AN) populations have substantial health inequities, and most of their disease entities begin in childhood. In addition, AI/AN children and adolescents have excessive disease rates compared with the general pediatric population. Because of this, providers of pediatric care are in a unique position not only to attenuate disease incidence during childhood but also to improve the health status of this special population as a whole. This policy statement examines the inequitable disease burden observed in AI/AN youth, with a focus on toxic stress, mental health, and issues related to suicide and substance use disorder, risk of and exposure to injury and violence in childhood, obesity and obesity-related cardiovascular risk factors and disease, foster care, and the intersection of lesbian, gay, bisexual, transgender, queer, and Two-Spirit and AI/AN youth. Opportunities for advocacy in policy making also are presented.

[a]Departments of Pediatrics and [b]Rehabilitation Medicine, School of Medicine, University of Washington and Seattle Children's Hospital, Seattle, Washington; and [c]Centers for American Indian and Alaska Native Health, Colorado School of Public Health, University of Colorado Anschutz Medical Campus, Aurora, Colorado

*Contributed equally as co-first authors

Drs Bell, Deen, Fuentes, and Moore were equally responsible for conceptualizing, writing, and revising the manuscript, while also considering input from all reviewers; and all authors approved the final manuscript as submitted.

Policy statements from the American Academy of Pediatrics benefit from expertise and resources of liaisons and internal (AAP) and external reviewers. However, policy statements from the American Academy of Pediatrics may not reflect the views of the liaisons or the organizations or government agencies that they represent.

The guidance in this statement does not indicate an exclusive course of treatment or serve as a standard of medical care. Variations, taking into account individual circumstances, may be appropriate.

All policy statements from the American Academy of Pediatrics automatically expire 5 years after publication unless reaffirmed, revised, or retired at or before that time.

DOI: https://doi.org/10.1542/peds.2021-050498

Address correspondence to Shaquita Bell, MD. Email: shaquita.bell@seattlechildrens.org

To cite: Bell S, Deen JF, Fuentes M, et al. AAP COMMITTEE ON NATIVE AMERICAN CHILD HEALTH. Caring for American Indian and Alaska Native Children and Adolescents. *Pediatrics.* 2021;147(4):e2021050498

INTRODUCTION

We acknowledge that this policy statement was written together on Coast Salish and Pueblo lands, both diverse, strong, and enduring communities that uphold a sacred legacy of protecting future generations. As American Indian (AI) authors and physicians ourselves, we acknowledge that we intend to represent a diverse and far-reaching group of Indigenous peoples. We humbly submit that not all aspects of caring for our communities could be captured in our article. We ask that this policy statement be used to support and advocate for improved health outcomes and the well-being of children and youth from all tribal and urban AI communities. Many solutions to the problems illustrated below can be found within these very communities.[1]

American Indian and Alaska Native (AI/AN) children and adolescents are found throughout the United States, with more now living in urban rather than rural areas.[2] Many tribal nations have their own languages, and all have rich histories, but most AI/AN people now live in metropolitan areas that may include many different tribal groups. Care for this special population presents a unique and complex clinical opportunity for pediatricians, other providers of pediatric care, and pediatric care organizations because of the high level of documented health inequities within a sociocultural context unfamiliar to most practicing providers of pediatric care. Not only do AI/AN youth face medical access barriers, but they also have a higher prevalence of chronic stress and adverse childhood experiences (ACEs) and exposure to environmental hazards resulting in poorer health outcomes[3] when compared with the general population.[4] In addition, several other significant barriers to care deserve mention. These include conventional barriers for underresourced families, such as lack of transportation, difficulty finding child care, inability to miss work, caring for elders, and other family and work obligations, as well as other socioeconomic challenges. Moreover, less well-recognized issues exist, such as long-standing mistrust of governmental agencies, discrimination in clinical settings attributable to implicit and explicit bias leading to mistrust of health care and of health care–related research, and the cumulative burden of generations of unresolved traumas and racism.[5-8] This policy statement explores the roles historical trauma and health inequities have played in shaping the current socioeconomic and health status of AI/AN youth. Disproportionate needs in mental and cardiovascular health and disease processes that are overrepresented in AI/AN youth are discussed to provide a summary of salient issues for pediatric care providers. This statement also provides strategies for culturally sensitive family-centered care to mitigate morbidity and policy recommendations to facilitate institutional and system changes needed for improved health outcomes.

Of note, Native Hawaiians and Pacific Islanders are considered a unique population of Indigenous people who live within the territories discussed but are not considered AI. They have their own distinct cultural identity as well as distinct health outcomes and needs. In addition, they are not considered tribes by the US federal government, so they are not beneficiaries of the Indian Health Service (IHS) or eligible for funding from the Bureau of Indian Affairs. Given these differences and the need for them to be addressed fully, this policy statement does not address this population.

Many of the cited publications in this document compare AI/AN youth to non-Hispanic white youth; the authors would like to note that this phenomenon can lead to white centering. Where possible, we avoided comparing racial groups in this way but were somewhat limited by the available studies.

ACES

The call to pediatricians to employ strategies to mitigate toxic stress caused by ACEs is especially critical for AI/AN children.[9] In a landmark study of more than 13 000 adults, categories of childhood abuse, neglect, and other forms of household dysfunction were linked to adult mortality and morbidity. Risk was quantified by using an ACE score, or the number of categories experienced by an individual before age 18 years.[10] A higher ACE score's association with poor health outcomes is postulated to stem from altered neurodevelopment with subsequent social, emotional, and neurocognitive impairment, which in turn leads to detrimental health behavior and poor health outcomes. For example, compared with those without ACEs, adults with an ACE score of 3 or more are twice as likely to smoke or have cardiovascular disease and 1.5 times more likely to

have severe obesity or diabetes.[11,12] AI adults and children experience a disparate number of ACEs compared with the general US population. A recent study of 516 AI adults from South Dakota revealed an ACE score of 3 or more in 45.4% of participants as compared with 17.4% of region-matched controls.[13] Among AI adults from 7 geographically diverse tribes, AI adults were 5 times more likely than non-AI adults to have had 4 or more ACEs.[14] According to the National Survey of Children's Health data collected in 2011 and 2012, 1453 AI children and adolescents aged 0 to 17 years were more likely to have had multiple ACEs compared with non-Hispanic white (NHW) children.[15] In that study, >25% of AI youth had 3 or more ACEs, compared with only 11.5% of NHW children. Regarding the types of ACEs endured, AI populations suffer from a disproportionate prevalence of emotional and physical neglect, substance use disorder, and incarceration among family members, as well as witnessed intimate partner violence, when compared with the general population.[13-16] The authors of another study of AI adolescents and young adults also found that historical loss–associated symptoms and perceived discrimination are relevant factors in considering ACEs for Indigenous children and youth, suggesting the importance of considering loss of culture and structural racism as contributors to childhood adversity in this population.[16]

OBESITY

Obesity prevalence in AI/AN youth is among the highest of all races and ethnicities.[17-19] Obesity onset occurs at a younger age compared with other racial and ethnic groups in the United States; AI children between 2 and 5 years of age have a higher combined prevalence of overweight and obesity (58.8%) than children of all other races or ethnicities (30%).[17,20,21]

Moreover, AI/AN children experienced an increase in obesity prevalence between 2003 and 2008, whereas the prevalence for other US racial groups declined. Recent data have revealed an alarmingly high prevalence of obesity compared with the general US population but suggest that obesity prevalence (29.7%) in AI/AN children 2 to 19 years of age may have stabilized.[22,23] Although recent research from 2010–2014 suggests a decline in severe obesity among children 2 to 4 years of age from low-income families, severe obesity remains high for young AI/AN children and is among the highest of all racial and/or ethnic groups receiving benefits through the Special Supplemental Nutrition Program for Women, Infants, and Children.[24] It follows that a significant portion of AI children with obesity have significantly abnormal blood lipid levels, higher blood glucose levels, and higher abdominal adiposity compared with children with normal-weight.[25]

Obesity may largely be determined in infancy, with excess prenatal maternal weight gain, macrosomia, and premature cessation of breastfeeding significantly predicting BMI at 1 year of age in a previous study.[26] In the same children, overweight or obesity status at age 1 year persisted to ages 5 to 8 years and was associated with unhealthy levels of low-density lipoprotein. In AI children, once obesity is established, it likely persists into adulthood and increases the risk of chronic disease.[27,28] The prevalence of disproportionate rates of obesity emerge in early childhood[17,20,29]; thus, tailored prevention and intervention strategies are needed for young AI/AN children.

Given the high rates of obesity, AI/AN youth also experience high rates of type 2 diabetes mellitus (T2DM). Testing, as recommended by the American Diabetes Association, for prediabetes and T2DM should be considered in AI/AN children and adolescents with overweight or obesity.[30,31] Further information is available in American Academy of Pediatrics technical and clinical reports on management of T2DM for children[32] and specifically for AI/AN youth.[33]

BREASTFEEDING

The benefits of human milk nutrition for infants are well documented and include wide-ranging effects, such as the reduction of respiratory tract infections, obesity and diabetes incidence, atopic disease, and infant mortality.[34] Although the breastfeeding initiation rate for the general US population is 75%, minority populations experience significant disparities in initiating and continuing breastfeeding at 6 and 12 months.[35] AI/AN women have the second-lowest prevalence of breastfeeding initiation, duration, and exclusivity compared with all other US racial and ethnic groups. In a previous study, only 59% of AI women initiated breastfeeding, and most of those (76%) stopped breastfeeding within 4 months.[26] Encouragingly, those who continued to breastfeed for 6 months tended to continue through infancy.[36] Health benefits of breastfeeding have been demonstrated in all populations, including AI/AN populations. For example, in a retrospective cohort study, a lower BMI was reported among AI/AN adolescents breastfed for >6 months.[37] Breastfeeding promotion is needed in AI/AN tribal communities and would ideally be coordinated by tribal entities and would involve community members, elders, and health care providers, including paraprofessionals.[38,39]

CHILDREN AND YOUTH WITH SPECIAL HEALTH CARE NEEDS

AI/AN children and youth with special health care needs (CYSHCN) are at particular risk of health disparities. Although there is no evidence of a higher prevalence of special health care needs among AI/AN children compared with NHW children, AI/AN children are more likely than NHW children to meet criteria for special health care needs on the basis of functional difficulties.[40] In addition, AI/AN CYSHCN are more likely than NHW CYSHCN to have 3 or more functional difficulties,[40] which can be interpreted as AI/AN CYSHCN likely having more disability. Although there are no studies on the prevalence of developmental delay, functional difference, or disability among AI/AN children, it is possible that there is a higher prevalence in AI/AN children, compared with the general population, because of a disproportionate burden of injury,[41] inadequate prenatal care,[42,43] preterm birth,[43] environmental stressors,[42,44] and other social determinants of health and function.

CYSHCN benefit from the accessible, comprehensive, and coordinated care provided by a medical home, but AI/AN CYSHCN are significantly less likely than children without special health care needs to receive care meeting the medical home definition (odds ratio 0.2; 95% confidence interval 0.1–0.4).[7] In addition to difficulties receiving medical home–based primary care, AI/AN CYSHCN may have challenges accessing subspecialty medical care or pediatric rehabilitation therapies; those who live in rural or remote communities may have to travel many hours to access specialized care. Even among urban AI/AN CYSHCN, there may still be barriers related to transportation,[45,46] funding, and wait times.[47] The care used by AI/AN CYSHCN may not be sensitive to the family's values[7] or address the child's functional needs related to their tribal culture.[48] Efforts should be made to identify CYSHCN in a timely manner, implement culturally sensitive medical home–based care for AI/AN

TABLE 1 Risk Behaviors and Emotional Distress Reported by Ninth- and 11th-Grade Students in a Minnesota Student Survey Sample

Reported	AI/AN LGBTQ (n = 149 Ninth- and 11th-Graders)	Full MSS Sample (n = 81 885 Ninth- and 11th-Graders)	All LGBTQ (n = 8758 Ninth- and 11th-Graders)
Substance use			
Smoked cigarettes (past 30 d)	32.9	6.1	14.1
Drank alcohol (past 30 d)	25.2	17.2	22.3
Binge drinking (past 30 d)	16.8	8.4	10.7
Smoked marijuana (past 30 d)	33.1	10.8	17.0
Sexual behaviors			
Ever had sex	33.8	22.1	28.8
≥2 partners (past year)[a]	18.3	8.7	14.7
Emotional distress			
Depressive symptoms	51.7	22.3	48.1
Self-harm (past year)	52.1	15.4	43.7
Suicidal ideation (ever)	60.5	21.0	53.6
Suicide attempt (ever)	37.7	7.7	24.4

Minnesota Student Survey (MSS) data were provided by public school students in Minnesota via local public school districts and are managed by the Minnesota Student Survey Interagency Team (M. Eisenberg, ScD, MPH, personal communication, 2018). LGBTQ, lesbian, gay, bisexual, transgender, and queer.
[a] Among sexually active ninth- and 11th-grade students only.

CYSHCN, and facilitate access to services that will help AI/AN CYSHCN achieve their full functional potential and be included in their communities.

SUICIDE AND MENTAL HEALTH

Suicide is the second-leading cause of death for AI/AN and non-AI/AN youth 10 to 24 years of age,[49,50] but the 2016 age-adjusted suicide mortality rate among AI/AN youth (15.59 per 100 000) is more than 1.5 times higher than that of the general population (9.60 per 100 000).[51] There is significant regional and intertribal variation in AI/AN youth suicide mortality, with some tribes having youth suicide rates 7 times higher than the national AI/AN rate and 12 times higher than the general population rate.[52,53]

In previous studies, differences in risk and protective factors that may attenuate that risk (such as having a connectedness to family and having the ability to discuss problems with family and friends[54]) explained the higher prevalence of suicidal behaviors among AI/AN students compared with other students.[55,56] ACEs were also associated with suicide attempts; after controlling for multiple factors, each additional ACE

increased the risk of lifetime suicide attempt by 37% for AI youth.[16] AI/AN individuals of all ages who died by suicide were less likely than NHW individuals to have received mental health diagnoses or treatments and were more likely to have a family member or friend's death precipitate suicide.[57]

Suicide prevention initiatives that are strengths based, community driven, and culturally centered have been used in several AI/AN communities to reduce youth suicide behaviors.[57,58] For AI/AN youth who do not have access to a community-specific suicide prevention program, efforts should be made to identify youth with an increased burden of suicide risk factors and to strengthen protective factors, particularly cultural protective factors.[55] If available, school-based health centers may be used for adjunctive mental health care.[59]

INTERSECTIONS OF HEALTH AND IDENTITY

Lesbian, gay, pansexual, bisexual, transgender, gender queer, intersex, and Two-Spirit AI/AN youth experience exponential increases in risk for health disparities.[60–63] "Two-Spirit" is a unifying term that

encompasses both gender identity and traditional Indigenous understandings of identity and is a widely used term in Indigenous communities across North America. In the 2015 US National Transgender Health Survey, AI/AN transgender respondents reported having experienced harassment (86%), physical assault (51%), and sexual assault (21%). Fifty-seven percent of AI/AN youth identifying as transgender have attempted or contemplated suicide, compared with 4.6% of the general US population and 33.7% of transgender youth as a whole.[64,65] In this same study, 23% of transgender respondents (all ages) identifying as AI/AN experienced unemployment in the last year.[66] In another study, youth at the intersection of gender and racial identity had higher rates of risk behaviors and emotional distress (Table 1). Careful attention to gender-affirming care and risk assessments may mitigate these effects.[67]

VIOLENCE

Violence affects AI/AN youth in unique but disproportionate ways. In a study using data from the National Trauma Data Bank, 11.8% of AI/AN children hospitalized for traumatic injury experienced injury as a result of violent assaults, compared with only 4.2% of NHW children.[68] Many communities have started to focus on the crisis of missing and murdered Indigenous women and girls. Although limited data exist on rates of missing and murdered Indigenous women and girls and underreporting is extremely likely, a recent study completed by the Urban Indian Health Institute reveals staggering rates of violence toward Indigenous women and girls.[69] Pediatricians have an opportunity to advocate for better data collection and unbiased media coverage. The Urban Indian Health Institute has created a tool kit (https://www.uihi.org/resources/mmiwg-we-demand-more-partner-toolkit/) on how further work in this area can be tailored in a culturally appropriate manner.[69]

AI/AN youth and communities are also vulnerable to sex trafficking.[70] It is estimated that 30% of AI girls between 11 and 17 years old have a history of sexual abuse, and 11% have reported being raped.[71,72] Alaska Native women and girls make up 8% of the population in Alaska but represent 33% of sex-trafficking victims.[73] In turn, AI/AN girls are 5 times more likely to be incarcerated for prostitution than NHW girls.[73] It is important to recognize that men and nonbinary-gendered youth can also experience trafficking, and often times, finding data on these groups proves to be challenging. Identifying, preventing, and addressing trafficking and reducing violence is an integral part of caring for AI/AN communities.[74]

FOSTER CARE

The National Child Abuse and Neglect Data System, the Bureau of Indian Affairs, and the IHS report high rates of child protective services referrals for AI/AN youth.[75,76] In a previous study, AI/AN youth in foster care

were more likely to have special health care needs compared with others in foster care.[77] Historically, AI/AN children were systematically removed from their homes in an effort to assimilate them into mainstream culture and to terminate the existence of tribal culture. Rates of ongoing referrals reflect both historical trauma and ongoing social and environmental determinants of inequities at work. The Indian Child Welfare Act was ratified in 1978 after decades of fierce advocacy by tribes for the right to keep their children within families that identify as AI/AN. Often used as a leverage point to threaten the sovereignty of tribal nations, the Indian Child Welfare Act remains an opportune protection for AI/AN children and adolescents.[78]

OTHER HEALTH DISPARITIES

The poor oral health status of AI/AN children is a major public health concern. AI/AN children have the highest rates of tooth decay among any racial and ethnic group in the United States.[79] The prevalence of tooth decay among AI/AN children between 2 and 4 years of age is 5 times greater than the average US rate.[79,80] AI/AN children also have limited access to dental services because of ongoing difficulties with recruitment and retention of qualified dentists in the IHS.[79] More severe early childhood caries frequently requires extensive treatment under general anesthesia, creating an additional health care access barrier for AI/AN children. More information is available in the joint American Academy of Pediatrics and Canadian Paediatric Society policy statement on early childhood caries and its impact on Indigenous communities.[81] In addition to oral health conditions, chronic otitis media and many other conditions disproportionally and inequitably affect AI/AN children and adolescents.[82,83] The authors have chosen some of the most prominent

to focus on but do not consider this an exhaustive list.

GOVERNMENTAL AND POLITICAL INFLUENCES

The delivery of health care to AI/AN children is influenced by governmental policy at the federal, state, and tribal level. Treaties between the federal government and sovereign tribal nations established a trust relationship for health care. Although these treaties are unique agreements between tribal nations and the US government, failure of the government to honor them has also shaped mistrust among many AI/AN people and communities. Today, that treaty-based health care system is organized through the IHS, an agency within the US Department of Health and Human Services. Many health care settings serving AI/AN people receive funding through the IHS, including IHS federally operated clinics and hospitals, tribally operated clinics and hospitals, and urban AI clinics run by urban AI health organizations in metropolitan areas. Yet many AI/AN children receive health care services at clinics that are not associated with the IHS, including private clinics and federally qualified health centers.

Not all people who identify as AI/AN are members of tribes that have been federally recognized. Tribes that are not federally recognized are not eligible for federal funding from the IHS or the Bureau of Indian Affairs.

The IHS is chronically underfunded, with the budget determined by annual federal appropriations. By way of comparison, in 2017 the IHS was funded at $4078 per person, whereas the US government spent $10 692 per person in the Veterans Affairs system.[80] An underfunded IHS results in workforce instability and reduced ability to effectively deliver a full spectrum of necessary health care. Chronic underfunding leads to infrastructure issues as well. Many facilities are overdue for updates, many locations have trouble providing housing for staff and providers, and much of the equipment is outdated. Furthermore, funding shortages lead to challenges in providing specialty care through contract health services.

Medicaid payment rates are directly tied to the likelihood of a practice accepting Medicaid patients, which is subsequently correlated with access to health care for children with Medicaid.[84,85] It follows, therefore, that increasing Medicaid payment rates and access to Medicaid coverage would potentially improve health care access for AI/AN youth. With more than 300 000 AI/AN children covered by Medicaid, there is an obvious need for continued and improved access to health services.[86,87] Continuing to expand access to Medicaid coverage for AI/AN children is essential for ensuring access to needed services.

Another complicating factor for many AI/AN communities is the inconsistent and overenforcement of punitive drug laws targeting pregnant women. Punitive drug screening practices for pregnant women lead to a decrease in prenatal visits, which, in turn, increases the risk of preterm birth.[88,89] Often, tribal laws differ from state and local laws, and in some instances, tribal jurisdictional boundaries may cross multiple states. Federally operated IHS facilities are bound by federal laws and policies. This overlap of governing bodies often results in confusing policies and a lack of standard and universal screening of pregnant AI/AN women, leading to late or inadequate detection of infants with a history of in utero substance exposure, including infants with neonatal opioid withdrawal syndrome.

RECOMMENDATIONS

Opportunities for Pediatric Care Providers in Practice

Pediatric care providers, because of their early interaction with AI/AN youth and their families, have a distinct opportunity to promote resilience and improve the health of these children, which will have far-reaching benefits as they age and raise their own children. Pediatricians and other pediatric care providers can implement systems in their practice that can help all patients and families, including AI/AN families, feel that they are welcome and will be treated respectfully and that high-quality family- and patient-centered care will be delivered regardless of social class, personal history, or cultural, spiritual, gender, racial, or ethnic identity. These strategies include providing trauma-informed care,[90–92] screening for substance use[93] and social determinants of health,[94–96] connecting to substance use prevention and treatment programs,[93] home visiting,[97] literacy programs,[98,99] and leveraging school-based health centers if available.[59] Addressing social determinants of health also includes addressing housing insecurity[100] and food insecurity.[101] The inclusion of the AI/AN perspective and disaggregated data in early childhood initiatives should be sought to improve outcomes within broader systems-based efforts. When implementing these strategies, pediatricians are encouraged to seek programs and interventions that incorporate AI/AN culture, tradition, and practices.[102] The following recommendations reflect the issues raised above and provide opportunities for pediatricians and others who provide care to AI/AN pediatric patients:

- Partner with local tribes and communities to set health priorities, understand historical experiences, and combine efforts already underway, such as cultural enrichment and preservation programs.

- Provide opportunities for adequate training of clinical and office staff in culturally sensitive care practices. Advocate for local and regional models that incorporate culturally and linguistically appropriate services tailored for local tribes.

- Provide evidence-based supports for parents and young children by promoting the use of home visiting models, high-quality child care, and early childhood programs, such as Early Head Start, Head Start, and Nurse-Family Partnership (https://www.nursefamilypartnership.org).[103]

- Start a Reach Out and Read program in AI/AN clinics and any clinic serving these families. Include books representing AI/AN and Indigenous children and families.

- Assess patients for ACEs and social determinants of health (eg, poverty, food insecurity, homelessness, lack of neighborhood safety, incarceration of parents or other family members, mental health conditions of parents or other household family members, housing inequity, access to schools, academic achievement, intimate partner violence, child abuse and neglect, and involvement with the juvenile legal system) to help families identify and implement practical solutions.

- Identify strengths and screen youth and families for protective factors to promote positive youth development.

- Create efforts to promote and strengthen protective factors for youth, focusing on cultural preservation–based efforts.

- Consider testing for prediabetes and T2DM in AI/AN children and adolescents with overweight or obesity, as recommended by the American Diabetes Association.

- Promote breastfeeding in AI/AN tribal communities, ideally coordinated by tribal entities and involving community members, elders, and health care providers, including paraprofessionals.

- Include early childhood oral health as part of overall childhood health and well-being. Perform oral health screening during early childhood health assessments and provide referrals as needed to dental health providers. Be knowledgeable of fluoride levels in the drinking water for local tribal communities in your area.[81]

- Create a medical home that acknowledges and is sensitive to discrimination in clinical settings and generations of unresolved traumas and racism that AI/AN children and families experience. Work with local community hospitals and pediatric emergency departments, which may serve as a referral source, to become a medical home for AI/AN children whose families use emergency departments rather than seek primary care.

- Create a medical home model that facilitates access to services that will help AI/AN CYSHCN achieve their functional potential. Identify AI/AN CYSHCN, engaging staff, including care coordinators, in cultural competency training and partnering with the community.

- Assess patients for mental health conditions, including signs of posttraumatic stress, anxiety, grief, depressive symptoms, and suicidality, as well as their mothers for perinatal depression[104] using validated screening tools and a trauma-informed approach. Participate in strengths-based, community-driven, and culturally centered suicide prevention programs.[58]

- Screen AI/AN youth for substance use, and if identified, conduct a brief intervention and then refer for ongoing treatment.[105–107]

- Work with local schools to identify AI/AN students in need of mental health and educational services.

- Offer gender-affirming care in line with the previously published American Academy of Pediatrics policy statement.[67]

- Work to prevent, identify, and address sex trafficking in AI/AN youth.

Opportunities for Public Policy Advocacy

Pediatricians also have an opportunity to advocate for systems change that addresses health inequities and other systemic factors that contribute to ongoing health disparities experienced by AI/AN children and youth. The following recommendations are intended to support the policies and systems needed to promote and protect the health of AI/AN children and youth:

- Advocate for community initiatives and develop partnerships to address health disparities, such as altering practices of frequent consumption of sugar-sweetened beverages through education and improving the selection of foods locally available, to address healthy weight and oral health.

- Share information with the US Congress, state legislatures, foundations, and other appropriate advocacy groups about the inequities and tremendous health disparities that exist between AI/AN populations and the general US population.

- Invest in new research and clinical pathways to create culturally relevant screening and interventions for ACEs.

- Advocate for federal, state, and local policy to end AI/AN homelessness through consultation and engagement with tribal leaders, AI/AN communities, and AI/AN young people with lived experience of homelessness. Advocate for the investment in improved data collection on homelessness among both rural and urban AI/AN youth and culturally responsive interventions to address homelessness among diverse tribal nations.

- Work with local tribes and communities to address the need for research and advocacy around missing and murdered Indigenous women and girls.[69]

- Advocate for the protection and enforcement of the Indian Child Welfare Act.

- Advocate for increased Medicaid coverage for children and families as well as increased payment for services.

- Advocate for improved IHS budget and funding, which is chronically underfunded. IHS expenditures are among the lowest per capita compared with other federal health care expenditures, such as Medicare and the Veterans Health Administration. This disparity contributes significantly to the ongoing health inequities experienced by AI/AN people. Advocate for policies such as advanced appropriations or mandatory funding to provide the IHS with predictable and continuous funding.

- Work with local government and tribal communities to understand and mitigate the negative effects of punitive drug laws for pregnant women.

LEAD AUTHORS

Shaquita Bell, MD, FAAP
Jason F. Deen, MD, FAAP
Molly Fuentes, MD, MS
Kelly Moore, MD, FAAP

ABBREVIATIONS

ACE: adverse childhood experience
AI: American Indian
AI/AN: American Indian and Alaska Native
CYSHCN: children and youth with special health care needs
IHS: Indian Health Service
NHW: non-Hispanic white
T2DM: type 2 diabetes mellitus

PEDIATRICS (ISSN Numbers: Print, 0031-4005; Online, 1098-4275).

Copyright © 2021 by the American Academy of Pediatrics

FINANCIAL DISCLOSURE: Dr Moore was a paid consultant for the Public Health Institute (Oakland, CA); and Drs Bell, Deen, and Fuentes have indicated they have no financial relationships relevant to this article to disclose.

FUNDING: No external funding.

POTENTIAL CONFLICT OF INTEREST: Dr Moore was a paid consultant for the Public Health Institute (Oakland, CA); and Drs Bell, Deen, and Fuentes have indicated they have no potential conflicts of interest to disclose.

REFERENCES

1. Brave Heart MY. The historical trauma response among natives and its relationship with substance abuse: a Lakota illustration. *J Psychoactive Drugs*. 2003;35(1):7–13

2. US Census Bureau. Facts for Features: American Indian and Alaska Native Heritage Month: November 2018. Available at: https://www.census.gov/newsroom/facts-for-features/2018/aian.html. Accessed February 25, 2021

3. Hoover E, Cook K, Plain R, et al. Indigenous peoples of North America: environmental exposures and reproductive justice. *Environ Health Perspect*. 2012;120(12):1645–1649

4. Sarche M, Spicer P. Poverty and health disparities for American Indian and Alaska native children: current knowledge and future prospects. *Ann N Y Acad Sci*. 2008;1136:126–136

5. Call KT, McAlpine DD, Johnson PJ, Beebe TJ, McRae JA, Song Y. Barriers to care among American Indians in public health care programs. *Med Care*. 2006;44(6):595–600

6. Puumala SE, Burgess KM, Kharbanda AB, et al. The role of bias by emergency department providers in care for American Indian children. *Med Care*. 2016;54(6):562–569

7. Barradas DT, Kroelinger CD, Kogan MD. Medical home access among American Indian and Alaska native children in 7 states: National Survey of Children's Health. *Matern Child Health J*. 2012;16(suppl 1):S6–S13

8. Trent M, Dooley DG, Dougé J; Section on Adolescent Health; Council on Community Pediatrics; Committee on Adolescence. The impact of racism on child and adolescent health. *Pediatrics*. 2019;144(2):e20191765

9. Garner AS, Shonkoff JP; Committee on Psychosocial Aspects of Child and Family Health; Committee on Early Childhood, Adoption, and Dependent Care; Section on Developmental and Behavioral Pediatrics. Early childhood adversity, toxic stress, and the role of the pediatrician: translating developmental science into lifelong health. *Pediatrics*. 2012;129(1). Available at: www.pediatrics.org/cgi/content/full/129/1/e224

10. Felitti VJ, Anda RF, Nordenberg D, et al. Relationship of childhood abuse and household dysfunction to many of the leading causes of death in adults. The

Adverse Childhood Experiences (ACE) Study. *Am J Prev Med*. 1998;14(4):245–258

11. Dong M, Anda RF, Felitti VJ, et al. The interrelatedness of multiple forms of childhood abuse, neglect, and household dysfunction. *Child Abuse Negl*. 2004;28(7):771–784

12. Anda RF, Felitti VJ, Bremner JD, et al. The enduring effects of abuse and related adverse experiences in childhood. A convergence of evidence from neurobiology and epidemiology. *Eur Arch Psychiatry Clin Neurosci*. 2006;256(3):174–186

13. Warne D, Dulacki K, Spurlock M, et al. Adverse childhood experiences (ACE) among American Indians in South Dakota and associations with mental health conditions, alcohol use, and smoking. *J Health Care Poor Underserved*. 2017;28(4):1559–1577

14. Koss MP, Yuan NP, Dightman D, et al. Adverse childhood exposures and alcohol dependence among seven Native American tribes. *Am J Prev Med*. 2003;25(3):238–244

15. Kenney MK, Singh GK. Adverse childhood experiences among

American Indian/Alaska native children: the 2011-2012 National Survey of Children's Health. *Scientifica (Cairo)*. 2016;2016:7424239

16. Brockie TN, Dana-Sacco G, Wallen GR, Wilcox HC, Campbell JC. The relationship of adverse childhood experiences to PTSD, depression, poly-drug use and suicide attempt in reservation-based Native American adolescents and young adults. *Am J Community Psychol*. 2015;55(3–4): 411–421

17. US Department of Health and Human Services. Obesity and American Indians/Alaska natives. Available at: https://aspe.hhs.gov/basic-report/ obesity-and-american-indiansalaska-natives. Accessed December 2, 2016

18. Lindsay RS, Cook V, Hanson RL, Salbe AD, Tataranni A, Knowler WC. Early excess weight gain of children in the Pima Indian population. *Pediatrics*. 2002;109(2):E33

19. Salbe AD, Weyer C, Lindsay RS, Ravussin E, Tataranni PA. Assessing risk factors for obesity between childhood and adolescence: I. Birth weight, childhood adiposity, parental obesity, insulin, and leptin. *Pediatrics*. 2002;110(2 pt 1): 299–306

20. Dalenius K, Borland E, Smith B, Polhamus B, Grummer-Strawn L. *Pediatric Nutrition Surveillance 2010 Report*. Atlanta, GA: Centers for Disease Control and Prevention; 2012

21. Schell LM, Gallo MV. Overweight and obesity among North American Indian infants, children, and youth. *Am J Hum Biol*. 2012;24(3):302–313

22. Centers for Disease Control and Prevention (CDC). Obesity prevalence among low-income, preschool-aged children - United States, 1998-2008. *MMWR Morb Mortal Wkly Rep*. 2009; 58(28):769–773

23. Bullock A, Sheff K, Moore K, Manson S. Obesity and overweight in American Indian and Alaska native children, 2006-2015. *Am J Public Health*. 2017;107(9): 1502–1507

24. Pan L, Park S, Slayton R, Goodman AB, Blanck HM. Trends in severe obesity among children aged 2 to 4 years enrolled in Special Supplemental Nutrition Program for Women, Infants,

and Children from 2000 to 2014. *JAMA Pediatr*. 2018;172(3):232–238

25. Tomayko EJ, Prince RJ, Cronin KA, Adams AK. The Healthy Children, Strong Families intervention promotes improvements in nutrition, activity and body weight in American Indian families with young children. [published correction appears in Public Health Nutr. 2017;20(2):380]. *Public Health Nutr*. 2016;19(15):2850–2859

26. Lindberg SM, Adams AK, Prince RJ. Early predictors of obesity and cardiovascular risk among American Indian children. *Matern Child Health J*. 2012;16(9):1879–1886

27. Institute of Medicine. *Early Childhood Obesity Prevention Policies*. Washington, DC: National Academies Press; 2011

28. Whitaker RC, Wright JA, Pepe MS, Seidel KD, Dietz WH. Predicting obesity in young adulthood from childhood and parental obesity. *N Engl J Med*. 1997; 337(13):869–873

29. Pan L, May AL, Wethington H, Dalenius K, Grummer-Strawn LM. Incidence of obesity among young U.S. children living in low-income families, 2008-2011. *Pediatrics*. 2013;132(6):1006–1013

30. American Diabetes Association. Type 2 diabetes in children and adolescents. *Diabetes Care*. 2000;23(3):381–389

31. American Diabetes Association. 2. Classification and diagnosis of diabetes: *Standards of Medical Care in Diabetes-2018. Diabetes Care*. 2018; 41(suppl 1):S13–S27

32. Springer SC, Silverstein J, Copeland K, et al; American Academy of Pediatrics. Management of type 2 diabetes mellitus in children and adolescents. [published correction appears in Pediatrics. 2013; 131(5):1014]. *Pediatrics*. 2013;131(2). Available at: www.pediatrics.org/cgi/ content/full/131/2/e648

33. Gahagan S, Silverstein J; American Academy of Pediatrics Committee on Native American Child Health; American Academy of Pediatrics Section on Endocrinology. Prevention and treatment of type 2 diabetes mellitus in children, with special emphasis on American Indian and Alaska native children. *Pediatrics*. 2003;112(4).

Available at: www.pediatrics.org/cgi/ content/full/112/4/e328

34. Section on Breastfeeding. Breastfeeding and the use of human milk. *Pediatrics*. 2012;129(3). Available at: www.pediatrics.org/cgi/content/full/ 129/3/e827

35. Jones KM, Power ML, Queenan JT, Schulkin J. Racial and ethnic disparities in breastfeeding. *Breastfeed Med*. 2015; 10(4):186–196

36. Sparks PJ. Racial/ethnic differences in breastfeeding duration among WIC-eligible families. *Womens Health Issues*. 2011;21(5):374–382

37. Zamora-Kapoor A, Omidpanah A, Nelson LA, Kuo AA, Harris R, Buchwald DS. Breastfeeding in infancy is associated with body mass index in adolescence: a retrospective cohort study comparing American Indians/Alaska natives and non-Hispanic whites. *J Acad Nutr Diet*. 2017;117(7):1049–1056

38. Houghtaling B, Byker Shanks C, Ahmed S, Rink E. Grandmother and health care professional breastfeeding perspectives provide opportunities for health promotion in an American Indian community. *Soc Sci Med*. 2018;208: 80–88

39. Walkup JT, Barlow A, Mullany BC, et al. Randomized controlled trial of a paraprofessional-delivered in-home intervention for young reservation-based American Indian mothers. *J Am Acad Child Adolesc Psychiatry*. 2009; 48(6):591–601

40. Kenney MK, Thierry J. Chronic conditions, functional difficulties, and disease burden among American Indian/Alaska native children with special health care needs, 2009-2010. *Matern Child Health J*. 2014;18(9): 2071–2079

41. Wong CA, Gachupin FC, Holman RC, et al. American Indian and Alaska native infant and pediatric mortality, United States, 1999-2009. *Am J Public Health*. 2014;104(suppl 3):S320–S328

42. Cappiello MM, Gahagan S. Early child development and developmental delay in indigenous communities. *Pediatr Clin North Am*. 2009;56(6):1501–1517

43. MacDorman MF. Race and ethnic disparities in fetal mortality, preterm birth, and infant mortality in the United

States: an overview. *Semin Perinatol.* 2011;35(4):200–208

44. Barros N, Tulve NS, Heggem DT, Bailey K. Review of built and natural environment stressors impacting American-Indian/Alaska-native children. *Rev Environ Health.* 2018;33(4):349–381

45. Itty TL, Hodge FS, Martinez F. Shared and unshared barriers to cancer symptom management among urban and rural American Indians. *J Rural Health.* 2014;30(2):206–213

46. Call KT, McAlpine DD, Garcia CM, et al. Barriers to care in an ethnically diverse publicly insured population: is health care reform enough? *Med Care.* 2014; 52(8):720–727

47. Fuentes MM, Thompson L, Quistberg DA, et al. Auditing access to outpatient rehabilitation services for children with traumatic brain injury and public insurance in Washington State. *Arch Phys Med Rehabil.* 2017;98(9): 1763–1770.e7

48. Fuentes M, Lent K. Culture, health, function, and participation among American Indian and Alaska native children and youth with disabilities: an exploratory qualitative analysis. *Arch Phys Med Rehabil.* 2019;100(9): 1688–1694

49. Centers for Disease Control and Prevention. Web-based Injury Statistics Query and Reporting System (WISQARS) [online]. Details of leading cause of death: 2016, United States, suicide, ages 10-24, American Indian/Alaska native, both sexes. Available at: www.cdc.gov/injury/wisqars. Accessed November 29, 2018

50. Centers for Disease Control and Prevention. Web-based Injury Statistics Query and Reporting System (WISQARS) [online]. Details of leading cause of death: 2016, United States, suicide ages 10-24, all races, both sexes. Available at: www.cdc.gov/injury/wisqars. Accessed November 29, 2018

51. Centers for Disease Control and Prevention. Web-based Injury Statistics Query and Reporting System (WISQARS) [online]. 2016, United States, suicide injury deaths and rates per 100,000, all races, both sexes, ages 10-24. Available at: www.cdc.gov/injury/wisqars. Accessed November 29, 2018

52. Herne MA, Bartholomew ML, Weahkee RL. Suicide mortality among American Indians and Alaska natives, 1999-2009. *Am J Public Health.* 2014;104(suppl 3): S336–S342

53. Mullany B, Barlow A, Goklish N, et al. Toward understanding suicide among youths: results from the White Mountain Apache tribally mandated suicide surveillance system, 2001-2006. *Am J Public Health.* 2009;99(10): 1840–1848

54. Borowsky IW, Resnick MD, Ireland M, Blum RW. Suicide attempts among American Indian and Alaska native youth: risk and protective factors. *Arch Pediatr Adolesc Med.* 1999;153(6): 573–580

55. Mackin J, Perkins T, Furrer C. The power of protection: a population-based comparison of native and non-native youth suicide attempters. *Am Indian Alsk Native Ment Health Res.* 2012;19(2): 20–54

56. Qiao N, Bell TM. Indigenous adolescents' suicidal behaviors and risk factors: evidence from the National Youth Risk Behavior Survey. *J Immigr Minor Health.* 2017;19(3):590–597

57. Leavitt RA, Ertl A, Sheats K, Petrosky E, Ivey-Stephenson A, Fowler KA. Suicides among American Indian/Alaska natives - National Violent Death Reporting System, 18 states, 2003-2014. *MMWR Morb Mortal Wkly Rep.* 2018;67(8): 237–242

58. Allen J, Rasmus SM, Fok CCT, Charles B, Henry D; Qungasvik Team. Multi-level cultural intervention for the prevention of suicide and alcohol use risk with Alaska native youth: a nonrandomized comparison of treatment intensity. *Prev Sci.* 2018;19(2):174–185

59. Koenig KT, Ramos MM, Fowler TT, Oreskovich K, McGrath J, Fairbrother G. A statewide profile of frequent users of school-based health centers: implications for adolescent health care. *J Sch Health.* 2016;86(4):250–257

60. Almeida J, Johnson RM, Corliss HL, Molnar BE, Azrael D. Emotional distress among LGBT youth: the influence of perceived discrimination based on sexual orientation. *J Youth Adolesc.* 2009;38(7):1001–1014

61. Kessler RC, Borges G, Walters EE. Prevalence of and risk factors for lifetime suicide attempts in the National Comorbidity Survey. *Arch Gen Psychiatry.* 1999;56(7):617–626

62. Institute of Medicine Committee on Lesbian, Gay, Bisexual, and Transgender Health Issues and Research Gaps and Opportunities. *The Health of Lesbian, Gay, Bisexual, and Transgender People: Building a Foundation for Better Understanding.* Washington, DC: National Academies Press; 2011

63. Angelino A, Evans-Campbell T, Duran B. Assessing health provider perspectives regarding barriers American Indian/Alaska native transgender and two-spirit youth face accessing healthcare. *J Racial Ethn Health Disparities.* 2020; 7(4):630–642

64. Perez-Brumer A, Day JK, Russell ST, Hatzenbuehler ML. Prevalence and correlates of suicidal ideation among transgender youth in California: findings from a representative, population-based sample of high school students. *J Am Acad Child Adolesc Psychiatry.* 2017;56(9):739–746

65. Bostwick WB, Meyer I, Aranda F, et al. Mental health and suicidality among racially/ethnically diverse sexual minority youths. *Am J Public Health.* 2014;104(6):1129–1136

66. James SE, Herman JL, Rankin S, Keisling M, Mottet L, Anafi M. *The Report of the 2015 U.S. Transgender Survey.* Washington, DC: National Center for Transgender Equality; 2016

67. Rafferty J; Committee on Psychosocial Aspects of Child and Family Health; Committee on Adolescence; Section on Lesbian, Gay, Bisexual, and Transgender Health and Wellness. Ensuring comprehensive care and support for transgender and gender-diverse children and adolescents. *Pediatrics.* 2018;142(4):e20182162

68. Fuentes MM, Moore M, Qiu Q, Quistberg A, Frank M, Vavilala MS. Differences in injury characteristics and outcomes for American Indian/Alaska native people hospitalized with traumatic injuries: an analysis of the National Trauma Data Bank. *J Racial Ethn Health Disparities.* 2019;6(2):335–344

69. Urban Indian Health Institute. *Missing and Murdered Indigenous Women &*

Girls: A Snapshot of Data from 71 Urban Cities in the United States. Seattle, WA: Urban Indian Health Institute; 2018

70. Greenbaum J, Bodrick N; Committee on Child Abuse and Neglect; Section on International Child Health. Global human trafficking and child victimization. *Pediatrics.* 2017;140(6): e20173138

71. National Center on Domestic and Sexual Violence. Sexual violence/assault. 2012. Available at: www.ncdsv.org/publications_Sexual-Violence-Assault.html. Accessed November 11, 2019

72. Pierce A. *Shattered Hearts: The Commercial Sexual Exploitation of American Indian Women and Girls in Minnesota.* Minneapolis, MN: Minnesota Indian Women's Resource Center; 2009

73. Wiltz T. *American Indian Girls Often Fall Through the Cracks.* Philadelphia, PA: The Pew Charitable Trusts; 2016. Available at: https://www.pewtrusts.org/en/research-and-analysis/blogs/stateline/2016/03/04/american-indian-girls-often-fall-through-the-cracks. Accessed November 11, 2019

74. Administration for Children and Families. Combating Trafficking: Native Youth Toolkit on Human Trafficking. Washington, DC: Administration for Children and Families; 2017. Available at: https://www.acf.hhs.gov/blog/2018/01/combating-trafficking-native-youth-toolkit-on-human-trafficking. Accessed November 11, 2019

75. Children's Bureau. Child maltreatment 2017. Available at: https://www.acf.hhs.gov/cb/resource/child-maltreatment-2017. Accessed November 11, 2019

76. Williams SC. State-level data for understanding child welfare in the United States. Available at: https://www.childtrends.org/publications/state-level-data-for-understanding-child-welfare-in-the-united-states. Accessed November 11, 2019

77. Hill KM. The prevalence of youth with disabilities among older youth in out-of-home placement: an analysis of state administrative data. *Child Welfare.* 2012;91(4):61–84

78. Earle K, Cross A. *Child Abuse and Neglect Among American Indian/Alaska Native Children: An Analysis of Existing Data.* Seattle, WA: Casey Family Programs; 2001

79. Nash DA, Nagel RJ. Confronting oral health disparities among American Indian/Alaska native children: the pediatric oral health therapist. *Am J Public Health.* 2005;95(8):1325–1329

80. Indian Health Service. *The 1999 Oral Health Survey of American Indian and Alaska Native Dental Patients: Findings, Regional Differences and National Comparisons.* Rockville, MD: US Department of Health and Human Services; 2001

81. Holve S, Braun P, Irvine JD; American Academy of Pediatrics Committee on Native American Child Health and Section on Oral Health; Canadian Paediatric Society First Nations, Inuit and Métis Committee. Early childhood caries in indigenous communities. *Pediatrics.* 2021, In press

82. Ochi JW, Wheelbarger L, Dautenhahn LW. Chronic otitis media in ancient American Indians. *Pediatrics.* 2018; 141(4):e20172308

83. Curns AT, Holman RC, Shay DK, et al. Outpatient and hospital visits associated with otitis media among American Indian and Alaska native children younger than 5 years. *Pediatrics.* 2002;109(3). Available at: www.pediatrics.org/cgi/content/full/109/3/e41

84. Atherly A, Mortensen K. Medicaid primary care physician fees and the use of preventive services among Medicaid enrollees. *Health Serv Res.* 2014;49(4):1306–1328

85. Polsky D, Richards M, Basseyn S, et al. Appointment availability after increases in Medicaid payments for primary care. *N Engl J Med.* 2015;372(6):537–545

86. Alker J, Wagnerman K, Schneider A. *Coverage Trends for American Indian and Alaska Native Children and Families.* Washington, DC: Georgetown University Health Policy Institute; 2017

87. Artiga S, Ubri U, Foutz J. *Medicaid and American Indians and Alaska Natives.* San Francisco, CA: Henry J. Kaiser Family Foundation; 2017

88. Vintzileos AM, Ananth CV, Smulian JC, Scorza WE, Knuppel RA. The impact of prenatal care in the United States on preterm births in the presence and absence of antenatal high-risk conditions. *Am J Obstet Gynecol.* 2002; 187(5):1254–1257

89. Stone R. Pregnant women and substance use: fear, stigma and barriers to care. *Health Justice.* 2015;3:2

90. Soleimanpour S, Geierstanger S, Brindis CD. Adverse childhood experiences and resilience: addressing the unique needs of adolescents. *Acad Pediatr.* 2017;17(suppl 7):S108–S114

91. Marsac ML, Kassam-Adams N, Hildenbrand AK, et al. Implementing a trauma-informed approach in pediatric health care networks. *JAMA Pediatr.* 2016;170(1):70–77

92. Ginsburg KR, Kinsman SB, eds.. *Reaching Teens: Strength-Based Communication Strategies to Build Resilience and Support Healthy Adolescent Development.* Elk Grove Village, IL: American Academy of Pediatrics; 2014

93. Swaim RC, Stanley LR. Substance use among American Indian youths on reservations compared with a national sample of US adolescents. *JAMA Netw Open.* 2018;1(1):e180382

94. American Academy of Family Physicians. The EveryONE project toolkit. Available at: https://www.aafp.org/patient-care/social-determinants-of-health/everyone-project/eop-tools.html. Accessed December 5, 2018

95. Giuse NB, Koonce TY, Kusnoor SV, et al. Institute of Medicine measures of social and behavioral determinants of health: a feasibility study. *Am J Prev Med.* 2017; 52(2):199–206

96. Arthur KC, Lucenko BA, Sharkova IV, Xing J, Mangione-Smith R. Using state administrative data to identify social complexity risk factors for children. *Ann Fam Med.* 2018;16(1):62–69

97. Duffee JH, Mendelsohn AL, Kuo AA, Legano LA, Earls MF; Council on Community Pediatrics; Council on Early Childhood; Committee on Child Abuse and Neglect. Early childhood home visiting. *Pediatrics.* 2017;140(3): e20172150

98. Klass P, Dreyer BP, Mendelsohn AL. Reach out and read: literacy promotion in pediatric primary care. *Adv Pediatr.* 2009;56:11–27

99. American Indian Library Association. American Indian youth literature award. Available at: https://ailanet.org/activities/american-indian-youth-literature-award/. Accessed December 5, 2018

100. Morton MH, Chávez R, Moore K. Prevalence and correlates of homelessness among American Indian and Alaska native youth. *J Prim Prev.* 2019;40(6):643–660

101. Thomas MMC, Miller DP, Morrissey TW. Food insecurity and child health. *Pediatrics.* 2019;144(4):e20190397

102. Blue Cross Complete of Michigan. Culturally and Linguistically Appropriate Services (CLAS) provider cultural competency. Available at: https://www.bcbsm.com/content/dam/microsites/blue-cross-complete/blue-cross-complete-clas-training-presentation.pdf. Accessed January 15, 2019

103. Donoghue EA; Council on Early Childhood. Quality early education and child care from birth to kindergarten. *Pediatrics.* 2017;140(2):e20171488

104. Earls MF, Yogman MW, Mattson G, Rafferty J; Committee on Psychosocial Aspects of Child and Family Health. Incorporating recognition and management of perinatal depression into pediatric practice. *Pediatrics.* 2019;143(1):e20183259

105. Committee on Substance Use and Prevention. Substance use screening, brief intervention, and referral to treatment. *Pediatrics.* 2016;138(1):e20161210

106. Levy SJ, Williams JF; Committee on Substance Use and Prevention. Substance use screening, brief intervention, and referral to treatment. *Pediatrics.* 2016;138(1):e20161211

107. Patrick SW, Schiff DM; Committee on Substance Use and Prevention. A public health response to opioid use in pregnancy. *Pediatrics.* 2017;139(3):e20164070

POLICY STATEMENT Organizational Principles to Guide and Define the Child Health
Care System and/or Improve the Health of all Children

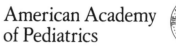

American Academy
of Pediatrics

DEDICATED TO THE HEALTH OF ALL CHILDREN®

Truth, Reconciliation, and Transformation: Continuing on the Path to Equity

American Academy of Pediatrics Board of Directors

One year ago, the American Academy of Pediatrics (AAP) published a landmark policy statement identifying racism as a core social determinant of health and a driver of health inequities.[1] Seventy-five years ago, the AAP admitted its first Black members, Drs Alonzo deGrate Smith and Roland Boyd Scott. As the AAP continues to evolve its equity agenda, it is essential that the tortuous experiences of Drs deGrate Smith and Scott on their pathway to AAP membership be truthfully acknowledged and reckoned with.

At the time of their initially rejected applications in 1939, both Drs deGrate Smith and Scott were busy clinicians and well-established leaders in the pediatric academic community as faculty at the Howard University College of Medicine in Washington, DC. Dr deGrate Smith, through the practice pathway, and Dr Scott, via examination, were among the earliest pediatricians to achieve certification under the Advisory Board of Medical Specialties (ABMS) when the American Board of Pediatrics (ABP) was established in 1933. However, the ABMS required American Medical Association (AMA) membership to honor certification, and the local AMA chapter, the Medical Society of the District of Columbia, was segregated.[2] According to the oral history interview of Dr Melvin E. Jenkins Jr, advocacy on the part of the inaugural ABP president, Dr Borden Veeder, was necessary to permanently eliminate this exclusionary barrier and to make certification possible for all eligible candidates regardless of race or ethnicity.[3] Drs deGrate Smith and Scott faced other systemic barriers, including the inability to gain admitting privileges to care for even their own patients at local hospitals in the District of Columbia. This was a hurdle that Dr Scott was not able to overcome until 1955, fully 6 years after he had already been appointed Chair of Pediatrics at Howard University.[4]

Although AAP bylaws did not explicitly prohibit physicians of color from membership, and Drs deGrate Smith and Scott were finally admitted in 1945, it is clear that the AAP Executive Board struggled with unbiased consideration of their applications. The characterizations related to Drs deGrate Smith and Scott in the following passages excerpted directly from meeting transcripts of AAP Executive Board meetings in November 1939,

DOI: https://doi.org/10.1542/peds.2020-019794

Address correspondence to President@aap.org.

PEDIATRICS (ISSN Numbers: Print, 0031-4005; Online, 1098-4275).

To cite: American Academy of Pediatrics Board of Directors. Truth, Reconciliation, and Transformation: Continuing on the Path to Equity. *Pediatrics.* 2020;146(3): e2020019794

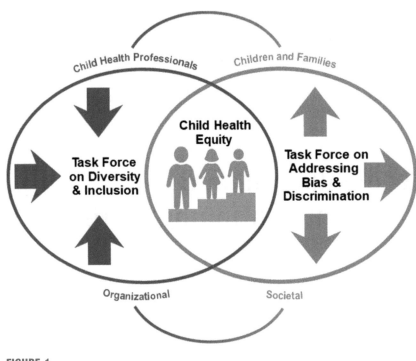

FIGURE 1
AAP Equity Agenda.

November 1944, and June 1945 are elucidating, instructive, and painful to read. The verbatim dialogue and proceedings highlight the racist attitudes and beliefs from which early AAP leaders were clearly not immune.

November 1939—American Academy of Pediatrics Executive Board

[Region I Chairman] then presented the application of Dr Alfred [sic] deGrate Smith. Motion made by [Region I Chairman] that this application not be accepted and that a letter be sent to his sponsor outlining the educational advancements being outlined by the American Academy of Pediatrics for negro physicians; motion seconded by [Region I Associate Chairman] and carried.[5]

[Region III Chairman] moved that all of these [Region III] applications, with the exception of Dr Scott, be accepted into membership; motion duly seconded and carried. Motion made by [Region I Chairman] that the same action be taken on Dr Scott as had been taken on Dr Smith; motion seconded and carried.[5]

November 1944—American Academy of Pediatrics Executive Board

"I know Smith and he is a very nice fellow. Scott has for a year or two attended the Sunday morning clinical

conferences at Children's Hospital. He has taken part in the discussion of cases at Freedman's Hospital. I think the local men in Washington would like to have something to say about men taken into the Academy from that particular location. I think they would rather resent an effort being made to put these men in. I would like to hear what [Region II Chairman] has to say."[5]

"We allow negroes to come to our meeting and we fix a separate place for them to sit. They do not become members. If they became members they would want to come and eat with you at the table. You cannot hold them down."[5]

June 1945—American Academy of Pediatrics Executive Board

"We talked with them for about a half hour and they conducted themselves as gentlemen. They said their only interest in wishing to join the Academy was for educational purposes. They said they would not attend any meetings held South of the Mason and Dixon line. They would attend meetings in other parts of the country, but under no circumstances enter into the social side for the reason that they did not want to get hurt themselves. I impressed upon them the importance should they be elected, of their being leaders and not pushers, and their acceptance in the Academy would be guidance for those who would come at a later time."[6]

"I think the problem is of much more concern to us than it needs to be. In the first place, we have a definite responsibility to these negro representatives and to the negro population of the country. The only trouble is the social implication. The burden lies much heavier upon Smith and Scott than upon us. As the President (of the Academy) says, we have the authority to say who will not be admitted. In the event that either of these men transgress the social lines, they completely stop the advancement of the negro."[6]

In the United States there is a tendency to be ahistorical when it comes to race. The lack of acknowledgment, or worse, the intentional whitewashing of history and the longitudinal relationship of 400 years of oppression on the present-day expression of racism is not uncommon. As the AAP turns the corner toward the 2030 centennial anniversary of its founding, we cannot do so without authentically acknowledging, owning, and reconciling past discriminatory transgressions like the shameful gauntlet to membership experienced by Drs Alonzo deGrate Smith and Roland Boyd Scott.

In honoring the memory of these two trailblazers and their contributions to pediatrics and the AAP,[7] be it resolved that, we, the Board of Directors of the AAP:

1) Apologize for the racism that contributed to the inequities that Drs deGrate Smith, Scott, and other pediatricians have endured, and;

2) Commit to a bylaws referendum to explicitly codify that AAP membership does not discriminate on the basis of race, ethnicity, religion, sex, sexual orientation, gender identity, disability, or national origin.

The AAP as an organization is on a firm pathway to broadly establishing an equity agenda through meaningful diversity and inclusion and a societal commitment to combating bias and discrimination in all its forms, including structural and systemic anti-Black racism (Fig 1). This country is already majority represented by children of color when it comes to the pediatric population.

Embracing racial and ethnic socialization is critical for *all* children and families as well as for the pediatricians who care for them. Healing starts at home with truth, reckoning, and honest reconciliation.

The AAP is proud to transparently acknowledge, proud to publicly reconcile, and proud to continue to lead on behalf of the best interests of children, adolescents, and young adults and the people who care for them.

AMERICAN ACADEMY OF PEDIATRICS BOARD OF DIRECTORS EXECUTIVE COMMITTEE

PRESIDENT

Sara H. Goza, MD, FAAP

PRESIDENT-ELECT

Lee Savio Beers, MD, FAAP

IMMEDIATE PAST PRESIDENT

Kyle E. Yasuda, MD, FAAP

SECRETARY/TREASURER

Warren M. Seigel, MD, FAAP

CEO/EXECUTIVE VICE PRESIDENT

Mark Del Monte, JD

BOARD OF DIRECTORS

DISTRICT I

Wendy S. Davis, MD, FAAP

DISTRICT II

Warren M. Seigel, MD, FAAP

DISTRICT III

Margaret C. Fisher, MD, FAAP

DISTRICT IV

Michelle D. Fiscus, MD, FAAP

DISTRICT V

Richard H. Tuck, MD, FAAP

DISTRICT VI

Dennis M. Cooley, MD, FAAP

DISTRICT VII

Gary W. Floyd, MD, FAAP

DISTRICT VIII

Martha C. Middlemist, MD, FAAP

DISTRICT IX

Yasuko Fukuda, MD, FAAP

DISTRICT X

Lisa A. Cosgrove, MD, FAAP

AT LARGE

Charles G. Macias, MD, FAAP

AT LARGE

Constance S. Houck, MD, FAAP

AT LARGE

Joseph L. Wright, MD, FAAP

REFERENCES

1. Trent M, Dooley DG, Dougé J; Section on Adolescent Health; Council on Community Pediatrics; Committee on Adolescence. The impact of racism on child and adolescent health. *Pediatrics.* 2019;144(2):e20191765

2. Negro doctor addresses DC medical society. *Jet.* April 16, 1953

3. Interview of Melvin E. Jenkins Jr, MD. American Academy of Pediatrics Oral History Project, August 12, 2008

4. DC hospital admits 3 Negro physicians. *Jet.* March 10, 1955

5. AAP Gartner Pediatric History Center. Archived Executive Board Meeting Minutes. Accessed June 28, 2020

6. Wyckoff AS. First Black AAP members rose in prominence but faced scrutiny. *AAP News.* 2019. Available at: https://www.aappublications.org/news/2019/02/04/dyk020419. Accessed July 13, 2020

7. Parrott RH, Jenkins ME. Howland Award presentation to Roland B. Scott. *Pediatr Res.* 1991;30(6):626–627

POLICY STATEMENT Organizational Principles to Guide and Define the Child Health Care System and/or Improve the Health of all Children

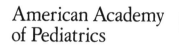

American Academy of Pediatrics

DEDICATED TO THE HEALTH OF ALL CHILDREN™

The Impact of Racism on Child and Adolescent Health

Maria Trent, MD, MPH, FAAP, FSAHM,[a] Danielle G. Dooley, MD, MPhil, FAAP,[b] Jacqueline Dougé, MD, MPH, FAAP,[c] SECTION ON ADOLESCENT HEALTH, COUNCIL ON COMMUNITY PEDIATRICS, COMMITTEE ON ADOLESCENCE

The American Academy of Pediatrics is committed to addressing the factors that affect child and adolescent health with a focus on issues that may leave some children more vulnerable than others. Racism is a social determinant of health that has a profound impact on the health status of children, adolescents, emerging adults, and their families. Although progress has been made toward racial equality and equity, the evidence to support the continued negative impact of racism on health and well-being through implicit and explicit biases, institutional structures, and interpersonal relationships is clear. The objective of this policy statement is to provide an evidence-based document focused on the role of racism in child and adolescent development and health outcomes. By acknowledging the role of racism in child and adolescent health, pediatricians and other pediatric health professionals will be able to proactively engage in strategies to optimize clinical care, workforce development, professional education, systems engagement, and research in a manner designed to reduce the health effects of structural, personally mediated, and internalized racism and improve the health and well-being of all children, adolescents, emerging adults, and their families.

abstract

[a]Division of Adolescent and Young Adult Medicine, Department of Pediatrics, School of Medicine, Johns Hopkins University, Baltimore, Maryland; [b]Division of General Pediatrics and Community Health and Child Health Advocacy Institute, Children's National Health System, Washington, District of Columbia; and [c]Medical Director, Howard County Health Department, Columbia, Maryland

Drs Trent, Dooley, and Dougé worked together as a writing team to develop the manuscript outline, conduct the literature search, develop the stated policies, incorporate perspectives and feedback from American Academy of Pediatrics leadership, and draft the final version of the manuscript; and all authors approved the final manuscript as submitted.

Policy statements from the American Academy of Pediatrics benefit from expertise and resources of liaisons and internal (AAP) and external reviewers. However, policy statements from the American Academy of Pediatrics may not reflect the views of the liaisons or the organizations or government agencies that they represent.

The guidance in this statement does not indicate an exclusive course of treatment or serve as a standard of medical care. Variations, taking into account individual circumstances, may be appropriate.

All policy statements from the American Academy of Pediatrics automatically expire 5 years after publication unless reaffirmed, revised, or retired at or before that time.

DOI: https://doi.org/10.1542/peds.2019-1765

Address correspondence to Maria Trent, MD. E-mail: mtrent2@jhmi.edu

To cite: Trent M, Dooley DG, Dougé J, AAP SECTION ON ADOLESCENT HEALTH, AAP COUNCIL ON COMMUNITY PEDIATRICS, AAP COMMITTEE ON ADOLESCENCE. The Impact of Racism on Child and Adolescent Health. *Pediatrics.* 2019;144(2):e20191765

STATEMENT OF THE PROBLEM

Racism is a "system of structuring opportunity and assigning value based on the social interpretation of how one looks (which is what we call 'race') that unfairly disadvantages some individuals and communities, unfairly advantages other individuals and communities, and saps the strength of the whole society through the waste of human resources."[1] Racism is a social determinant of health[2] that has a profound impact on the health status of children, adolescents, emerging adults, and their families.[3–8] Although progress has been made toward racial equality and equity,[9] the evidence to support the continued negative impact of racism on health and well-being through implicit and explicit biases, institutional structures, and interpersonal relationships is clear.[10] Failure to address racism will

POLICY STATEMENT Organizational Principles to Guide and Define the Child Health
Care System and/or Improve the Health of all Children

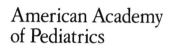

American Academy
of Pediatrics

DEDICATED TO THE HEALTH OF ALL CHILDREN™

This Policy Statement was reaffirmed September 2022.

Race, Ethnicity, and Socioeconomic Status in Research on Child Health

Tina L. Cheng, MD, MPH, FAAP, Elizabeth Goodman, MD, FAAP, THE COMMITTEE ON PEDIATRIC RESEARCH

abstract

An extensive literature documents the existence of pervasive and persistent child health, development, and health care disparities by race, ethnicity, and socioeconomic status (SES). Disparities experienced during childhood can result in a wide variety of health and health care outcomes, including adult morbidity and mortality, indicating that it is crucial to examine the influence of disparities across the life course. Studies often collect data on the race, ethnicity, and SES of research participants to be used as covariates or explanatory factors. In the past, these variables have often been assumed to exert their effects through individual or genetically determined biologic mechanisms. However, it is now widely accepted that these variables have important social dimensions that influence health. SES, a multidimensional construct, interacts with and confounds analyses of race and ethnicity. Because SES, race, and ethnicity are often difficult to measure accurately, leading to the potential for misattribution of causality, thoughtful consideration should be given to appropriate measurement, analysis, and interpretation of such factors. Scientists who study child and adolescent health and development should understand the multiple measures used to assess race, ethnicity, and SES, including their validity and shortcomings and potential confounding of race and ethnicity with SES. The American Academy of Pediatrics (AAP) recommends that research on eliminating health and health care disparities related to race, ethnicity, and SES be a priority. Data on race, ethnicity, and SES should be collected in research on child health to improve their definitions and increase understanding of how these factors and their complex interrelationships affect child health. Furthermore, the AAP believes that researchers should consider both biological and social mechanisms of action of race, ethnicity, and SES as they relate to the aims and hypothesis of the specific area of investigation. It is important to measure these variables, but it is not sufficient to use these variables alone as explanatory for differences in disease, morbidity, and outcomes without attention to the social and biologic influences they have on health throughout the life course. The AAP recommends more research, both in the United States and internationally, on measures of race, ethnicity, and SES and how these complex constructs affect health care and health outcomes throughout the life course.

www.pediatrics.org/cgi/doi/10.1542/peds.2014-3109

DOI: 10.1542/peds.2014-3109

PEDIATRICS (ISSN Numbers: Print, 0031-4005; Online, 1098-4275).

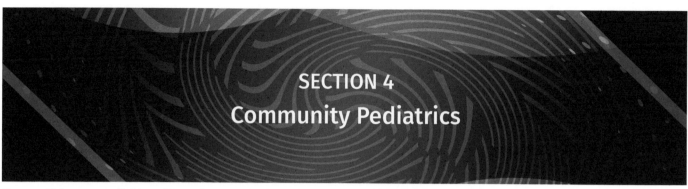

SECTION 4
Community Pediatrics

Some articles are available online only; scan the QR code to access online content.

POLICY STATEMENT
Organizational Principles to Guide and Define the Child Health
Care System and/or Improve the Health of all Children

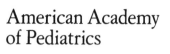

American Academy
of Pediatrics

DEDICATED TO THE HEALTH OF ALL CHILDREN™

Pediatric Primary Health Care: The Central Role of Pediatricians in Maintaining Children's Health in Evolving Health Care Models

Alexy Boudreau, MD, FAAP,[a] Alex Hamling, MD, FAAP,[b] Edward Pont, MD, FAAP,[c] Thomas W. Pendergrass, MD, MSPH, FAAP,[d] Julia Richerson, MD, FAAP,[e] COMMITTEE ON PEDIATRIC WORKFORCE, COMMITTEE ON PRACTICE AND AMBULATORY MEDICINE

abstract

Pediatric primary health care (PPHC) is of principal importance to the health and development of all children, helping them reach their true potential. Pediatricians, as the clinicians most intensively trained and experienced in child health, are the natural leaders of PPHC within the context of the medical home. Given the rapidly evolving models of pediatric health care delivery, including the explosion of telehealth in the wake of the COVID-19 pandemic, pediatricians, together with their representative national organizations such as the American Academy of Pediatrics (AAP), are the most capable clinicians to guide policy innovations on both the local and national stage.

[a]Primary Care, Massachusetts General Hospital, Boston, Massachusetts; [b]Pediatrics, Pacific Medical Centers, Seattle, Washington; [c]Pediatrics, DuPage Medical Group, Elmhurst, Illinois; [d]Department of Pediatrics, University of Washington, Seattle, Washington; and [e]Pediatrics, Family Health Centers, Louisville, Kentucky

Drs Boudreau, Hamling, Pont, Pendergrass, and Richerson were each responsible for all aspects of writing and editing the document and reviewing and responding to questions and comments from reviewers and the board of directors; and all authors approved the final manuscript as submitted and agree to be accountable for all aspects of the work.

To cite: Boudreau A, Hamling A, Pont E, et al; AAP Committee on Pediatric Workforce, AAP Committee on Practice and Ambulatory Medicine. Pediatric Primary Health Care: The Central Role of Pediatricians in Maintaining Children's Health in Evolving Health Care Models. *Pediatrics.* 2022;149(2):e2021055553

WHAT IS PEDIATRIC PRIMARY HEALTH CARE?

Pediatric primary health care (PPHC) always aspires to be continuous, comprehensive, and coordinated care that is accessible and affordable to meet the health needs of the infant, child, adolescent, and young adult by providing family-centered care. PPHC encompasses comprehensive care across the life cycle, from infancy to young adulthood. PPHC includes health supervision, with a focus on prevention of physical and mental health conditions; anticipatory guidance and promotion of wellness including mental health and monitoring physical, cognitive, and social growth and development; and age-appropriate screening for health promotion and disease prevention.[1] Although 1 in 5 children have an identified special health care need or chronic illness, these illnesses are diverse with a relatively low but increasing prevalence. Board-certified and board-eligible pediatricians have the ongoing challenge of identifying and addressing significant clinical concerns in a typically healthy population.[2] Therefore, PPHC also encompasses diagnosis and treatment of acute and chronic health disorders; management of serious and life-threatening illnesses; and when appropriate, referral of patients with more complex conditions for medical subspecialty or surgical specialty care. To achieve optimal health outcomes, PPHC also involves coordinated management of health problems that require multiple professional services and well-planned transitioning of all children, especially those with chronic illness, to adult care. Finally, PPHC ideally strives to be both patient- and family-centered and to incorporate community resources and strengths, risk and protective factors, and sociocultural effectiveness into strategies for care delivery and clinical practice.[1]

WHAT IS THE UNIQUE ROLE OF THE PEDIATRICIAN IN PEDIATRIC PRIMARY CARE?

Pediatricians have received comprehensive education and training devoted to all aspects of pediatric health care.[3] This education and training is coupled with a demonstrated interest in and total professional commitment to the health care of infants, children, adolescents, and young adults. Because of these unique qualifications, the pediatrician is a highly skilled and qualified supervisor of PPHC delivery, often partnering with other professionals to support team-based care. Within all of medicine, pediatrics is the only specialty for which training focuses exclusively on the care and unique health needs of infants, children, adolescents, and young adults. Given the continuity that pediatricians typically establish with their patients, often spanning their entire childhood and adolescence, pediatricians are uniquely able to

monitor normal growth and development and flag concerns when their patients deviate from their expected developmental path. In this way, pediatricians have a singular role in maintaining their patients' physical and mental health, with benefits that extend well into their adulthood.

PPHC is best delivered within the context of a patient- and family-centered medical home that provides comprehensive, continuous, coordinated, compassionate, and culturally effective care that is accessible, affordable, and delivered or directed by board-certified or board-eligible pediatricians.[4] Advanced practice providers (ie, nurse practitioners, physician assistants, and other trained pediatric professionals) best support the medical home when they work in collaboration with pediatricians.[5,6]

Team-based care, with physician supervision, limits the occurrence of fragmented care, such as that received from freestanding or retail-based clinics outside the medical neighborhood.[7] Indeed, the medical home best serves as the "hub" of the entire medical neighborhood, placing the pediatrician at the hub's center.[8] In some instances, the pediatric medical subspecialist or pediatric surgical specialist will be the leader of the child's health care team while managing complex conditions and will coordinate the delivery of care among the entire health care team.[9] Collaboration among all providers of PPHC, guided by the pediatrician, is critical to the maximal efficiency, accuracy, and effectiveness of the care of the patient, the family, the community, and the population.

EVOLVING HEALTH CARE DELIVERY MODELS

Because of their training and holistic outlook, pediatricians are uniquely

prepared to move PPHC into integrated health systems that "allow children to develop and realize their potential."[10] Of all health professionals who care primarily for children, pediatricians have a unique mandate to maintain awareness of the larger health policy landscape to ensure it addresses the unique needs of children's health.[11] Pediatricians are also frequently leaders of larger health organizations such as accountable care organizations (ACOs), which have been shown to improve health care quality while also containing costs.[12] With the increased use of telehealth platforms as a result of the COVID-19 pandemic, pediatricians' experience and training will be vital to appropriately integrating this new care pathway into established medical homes. Pediatricians are also best positioned to keep abreast of issues beyond the medical home that can affect the care of children. By participating in the larger health care and policy arena—with state legislators, agency administrators, and other advocacy groups—pediatricians can enhance their patients' health as well as the soundness of public policy regarding children.

RECOMMENDATIONS FOR POLICYMAKERS*:

1. Recognize that the pediatrician is the best expert to navigate the myriad children's health issues that come before health systems, legislatures, executive agencies, and courts. Although other health care professionals should lend their expertise, pediatricians' training and experience are vital to informing policy and understanding how best to promote the health of children.

---

*Policymakers refers to federal and state executive branches, Congress and state legislatures, health insurers and health systems, courts, and other entities that influence pediatric health policy.

2. Include the American Academy of Pediatrics (AAP) and its relevant state chapters in policy decision-making. As the nation's flagship pediatric organization, the AAP has access to pediatricians, pediatric medical subspecialists and pediatric surgical specialists, policy experts, and decades of experience regarding pediatric health care.

3. Always consider the impact of any policy change on children's health and well-being. As our nation's most vulnerable population, children, especially those experiencing health inequity, are unable to advocate for themselves—their well-being depends on astute policy-makers who not only understand their needs but can take them into account as they consider a given policy.

LEAD AUTHORS

Alexy Boudreau, MD, FAAP
Alex Hamling, MD, FAAP
Edward Pont, MD, FAAP
Thomas W. Pendergrass, MD, MSPH, FAAP
Julia Richerson, MD, FAAP

COMMITTEE ON PEDIATRIC WORKFORCE, 2020–2021

Harold K. Simon, MD, MBA, FAAP, Chairperson
Julie S. Byerley, MD, MPH, FAAP
Nancy A. Dodson, MD, FAAP
Eric N. Horowitz, MD, FAAP
Thomas W. Pendergrass, MD, MSPH, FAAP
Edward A. Pont, MD, FAAP
Kristin N. Ray, MD, FAAP

LIAISONS

Laurel K. Leslie, MD, MPH, FAAP – American Board of Pediatrics

STAFF

Lauren F. Barone, MPH

COMMITTEE ON PRACTICE AND AMBULATORY MEDICINE, 2020–2021

Jesse M. Hackell, MD, FAAP, Chairperson
Joseph J. Abularrage, MD, MPH, MPhil, FAAP
Yvette M. Almendarez, MD, FAAP

Alexy D. Arauz Boudreau, MD, MPH, FAAP
Abeba M. Berhane, MD, FAAP
Patricia E. Cantrell, MD, FAAP
Lisa M. Kafer, MD, FAAP
Katherine S. Schafer, DO, FAAP
Robin Warner, MD, FAAP

FORMER COMMITTEE MEMBERS

Alex Hamling, MD, FAAP
Julia Richerson, MD, FAAP

FAMILY LIAISON

Alisa Skatrud

STAFF

Elisha Ferguson

ABBREVIATIONS

AAP: American Academy of Pediatrics
PPHC: pediatric primary health care

All policy statements from the American Academy of Pediatrics automatically expire 5 years after publication unless reaffirmed, revised, or retired at or before that time.

DOI: https://doi.org/10.1542/peds.2021-055553

Address correspondence to Edward Pont, MD, FAAP. E-mail: edpont122@gmail.com

PEDIATRICS (ISSN Numbers: Print, 0031-4005; Online, 1098-4275).

Copyright © 2022 by the American Academy of Pediatrics

FINANCIAL DISCLOSURE: The authors have indicated they do not have a financial relationship relevant to this article to disclose.

FUNDING: No external funding.

POTENTIAL CONFLICT OF INTEREST: The authors have indicated they have no potential conflicts of interest relevant to this article to disclose.

REFERENCES

1. Hagan JF, Shaw JS, Duncan PM, eds. *Bright Futures: Guidelines for Health Supervision of Infants, Children, and Adolescents*, 4th ed. Itasca, IL: American Academy of Pediatrics; 2017

2. Child and Adolescent Health Measurement Initiative, Data Resource Center on Child and Adolescent Health. National Survey of Children's Health 2018. Available at: https://www.childhealthdata.org/learn-about-the-nsch/NSCH. Accessed September 17, 2020

3. American Academy of Pediatrics, Committee on Pediatric Workforce. Definition of a pediatrician. *Pediatrics.* 2015;135(4):780–781

4. Medical Home Initiatives for Children With Special Needs Project Advisory Committee. American Academy of Pediatrics. The medical home. *Pediatrics*. 2002;110(1 Pt 1):184–186

5. Agiro A, Gautam S, Wall E, et al. Variation in outpatient antibiotic dispensing for respiratory infections in children by clinician specialty and treatment setting. *Pediatr Infect Dis J*. 2018;37(12):1248–1254

6. Frost HM, McLean HQ, Chow BDW. Variability in antibiotic prescribing for upper respiratory illnesses by provider specialty. *J Pediatr*. 2018;203:76–85.e8

7. Ray KN, Shi Z, Gidengil CA, Poon SJ, Uscher-Pines L, Mehrotra A. Antibiotic prescribing during pediatric direct-to-consumer telemedicine visits. *Pediatrics*. 2019;143(5):e20182491

8. Patient Centered Primary Care Collaborative. Definition of medical neighborhood. Available at: https://www.pcpcc.org/content/medical-neighborhood. Accessed September 17, 2020

9. Katkin JP, Kressly SJ, Edwards AR, et al; Task Force on Pediatric Practice Change. Guiding principles for team-based pediatric care. *Pediatrics*. 2017;140(2):e20171489

10. Halfon N, DuPlessis H, Inkelas M. Transforming the U.S. child health system. *Health Aff (Millwood)*. 2007;26(2):315–330

11. Kuo AA, Thomas PA, Chilton LA, Mascola L; Council on Community Pediatrics; Section on Epidemiology, Public Health, and Evidence. Pediatricians and Public Health: Optimizing the Health and Wellbeing of the Nation's Children. *Pediatrics*. 2018;141(2):e20173848

12. Kelleher KJ, Cooper J, Deans K, et al. Cost saving and quality of care in a pediatric accountable care organization. *Pediatrics*. 2015;135(3):e582–e589

American Academy
of Pediatrics
DEDICATED TO THE HEALTH OF ALL CHILDREN™

Organizational Principles to Guide and Define the Child
Health Care System and/or Improve the Health of all Children

This Policy Statement was reaffirmed October 2016 and December 2023.

POLICY STATEMENT

Community Pediatrics: Navigating the Intersection of Medicine, Public Health, and Social Determinants of Children's Health

COUNCIL ON COMMUNITY PEDIATRICS

KEY WORDS
community pediatrics, child advocacy, public health, social determinants of health

www.pediatrics.org/cgi/doi/10.1542/peds.2012-3933

doi:10.1542/peds.2012-3933

PEDIATRICS (ISSN Numbers: Print, 0031-4005; Online, 1098-4275).

Copyright © 2013 by the American Academy of Pediatrics

abstract

This policy statement provides a framework for the pediatrician's role in promoting the health and well-being of all children in the context of their families and communities. It offers pediatricians a definition of community pediatrics, emphasizes the importance of recognizing social determinants of health, and delineates the need to partner with public health to address population-based child health issues. It also recognizes the importance of pediatric involvement in child advocacy at local, state, and federal levels to ensure all children have access to a high-quality medical home and to eliminate child health disparities. This statement provides a set of specific recommendations that underscore the critical nature of this dimension of pediatric practice, teaching, and research. *Pediatrics* 2013;131:623–628

Environmental and social factors contribute significantly to the health and well-being of children in the contexts of families, schools, and communities. Over the past decade, the Institute of Medicine recognized and quantified the effects of external factors on early brain development and the health of children in 2 seminal reports, *Neurons to Neighborhoods*[1] in 2000 and *Children's Health, the Nation's Wealth*[2] in 2004. As understanding of the mechanisms and impact of biological, behavioral, cultural, social, and physical environments on healthy development deepens and expands, the long-standing role of pediatricians in promoting the physical, mental, and social health and well-being of all children must also evolve.[3] The field of pediatrics must address the problems facing children in the 21st century by influencing these critical determinants of child health and well-being.[4] To do so, pediatricians must successfully merge their traditional clinical skills with public health, population-based approaches to practice, and advocacy.

DEFINITION OF COMMUNITY PEDIATRICS

The American Academy of Pediatrics (AAP) offers a definition of community pediatrics to remind all pediatricians, pediatric medical subspecialists, and pediatric surgical specialists alike of the profound importance of the community dimension in pediatric practice. Community pediatrics is the practice of promoting and integrating the

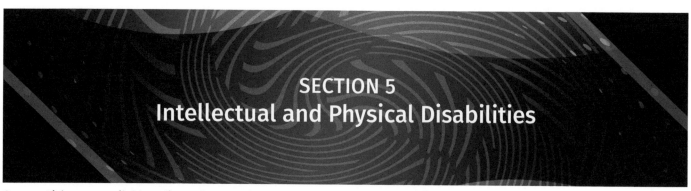

SECTION 5
Intellectual and Physical Disabilities

Some articles are available online only; scan the QR code to access online content.

CLINICAL REPORT Guidance for the Clinician in Rendering Pediatric Care

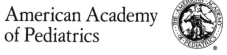

American Academy
of Pediatrics

DEDICATED TO THE HEALTH OF ALL CHILDREN™

Health Supervision for Children and Adolescents With Down Syndrome

Marilyn J. Bull, MD, FAAP,[a] Tracy Trotter, MD, FAAP,[b] Stephanie L. Santoro, MD, FAAP,[c] Celanie Christensen, MD, MS, FAAP,[a] Randall W. Grout, MD, MS, FAAP,[d] THE COUNCIL ON GENETICS

This clinical report is designed to assist the pediatrician in caring for the child, adolescent, and family in whom a diagnosis of Down syndrome has been confirmed by chromosome analysis or suspected by prenatal screening. Although a pediatrician's initial contact with the child is usually during infancy, occasionally the pregnant woman who has been given a prenatal diagnosis of Down syndrome will be referred for review of the condition and genetic counseling; this report offers guidance for this situation, as well. Age-specific guidance for the clinician is provided in Supplemental Fig 1.

Pediatricians play an important role in the care of children and adolescents with Down syndrome and their families. Down syndrome is the most common chromosomal cause of intellectual disability, and there has been a significant improvement in quality of life for affected people. Awareness of the issues important to affected children, adolescents, and their caregivers can make a great difference in outcomes across the lifespan.

Children with Down syndrome may have many cooccurring medical conditions and cognitive impairment because of the presence of extra genetic material from chromosome 21 (Table 1).[1,2] Although the phenotype is variable, there typically are multiple features that enable the experienced clinician to suspect the diagnosis. Among the more common physical findings are hypotonia, small brachycephalic head, epicanthal folds, flat nasal bridge, upward-slanting palpebral fissures, Brushfield spots, small mouth, small ears, excessive skin at the nape of the neck, single transverse palmar crease, short fifth finger with clinodactyly, and wide spacing between the first and second toes, often with a deep plantar groove. The degree of cognitive impairment is variable and may be mild (IQ of 50–70), usually is moderate (IQ of 35–50), or occasionally is severe (IQ of 20–35).

Medical conditions common in children with Down syndrome include hearing loss (75%), obstructive sleep apnea (50%–79%), otitis media

[a]Department of Pediatrics, Division of Developmental Medicine, Indiana University School of Medicine, Riley Hospital for Children, Indianapolis, Indiana; [b]San Ramon Valley Primary Care Medical Group, San Ramon, California; [c]Department of Pediatrics, Division of Medical Genetics and Metabolism, Massachusetts General Hospital, Boston, Massachusetts; and [d]Division of Children's Health Services Research, Department of Pediatrics, Indiana University School of Medicine, Indianapolis, Indiana

Drs Bull, Trotter, Santoro, Christensen, and Grout were directly involved in the planning, researching, and writing of this report, approved the final manuscript as submitted, and agree to be accountable for all aspects of the work.

All clinical reports from the American Academy of Pediatrics automatically expire 5 years after publication unless reaffirmed, revised, or retired at or before that time.
DOI: https://doi.org/10.1542/peds.2022-057010

Address correspondence to Marilyn J. Bull, MD, FAAP. E-mail: mbull@iu.edu

PEDIATRICS (ISSN Numbers: Print, 0031-4005; Online, 1098-4275).

To cite: Bull MJ, Trotter T, Santoro SL, et al; AAP Council on Genetics. Health Supervision for Children and Adolescents With Down Syndrome. *Pediatrics.* 2022;149(5):e2022057010

TABLE 1 Medical Problems Common in Down Syndrome

Condition	%
Hearing problems	75
Vision problems	60–80
Nystagmus	3–33
Glaucoma	<1–7
Nasolacrimal duct occlusion	3–36
Cataracts	3
Strabismus	36
Refractive errors	36–80
Keratoconus	1–13
Obstructive sleep apnea	50–79
Otitis media with effusion	50–70
Congenital heart disease	40–50
Feeding difficulty	31–80
Respiratory infection	20–36
Dermatologic problems	56
Hypodontia and delayed dental eruption	23
Congenital hypothyroidism	2–7
Antithyroid antibody positive (Hashimoto thyroiditis; incidence dependent on age)	13–39
Hyperthyroidism	0.65–3
Thyroid disease by adulthood	50
Gastrointestinal atresias	12
Seizures	1–13
Hematologic problems	
Anemia	1.2
Iron deficiency	6.7
Transient abnormal myelopoiesis	10
Leukemia	1
Autoimmune conditions	
Hashimoto thyroiditis	13–39
Graves' disease	1
Celiac disease	1–5
Type 1 diabetes	1
Juvenile idiopathic arthritis	<1
Alopecia	5
Symptomatic atlantoaxial instability	1–2
Autism	7–19
Hirschsprung disease	<1
Moyamoya disease	Down syndrome 26 times greater in patients with Moyamoya than Down syndrome in live births

(50%–70%), eye problems (60%–80%), including cataracts (<1%–3%),[3] nasolacrimal duct obstruction (3%–36%), and strabismus and severe refractive errors (36%–80%), congenital heart defects (50%), neurologic dysfunction (1%–13%), gastrointestinal atresia (12%), hip dislocation and hip abnormalities (2%–8%),[4,5] symptomatic atlantoaxial instability (1%–2%),[6,7] thyroid disease (24%–50%)[2,8] and, less commonly, transient abnormal myelopoiesis (4%–10%) and later leukemia (1%), autoimmune diseases,[2,8–10] including Hashimoto thyroiditis (13%–39%), with incidence dependent on age, celiac disease (1%–5%), Hirschsprung disease (<1%),[3] and autism (7%–19%).[11,12]

People with Down syndrome often function more effectively in social situations than would be predicted based on cognitive assessment results, unless there is presence of cooccurring autism. Although the level of social–emotional functioning may vary, these skills may be improved with early intervention and therapy through early adulthood.

In ~96% of children with Down syndrome, the condition is sporadic because of nonfamilial trisomy 21, in which there are 47 chromosomes with the presence of a free extra chromosome 21. In ~3% to 4% of people with the Down syndrome phenotype, the extra chromosomal material is the result of an unbalanced translocation between chromosome 21 and another acrocentric chromosome, usually chromosome 14 or 21. Approximately three-quarters of these unbalanced translocations are de novo, and the remainder result from translocation inherited from a parent. If the child has a translocation, the parents should be offered a karyotype to determine whether the translocation is familial or de novo. In the remaining 1% to 2% of people with the Down syndrome phenotype, a mix of 2 cell lines is present: 1 normal and the other with trisomy 21. This condition is called mosaicism. People with mosaicism may be more mildly affected than people with complete trisomy 21 or translocation chromosome 21, but this is not always the case, and their condition may include any of the associated medical problems and may be indistinguishable from trisomy 21. The chance of recurrence for families with an affected child depends on many factors and vary greatly, from 1% in most families to 100% in some circumstances. Table 2 describes the different chromosomal characteristics of Down syndrome.

Formal counseling by a clinical geneticist or genetic counselor is recommended for all families.

Several areas require ongoing assessment throughout childhood and should be reviewed at every

TABLE 2 Chromosomal Basis of Down Syndrome

Percentage	Chromosomal Basis
96	Meiotic nondisjunction (95% occur in egg, with recurrence risk of 1% until mother's age risk exceeds 1% at age 40, and it then increases according to maternal age)
3–4	Translocation (usually occurs with 1 chromosome 21 attached to chromosome 14, 21, or 22)
	14/21 translocation (1/3 of patients have a parent carrier with balanced karyotype)
	90% have mother as the carrier parent, with a recurrence chance of 10%–15%
	10% have father as the carrier, with a recurrence chance of 2%–5%
	21/21 translocation (1/14 of patients have parent carrier with a balanced karyotype); carrier parent equally likely mother or father, with recurrence chance of 100%[13]
1–2	Mosaicism: number of affected cells vary between individuals; clinical findings vary widely
	Medical complications fewer and intellectual disability often less severe
	Partial trisomy: duplication of delimited segment of chromosome 21 present; extremely rare

Adapted from Bull MJ. Down syndrome.[14]
Information regarding meiotic nondisjunction and translocation is from Hook,[13] information regarding mosaicism is from Papavassiliou et al,[15] and information regarding partial trisomy is from Pelleri et al.[16]

health supervision visit and at least annually. These areas include:

- personal support available to family;
- participation in a family-centered medical home;
- age-specific Down syndrome-related medical and developmental conditions;
- financial and medical support programs and long-term financial planning for which the child and family may be eligible;
- injury and abuse prevention, with special consideration of developmental skills and intellectual ability; and
- nutrition and activity to maintain appropriate weight.

THE PRENATAL VISIT

The American College of Obstetricians and Gynecologists recommends that all pregnant women, regardless of age or risk status, be offered the option of screening and diagnostic testing for Down syndrome.[17,18]

A wide variety of screening test options exist in the first and second trimester using maternal serum and ultrasonography. Each offers varying levels of sensitivity and specificity. No 1 screening test is superior to other screening tests in all characteristics. In recent years, noninvasive prenatal testing by cell-free DNA (cfDNA) has become available and is the most sensitive method for screening for Down syndrome. cfDNA screening for Down syndrome is significantly more sensitive and specific than conventional screening methods, with a 2017 meta-analysis reporting a detection rate of 99.7%, with a false-positive rate of 0.04% in singleton pregnancies.[19] cfDNA uses a maternal blood sample to analyze free-floating small fragments of DNA from the placenta. Because cfDNA is from the placenta and not directly from the fetus, it is a screening test and not diagnostic. cfDNA analysis can be performed as early as 9 to 10 weeks' gestation depending on the laboratory, and a high-risk result from cfDNA would require confirmation by diagnostic testing with chorionic villus sampling (CVS) or amniocentesis. Screening for trisomy 21 by cfDNA in twin pregnancies can be performed, but total number of reported cases is small.[20]

Other screening tests for Down syndrome include first-trimester screening, which incorporates maternal age, nuchal translucency ultrasonography, and measurement of maternal serum β human chorionic gonadotropin and pregnancy-associated plasma protein A. Second-trimester screening is available for patients who first seek medical care in the second trimester or in locations where first-trimester screening is not available. The second-trimester serum screening, often called the quad screen, incorporates maternal age risk with measurement of maternal serum β human chorionic gonadotropin, unconjugated estriol, α-fetoprotein, and inhibin concentrations. The detection rate of Down syndrome by first-trimester screening is 82% to 87%, by second trimester screening is 80%, and by combined first- and second-trimester screening (referred to as integrated screening) is ~95%. These screening tests are reported to have a 5% false-positive rate.[21-24]

Ultrasonography is an additional screening tool for Down syndrome because structural changes, including congenital heart defects, increased nuchal skin fold, "double bubble" sign suggestive of duodenal atresia, ventriculomegaly, and short–long bones, may be identified by prenatal imaging. Although ultrasonography is an additional screening tool, it is not diagnostic for Down syndrome.

Diagnostic testing for Down syndrome includes CVS or amniocentesis. CVS has the benefit of being performed earlier in pregnancy, between 10 and 14 completed weeks' gestation. A placental sample is obtained either transabdominally or transcervically, depending on provider preference and placental location. Amniocentesis is a transabdominal procedure to remove a sample of amniotic fluid performed after 15 weeks' gestational age. Risk for procedure-related loss of pregnancy from CVS or amniocentesis is comparable in recent studies when performed by providers with expertise, 0.22% for amniocentesis and 0.11% for CVS.[25,26]

Pediatricians may be asked to counsel a family whose fetus has been identified with or is at increased chance of having Down syndrome. Families may have a great number of questions during any pregnancy and especially when the child will have Down syndrome. They may have received counseling from a certified genetic counselor, a clinical geneticist, maternal–fetal medicine specialist, obstetrician, or developmental specialist. In addition, parents may have received information and support from a family-led organization such as Parent to Parent USA, a local Down syndrome group, a national Down syndrome organization, social media, or possibly an Internet site with inaccurate information. Pediatricians who often have a previous relationship with the family may be the natural source of support for and guidance in the context of the medical home. The clinician should be prepared to respond to questions, review information the family has received, and assist in the decision-making process.[27] When asked, the pediatrician should discuss the following topics with the family:

1. The prenatal laboratory studies and any confirmatory testing that led to the diagnosis and any fetal imaging studies that have been or will be performed. Many families find it important to have the diagnosis confirmed before they can consider what it will mean to their infant and their family.

2. Families benefit from hearing a fair and balanced perspective, including the many positive outcomes of children with Down syndrome and their effects on the family. Families usually have questions about prognosis and phenotypic manifestations, including the wide range of variability seen in infants and children with Down syndrome. The prenatal visit is a good time to offer a connection to a peer-to-peer organization for support (see Family Resources).

3. Discuss any additional studies performed that may refine the estimation of the prognosis (eg, fetal echocardiography, ultrasonography for gastrointestinal tract malformations). Consultation with an appropriate medical subspecialist, such as a pediatric cardiologist or a pediatric surgeon, may occur prenatally if abnormal findings are detected.

4. Discuss currently available treatments and interventions. Families need to hear that they are not alone and that there are supports and services for them after the infant is born. Discuss early intervention resources, parent-support programs, and any appropriate future treatments.

5. Discuss extended life expectancy that has increased from 30 years in 1973 to 60 years in 2002. This increase has resulted from improved medical care, educational options, and enhanced social adaptation. Potential complications and adverse effects, costs and financial supports available, and other challenges associated with comprehensive management and care should also be discussed. The pediatrician can explain that they will be supported best in the context of a patient-centered medical home.

6. There are many issues for the family learning that their child will have Down syndrome to consider. These issues should be discussed using a nondirective approach. In cases of prenatal diagnosis, this may include discussion of pregnancy continuation or termination, raising the child in the family, foster care placement, and adoption.[28]

7. The mechanism for occurrence of Down syndrome in the fetus and the potential recurrence rate for the family, as provided by genetic counseling, should be shared. Discuss availability of genetic counseling or meeting with a genetics professional.

As the pregnancy continues, the pediatrician may:

1. Develop a plan for delivery and neonatal care with the obstetrician and the family. As the pregnancy progresses, additional studies should be performed if available, if recommended by medical subspecialists and/or if desired by the family. These studies (eg, detection of a complex heart defect by fetal echocardiography) may help direct development of a management plan and improve outcome for the mother and infant.[29]

2. Offer parent-to-parent contact and information about local and national support organizations because communication with experienced parents is often a very helpful resource for caregiver decision-making.

3. Offer referral to a clinical geneticist or genetic counselor for a more extended discussion of clinical outcomes and variability, recurrence rates, future reproductive options, and evaluation of the risks for other family members.

HEALTH SUPERVISION FROM BIRTH TO 1 MONTH: NEWBORN INFANTS

It is recognized that the medical needs of newborn infants with Down syndrome vary, and the timing of each intervention depends on the infant's needs, but that it is important that all interventions are addressed and that careful transfer of care occurs at the time of discharge from the hospital.

Examination

The first step in evaluating a newborn infant for trisomy 21 is a careful review of the family history and prenatal information, to include:

- results of prenatal chromosome studies, if performed; and
- family history of previous children born with trisomy 21 or developmental differences or pregnancies that ended in miscarriage. (These may be significant clues that a family may carry a balanced translocation that predisposes them to having children with trisomy 21.)

For children who have had the diagnosis made prenatally, a formal copy of the chromosome report from an amniocentesis or CVS should be obtained. This report allows the clinician to confirm the diagnosis, review the results with the family, and add the formal diagnosis to the child's medical record. If the results of prenatal testing are not available or if cfDNA alone was performed, a sample of cord or peripheral blood should be obtained for postnatal karyotype to confirm the diagnosis and rule out a chromosome translocation.

A physical examination is the most sensitive test in the first 24 hours of life to diagnose trisomy 21 in an infant. If the clinician believes that criteria for Down syndrome are present on physical examination, then a blood sample should be sent

for a karyotype. The clinician should alert the laboratory and request rapid results. A study that uses fluorescent in situ hybridization (FISH) technology, in addition, should be available within 24 to 48 hours, if necessary, to facilitate diagnosis and parent counseling. A FISH study, however, can only indicate that an extra copy of chromosome 21 is present and does not determine the presence or absence of a translocation. Therefore, a positive FISH result should be confirmed by a karyotype to identify translocations that may have implications for further reproductive counseling for the parents and possibly other family members. A chromosomal microarray analysis is not appropriate because it will not differentiate trisomy 21 caused by nondisjunction versus an unbalanced translocation.

When delivering a diagnosis of Trisomy 21 (Table 3):

- the mother should be allowed to recover from the immediate delivery of the infant and have her partner or support person present before the diagnosis is given;
- the information should be relayed in a private setting by the physicians involved, optimally by the primary care provider for the infant and the delivering physician[30]; and
- it is recommended that hospitals coordinate the delivery of the information and offer a private hospital room pending confirmation of the diagnosis.

When providing information about Down syndrome to families, the physician should first congratulate parents on the birth of their infant. Obstetricians and pediatricians should coordinate their messaging and inform parents of their suspicion immediately, in a private setting, and when appropriate, with both parents together. Physicians should use their experience and

TABLE 3 Communicating With Families[31]

At diagnosis, immediate advice remains pertinent regarding the need to:
- first, congratulate the family
- have infant present; refer to infant by name
- use a respectful bedside manner
- time discussion after labor is complete and as soon as diagnosis is suspected (not necessarily confirmed)
- have a support person present for mother, father, and family members as appropriate
- use a cohesive, physician-led team approach

Helpful discussion will include:
- up-to-date, accurate information
- a balanced approach rather than relying on personal opinions and experience
- person-first language (ie, child *with* Down syndrome)[32];
- connection to other parents and resource groups
- discussion of life potentials for people with Down syndrome

Share with families the interplay within families and individual perspectives:
- individuals with Down syndrome: nearly 99% indicated that they were happy with their lives, and 97% liked who they are and encouraged health care professionals to value them, emphasizing that they share similar hopes and dreams as people without Down syndrome[33];
- parents: 79% felt their outlook on life was more positive because of people with Down syndrome[31];
- siblings: 88% felt that they were better people because of their siblings with Down syndrome[33];
- a majority of families report unanimous feelings of love and pride
- positive themes dominate modern families[34]

expertise in providing support and guidance for families. Clinicians should ensure a balanced approach that reflects the variability and broad range of current outcomes, rather than their personal opinions or experience, give current printed materials, and offer access to other families who have children with Down syndrome and support organizations if locally available. It is important that clinicians be cognizant of the realities and possibilities for people with Down syndrome to have healthy, productive lives.[30]

The laboratory diagnosis of Down syndrome should be confirmed, and the karyotype should be reviewed with the parents when the final result is available. The specific findings should be discussed with both parents whenever possible, including the potential clinical manifestations associated with the syndrome. These topics should be reviewed again at a subsequent meeting. Families should be offered referral for genetic counseling if it was not conducted prenatally.

Newborn care is often provided in a hospital setting by a physician who will not be the primary care pediatrician. If the physician providing newborn care will not be the primary care pediatrician, he or she should ensure that there is a smooth transition by transferring medical records and ensuring that an early newborn follow-up appointment is scheduled.

Characteristics attributable to Down syndrome, as well as those that are familial, should be discussed.

Discuss and Review
- Hypotonia.
- Facial appearance and acknowledge the presence of familial characteristics.
- Cutis marmorata; explain that this is common in infants with

Down syndrome and provide reassurance to family about this finding.

Evaluate For
- Heart defects (∼50% risk). Perform an echocardiogram, to be read by a pediatric cardiologist, regardless of whether a fetal echocardiogram was performed. Refer to a pediatric cardiologist for evaluation any infant whose postnatal echocardiogram results are abnormal.
- Feeding problems. Feeding difficulties including gastroesophageal reflux and dysphagia are extremely common (31%–80% in Down syndrome).[35,36] Dysphagia can result from both oromotor problems and oropharyngeal dysfunction. Hypotonia, relative macroglosia with a relatively small oral cavity, decreased jaw strength, and poor tongue control contribute to the problems. Symptoms of feeding difficulty include slow feeding, choking with feeds, and slow weight gain. Up to 90% of patients with Down syndrome who aspirate do so silently without cough or overt symptoms, and symptoms often are not recognized during a clinical feeding evaluation.[35,37] Feeding difficulty occurs with increased frequency in all infants with Down syndrome, but especially those who are born preterm, have marked hypotonia, are underweight, or have desaturation with feeds. Infants who (1) have marked hypotonia as judged by the pediatrician, (2) are underweight, (3) have slow feeds, (4) have choking with feeds, (5) have recurrent or persistent respiratory symptoms, or (6) desaturate with feeds should be referred promptly for skilled feeding assessment or possible video feeding study.[37,38] Video feeding studies can be helpful for determining which infants require intervention.

Nonradiologic videofluoroscopic swallow studies, where available, may be performed for infants, including those who are breastfed. Feeding function changes over infancy and early childhood, and repeat studies may be indicated, especially if respiratory symptoms persist.[39] If untreated, aspiration is an overlooked cause of recurrent respiratory symptoms.[40] Infants with Down syndrome can breastfeed successfully, but some may need early support until a successful nursing pattern is established. Some infants may sleep for prolonged periods and if not gaining weight adequately, need to be awakened for feeds to maintain adequate calorie intake.

- Cataracts at birth by looking for a red reflex. Cataracts may progress slowly and, if detected, require prompt evaluation and treatment by an ophthalmologist with experience in managing the child with Down syndrome, because surgical outcomes in these cases are reassuring.[41,42]
- Congenital hearing loss, with objective testing, such as brainstem auditory evoked response or otoacoustic emission. If the infant did not pass newborn screening studies, refer to an otolaryngologist who is experienced in examining infants with stenotic external canals to determine whether a middle-ear abnormality is present. Tympanometry may be necessary if the tympanic membrane is poorly visualized.[42,43] Refer to early intervention within 48 hours of confirmation that the infant is deaf or hard of hearing.[43,44]
- Duodenal atresia or anorectal atresia/stenosis by obtaining a history and performing a clinical examination.
- Evaluation for apnea, bradycardia, or oxygen desaturation should occur with the infant in a

car safety seat, because all infants with Down syndrome are at increased risk attributable to hypotonia, upper airway obstruction, or having had cardiac surgery. A car safety seat screen should be conducted before hospital discharge.[45]

- Constipation. If constipation is present, evaluate for restricted diet or limited fluid intake, hypotonia, hypothyroidism, or gastrointestinal tract malformation, including stenosis or Hirschsprung disease, for which there is an increased risk. Review the timing of the passing of meconium because a delay may indicate Hirschsprung disease and other considerations.
- Gastroesophageal reflux, which is usually diagnosed and managed clinically. If contributing to cardiorespiratory problems or failure to thrive, refer for subspecialty intervention.
- Stridor, wheezing, or noisy breathing. If contributing to cardiorespiratory problems or feeding difficulty, refer to an otolaryngologist, pediatric pulmonologist, or aerodigestive program to assess for airway anomalies. Small nasal passages and nasal congestion often contribute to stridor. Tracheal anomalies and small tracheal size may also make intubation more difficult. Hypotonia and small tracheal size also increase the risk of recurrent episodes of croup.
- Hematologic abnormalities. Obtain a complete blood cell count with differential by 3 days of age to evaluate for transient abnormal myelopoiesis (TAM) (formerly called transient myeloproliferative disorder), polycythemia, and other hematologic abnormalities. Leukocytosis or TAM is relatively common in this population (9%) and can present with pericardial and pleural effusions, but can be silent without

hepatosplenomegaly, jaundice, or rash.[46,47] Although leukocytosis or TAM usually regresses spontaneously within the first 3 months of life, infants with TAM may require chemotherapy and are at risk for death in the first 6 months of life (up to 20%), and have an increased risk of acute myeloid leukemia in the first 4 years of life (~30%). All infants with Down syndrome and TAM should be evaluated by pediatric hematology/oncology as soon as they are diagnosed. Numerous hematologic abnormalities other than >10% blasts are commonly reported in newborn infants with trisomy 21, including neutrophilia (80%), thrombocytopenia (66%), and thrombocytosis, which generally resolve in the first week of life, whereas macrocytosis is also common but often does not resolve.[48] Infants with numeric abnormalities other than macrocytosis that persist after the first week of life should be referred to a hematologist. Leukemia is more common in children with Down syndrome than in the general population but is still rare (1%).[49]
- Caregivers of infants with TAM should be counseled regarding the risk of leukemia and made aware of the signs, including easy bruising, recurring fevers, bone pain, easy bruising or bleeding, petechiae, onset of lethargy, or change in feeding patterns. Although leukemia is rare, children with Down syndrome are at increased risk to develop both acute lymphoblastic leukemia and acute myeloid leukemia, even without a history of TAM as a newborn infant.
- Polycythemia. Unrelated to congenital heart disease, polycythemia is common in the first week of life in Down syndrome (33%) and may persist for several months. Persistent polycythemia

requires regular follow-up with blood counts until resolution.
- Congenital hypothyroidism (2%–7% risk).[8,50] Obtain thyroid-stimulating hormone (TSH) concentration if state's newborn screening measures only free thyroxine (T4); congenital hypothyroidism can be missed if only the T4 concentration is obtained in the newborn screening. Many children with Down syndrome (25%–60%) have mildly elevated TSH and normal free T4 concentration (subclinical hypothyroidism), and hyperthyroidism occurs in 0.65% to 3%.[51] Elevated antithyroid antibodies occur frequently and, when present, increase the risk of later hypothyroidism.[50] By late childhood, the incidence of thyroid abnormality is 50%.[8,50] Management of children with abnormal TSH or T4 concentrations should be discussed with a pediatric endocrinologist.

Anticipatory Guidance Given Between Birth and 1 Month of Age

- Discuss the strengths of the child and positive family experiences.
- Discuss the individual resources for support, such as family, religion, and friends.
- Talk about how and what to tell siblings, other family members, and friends. Review methods of coping with long-term disabilities (see "Resources for Families").
- Discuss efficacy of early intervention and availability of early intervention services and therapies in the community. Initiate referral for speech, fine motor, or gross motor therapies, unless medically contraindicated. Encourage families to participate in selection of therapies and therapists. Counsel families to share their impressions of their infant's strengths and progress with therapists and to actively participate in therapy sessions.

- Share information for local Down syndrome family and support groups, current books and pamphlets, and referrals for community and financial resources (see Resources for Families).
- Discuss increased susceptibility to respiratory tract infection. Children with signs and symptoms of lower respiratory tract infection should be evaluated acutely by a medical provider, and in the presence of cardiac or chronic respiratory disease, prompt diagnosis and treatment should be instituted.[40,52]
- Children with cooccurring conditions including qualifying congenital heart disease, airway clearance issues, or prematurity (born at <29 weeks, 0 days' gestation) may be considered for administration of respiratory syncytial virus prophylaxis.[53]
- Discuss with families the importance of cervical spine-positioning precautions to avoid excessive extension or flexion during any anesthetic, surgical, or radiographic procedure.
- Using the previously obtained karyotype, review the chance of recurrence in subsequent pregnancies and the availability of prenatal testing options, as discussed in previous genetic counseling.
- Discuss treatments that are considered complementary or alternative. Families need an opportunity to learn objectively which therapies are safe and which are potentially dangerous (eg, cell therapy that may transmit slow viruses and high doses of fat-soluble vitamins that can cause toxicity).
- Determine whether the child receives supplements, herbs, teas, or other treatments or supplements not previously discussed. Approximately 38% of parents of children with Down syndrome report using dietary

supplements in their children, and 20% report they have not informed their pediatrician, usually because they have not been asked.[54] Several articles and websites provide useful information for clinicians and families.[54–55]

- Renal and urinary tract anomalies have been reported to occur at increased frequency among people with Down syndrome.[56] Although routine postnatal screening for renal anomalies is not currently recommended, if renal abnormalities are detected on prenatal ultrasonography, standard assessment would be required.

HEALTH SUPERVISION FROM 1 MONTH TO 1 YEAR: INFANCY

Physical Examination and Laboratory Studies

Follow *Bright Futures* schedule or more frequently if indicated.

- Obtain a history and perform a physical examination.
- Monitor weight and follow weight-for-length trends at each health care visit. Review the infant's growth and plot it on the Down syndrome-specific charts for weight, length, weight for length, and head circumference (available at www.cdc.gov).[57,58]
- Review feeding at every health supervision visit, ensure adequate iron intake, and inquire about any changes in respiratory symptoms with feeding (see "Health Supervision From Birth to 1 Month" for discussion).
- Review the previous hearing evaluation (brainstem auditory evoked response [BAER] or otoacoustic emission). If the infant passed the newborn screening study, rescreen at 6 months of age for confirmation.
- Risk of otitis media with effusion is 50% to 75%.[43] Middle-ear

disease should be treated immediately when diagnosed. As soon as a clear ear is established, a diagnostic BAER should be performed to accurately establish hearing status.

- In children with stenotic canals in which the tympanic membranes cannot be seen, refer to an otolaryngologist as soon as possible for examination under an office microscope. Interval ear examinations should be performed by the otolaryngologist every 3 to 6 months until the tympanic membrane can be visualized by the pediatrician and tympanometry can be performed reliably.[43]
- A behavioral audiogram may be attempted at 1 year of age, but many children will not be able to complete the study. If unable to complete a behavioral audiogram, additional testing by BAER should be performed at 1 year.
- Ear anomalies also place child at risk for sensorineural hearing loss and vestibular problems that may affect balance, making the thorough audiologic assessment additionally important.[59–61]
- Within the first 6 months of life, refer to a pediatric ophthalmologist or ophthalmologist with expertise and experience with infants with disabilities to evaluate for strabismus, cataracts, nasolacrimal duct obstruction, refractive errors, glaucoma, and nystagmus.[16,62–64]
- Check the infant's vision at each visit and use developmentally appropriate subjective and objective criteria. If lacrimal duct obstruction is present, refer for evaluation for surgical repair of drainage system if not resolved by 9 to 12 months of age.[65]
- Verify results of newborn thyroid-function screen if not previously reviewed. Because of increased risk of acquired thyroid disease, repeat

measurement of TSH at 6 and 12 months of age and then annually (see Health Supervision From Birth to 1 Month for discussion).

- Monitor infants with cardiac defects at all well-child visits, typically ventricular or atrioventricular septal defects that cause intracardiac left-to-right shunts, for symptoms and signs of congestive heart failure as pulmonary vascular resistance decreases and pulmonary blood flow increases. Tachypnea, feeding difficulties, and poor weight gain may indicate heart failure. Medical management, including nutritional support, may be required until the infant is in optimal condition to undergo cardiac surgery to repair the defects to limit the potential for development of pulmonary hypertension and associated complications.[66] Infants and children with Down syndrome are also at increased risk of pulmonary hypertension even in the absence of intracardiac structural defects. Close coordination of care between the primary care physician and the subspecialist is important for these infants.
- Anemia/iron deficiency: Obtain a complete blood cell count (CBC) with differential and either (1) a combination of ferritin and C-reactive protein (CRP), or (2) a combination of serum iron and total iron-binding capacity (TIBC), beginning at 1 year of age and annually thereafter.

Children with Down syndrome have been shown to have a similar risk for iron-deficiency anemia as the typical population, but it may be missed because of macrocytosis.[67] Iron insufficiency may precede iron-deficiency anemia and also can have long-term neurologic effects.[67,68] Macrocytosis, with increased erythrocyte mean corpuscular

volume, is present in up to one-third of patients with Down syndrome.[69] Thus, a low mean corpuscular volume is not a useful screen for the diagnoses of iron deficiency/insufficiency, lead toxicity, or thalassemia in children with Down syndrome. Screening by hemoglobin concentration identifies iron deficiency anemia but misses iron deficiency/iron insufficiency. Using the CBC parameter of an elevated relative distribution width with ferritin or transferrin saturation or serum iron divided by TIBC leads to 100% sensitivity in identifying iron insufficiency, iron deficiency, or anemia. Serum ferritin concentration is an acute-phase reactant and is not useful if inflammation is present or CRP is elevated: subsequent evaluation with iron concentration and TIBC may be needed to confirm diagnosis.

- Although not unique to children with Down syndrome, low ferritin is also associated with sleep problems, and iron deficiency may be considered in differentials for children with sleep difficulty.[70] A physician may prescribe iron supplementation for children with sleep problems and a ferritin concentration <50 µg/L.[70,71]
- Pediatricians should be alert to the signs and symptoms of leukemia discussed in Health Supervision From Birth to 1 Month and obtain an extra CBC with differential if symptoms occur. Children with Down syndrome who develop acute leukemia can be treated successfully with similar acute lymphocytic leukemia therapy or de-intensified acute myeloid leukemia chemotherapy regimens with outcomes superior to other children.[72,73]
- Assess with complete neurologic history and examination and

consult with neurology as needed for signs of neurologic dysfunction that may occur. Children with Down syndrome have an increased risk of seizures, including infantile spasms (1%–13%)[74,75] and other conditions, including moyamoya disease[76,77] and benign movement disorders such as shuddering.

- Administer immunizations, including influenza vaccine, respiratory syncytial virus vaccine for infants with cooccurring qualifying conditions, and other vaccines recommended for all children, unless there are specific contraindications.[78]
- Assess for dermatologic findings and advise parents that xerosis (dry skin) and cutis marmorata are common.
- At least once during the first 6 months of life, discuss with family symptoms of obstructive sleep apnea, including heavy breathing, snoring, uncommon sleep positions, frequent night awakening, daytime sleepiness, apneic pauses, and behavior problems that could be associated with poor sleep. Refer to a physician with expertise in pediatric sleep disorders for examination and further evaluation of a possible sleep disorder if any of the previously mentioned symptoms occur.[79,80]
- At each well-child visit, discuss with parents the importance of maintaining the cervical spine in a neutral position during any anesthetic, surgical, or radiographic procedure to minimize the risk of spinal cord injury and review the signs and symptoms of myelopathy, which include asymmetry of movement, weakness, and, on examination, increased deep tendon reflexes. Obtain history and carefully perform a physical examination, paying attention for myelopathic signs and symptoms.

Anticipatory Guidance From 1 Month to 1 Year

- Review availability of resources, including Down syndrome support groups and organizations that help with navigation of community and financial resources, at least once in the first year of life (see Resources for Families).
- Assess the emotional status of caregivers and intrafamilial relationships at each well-child visit. Share information for support, including respite care and caregiver counseling, as desired. Inquire about how siblings are adjusting to the new baby and offer education to support the siblings as needed.
- Review connection to early intervention services and their relationship to the strengths and needs of the infant and family at each well-child visit. Ensure that the family knows how to implement early intervention therapy recommendations on a daily basis.
- Review the family's understanding of the chance of recurrence of Down syndrome and the availability of prenatal diagnosis and/or screening at least once in the first year of life, and more often if judged necessary by the clinician. Offer referral for genetic counseling if desired by the family.
- Be prepared to discuss and answer questions about treatments that are considered complementary and alternative at each well-child visit.

HEALTH SUPERVISION FROM 1 TO 5 YEARS: EARLY CHILDHOOD

Follow *Bright Futures* schedule or more frequently if indicated.

- Obtain a history and perform a physical examination.
- Monitor weight and follow weight-for-height trends at each health care visit. Review the infant's growth and plot it on the Down syndrome-specific charts for weight, length, weight for length <2 years of age, BMI for age 2 to 10 years, and head circumference (available at www.cdc.gov).[58]
- Ask about changes in feeding or any changes in respiratory symptoms with feeding and ensure adequate iron intake (see Health Supervision From Birth to 1 Month for discussion).
- Anemia/iron deficiency: Obtain a CBC with differential and either (1) a combination of ferritin and CRP, or (2) a combination of serum iron and TIBC, beginning at 1 year of age and annually thereafter[69] (see "Health Supervision From 1 Month to 1 Year" for discussion).
- Low ferritin is also associated with sleep problems, particularly restless leg syndrome, and iron deficiency may be considered in the differential diagnosis for children with sleep difficulty.[70] A physician may prescribe iron supplementation for children with restless sleep and a ferritin concentration <50 µg/L.[70,71]
- Solid tumors: In contrast to the increased risk of leukemia, compared with the general population, the overall risk for solid tumors is not increased in Down syndrome. Although rare, solid tumors may occur, and clinicians should remain alert to this possibility.[81] Some are very rare (breast cancers, neuroblastoma, and medulloblastoma), and some do not differ significantly from the general population (gastric, colon, and ovarian cancers and gliomas).[82] Importantly, testicular cancer is the only solid tumor that is more common in Down syndrome.[83] Clinicians should palpate the testes during routine health supervision examinations for any changes, including development of a lump or swelling. Patients with Down syndrome may not recognize testicular changes that could be a sign of testicular cancer. Although there is not clear evidence that screening is beneficial, the physician may recommend routine screening for testicular cancer by a trusted adult.[84]
- Review the risk of hearing loss associated with otitis media with effusion.
  - For a child who passed diagnostic hearing testing, behavioral audiogram and tympanometry should be performed every 6 months until normal hearing levels are established bilaterally by ear-specific testing (usually after 4 years of age).
  - Subsequently, behavioral hearing tests should be performed annually. If normal hearing is not established by behavioral testing, additional screening by otoacoustic emissions or diagnostic BAER should be performed, with sedation if necessary.
  - Children who demonstrate hearing loss should be referred to an otolaryngologist who is comfortable with the examination of children with stenotic ear canals. The risk of otitis media with effusion between 3 and 5 years of age is ~50% to 70%. If middle ear disease occurs, obtain developmentally appropriate hearing evaluation after treatment.
  - Discuss with caregivers the importance of optimal hearing for speech development and learning.
- Check the child's vision, and use developmentally appropriate subjective and objective criteria, including photoscreening if available, at each well-child visit.[85] Refer the child with abnormal findings on photoscreening or annually if photoscreening is not available to a pediatric

ophthalmologist or ophthalmologist with special expertise and experience with children with disabilities. Children with Down syndrome have a 50% risk of refractive errors that lead to amblyopia between 3 and 5 years of age. Addressing refractive errors and strabismus at an early age can help prevent amblyopia and encourage normal visual development.[63,85,86]

- Atlantoaxial instability: Discuss with parents, at least biennially, the importance of cervical spine–positioning precautions for protection of the cervical spine during any anesthetic, surgical, or radiographic procedure. Perform careful history and physical examination with attention to myelopathic signs and symptoms at every well-child visit or when symptoms possibly attributable to spinal cord impingement are reported. Parents should also be instructed to contact their physician for new onset of symptoms of change in gait or use of arms or hands, change in bowel or bladder function, neck pain, stiff neck, head tilt, torticollis, how the child positions his or her head, change in general function, or weakness.

The Child Without Symptoms of Atlantoaxial Instability

- Children with Down syndrome are at slightly increased risk of symptomatic atlantoaxial subluxation.[6,7] However, the child <3 years does not have adequate vertebral mineralization and epiphyseal development for accurate radiographic evaluation of the cervical spine.[87] Plain radiographs do not predict well which children are at increased risk of developing spine problems, and normal radiographs do not provide assurance that a child will not develop spine problems later.[88,89] For these reasons, routine radiologic evaluation of the

cervical spine in asymptomatic children is not recommended. Current evidence does not support performing routine screening radiographs for assessment of potential atlantoaxial instability in asymptomatic children.[7,90–93]

- Special Olympics requires documentation of physical examination of all athletes for participation in sports.[94]

The Child With Symptoms of Possible Atlantoaxial Instability

- Any child who has significant neck pain, radicular pain, weakness, spasticity or change in tone, gait difficulties, hyperreflexia, change in bowel or bladder function, or other signs or symptoms of myelopathy must undergo plain cervical spine radiography in the neutral position.[95] If significant radiographic abnormalities are present in the neutral position, no further radiographs should be taken and the patient should be referred as quickly as possible to a pediatric neurosurgeon or pediatric orthopedic surgeon with expertise in evaluating and treating atlantoaxial instability. If no significant radiographic abnormalities are present, flexion and extension radiographs may be obtained in collaboration with the subspecialist before the patient is promptly referred.[92,93,95]

- Discuss with caregivers that trampoline use should be avoided by all children, with or without Down syndrome, unless part of a structured training program with appropriate supervision and safety measures in place.[96] Parents can be advised that participation in contact sports, such as football, soccer, and gymnastics, places children at risk for spinal cord injury.[97]

- Measure TSH annually or sooner if child has symptoms that could be related to thyroid dysfunction

(see Health Supervision From Birth to 1 Month for discussion). Measure TSH every 6 months if antithyroid antibodies were previously detected.

- For children on a diet that contains gluten, review for symptoms potentially related to celiac disease at each health supervision visit because children with Down syndrome are at increased risk. These symptoms include diarrhea or protracted constipation, slow growth, unexplained failure to thrive, anemia, abdominal pain or bloating, or refractory developmental or behavioral problems.[97–99] For those with symptoms, obtain a tissue transglutaminase immunoglobulin A (TTG IgA) concentration and simultaneous quantitative IgA. The quantitative IgA is important, because an IgA deficiency renders the TTG IgA unreliable. Refer patients with abnormal laboratory values for specialty assessment. Do not institute a gluten-free diet before confirmation of the diagnosis, because lack of gluten can make interpretation of endoscopic results difficult. There is no evidence that routine screening of asymptomatic individuals would be beneficial. There are neither data nor consensus that would indicate whether patients with persistent symptoms who had normal laboratory values on initial evaluation should have further laboratory tests.

- Discuss symptoms of sleep-disordered breathing, including heavy breathing, snoring, restless sleep, uncommon sleep positions, frequent night awakening, daytime sleepiness, apneic pauses, and behavior problems that could be associated with poor sleep at each well-child visit. There is poor correlation between negative parent-report of symptoms and polysomnogram results.[80,100]

Therefore, referral to a pediatric sleep laboratory for a sleep study or polysomnogram for all children with Down syndrome between ages 3 and 4 years is recommended. Refer to a physician with expertise in pediatric sleep any child with signs or symptoms of obstructive sleep apnea or abnormal sleep-study results. Children who have adenotonsillectomy for treatment of obstructive sleep apnea should have a repeat polysomnogram after surgical intervention, because there is significant incidence of persistent air obstruction that requires additional evaluation and intervention.[101,102] It is recognized that access to a pediatric sleep laboratory or specialist may be limited for some populations and geographic areas.

- Discuss obesity as a risk factor for sleep apnea.[103]
- Recognize that sleep disturbance is extremely distressful to families. Low ferritin is also associated with sleep problems, particularly restless leg syndrome, and iron deficiency may be considered in the differential diagnosis for children with sleep difficulty.[70] A physician may elect to prescribe iron supplementation for children with restless sleep and a ferritin concentration <50 µg/L.[70,71]
- Remind the family to maintain follow-up with a pediatric cardiologist, per specialist recommendation, for patients with cardiac lesions, even after complete repair to monitor for recurrent/residual lesions, as well as possible development of pulmonary hypertension.
- Discuss with caregivers at every health supervision visit the child's behavioral and social progress. Encourage families to teach self-help skills and counsel to prevent wandering. Refer

children who may have autism spectrum disorder, attention-deficit/hyperactivity disorder, or other psychiatric or behavioral problems for appropriate evaluation and intervention as soon as suspected.[104] Autism and other behavioral problems occur with increased frequency in children with Down syndrome, and symptoms may manifest as early as 2 or 3 years of age.[11,12,105–107]

- A variety of screening tools have been used to identify children who may have a dual diagnosis of Down syndrome with autism spectrum disorder, although none have been studied in a large population. Examples (not an exhaustive list) include the Childhood Autism Rating Scale, the Social Communication Questionnaire, the Aberrant Behavior Checklist, and the Autism Behavior Checklist.[11,12,108,109]

- The diagnosis of autism spectrum disorder in children with Down syndrome is often delayed, because presentation can be subtly different from children with idiopathic autism spectrum disorder. Children with Down syndrome and autism spectrum disorder have better imitation, relating, and receptive skills when compared with children with autism spectrum disorder without Down syndrome. However, these adaptive skills are impaired in children with a dual diagnosis when compared with children with Down syndrome alone.[110] Also, when compared with children with Down syndrome alone, children with dual diagnosis exhibit more stereotypies, repetitive language, overactivity, social withdrawal, anxiety, and self-injury.[12,109] There is also decreased receptive and

expressive language skills, as well as cognitive skills in children with a dual diagnosis.[105] Given these differences, specialty evaluation is needed to make an appropriate diagnosis of autism spectrum disorder in children with Down syndrome. The pediatrician should screen all children with Down syndrome for autism, as they would other children, between 18 and 24 months of age, and refer those with a concerning screen for specialty evaluation.[111] It is important to avoid assuming symptoms of autism are the known delays related to Down syndrome, referred to as overshadowing. Referral as soon as an autism diagnosis is suspected is critical, because early treatment is important in all children with autism spectrum disorder, including those with Down syndrome.

- Inquire about symptoms of neurologic dysfunction, including seizures, and perform a neurologic examination. Pediatricians should be aware of symptoms referred to as "acute regression in Down syndrome," "catatonia," or "disintegrative disorder" occurring in late childhood, adolescence, or early adulthood. Patients who experience loss of skills, marked mood changes, or catatonia, or who develop repetitive thoughts or behaviors that interfere with usual life activity, should be referred to specialists familiar with diagnosis and treatment of the disorder.[112,113]
- Skin problems are particularly common in patients with Down syndrome. Xerosis (very dry skin) or hair thinning may be a sign of hypothyroidism and warrant an interim TSH. Be attentive to dermatologic issues that may have an autoimmune etiology and are prevalent among children with Down syndrome, such as alopecia areata and vitiligo.

Folliculitis and keratosis pilaris are also commonly seen in children with Down syndrome. Assess for skin findings, discuss them with the patient and family, and consider referral to a dermatologist if needed.[114,115]

Anticipatory Guidance From 1 to 5 Years

- Review early intervention, including physical therapy, occupational therapy, and speech therapy, at all health supervision visits.
- Discuss at the 30-month visit the transition from early intervention to preschool, which occurs at 36 months of age. Help the family understand the change from the Individualized Family Service Plan in early intervention to the Individualized Education Program through public education (see Resources for Families).
- Review availability of resources, including Down syndrome support groups and organizations that help with navigation of community and financial resources, including child care (see Resources for Families).
- Provide influenza vaccine annually. Respiratory syncytial virus prophylaxis may be considered for children <2 years who have cooccurring qualifying conditions. Children with chronic cardiac or pulmonary disease should be given the 23-valent pneumococcal polysaccharide vaccine at 2 years of age or older.[53]
- Reassure parents that delayed and irregular dental eruption patterns are common and that hypodontia occurs with increased frequency (23%).[116,117]
- Encourage and model use of accurate terms for genitalia and other private body parts (penis, vulva) anytime these body parts are discussed or examined. Model respect for body rights by reminding patients that their body is their own and explain what you will do before moving

into their personal space or performing a procedure. Remind patient and family that the only reason anyone should be looking at or touching private body parts is for health (doctor office visits) or hygiene (bathing or showering).[118]

- On at least 1 well-child visit, educate the family about increased risk of sexual exploitation, and remind them that people their child knows and trusts are more likely than strangers to be perpetrators.
- At least once between 1 and 5 years of age, discuss future parental pregnancy planning and review chance of recurrence of Down syndrome and availability of prenatal testing options. Offer referral for genetic counseling if desired by the family.
- Assess the child's behavior and talk about behavioral management, sibling adjustments, socialization, and recreational skills.[119]
- Encourage families to establish optimal dietary and physical exercise patterns that will prevent obesity.
- Be prepared to discuss and answer questions about treatments that are considered complementary or alternative (see Health Supervision From Birth to 1 Month for discussion).

HEALTH SUPERVISION FROM 5 TO 12 YEARS: LATE CHILDHOOD

Follow *Bright Futures* schedule or more frequently as indicated.

- Obtain a history and perform a physical examination.
- Monitor weight and follow BMI trends at each health care visit. Review the child's growth and plot it on the Down syndrome-specific charts for weight, height, and head circumference.[120] These charts should be used in conjunction with the Down syndrome-specific BMI chart for

children up to age 10 and with the BMI chart from the Centers for Disease Control and Prevention, which is a better indicator of excess adiposity for children with Down syndrome over the age of 10.[58]

- Review feeding. Ask about any changes in respiratory symptoms with feeding and ensure adequate iron intake (see Health Supervision From Birth to 1 Month for discussion).
- Emphasize healthy diet and lifestyle for preventing obesity.
- Obtain annual ear-specific audiologic evaluation (see Health Supervision From 1 Month to 1 Year for discussion). If middle ear disease occurs, obtain developmentally appropriate hearing evaluation after treatment.
- Obtain ophthalmologic evaluation by photoscreening, if available, at every health supervision visit or by a pediatric ophthalmologist or ophthalmologist with expertise in children with disabilities every 2 years[63,85] (see Health Supervision From 1 Month to 1 Year for discussion).
- Measure TSH annually; the risk of hypothyroidism increases with age (See "Health Supervision From 1 to 5 Years" for discussion). Measure TSH every 6 months if antithyroid antibodies have been detected.
- Individualize cardiology follow-up on the basis of history of cardiac defects.
- Obtain a CBC and either (1) a combination of ferritin and CRP, or (2) a combination of serum iron and TIBC, beginning at 1 year of age and annually thereafter (see Health Supervision From 1 Month to 1 Year for discussion).
- A physician may prescribe iron supplementation for children with sleep problems and a ferritin concentration <50 μg/L (see Health Supervision From 1 to 5 Years for discussion).

- Palpate testes at each health supervision visit (see Health Supervision From 1 to 5 Years for discussion).
- For children on a diet that contains gluten, review for symptoms potentially related to celiac disease at every health maintenance visit and evaluate if indicated (see Health Supervision From 1 to 5 Years for discussion).
- At each well-child visit, discuss with family the importance of universal precautions for protection of the cervical spine during any anesthetic, surgical, or radiographic procedure. Perform careful history and physical examination, with attention to myelopathic signs and symptoms. Caregivers should also be instructed to contact their physician immediately for new onset of symptoms of myelopathy (see Health Supervision From 1 to 5 Years for discussion).
- Discuss skin, hair, and scalp care at each preventive health care visit and refer to dermatologist if needed (see Health Supervision From 1 to 5 Years for discussion).
- Encourage caregivers to promote self-help skills and assume developmentally appropriate responsibilities in the home. Monitor for behavior problems that interfere with function in the home, community, or school. Attention problems, attention-deficit/hyperactivity disorder, obsessive-compulsive behaviors, noncompliant behavior, and wandering off are some of the common behavior concerns reported. Psychiatric disorders affecting typically developing children may also occur. Evaluate for medical problems that can be associated with behavior changes, including thyroid abnormalities, celiac disease, sleep-disordered breathing, gastroesophageal reflux, and

constipation. Intervention strategies depend on the child's age, the severity of the problem, and the setting in which the problem occurs. When symptoms interfere with daily activities, refer to community treatment programs, psychosocial services for consultative care, or behavioral specialists experienced in working with children with special needs. Refer patients who have chronic behavioral problems or manifest acute deterioration in function for specialized evaluation and intervention[112,113,121] (see Health Supervision From 1 to 5 Years for discussion).
- Be aware that children with Down syndrome are frequently more sensitive to certain medications. Before initiating medication for behavior management, the process should be discussed between the primary care physician and specialists involved in the child's care. Although there has been little research to directly address the use of psychotropic medications among children with Down syndrome, anecdotal reports indicate that these children may differ in their response to medications. Experience has led to the recommendation to start medications at the lowest recommended dose and increase or decrease the dose according to the child's response.[122]
- Inquire regarding symptoms of neurologic dysfunction, including seizures, and perform a neurologic examination.
- Discuss symptoms related to sleep-disordered breathing at every well-child visit, including snoring, restless sleep, daytime sleepiness, nighttime awakening, behavior problems, and abnormal sleep position. Refer to a physician with expertise in pediatric sleep, otolaryngologist, or a pediatric sleep medicine

specialist any child with signs or symptoms of sleep-disordered breathing or abnormal sleep-study results. Children with sleep problems and a ferritin concentration <50 μg/L may benefit from iron supplementation.[70,71] Discuss obesity as a risk factor of sleep apnea and review need to implement healthy diet and activity in affected patients (see Health Supervision From 1 to 5 Years for discussion).

Anticipatory Guidance From 5 to 12 Years at Every Health Supervision Visit, Unless Otherwise Indicated

- Review the child's development and appropriateness of transition to elementary school placement and any additional developmental intervention.
- Discuss socialization, family status, and relationships, including financial arrangements, health insurance, and guardianship, incorporating supported decision-making where recognized (see Resources for Families).
- Encourage development of age-appropriate social skills, self-help skills, and development of a sense of responsibility.
- Counsel families regarding the transition from elementary to middle school, when major change often occurs, from 1 teacher to several and from 1 class to changing classes. Prepare them to facilitate adjustment at a time when the academic disparity becomes greater and full inclusion becomes more difficult. Although transition to work-environment planning occurs formally at age 14 in the individualized education program, the discussion and participation in community resources may begin at a much earlier age, approximately age 10, and all subsequent visits.
- Refer patients with behavior or history concerning for autism for appropriate evaluation (see

Health Supervision From 1 to 5 Years for discussion).

- Continue to assess, monitor, and encourage independence with hygiene and self-care. Encourage family to teach, model, and respect privacy at home and in the community. Discuss appropriate management of sexual behaviors such as masturbation.
- Discuss progression of physical and psychosocial changes through puberty and issues of fertility and contraception.[118] Remind family that pubertal development usually follows patterns similar to those found in the general population, but the child with Down syndrome will likely need more preparation in understanding and managing these changes.[123]
- On at least 1 health supervision visit, educate family about increased risk of sexual exploitation (see "Anticipatory Guidance From 1 to 5 Years" for discussion).
- Discuss the need for gynecologic care in the pubescent girl. Provide developmentally appropriate discussion about puberty and include menses and dysmenorrhea (see Resources for Families). When developmentally appropriate on at least 1 visit, talk with the patient and her family about the chance of Down syndrome in her children (50%) if she were to become pregnant.[124]
- Although males with Down syndrome are usually infertile, there have been rare instances in which a male has reproduced.[125,126]
- When developmentally appropriate, birth control and prevention of sexually transmitted infections should be discussed with patients and their families.[123] Advocate for and offer long-acting, reversible contraception. Be familiar with local law and resources to

assist the family in their decision-making regarding questions about long-term and reversible birth control.[123,127,128]

- At least once between 5 and 12 years of age, as with discussion in the first year of life, discuss future parental pregnancy planning and review risk possibility of recurrence of Down syndrome, as well as availability of prenatal testing options. Offer referral for genetic counseling if desired by the family.
- Parents should be advised that trampoline use should be avoided by all children, with or without Down syndrome, unless part of a structured training program with appropriate supervision and safety measures in place. Parents can be advised that participation in contact sports, such as football, soccer, and gymnastics, places children at risk for spinal cord injury.[96,129]
- Special Olympics requires documentation of physical examination of all athletes for participation in sports.[94]
- Be prepared to discuss and answer questions regarding treatments that are considered complementary or alternative (see Health Supervision From 1 Month to 1 Year for discussion).

HEALTH SUPERVISION FROM 12 TO 21 YEARS OR OLDER: ADOLESCENCE TO EARLY ADULTHOOD

Follow *Bright Futures* schedule or more frequently as indicated.

Physical Examination and Laboratory Values

- Obtain a history and perform a physical examination.
- Monitor weight and follow BMI trends at each health care visit. Review the adolescent/young adult's weight and height and plot it on the Down-syndrome specific charts for weight, height,

and head circumference. These should be used in conjunction with the Centers for Disease Control BMI chart[58,120] (see "Health Supervision From 5 to 12 Years" for discussion). Counsel regarding healthy diet and a structured exercise program.

- Review feeding, ask if there have been any changes in eating patterns or respiratory symptoms with feeding, and ensure adequate iron intake (see Health Supervision From Birth to 1 Month for discussion).
- Emphasize healthy diet and lifestyle for preventing obesity.
- Obtain a CBC with differential and either (1) a combination of ferritin and CRP, or (2) a combination of serum iron and TIBC, beginning at 1 year of age and annually thereafter.
- A physician may elect to prescribe iron supplementation for adolescents/early adults with restless sleep and a ferritin concentration <50 μg/L for children or 75 for adults[71], (see Health Supervision From 1 to 5 Years for discussion).
- Palpate testes at each health supervision visit (see Health Supervision From 1 to 5 Years for discussion).
- Measure TSH concentration annually and obtain TSH sooner if there are symptoms of thyroid dysfunction (see Health Supervision From Birth to 1 Month for discussion). Measure TSH every 6 months if antithyroid antibodies have been detected.
- Obtain annual ear-specific audiologic evaluation (see Health Supervision From 1 Month to 1 Year for discussion). If middle ear disease occurs, obtain developmentally appropriate hearing evaluation after treatment.
- For adolescents/early adults on a diet that contains gluten, review for symptoms potentially related to celiac disease at every health

supervision visit and evaluate if indicated (see Health Supervision From 1 to 5 Years for discussion).

- Individualize cardiology follow-up on the basis of history of cardiac defects.
- Discuss symptoms related to sleep-disordered breathing, including snoring, restless sleep, daytime sleepiness, nighttime awakening, behavior problems, and sleep position, at every health supervision visit. Refer to a physician with expertise in pediatric sleep any child with signs or symptoms of sleep-disordered breathing or an abnormal sleep-study result. Discuss the risk factor of obesity for sleep apnea and counsel regarding healthy diet and activity if needed.
- Discuss with caregivers and the patient at every health supervision visit the importance of cervical spine-positioning precautions for protection of the cervical spine during any anesthetic, surgical, or radiographic procedure. Perform careful history and physical examination with attention to myelopathic signs and symptoms. Caregivers and patients should also be instructed to contact their physician immediately for new onset of symptoms of myelopathy (see Health Supervision From 1 to 5 Years for discussion).
- Inquire regarding symptoms of neurologic dysfunction, including seizures, and perform neurologic examination.
- Discuss behavioral and social status and refer patients who have depression,[130] chronic behavioral problems, or acute deterioration in function for specialized evaluation and intervention.[112,113,121]
- Inquire regarding symptoms of acute regression (see Health Supervision From 1 to 5 Years for discussion).

- Skin problems are particularly common in people with Down syndrome. Discuss skin, hair, and scalp care at each preventive health care visit and consider referral to a dermatologist if needed (see Health Supervision From 1 to 5 Years for discussion). In addition, inflammatory disorders such as hidradenitis suppurativa may present at an older age.[131]
- Perform visual acuity testing or photoscreening, if available, at every health supervision visit or ensure adolescent/young adult is under care of a pediatric ophthalmologist or ophthalmologist experienced in care of people with disabilities who will determine the frequency of assessment. Assessment for onset of cataracts, refractive errors, and keratoconus, which can cause blurred vision, corneal thinning, or corneal haze and is typically diagnosed after puberty, is important.[63,85]
- Examine annually for acquired mitral and aortic valvular disease in older patients with Down syndrome. An echocardiogram should be obtained if there is a history of increasing fatigue, shortness of breath, exertional dyspnea, or a new murmur or gallop.
- Refer patients with behavior or history concerning for autism spectrum disorder for appropriate evaluation and therapy (see Anticipatory Guidance From 1 to 5 Years for discussion).

Anticipatory Guidance From 12 to 21 Years and Older at Every Health Supervision Visit, Unless Otherwise Indicated

- Issues related to transition into adulthood, including educational goals, work, independence, and transition of medical care. Continue these discussions and include guardianship incorporating supported decision-making,

where recognized, and long-term financial planning from early adolescence (see Resources for Families).[132,133] Potential adult morbidities, including apparent tendency toward premature aging and increased risk of Alzheimer disease, may also be discussed.[134]

- Discuss appropriateness of school placement and vocational planning as early as possible in the school setting and emphasize planning for transition to adulthood and adequate vocational training within the school curriculum.
- Patients/caregivers should be advised that trampoline use should be avoided by all children, with or without Down syndrome, unless part of a structured training program with appropriate supervision and safety measures in place. Parents can be advised that participation in contact sports, such as football, soccer, and gymnastics, places children at risk for spinal cord injury.[129]
- Special Olympics requires documentation of physical examination of all athletes for participation in sports.[94] Be prepared to discuss and answer questions regarding treatments that are considered complementary or alternative (see Health Supervision From 1 Month to 1 Year for discussion).
- On at least 1 health supervision visit, educate family about increased risk of sexual exploitation (see Anticipatory Guidance From 1 to 5 Years for discussion).
- Continue to assess, monitor, and encourage independence with hygiene and self-care. Provide guidance on healthy, normal, and typical sexual development and behaviors. Provide education and guidance about normal masturbation behaviors and personal boundaries. Emphasize the need

for understandable information and encourage opportunities for advancing comprehension of sexuality (see Resources for Families). Discuss the need for contraception and prevention of sexually transmitted infections and the degree of supervision required. Advocate for and offer use of long-acting, reversible contraception and be familiar with local laws and resources to assist the family in their decision-making regarding questions about long-term and reversible birth control.[123]

- Make recommendations and provide or refer for routine gynecologic care as needed for long-acting, reversible contraception or other indications if not already provided. Discuss premenstrual behavioral problems and management of menses, including caregiver concerns regarding menstrual suppression for hygiene purposes.[128,135,136]

- At least at 1 visit, talk with the female patient and her family about the chance that she could have a child with Down syndrome if she were to become pregnant.[123–124]

- Discuss independent living opportunities, group homes, options for postsecondary education, workshop settings, and other community-supported employment.

- Discuss intrafamily relationships, financial planning including the Achieving a Better Life Experience Act (see Resources for Families), and guardianship including supported decision-making where recognized.[132]

- Facilitate transition and provide coordination to adult medical primary and subspecialty care.[137] It is recognized that many young adults receive care from pediatricians, and providers will want to be aware of the newly developed health supervision for adults.[138]

FUTURE CONSIDERATIONS

Many issues related to the development and health of people with Down syndrome remain to be evaluated, and research agendas for addressing both public health and basic science topics have been developed. Knowledge in several topics of great importance to the care of children with Down syndrome could be enhanced through population-based research. A rigorous, evidence-based review of screening and treatment of atlantoaxial instability, for example, is needed, and continuing research is critical for directing the care for optimal outcomes of people with Down syndrome.[1,139–141]

RESOURCES FOR FAMILIES

Prenatal and Infancy

- Brighter Tomorrows Supporting Families: https://hdi.uky.edu/project/brighter-tomorrows-supporting-families-with-accurate-information-about-down-syndrome. Supporting families with accurate information about Down syndrome (includes Lettercase resources). Interdisciplinary Human Development Institute, University of Kentucky.

- Lettercase resources: www.lettercase.org. Provides prenatal and postnatal counseling for families. One copy provided free to professionals and family.

- Down Syndrome Diagnosis Network: www.dsdiagnosisnetwork.org. Cohorts of families with similar due dates or birthdates connected in moderated Facebook groups.

- Skallerup SJ. *Babies With Down Syndrome: A New Parents Guide*, 3rd ed. Bethesda, MD: Woodbine House; 2009. (English and Spanish editions available at www.woodbinehouse.com.) Provides guidance for raising and caring for a child with Down syndrome through age 5.

Childhood

- Pueschel SM, ed. *A Parent's Guide to Down Syndrome: Toward a Brighter Future*. Bethesda, MD: Brookes Publishing; 2001.

- Stein DS. *Supporting Positive Behavior in Children and Teens with Down Syndrome: The Respond but Don't React Method*. Bethesda, MD: Woodbine House; 2016.

- www.woodbinehouse.com. Variety of books for families, therapists, and teachers of children with Down syndrome.

Adolescence

- Got Transition: http://www.gottransition.org/. Provides resources and guidance for transition.

- Couwenhoven T. *Boys Guide to Growing Up–Choices & Changes During Puberty Written for Persons with Intellectual Disability*. Bethesda, MD: Woodbine House; 2012.

- Couwenhoven T. *Girls Guide to Growing Up–Choices & Changes During Puberty Written for Persons with Intellectual Disability*. Bethesda, MD: Woodbine House; 2012.

- Simmons J. *The Down Syndrome Transition Handbook: Charting Your Child's Course to Adulthood*. Bethesda, MD: Woodbine House; 2010. Available at: www.woodbinehouse.com.

Across the Lifespan

- DS-Connect: The Down Syndrome Registry: https://DSConnect.nih.gov. Families and patients connect with researchers and health care providers and may participate in clinical studies and take confidential health-related surveys that help achieve better understanding of people with Down syndrome across the lifespan.

- National Down Syndrome Congress: www.ndsccenter.org. Information, advocacy, education, and support for persons with Down syndrome, siblings, and families in English and Spanish.

- National Down Syndrome Society: www.ndss.org. Advocacy and information regarding Down syndrome across the lifespan.
- Family Voices: https://familyvoices.org/affiliates/. Family-to-family health information centers that help families navigate systems needed by children with special health care needs.
- Parent to Parent USA: https://www.p2pusa.org/parents. Provides support to deal with challenges of raising children with special health care needs.
- Parent Training and Information Centers: https://www.parentcenterhub.org. Resources in each state that inform, prepare, and assist families with navigation of the education system.
- March of Dimes: www.marchofdimes.com. Information for parents on health issues related to pregnancy and birth defects.
- Down Syndrome Education International: www.downsed.org. Resources for educators and parents relevant to communication, numeracy, speech, and supporting inclusion.
- Canadian Down Syndrome Society: www.cdss.ca. Resources for families on a variety of issues related to Down syndrome.
- ABLE ACT 2014: https://www.irs.gov/government-entities/federal-state-local-governments/able-accounts-tax-benefit-for-people-with-disabilities. Tax benefit for people with disabilities: allow states to create

tax-advantage savings programs for eligible people with disabilities (designated beneficiaries) and can help pay for qualified disability expenses.

- DSC2U Down syndrome clinic to you: www.dsc2u.org. Provides personalized health and wellness information about Down syndrome to caregivers and primary care physicians.

Lead Authors

Marilyn J. Bull, MD, FAAP
Tracy Trotter, MD, FAAP
Stephanie L. Santoro, MD, FAAP
Celanie Christensen, MD, MS, FAAP
Randall W. Grout, MD, MS, FAAP

Council on Genetics Executive Committee, 2019–2020

Leah W. Burke, MD, FAAP; Chairperson
Susan A. Berry, MD, FAAP
Timothy A. Geleske, MD, FAAP
Ingrid Holm, MD, FAAP
Robert J. Hopkin, MD, FAAP
Wendy J. Introne, MD, FAAP
Michael J. Lyons, MD, FAAP
Danielle C. Monteil, MD, FAAP
Angela Scheuerle, MD, FAAP
Joan M. Stoler, MD, FAAP
Samantha A. Vergano, MD, FAAP

Former Executive Committee Members

Emily Chen, MD, PhD, FAAP, Co-Chairperson
Rizwan Hamid, MD, PhD, FAAP
Tracy L. Trotter, MD, FAAP, Co-Chairperson

Partnership for Policy Implementation Contributors

Stephen M. Downs, MD, MS, FAAP
Randall W. Grout, MD, MS, FAAP

Liaisons

Christopher Cunniff, MD, PhD, FAAP; American College of Medical Genetics
Melissa A. Parisi, MD, PhD, FAAP; Eunice Kennedy Shriver National Institute of Child Health and Human Development
Steven J. Ralston, MD; American College of Obstetricians and Gynecologists
Joan A. Scott, MS, CGC; Health Resources and Services Administration, Maternal and Child Health Bureau
Stuart K. Shapira, MD, PhD; Centers for Disease Control and Prevention

Staff

Paul Spire

ABBREVIATIONS

BAER: brainstem auditory evoked response
CBC: complete blood cell count
cfDNA: cell-free DNA
CRP: C-reactive protein
CVS: chorionic villus sampling
FISH: fluorescent in situ hybridization
IgA: immunoglobulin A
T4: free thyroxine
TAM: transient abnormal myelopoiesis
TIBC: total iron-binding capacity
TSH: thyroid-stimulating hormone
TTG: tissue transglutaminase

REFERENCES

1. Schieve LA, Boulet SL, Boyle C, Rasmussen SA, Schendel D. Health of children 3 to 17 years of age with Down syndrome in the 1997-2005 national health interview survey. *Pediatrics.* 2009;123(2):e253–e260

2. Roizen NJ, Magyar CI, Kuschner ES, et al. A community cross-sectional survey of medical problems in 440 children with Down syndrome in New York State. *J Pediatr.* 2014;164(4):871–875

3. Stoll C, Dott B, Alembik Y, Roth MP. Associated congenital anomalies among cases with Down syndrome. *Eur J Med Genet.* 2015;58(12):674–680

4. Shaw EDBR, Beals RK. The hip joint in Down syndrome. A study of its structure and associated disease. *Clin Orthop Relat Res.* 1992; (278): 101–107

5. Caird MS, Wills BP, Dormans JP. Down syndrome in children: the role of the orthopaedic surgeon. *J Am Acad Orthop Surg.* 2006;14(11):610–619

6. Pueschel SM, Findley TW, Furia J, Gallagher PL, Scola FH, Pezzullo JC. Atlantoaxial instability in Down syndrome: roentgenographic, neurologic, and somatosensory evoked potential studies. *J Pediatr.* 1987;110(4):515–521

7. Selby KA, Newton RW, Gupta S, Hunt L. Clinical predictors and radiological reliability in atlantoaxial subluxation in Down syndrome. *Arch Dis Child.* 1991;66(7):876–878

8. Pierce MJ, LaFranchi SH, Pinter JD. Characterization of thyroid abnormalities in a large cohort of children with Down syndrome. *Horm Res Paediatr.* 2017;87(3):170–178

9. Juj H, Emery H. The arthropathy of Down syndrome: an underdiagnosed and under-recognized condition. *J Pediatr.* 2009;154(2):234–238

10. Bergholdt R, Eising S, Nerup J, Pociot F. Increased prevalence of Down syndrome in individuals with type 1 diabetes in Denmark: a nationwide population-based study. *Diabetologia.* 2006;49(6):1179–1182

11. Kent L, Evans J, Paul M, Sharp M. Comorbidity of autistic spectrum disorders in children with Down syndrome. *Dev Med Child Neurol.* 1999;41(3):153–158

12. Moss J, Richards C, Nelson L, Oliver C. Prevalence of autism spectrum disorder symptomatology and related behavioural characteristics in individuals with Down syndrome. *Autism.* 2013;17(4):390–404

13. Hook EB. *Epidemiology of Down Syndrome.* Cambridge: Ware Press; 1982

14. Bull MJ. Down syndrome. *N Engl J Med.* 2020;382(24):2344–2352

15. Papavassiliou P, Charalsawadi C, Rafferty K, Jackson-Cook C. Mosaicism for trisomy 21: a review. *Am J Med Genet A.* 2015;167A(1):26–39

16. Pelleri MC, Cicchini E, Locatelli C, et al. Systematic reanalysis of partial trisomy 21 cases with or without Down syndrome suggests a small region on 21q22.13 as critical to the phenotype. *Hum Mol Genet.* 2016;25(12):2525–2538

17. ACOG Committee on Practice Bulletins. ACOG practice bulletin no. 77: screening for fetal chromosomal abnormalities. *Obstet Gynecol.* 2007;109(1):217–227

18. American College of Obstetricians and Gynecologists. ACOG practice bulletin no. 88, December 2007. Invasive prenatal testing for aneuploidy. *Obstet Gynecol.* 2007;110(6):1459–1467

19. Gil MM, Accurti V, Santacruz B, Plana MN, Nicolaides KH. Analysis of cell-free DNA in maternal blood in screening for aneuploidies: updated meta-analysis. *Ultrasound Obstet Gynecol.* 2017;50(3):302–314

20. American College of Obstetricians and Gynecologists' Committee on Practice Bulletins–Obstetrics; Committee on Genetics; Society for Maternal-Fetal Medicine. Screening for fetal chromosomal abnormalities: ACOG Practice Bulletin, Number 226. *Obstet Gynecol.* 2020;136(4):e48–e69

21. Driscoll DA, Gross SJ. Screening for fetal aneuploidy and neural tube defects. *Genet Med.* 2009;11(11):818–821

22. Malone FD, Canick JA, Ball RH, et al. First- and Second-Trimester Evaluation of Risk (FASTER) Research Consortium. First-trimester or second-trimester screening, or both, for Down syndrome. *N Engl J Med.* 2005;353(19):2001–2011

23. Wald NJ, Rodeck C, Hackshaw AK, Walters J, Chitty L, Mackinson AM; SURUSS Research Group. First and second trimester antenatal screening for Down syndrome: the results of the Serum, Urine and Ultrasound Screening Study (SURUSS). *Health Technol Assess.* 2003;7(11):1–77

24. Spencer K, Spencer CE, Power M, Dawson C, Nicolaides KH. Screening for chromosomal abnormalities in the first trimester using ultrasound and maternal serum biochemistry in a one-stop clinic: a review of three years prospective experience. *BJOG.* 2003;110(3):281–286

25. [No authors listed] Practice bulletin no. 162: prenatal diagnostic testing for genetic disorders. *Obstet Gynecol.* 2016;127(5):e108–e122

26. Akolekar R, Beta J, Picciarelli G, Ogilvie C, D'Antonio F. Procedure-related risk of miscarriage following amniocentesis and chorionic villus sampling: a systematic review and meta-analysis. *Ultrasound Obstet Gynecol.* 2015;45(1):16–26

27. Adams RC, Levy SE. Council on Children With Disabilities. Shared decision-making and children with disabilities: pathways to consensus. *Pediatrics.* 2017;139(6):e20170956

28. Hornberger LL. Committee on Adolescence. Options counseling for the pregnant adolescent patient. *Pediatrics.* 2017;140(3):e20172274

29. Guseh SH, Little SE, Bennett K, Silva V, Wilkins-Haug LE. Antepartum management and obstetric outcomes among pregnancies with Down syndrome from diagnosis to delivery. *Prenat Diagn.* 2017;37(7):640–646

30. Skotko BG, Capone GT, Kishnani PS. Down Syndrome Diagnosis Study Group. Postnatal diagnosis of Down syndrome: synthesis of the evidence on how best to deliver the news. *Pediatrics.* 2009;124(4):e751–e758

31. Skotko BG, Levine SP, Goldstein R. Self-perceptions from people with Down syndrome. *Am J Med Genet A.* 2011;155A(10):2360–2369

32. Crocker AF, Smith SN. Person-first language: are we practicing what we preach? *J Multidiscip Healthc.* 2019;12:125–129

33. Skotko BG, Levine SP, Goldstein R. Having a brother or sister with Down syndrome: perspectives from siblings. *Am J Med Genet A.* 2011;155A(10):2348–2359

34. Skotko BG, Levine SP, Macklin EA, Goldstein RD. Family perspectives about Down syndrome. *Am J Med Genet A.* 2016;170A(4):930–941

35. Jackson A, Maybee J, Moran MK, Wolter-Warmerdam K, Hickey F. Clinical characteristics of dysphagia in children with Down syndrome. *Dysphagia.* 2016;31(5):663–671

36. Romano C, van Wynckel M, Hulst J, et al. European Society for Paediatric Gastroenterology, hepatology and nutrition guidelines for the evaluation and treatment of gastrointestinal and

nutritional complications in children with neurological impairment. *J Pediatr Gastroenterol Nutr.* 2017;65(2):242–264

37. Stanley MA, Shepherd N, Duvall N, et al. Clinical identification of feeding and swallowing disorders in 0–6-month-old infants with Down syndrome. *Am J Med Genet A.* 2019;179(2):177–182

38. Poskanzer SA, Hobensack VL, Ciciora SL, Santoro SL. Feeding difficulty and gastrostomy tube placement in infants with Down syndrome. *Eur J Pediatr.* 2020;179(6):909–917

39. Jackson A, Maybee J, Wolter-Warmerdam K, DeBoer E, Hickey F. Associations between age, respiratory comorbidities, and dysphagia in infants with Down syndrome. *Pediatr Pulmonol.* 2019;54(11):1853–1859

40. McDowell KM, Craven DI. Pulmonary complications of Down syndrome during childhood. *J Pediatr.* 2011;158(2):319–325

41. Santoro SL, Atoum D, Hufnagel RB, Motley WW. Surgical, medical and developmental outcomes in patients with Down syndrome and cataracts. *SAGE Open Med.* 2017;5:2050312117715583

42. Haargaard B, Fledelius HC. Down syndrome and early cataract. *Br J Ophthalmol.* 2006;90(8):1024–1027

43. Muse C, Harrison J, Yoshinaga-Itano C, et al. Joint Committee on Infant Hearing of the American Academy of Pediatrics. Supplement to the JCIH 2007 position statement: principles and guidelines for early intervention after confirmation that a child is deaf or hard of hearing. *Pediatrics.* 2013;131(4):e1324–e1349

44. Park AH, Wilson MA, Stevens PT, Harward R, Hohler N. Identification of hearing loss in pediatric patients with Down syndrome. *Otolaryngol Head Neck Surg.* 2012;146(1):135–140

45. Bull MJ, Engle WA. Committee on Injury, Violence, and Poison Prevention and Committee on Fetus and Newborn; American Academy of Pediatrics. Safe transportation of preterm and low birth weight infants at hospital discharge. *Pediatrics.* 2009;123(5):1424–1429

46. Roberts I, Alford K, Hall G, et al. Oxford-Imperial Down Syndrome Cohort Study Group. GATA1-mutant clones are frequent and often unsuspected in babies with Down syndrome: identification of a population at risk of leukemia. *Blood.* 2013;122(24):3908–3917

47. Tunstall O, Bhatnagar N, James B, et al. British Society for Haematology. Guidelines for the investigation and management of transient leukaemia of Down Syndrome. *Br J Haematol.* 2018;182(2):200–211

48. Kivivuori SM, Rajantie J, Siimes MA. Peripheral blood cell counts in infants with Down syndrome. *Clin Genet.* 1996;49(1):15–19

49. Hasle H, Clemmensen IH, Mikkelsen M. Risks of leukaemia and solid tumours in individuals with Down syndrome. *Lancet.* 2000;355(9199):165–169

50. Iughetti L, Predieri B, Bruzzi P, et al. Ten-year longitudinal study of thyroid function in children with Down syndrome. *Horm Res Paediatr.* 2014;82(2):113–121

51. Lagan N, Huggard D, Mc Grane F, et al. Multiorgan involvement and management in children with Down syndrome. *Acta Paediatr.* 2020;109(6):1096–1111

52. Santoro SL, Chicoine B, Jasien JM, et al. Pneumonia and respiratory infections in Down syndrome: a scoping review of the literature. *Am J Med Genet A.* 2021;185(1):286–299

53. American Academy of Pediatrics. Respiratory syncytial virus. In: Kimberlin DW, Barnett ED, Lynfield R, Sawyer MH, eds. *Red Book: Report of the Committee on Infectious Diseases 2021.* 32nd ed. Itasca, IL: American Academy of Pediatrics; 2021:628–636

54. Lewanda AF, Gallegos MF, Summar M. Patterns of dietary supplement use in children with Down syndrome. *J Pediatr.* 2018;201:100–105.e30

55. McClafferty H, Vohra S, Bailey M, et al. Section on Integrative Medicine. Pediatric Integrative Medicine. *Pediatrics.* 2017;140(3):e20171961

56. Kupferman JC, Druschel CM, Kupchik GS. Increased prevalence of renal and urinary tract anomalies in children with Down syndrome. *Pediatrics.* 2009;124(4):e615–e621

57. Zemel BS, Pipan M, Stallings VA, et al. Growth charts for children with Down syndrome in the United States. *Pediatrics.* 2015;136(5):e1204–e1211

58. Hatch-Stein JA, Zemel BS, Prasad D, et al. Body composition and BMI growth charts in children with Down syndrome. *Pediatrics.* 2016;138(4):e20160541

59. Shott SR. Down syndrome: common otolaryngologic manifestations. *Am J Med Genet C Semin Med Genet.* 2006;142C(3):131–140

60. De Schrijver L, Topsakal V, Wojciechowski M, Van de Heyning P, Boudewyns A. Prevalence and etiology of sensorineural hearing loss in children with down syndrome: a cross-sectional study. *Int J Pediatr Otorhinolaryngol.* 2019;116:168–172

61. Blaser S, Propst EJ, Martin D, et al. Inner ear dysplasia is common in children with Down syndrome (trisomy 21). *Laryngoscope.* 2006;116(12):2113–2119

62. American Academy of Ophthalmology. Trisomy 21/Down syndrome. Available at: https://eyewiki.aao.org/TGrisomy_21/Down_Syndrome. Accessed August 7, 2020

63. Umfress AC, Hair CD, Donahue SP. Prevalence of ocular pathology on initial screening and incidence of new findings on follow-up examinations in children with trisomy 21. *Am J Ophthalmol.* 2019;207:373–377

64. AAPOS. Vision screening recommendation. Available at: https://aapos.org/patients/patient-resources. 2019. Accessed August 7, 2020

65. Coats DK, McCreery KM, Plager DA, Bohra L, Kim DS, Paysse EA. Nasolacrimal outflow drainage anomalies in Down's syndrome. *Ophthalmology.* 2003;110(7):1437–1441

66. Martin T, Smith A, Breatnach CR, et al. Infants born with Down syndrome: burden of disease in the early neonatal period. *J Pediatr.* 2018;193:21–26

67. Dixon NE, Crissman BG, Smith PB, Zimmerman SA, Worley G, Kishnani PS. Prevalence of iron deficiency in children with Down syndrome. *J Pediatr.* 2010;157(6):967–971.e1

68. Georgieff MK. Long-term brain and behavioral consequences of early iron deficiency. *Nutr Rev.* 2011;69(Suppl 1):S43–S48

69. Hart SJ, Zimmerman K, Linardic CM, et al. Detection of iron deficiency in children with Down syndrome. *Genet Med.* 2020;22(2):317–325

70. Dosman C, Witmans M, Zwaigenbaum L. Iron's role in paediatric restless legs syndrome – a review. *Paediatr Child Health.* 2012;17(4):193–197

71. Allen RP, Picchietti DL, Auerbach M, et al. International Restless Legs Syndrome Study Group (IRLSSG). Evidence-based and consensus clinical practice guidelines for the iron treatment of restless legs syndrome/Willis-Ekbom disease in adults and children: an IRLSSG task force report. *Sleep Med.* 2018;41:27–44

72. Taub JW, Berman JN, Hitzler JK, et al. Improved outcomes for myeloid leukemia of Down syndrome: a report from the Children's Oncology Group AAML0431 trial. *Blood.* 2017;129(25): 3304–3313

73. Matloub Y, Rabin KR, Ji L, et al. Excellent long-term survival of children with Down syndrome and standard-risk ALL: a report from the Children's Oncology Group. *Blood Adv.* 2019;3(11):1647–1656

74. Goldberg-Stern H, Strawsburg RH, Patterson B, et al. Seizure frequency and characteristics in children with Down syndrome. *Brain Dev.* 2001;23(6):375–378

75. Kumada T, Ito M, Miyajima T, et al. Multi-institutional study on the correlation between chromosomal abnormalities and epilepsy. *Brain Dev.* 2005; 27(2):127–134

76. Jea A, Smith ER, Robertson R, Scott RM. Moyamoya syndrome associated with Down syndrome: outcome after surgical revascularization. *Pediatrics.* 2005;116(5):e694–e701

77. See AP, Ropper AE, Underberg DL, Robertson RL, Scott RM, Smith ER. Down syndrome and moyamoya: clinical presentation and surgical management. *J Neurosurg Pediatr.* 2015;16(1):58–63

78. Centers for Disease Control and Prevention. Immunization schedules. Available at: https://www.cdc.gov/vaccines/schedules. Accessed December 14, 2020

79. Fitzgerald DA, Paul A, Richmond C. Severity of obstructive apnoea in children with Down syndrome who snore. *Arch Dis Child.* 2007;92(5):423–425

80. Shott SR, Amin R, Chini B, Heubi C, Hotze S, Akers R. Obstructive sleep apnea: should all children with Down syndrome be tested? *Arch Otolaryngol Head Neck Surg.* 2006;132(4):432–436

81. Kobayashi T, Sakemi Y, Yamashita H. Increased incidence of retroperitoneal teratomas and decreased incidence of sacrococcygeal teratomas in infants with Down syndrome. *Pediatr Blood Cancer.* 2014;61(2):363–365

82. Satgé D, Vekemans M. Down syndrome patients are less likely to develop some (but not all) malignant solid tumours. *Clin Genet.* 2011;79(3): 289–290, author reply 291–292

83. Hasle H, Friedman JM, Olsen JH, Rasmussen SA. Low risk of solid tumors in persons with Down syndrome. *Genet Med.* 2016;18(11):1151–1157

84. Lin K, Sharangpani R. Screening for testicular cancer: an evidence review for the U.S. Preventive Services Task Force. *Ann Intern Med.* 2010;153(6): 396–399

85. Yanovitch T, Wallace DK, Freedman SF, et al. The accuracy of photoscreening at detecting treatable ocular conditions in children with Down syndrome. *J AAPOS.* 2010;14(6):472–477

86. Berk AT, Saatci AO, Erçal MD, Tunç M, Ergin M. Ocular findings in 55 patients with Down's syndrome. *Ophthalmic Genet.* 1996;17(1):15–19

87. Locke GR, Gardner JI, Van Epps EF. Atlas-dens interval (ADI) in children: a survey based on 200 normal cervical spines. *Am J Roentgenol Radium Ther Nucl Med.* 1966;97(1):135–140

88. Burke SW, French HG, Roberts JM, Johnston CE II, Whitecloud TS III, Edmunds JO Jr. Chronic atlanto-axial instability in Down syndrome. *J Bone Joint Surg Am.* 1985;67(9):1356–1360

89. Morton RE, Khan MA, Murray-Leslie C, Elliott S. Atlantoaxial instability in Down's syndrome: a five year follow up study. *Arch Dis Child.* 1995;72(2): 115–118, discussion 118–119

90. Hengartner AC, Whelan R, Maj R, Wolter-Warmerdam K, Hickey F, Hankinson

TC. Evaluation of 2011 AAP cervical spine screening guidelines for children with Down Syndrome. *Childs Nerv Syst.* 2020;36(11):2609–2614

91. Pueschel SM, Scola FH, Pezzullo JC. A longitudinal study of atlanto-dens relationships in asymptomatic individuals with Down syndrome. *Pediatrics.* 1992;89(6 Pt 2):1194–1198

92. Ferguson RL, Putney ME, Allen BL Jr. Comparison of neurologic deficits with atlanto-dens intervals in patients with Down syndrome. *J Spinal Disord.* 1997;10(3):246–252

93. Nader-Sepahi A, Casey AT, Hayward R, Crockard HA, Thompson D. Symptomatic atlantoaxial instability in Down syndrome. *J Neurosurg.* 2005;103(3 Suppl):231–237

94. Special Olympics. Athlete Medical Form – Health History. Available at: http://media.specialolympics.org/resources/health/disciplines/medfest/MedFest-Health-History-and-Physical-Exam-Form-NON-US-Programs-fillable.pdf. Accessed March 25, 2022

95. Brockmeyer D. Down syndrome and craniovertebral instability. Topic review and treatment recommendations. *Pediatr Neurosurg.* 1999;31(2):71–77

96. Briskin S, LaBotz M. Council on Sports Medicine and Fitness; American Academy of Pediatrics. Trampoline safety in childhood and adolescence. *Pediatrics.* 2012;130(4):774–779. Reaffirmed July 2015, March 2020

97. Hill ID, Dirks MH, Liptak GS, et al. North American Society for Pediatric Gastroenterology, Hepatology and Nutrition. Guideline for the diagnosis and treatment of celiac disease in children: recommendations of the North American Society for Pediatric Gastroenterology, Hepatology and Nutrition. *J Pediatr Gastroenterol Nutr.* 2005;40(1):1–19

98. Bonamico M, Mariani P, Danesi HM, et al. SIGEP (Italian Society of Pediatric Gastroenterology and Hepatology) and Medical Genetic Group. Prevalence and clinical picture of celiac disease in italian down syndrome patients: a multicenter study. *J Pediatr Gastroenterol Nutr.* 2001;33(2):139–143

99. Swigonski NL, Kuhlenschmidt HL, Bull MJ, Corkins MR, Downs SM. Screening for celiac disease in asymptomatic

children with Down syndrome: cost-effectiveness of preventing lymphoma. *Pediatrics.* 2006;118(2):594–602

100. Ng DK, Chan CH, Cheung JM. Children with Down syndrome and OSA do not necessarily snore. *Arch Dis Child.* 2007;92(11):1047–1048

101. Bassett EC, Musso MF. Otolaryngologic management of Down syndrome patients: what is new? *Curr Opin Otolaryngol Head Neck Surg.* 2017;25(6):493–497

102. Farhood Z, Isley JW, Ong AA, et al. Adenotonsillectomy outcomes in patients with Down syndrome and obstructive sleep apnea. *Laryngoscope.* 2017;127(6):1465–1470

103. Bertapelli F, Pitetti K, Agiovlasitis S, Guerra-Junior G. Overweight and obesity in children and adolescents with Down syndrome-prevalence, determinants, consequences, and interventions: A literature review. *Res Dev Disabil.* 2016;57:181–192

104. Wolraich ML, Hagan JF Jr, Allan C, et al. Subcommittee on Children and Adolescents With Attention-Deficit/Hyperactive Disorder. Clinical practice guideline for the diagnosis, evaluation, and treatment of attention-deficit/hyperactivity disorder in children and adolescents. *Pediatrics.* 2019;144(4):e20192528

105. Molloy CA, Murray DS, Kinsman A, et al. Differences in the clinical presentation of trisomy 21 with and without autism. *J Intellect Disabil Res.* 2009;53(2):143–151

106. Rasmussen P, Börjesson O, Wentz E, Gillberg C. Autistic disorders in Down syndrome: background factors and clinical correlates. *Dev Med Child Neurol.* 2001;43(11):750–754

107. Kielinen M, Rantala H, Timonen E, Linna SL, Moilanen I. Associated medical disorders and disabilities in children with autistic disorder: a population-based study. *Autism.* 2004;8(1):49–60

108. Capone GT, Grados MA, Kaufmann WE, Bernad-Ripoll S, Jewell A. Down syndrome and comorbid autism-spectrum disorder: characterization using the aberrant behavior checklist. *Am J Med Genet A.* 2005;134(4):373–380

109. Carter JC, Capone GT, Gray RM, Cox CS, Kaufmann WE. Autistic-spectrum disorders in Down syndrome: further delineation and distinction from other behavioral abnormalities. *Am J Med Genet B Neuropsychiatr Genet.* 2007;144B(1):87–94

110. Dressler A, Perelli V, Bozza M, Bargagna S. The autistic phenotype in Down syndrome: differences in adaptive behaviour versus Down syndrome alone and autistic disorder alone. *Funct Neurol.* 2011;26(3):151–158

111. Hyman SL, Levy SE, Myers SM. Council on Children With Disabilities, Section on Developmental and Behavioral Pediatrics. Identification, evaluation, and management of children with autism spectrum disorder. *Pediatrics.* 2020;145(1):e20193447

112. Prasher V. Disintegrative syndrome in young adults. *Ir J Psychol Med.* 2002;19(3):101

113. Worley G, Crissman BG, Cadogan E, Milleson C, Adkins DW, Kishnani PS. Down syndrome disintegrative disorder: new-onset autistic regression, dementia, and insomnia in older children and adolescents with Down syndrome. *J Child Neurol.* 2015;30(9):1147–1152

114. Pikora TJ, Bourke J, Bathgate K, Foley KR, Lennox N, Leonard H. Health conditions and their impact among adolescents and young adults with Down syndrome. *PLoS One.* 2014;9(5):e96868

115. Rork JF, McCormack L, Lal K, Wiss K, Belazarian L. Dermatologic conditions in Down syndrome: a single-center retrospective chart review. *Pediatr Dermatol.* 2020;37(5):811–816

116. Chow KM, O'Donnell D. Concomitant occurrence of hypodontia and supernumerary teeth in a patient with Down syndrome. *Spec Care Dentist.* 1997;17(2):54–57

117. Andersson EM, Axelsson S, Austeng ME, et al. Bilateral hypodontia is more common than unilateral hypodontia in children with Down syndrome: a prospective population-based study. *Eur J Orthod.* 2014;36(4):414–418

118. Couwenhoven T. *Teaching Children with Down Syndrome about Their Bodies, Boundaries, and Sexuality (Topics in Down Syndrome).* Bethesda, MD: Woodbine House, Inc.; 2007

119. Stein, DS. *Supporting Positive Behavior in Children and Teens With Syndrome: The Respond but Don't React Method.* Bethesda, MD: Woodbine House; 2016.

120. Centers for Disease Control and Prevention (CDC). Growth Charts for Children with Down Syndrome. Available at: https://www.cdc.gov/ncbddd/birthdefects/downsyndrome/growth-charts.html. Accessed March 25, 2022

121. Brodtmann A. Hashimoto encephalopathy and Down syndrome. *Arch Neurol.* 2009;66(5):663–666

122. Palumbo ML, McDougle CJ. Pharmacotherapy of Down syndrome. *Expert Opin Pharmacother.* 2018;19(17):1875–1889

123. Centers for Disease Control and Prevention. CDC Contraceptive Guidance for Health Care Providers. Available at: https://www.cdc.gov/reproductive-health/contraception/contraception_guidance.htm. Accessed March 25, 2022

124. Gardner RJMSG. *Chromosome Abnormalities and Genetic Counseling,* 3rd ed. New York, NY: Oxford University Press; 2004

125. Sheridan R, Llerena J Jr, Matkins S, Debenham P, Cawood A, Bobrow M. Fertility in a male with trisomy 21. *J Med Genet.* 1989;26(5):294–298

126. Pradhan M, Dalal A, Khan F, Agrawal S. Fertility in men with Down syndrome: a case report. *Fertil Steril.* 2006;86(6):1765.e1–1765.e3

127. Katz AL, Webb SA. Committee on Bioethics. Informed consent in decision-making in pediatric practice. *Pediatrics.* 2016;138(2):e20161485

128. Burke LM, Kalpakjian CZ, Smith YR, Quint EH. Gynecologic issues of adolescents with Down syndrome, autism, and cerebral palsy. *J Pediatr Adolesc Gynecol.* 2010;23(1):11–15

129. Carbone PSSP, Smith PJ, Lewis C, LeBlanc C. Promoting the participation of children and adolescents with disabilities in sports, recreation, and physical activity. *Pediatrics.* 2021;148(6):e2021054664

130. Zuckerbrot RA, Cheung A, Jensen PS, Stein REK, Laraque D. GLAD-PC Steering

Group. Guidelines for adolescent depression in primary care (GLAD-PC): part I. Practice preparation, identification, assessment, and initial management. *Pediatrics*. 2018;141(3): e20174081

131. Garg A, Strunk A, Midura M, Papagermanos V, Pomerantz H. Prevalence of hidradenitis suppurativa among patients with Down syndrome: a population-based cross-sectional analysis. *Br J Dermatol*. 2018;178(3):697–703

132. IRS. Able Act 2014. Available at: www. irs.gov/government-entities/ federal-state-local-governments. Accessed August 7, 2020

133. White PH, Cooley WC; Transitions Clinical Report Authoring Group; American Academy of Pediatrics; American Academy of Family Physicians; American College of Physicians. Supporting the health care transition from adolescence to adulthood in the medical home. *Pediatrics*. 2018;142(5): e20182587

134. Wiseman FK, Al-Janabi T, Hardy J, et al. A genetic cause of Alzheimer disease: mechanistic insights from Down syndrome. *Nat Rev Neurosci*. 2015;16(9): 564–574

135. American College of Obstetricians and Gynecologists' Committee on Adolescent Health Care. Committee opinion no. 668: menstrual manipulation for adolescents with physical and developmental disabilities. *Obstet Gynecol*. 2016;128(2):e20–e25

136. Kirkham YA, Allen L, Kives S, Caccia N, Spitzer RF, Ornstein MP. Trends in menstrual concerns and suppression in adolescents with developmental disabilities. *J Adolesc Health*. 2013;53(3): 407–412

137. Got Transition. Available at: https:// www.gottransition.org/six-core-elements/. Accessed March 25, 2022

138. Tsou AY, Bulova P, Capone G, et al. Global Down Syndrome Foundation Medical Care Guidelines for Adults with Down Syndrome Workgroup. Medical care of adults with Down syndrome: a clinical guideline. *JAMA*. 2020;324(15): 1543–1556

139. Rasmussen SA, Whitehead N, Collier SA, Frías JL. Setting a public health research agenda for Down syndrome: summary of a meeting sponsored by the Centers for Disease Control and Prevention and the National Down Syndrome Society. *Am J Med Genet A*. 2008;146A(23):2998–3010

140. Eunice Kennedy Shriver National Institute of Child Health and Human Development NIoH, Department of Health and Human Services. National Institutes of Health Research Plan on Down Syndrome (NA). Washington, DC: US Government Printing Office; 2007

141. National Institutes of Health. The INCLUDE Project. Available at: https:/ www.nih.gov/include-project. Accessed March 25, 2022

Supplemental Information

SUPPLEMENTAL FIGURE 1. Summary of Down syndrome-specific care.

Action	Prenatal	Birth up to 1 mo	1 mo up to 1 yr	1 yr up to 5 yr	5 yr up to 12 yr	12 yr up to 21 yr
1. Confirm DS diagnosis with either CVS or amniocentesis prenatally or karyotype postnatally	▓					
2. Review recurrence risk and offer the family referral to a clinical geneticist or genetic counselor.						
3. Offer parent-to-parent and support group information to the family.						
4. Use CDC DS-specific growth charts to monitor weight, length, weight-for-length, head circumference, or BMI. Use standard charts for BMI after age 10 years.		All healthcare visits				
5. Order an echo, to be read by a pediatric cardiologist.		▓				
6. Feeding assessment or video study if any: marked hypotonia, underweight (<5th %ile weight-for-length or BMI), slow feeding or choking with feeds, recurrent or persistent abnormal respiratory symptoms, desaturations with feeds		Any visit				
7. Obtain objective hearing assessment (may be in NBS protocols) and follow EHDI protocols.		▓	Up to 6 mo			
8. If TM can't be visualized, refer to otolaryngologist for exam with microscope until reliable TM and tympanometry exams are possible		Every 3-6 mo	‖‖			
9. Car safety seat evaluation before hospital discharge.		▓				
10. CBC with differential		By day 3				
11. If TAM, make caregivers aware of risk/signs of leukemia (e.g., easy bruising/bleeding, recurrent fevers, bone pain)		▓				
12. TSH		At birth (if not in NBS)	Every 5-7 mo	Annually, and every 6 mo if antithyroid antibodies ever detected		
13. RSV prophylaxis based on AAP guidelines.		Annually	Through 2 yr			
14. Discuss cervical spine-positioning for procedures and atlantoaxial stability precautions.		All HMV	Biennially			
15. Assess for CAM use, discourage any unsafe CAM practices.		All HMV				
16. Refer children to early intervention for speech, fine motor or gross motor therapy.		Any visit	Up to 3 yr			
17. If middle ear disease occurs, obtain developmentally-appropriate hearing evaluation.			When ear clear	After treatment		
18. Rescreen hearing with developmentally-appropriate methodology (BAER, behavioral, ear-specific).			Start at 6mo, every 6 mo until established normal bilaterally by ear-specific testing, then annually			
19. Refer to ophthalmologist with experience and expertise in children with disabilities.			By 6 mo			
20. CBC with differential if easy bruising or bleeding, recurrent fevers, or bone pain			Any visit			
21. Assess for sleep-disordered breathing; if present, refer to physician with expertise in pediatric sleep disorders.			At least once by 6 mo, then all subsequent HMV thereafter			
22. Ensure child is receiving developmental therapies, and family understands and is following therapy plan at home.		All HMV				
23. CBC with differential and either (1) a combination of ferritin and CRP, or (2) a combination of serum iron and Total Iron Binding Capacity				Annually		
24. If a child has sleep problems and a ferritin less than 50 mcg/L, the pediatrician may prescribe iron supplement.				Any visit		
25. Vision screening			All HMV, use developmentally-appropriate criteria	Photoscreen (all HMV); if unable, refer to ophthalmologist annually	Photoscreen (all HMV); if unable, refer to ophthalmologist biennially	Visual acuity or photoscreening at all HMV, or ophthalmology-determined schedule
26. If a child has myelopathic symptoms, obtain neutral C-spine plain films (see text for details).				Any visit		
27. Obtain polysomnogram.				Between 3-5 yr		
28. Prepare family for transition from early intervention to preschool.				At 30 mo		
29. Discuss sexual exploitation risks.				At least once	At least once	At least once
30. Make developmentally-appropriate plans for menarche, contraception (advocate/offer LARC), and STI prevention.					As developmentally-appropriate, then all subsequent HMV	
31. Discuss risk of DS if patient were to become pregnant.					At least once	At least once
32. Assess for any developmental regression.			All HMV			
33. Discuss and facilitate transitions: education, work, finance, guardianship, medical care, independent living					All HMV starting at 10 yr	

▓	Do once at this age	
░	Do if not done previously	
	Repeat at indicated intervals	
(border)	‖‖ See report for end point	

Abbreviations: DS, Down syndrome; CVS, Chorionic villus sampling; HMV, Health Maintenance Visit; BMI, Body mass index; CDC, Centers for Disease Control; EHDI, Early Hearing Detection and Intervention; NBS, Newborn screen; CAM, Complementary and alternative medicine; BAER, Brainstem auditory evoked response; TM, Tympanic membrane; TAM: transient abnormal myelopoiesis

CLINICAL REPORT Guidance for the Clinician in Rendering Pediatric Care

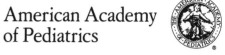

American Academy
of Pediatrics

DEDICATED TO THE HEALTH OF ALL CHILDREN™

Promoting Healthy Sexuality for Children and Adolescents With Disabilities

Amy Houtrow, MD, PhD, MPH, FAAP,[a] Ellen Roy Elias, MD, FAAP, FACMG,[b] Beth Ellen Davis, MD, MPH, FAAP,[c]
COUNCIL ON CHILDREN WITH DISABILITIES Dennis Z. Kuo, MD, MHS, FAAP Rishi Agrawal, MD, MPH, FAAP
Lynn F. Davidson, MD, FAAP Kathryn A. Ellerbeck, MD, FAAP Jessica E.A. Foster, MD, MPH, FAAP Ellen Fremion, MD, FAAP, FACP
Mary O'Connor Leppert, MD, FAAP Barbara S. Saunders, DO, FAAP Christopher Stille, MD, MPH, FAAP
Jilda Vargus-Adams, MD, MSc, FAAP Larry Yin, MD, MSPH, FAAP Kenneth NorwoodJr,MD, FAAP Cara Coleman, JD, MPH
Marie Y. Mann, MD, MPH, FAAP Edwin Simpser, MD, FAAP Jennifer Poon, MD, FAAP Marshalyn Yeargin-Allsopp, MD, FAAP, and
Alexandra Kuznetsov

This clinical report updates a 2006 report from the American Academy of Pediatrics titled "Sexuality of Children and Adolescents With Developmental Disabilities." The development of a healthy sexuality best occurs through appropriate education, absence of coercion and violence, and developmental acquisition of skills to navigate feelings, desires, relationships, and social pressures. Pediatric health care providers are important resources for anticipatory guidance and education for all children and youth as they understand their changing bodies, feelings, and behaviors. Yet, youth with disabilities and their families report inadequate education and guidance from pediatricians regarding sexual health development. In the decade since the original clinical report was published, there have been many advancements in the understanding and care of children and youth with disabilities, in part because of an increased prevalence and breadth of autism spectrum disorder as well as an increased longevity of individuals with medically complex and severely disabling conditions. During this same time frame, sexual education in US public schools has diminished, and there is emerging evidence that the attitudes and beliefs of all youth (with and without disability) about sex and sexuality are being formed through media rather than formal education or parent and/or health care provider sources. This report aims to provide the pediatric health care provider with resources and tools for clinical practice to address the sexual development of children and youth with disabilities. The report emphasizes strategies to promote competence in achieving a healthy sexuality regardless of physical, cognitive, or socioemotional limitations.

abstract

[a]Division of Pediatric Rehabilitation Medicine, Department of Physical Medicine and Rehabilitation, School of Medicine, University of Pittsburgh, Pittsburgh, Pennsylvania; [b]School of Medicine, University of Colorado and Special Care Clinic, Children's Hospital Colorado, Aurora, Colorado; and [c]School of Medicine, University of Virginia and University of Virginia Children's Hospital, Charlottesville, Virginia

Dr Houtrow reviewed the literature, drafted the manuscript, and critically edited the content; Drs Elias and Davis reviewed the literature, added content to the manuscript, and critically edited the content; and all authors approved the final manuscript as submitted.

This document is copyrighted and is property of the American Academy of Pediatrics and its Board of Directors. All authors have filed conflict of interest statements with the American Academy of Pediatrics. Any conflicts have been resolved through a process approved by the Board of Directors. The American Academy of Pediatrics has neither solicited nor accepted any commercial involvement in the development of the content of this publication.

Clinical reports from the American Academy of Pediatrics benefit from expertise and resources of liaisons and internal (AAP) and external reviewers. However, clinical reports from the American Academy of Pediatrics may not reflect the views of the liaisons or the organizations or government agencies that they represent.

The guidance in this report does not indicate an exclusive course of treatment or serve as a standard of medical care. Variations, taking into account individual circumstances, may be appropriate.

All clinical reports from the American Academy of Pediatrics automatically expire 5 years after publication unless reaffirmed, revised, or retired at or before that time.

To cite: Houtrow A, Elias E R, Davis B E, et al. Promoting Healthy Sexuality for Children and Adolescents With Disabilities. *Pediatrics.* 2021;148(1):e2021052043

INTRODUCTION

As stated by the World Health Organization, "Sexual health is a state of physical, emotional, mental and social well-being in relation to sexuality ... Sexual health requires a positive and respectful approach to sexuality and sexual relationships, as well as to the possibility of having pleasurable and safe sexual experiences, free of coercion, discrimination, and violence."[1] One's sexuality is experienced through one's thoughts and desires; attitudes, beliefs, and values; and actions, behaviors, and relationships.[1] Developing healthy sexuality is important for all individuals and depends, in part, on having evidenced-based and evidence-informed information to formulate attitudes and beliefs about sexual orientation, gender identity, relationships, and intimacy.[2-4] It is well known that sexual satisfaction and intimacy are directly related to quality of life,[5] and, thus, pediatric health care providers are encouraged to address the sexual health and education needs of their patients as they grow and develop to promote their patients' competence in achieving a healthy sexuality. Generally speaking, pediatric health care providers are an important resource for sexual education and counseling for children, adolescents, and young adults as well as for parents seeking anticipatory guidance.[6] Pediatric health care providers can help patients and their parents/caregivers understand their changing feelings, their changing bodies, their desires for relationships, and how to avoid risky sexual situations.[6] As is true for everyone, it is important that individuals with disabilities be provided experiences to acquire developmentally appropriate, relevant, and accurate sexual health knowledge to become competent. Youth with disabilities need regular opportunities to develop and use skills for negotiating sexual

desire, intimacy, and activity that supports healthy sexuality while limiting negative outcomes of sexual activity (such as sexually transmitted infections [STIs], unintended pregnancy or sexual coercion, violence, abuse, or exploitation) regardless of their intellectual capacity. Culturally responsive pediatric health care should include sexual health as a focus for all children and adolescents, including those with disabilities, and actively involve parents and caregivers, while respecting the youth's autonomy and rights to privacy.[2]

THE SEXUAL HEALTH NEEDS OF CHILDREN AND YOUTH WITH DISABILITIES

Children with disabilities are a growing subset of children with diverse needs that affect their functioning, health, and well-being. More than 10 million children in the United States have health conditions that moderately or consistently affect their daily activities at least some of the time.[7] This means that most pediatric primary care providers routinely care for children and youth with a broad range of developmental and acquired health conditions that affect their ability to function as children typically do or require special services such as Individualized Education Programs at school.[8] Disabilities experienced in childhood may be primarily physical in nature or associated with intellectual and/or social-communication impairments or may involve co-occurring conditions. The associated health condition or etiology of the disability or disabilities, the severity of the disability or disabilities, and what aspects of functioning are affected all influence how sexuality is addressed in the clinical setting.

Developing a healthy sexuality is a complex process for all children and youth, especially those with disabilities. Sexual development is not just physiologic changes of a

person's body but is a key part of social competency and should be considered in the context of basic human desires for connectedness and intimacy, beliefs, values, and aspirations. Sociosexual development is an essential part of growing up, and emphasis on this aspect of development is especially important for individuals with disabilities as they navigate changing bodies, expectations, and desires.[9] Individuals with all types of disabilities may have to negotiate varying and unique reproductive capacity and sexual intimacy issues, yet they routinely experience inadequate education and opportunities to develop competence.[10,11] Ample research indicates people with disabilities receive substandard sexual education and reproductive health care.[12-15] Families and/or caregivers of children with disabilities may be reluctant or feel that they are not empowered to acknowledge their child's potential as a sexual individual and may shelter them from the routine presexual social experiences of other children and underestimate their interest in sex and their risk for exploitation.[10,16] Helping families and/or caregivers understand their children's sexual development and how to support it may require additional time and counseling to address expectations of all involved around appropriate independence and autonomy through shared decision-making strategies.[17] In addition, children with disabilities are often limited in social participation and social networks outside of school,[10,18] which offer typical social experiences that form the developmental framework toward understanding one's own individual sexuality, interests, and behaviors. The lack of understanding about how disability affects sexual expression likely influences health care providers' willingness to address it, as does the more general stigmatization of people with disabilities as nonsexual beings.[19]

LIFECOURSE APPROACH TO SEXUALITY AND SEXUAL HEALTH FOR INDIVIDUALS WITH DISABILITIES

Bright Futures: Guidelines for Health Supervision of Infants, Children, and Adolescents, Fourth Edition, provides the foundation for pediatric health care providers to promote healthy sexual development.[20] Care and education should be delivered through a longitudinal, developmentally appropriate, culturally respectful relationship between health care providers and their patients and families, caregivers, and educators.[20] In the last 10 years, sexuality education resources specifically designed for individuals with specific health conditions have emerged (Table 1).[21] Routine health maintenance and chronic health care visits, including health care

TABLE 1 Sexuality Education Resources for Pediatric Health Care Providers

	Resource Information
For parents	
Center for Parent Information & Resources	www.parentcenterhub.org (also in Spanish)
Couwenhoven T. Boyfriends & Girlfriends: *A Guide to Dating for People With Disabilities*. Bethesda, MD: Woodbine House; 2015	—
Healthybodies.org (Vanderbilt) Boys/Girls	https://vkc.vumc.org/healthybodies/files/HealthyBodies-Boys-web.pdf; Includes a free online packet entitled "Healthy Bodies for Boys: A Parent's Guide for Boys with Disabilities" (and a separate one for girls); https://vkc.vumc.org/healthybodies/files/HealthyBodies-Girls-web.pdf
Bright Futures: Guidelines for Health Supervision of Infants, Children, and Adolescents, Fourth Edition	https://brightfutures.aap.org/Pages/default.aspx; Promoting Healthy Sexual Development and Sexuality; Adolescent Visits
Sexuality Resource Center for Parents	Teaching children across the age ranges 0–18; http://www.srcp.org/for_all_parents/development.html
AMAZE	https://amaze.org AMAZE uses digital media to provide young adolescents with medically accurate, age-appropriate, affirming, and honest sex education they can access directly online. AMAZE also strives to assist adults—parents, guardians, educators and health care providers—to communicate effectively and honestly about sex and sexuality with the children and adolescents in their lives. www.amaze.org
Condition-specific resources for pediatric health care providers	
ASD	AAP Autism Toolkit (Handout): Sexuality of Children and Youths with Autism Spectrum Disorder: https://toolkits.solutions.aap.org/autism/handout/504891; Autism Speaks: ATN/AIR-P Puberty and Adolescence Resource: https://www.autismspeaks.org/docs/family_services_docs/parentworkbook.pdf; Kate E. Reynolds books to help learn about puberty: *What's Happening to Ellie? A Book About Puberty for Girls and Young Women With Autism and Related Conditions* (2015); *What's Happening to Tom? A Book About Puberty for Boys and Young Men With Autism and Related Conditions* (2015)
Cerebral palsy	Glader L, Stevenson R. *Children and Youth with Complex Cerebral Palsy: Care and Management*. London, United Kingdom: Mac Keith Press; 2019. (chapters 17 and 18)
Spina bifida	The Spina Bifida Association: https://www.spinabifidaassociation.org/guidelines/; Centers for Disease Control and Prevention: https://www.cdc.gov/ncbddd/spinabifida/adult.html#sexual-health
Down syndrome	Chicoine B, McGuire D. *The Guide to Good Health for Teens and Adults with Down Syndrome*. Bethesda, MD: Woodbine House; 2010; Couwenhoven T. *Teaching Children with Down Syndrome About Their Bodies, Boundaries, and Sexuality: A Guide for Parents and Professionals*. Bethesda, MD: Woodbine House; 2005
Other	US National Library of Medicine, Genetics Home Reference: https://ghr.nlm.nih.gov/condition; An up-to-date genetic review of genetic conditions, easily searchable alphabetically, including rare microdeletions
For schools and educators	
Sexuality and Disabilities: A Guide for Professionals	https://www.routledge.com/Sexuality-and-Intellectual-Disabilities-A-Guide-for-Professionals/Triska/p/book/9781138231023 (2018). This book provides a concise overview of sexuality and gender identity in clients with intellectual disabilities for therapists, social workers, educators, and health care providers
Seattle and King County Sexual Health Education Curriculum	https://www.kingcounty.gov/depts/health/locations/family-planning/education/FLASH.aspx
Advocates for Youth	https://advocatesforyouth.org/wp-content/uploads/storage//advfy/documents/Factsheets/sexual--health-education-for-young-people-with-disabilities-educators.pdf

—, not applicable

transition preparation visits, afford opportunities for the pediatric health care provider to gather information, give guidance, provide education, and be a resource regarding sexuality for children and adolescents with disabilities as they develop their skills and competence.[6,20,22] Pediatric health care providers can introduce issues of psychosexual development to families and caregivers and their children in early childhood and have discussions at health maintenance visits throughout childhood, adolescence, and young adulthood.[2] Doing so, on a routine basis, helps normalize the topic and helps reinforce understanding. The education should go beyond the basics of anatomy and physiology of puberty and reproduction to incorporate education about gender identity, sexual orientation, interpersonal relationships, intimacy, the types of sexual expression, and body image.[23,24] Culturally responsive care recognizes that sexuality is influenced by personal and environmental factors, such as religion or ethnic background.[2] It is essential for developmentally appropriate sexuality education to start early in childhood, with families and/or caregivers and primary care providers helping young children to develop a safe, healthy, and positive attitude toward themselves and others. This healthy and safe attitude includes understanding respect, consent, and relationship building.[25]

ADDRESSING PUBERTAL DEVELOPMENT IN CHILDREN WITH DISABILITIES

Like any child, a child with disabilities may feel anxious and unhappy about how their body is changing during puberty. The timing of onset of puberty (Table 2) in a child with disabilities may be different from that of a typically developing child.[26] Some patients with severe nutritional issues may be late to go through puberty because of failure to thrive and low BMI and may achieve menarche late or have sparse menses that start at an older age than typical. Patients with certain genetic disorders or conditions associated with chromosome abnormalities[27] may require hormonal treatment to enter and proceed through puberty.

Conversely, patients with certain neurologic disorders, including myelomeningocele or hydrocephalus, have a greater chance of early adrenarche and pubarche, and girls may achieve menarche at younger than 10 years (Table 2).[28] Central precocious puberty is defined as the full activation of the hypothalamic-pituitary-gonadal axis before 8 years of age in genetic girls and before 9 years of age in genetic boys.[29,30] Central precocious puberty is more common in children with fragile X syndrome, congenital brain malformations, and a history of birth asphyxia, meningitis, or other acquired brain injury.[31]

Menstrual Manipulation and/or Suppression

Although menstruation is often not a barrier to care and well-being, there are a number of concerns that face the primary caregivers of individuals with disabilities once they achieve menarche.[32] These concerns may include hygiene issues (especially for individuals who cannot use a toilet independently), worsening seizures, worsening cyclical behavioral problems, discomfort for the child or adolescent (including breast tenderness and headaches), difficulty for a caregiver who is not comfortable dealing with menses, and difficulty coping at school.[33,34] Menstrual hygiene issues can be introduced early in puberty, even before menarche, and with caregiver shared decision-making, providers can help identify ways to foster independence and teach individuals with disabilities how to manage their menses or seek appropriate help, such as from the school nurse. It is important for caregivers to understand that amenorrhea is often not achieved immediately but that menstrual manipulation may be used to induce amenorrhea, better regulate cycles, or decrease the amount or duration of menstrual flow and minimize menstrual pain and/or dysmenorrhea.[35] Providers interested in understanding the myriad available options are encouraged to review the clinical report from the American Academy of Pediatrics (AAP) and the North American Society for Pediatric and

TABLE 2 Common Differences of Timing of Puberty in Patients with Disabilities

Early-Onset Puberty	Typical Puberty	Delayed Puberty
Congenital brain malformations	Varies by family, ethnic, and racial groups	Severe nutritional deficiency
Hydrocephalus	Attention-deficit/hyperactivity disorder	Hormonal abnormalities
Neural tube defects; myelomeningocele	Children with ASD with typical growth	Sex chromosome abnormalities
Epilepsy	Other behavioral and mental health issues	Chromosome abnormalities (ie, trisomy 21)
Severe cognitive disabilities	Mild and moderate cognitive disabilities	Complex disabilities
Brain injuries		Psychiatric medications causing high prolactin
Some genetic conditions such as fragile X, neurofibromatosis 1, tuberous sclerosis, and McCune-Albright syndrome		

Adolescent Gynecology, "Menstrual Management for Adolescents With Disabilities."[32] Surgical options for menstrual suppression are rarely indicated. Menstrual suppression before menarche and endometrial ablation are not recommended.[36] Permanent decisions regarding sterilization have ethical, legal, and medical implications, vary by state, and are beyond the scope of this report. There are also important ethical issues to consider such as patient autonomy and independent decision-making, separate from caregiver issues related to menstrual manipulation in general.[37] Having a conversation and physical examination performed in a confidential manner with appropriate chaperoning and consenting and the caregiver excused from the room is an important practice, especially for those patients with physical disabilities alone or cognitive disabilities requiring limited supports (mild intellectual disability). A confidential examination provides an opportunity to assess the individual's sexual health knowledge and risks or history of abuse or coercion.[6,35] Addressing menstruation can also foster a discussion regarding sexual activity, the risk of sexual victimization, and the need to prevent STIs and pregnancy.

STI and Pregnancy Prevention

Although individuals with disabilities may be delayed, compared with their peers, in terms of first sexual encounters, they are more likely to engage in unsafe sex practices, which is especially true for those with mild disabilities.[38,39] Some youth, such as youth with attention-deficit/hyperactivity disorder, are more likely than their peers to engage in sexual activity earlier and also engage in unsafe sex practices.[40,41] All sexually active

adolescents are at risk for STIs, including HIV, and, therefore, should be counseled about how to reduce their risks, including the use of barrier protection, in addition to long-acting reversible contraception, as appropriate.[2,6,42–44] Sexual minority youth often do not receive counseling appropriate for their sexuality; therefore, the pediatric health care provider should tailor counseling on the basis of the youth's specific needs when possible.[45] Providers should encourage and facilitate family-child communication about sexual health and confidentially ensure that any sexual activity is consensual for the youth.[6,45] Confidential family planning services and sexual health care should be made available to adolescents in accordance with legal obligations.[2,27,32,46] Effective counseling is characterized by compassion, respect, a nonjudgmental attitude, and using open-ended questions.[47] Shared decision-making strategies can be employed to enhance the autonomy of the individual with disabilities and can help ensure that all voices are heard during the decision-making process.[17]

Human Papillomavirus Vaccine

Vaccination against human papillomavirus (HPV) has become one of the most successful vaccination programs, not only to prevent this STI but also to significantly reduce certain cancers. Because of the efficacy and safety of the HPV vaccine, all pediatric patients, including those with disabilities, should receive a full course of this vaccine.[48,49] Patients with a history of sexual abuse or violence should receive the HPV series starting at 9 years of age.[50]

Counseling Regarding Genetic Reproductive Risks

Many patients with disabilities may have an underlying genetic disorder

as their primary diagnosis, which carries a recurrence risk.[51] Often, the diagnosis is made during infancy or early childhood and communicated with the family, but it is common that the diagnosis and recurrence risk may never have been formally discussed with the patient as he or she approaches reproductive age. Part of caring for patients with genetic disorders as they reach an age in which they may become sexually active or pregnant is to make sure that patients receive appropriate genetic counseling (such as with a genetic counselor) to understand contraception options and their reproductive risks.[52] Table 3 lists reproductive risks for some common genetic disorders. Extensive information regarding trisomy 21 is available in the health supervision guidance from the AAP.[53] There are thousands of genetic conditions that may be associated with disabilities for which the pediatric health care provider can find additional condition-specific information by searching https://ghr.nlm.nih.gov/condition. In addition, youth with disabilities may be taking medications that alter sexual function or have teratogenic effects. Screening and counseling regarding medication adverse effects are important aspects of ensuring optimal sexual and reproductive health.

ADDRESSING THE RISKS OF SEXUAL ABUSE AGAINST CHILDREN AND YOUTH WITH DISABILITIES

Children with disabilities of all types are nearly 3 times as likely as those without disabilities to be sexually abused, and the risks are increased further for children with intellectual disabilities.[54] Although overall lifetime sexual violence victimization is low for men, men with disabilities have 3 times higher rates of victimization than men without disabilities do (13.8% vs 3.7%, respectively).[55] Nearly 25% of

TABLE 3 Reproductive Risks in Common Genetic Disorders

Genetic Disorder	Reproductive Risks
Autosomal dominant disorders	
Achondroplasia: most common form of skeletal dysplasia caused by a mutation in FGFR3	A person with achondroplasia whose partner has normal stature has a 50% chance of having a child with achondroplasia. A pregnant woman with achondroplasia may have difficulty carrying the fetus to term.
	If both genetic parents have achondroplasia, there is a 25% chance of having an infant with a lethal disorder who has 2 copies of the FGFR3 mutation.
Deletion of 22q11: common, with wide spectrum of presentation including intellectual disabilities, mental health issues, congenital heart disease, immunodeficiency, and hypoparathyroidism (formerly called DiGeorge syndrome)	A parent with mild learning problems or mental health issues can have a child with more complex birth defects and severe developmental problems.
	Chromosomal abnormalities, such as microdeletions, are passed on in an autosomal dominant pattern and may have variable severity of the phenotype from one generation to the next.
OI: most forms of brittle bone disease are caused by mutations in COL1A1 or COL1A2.	Confirmation of the diagnosis of OI can now be made with DNA analysis in blood.
	Most severe cases of OI arise from de novo mutations, but patients with milder forms of OI have a 50% chance of passing on their mutation in each pregnancy. There are more rare forms of OI caused by autosomal recessive genes with a 25% recurrence risk.
EDS: there are now 14 types of EDS	The hypermobile type is the most common with an estimated incidence of 1:5000. The genes for this type are unknown. This type can be associated with gastrointestinal tract issues, immunologic changes, dysautonomia, pelvic floor dysfunction, prolapse of the rectum and/or uterine prolapse, and chronic pain and disability.
	The vascular form of EDS can be associated with severe, life-threatening issues including arterial rupture, intestinal rupture, and uterine rupture in pregnancy.
Autosomal recessive disorders	A history of consanguinity increases the chances of having a partner who carries mutations in the same gene.
	Genetic boys with cystic fibrosis are sterile.
	Patients of certain ethnic backgrounds have a higher carrier rate of having mutations in autosomal recessive disorders; there are now next-generation sequencing panels that screen for carriers of certain disorders so that patients can receive genetic counseling regarding their recurrence risks.
	Many patients with autosomal recessive disorders have more severe disabilities and are less likely to procreate.
X-linked disorders	Females who are carriers of FMR1, which causes fragile X syndrome, have an increased risk of premature ovarian failure. The maternal grandfather may develop a condition that mimics Parkinson disease, called FRAXTAS.
	The severity of symptoms in female carriers of X-linked disorders may be affected by skewed X-inactivation.
	A female carrying a mutation in an X-linked gene (eg, fragile X syndrome) may be normal or have just a mild phenotype but has a risk of having a male child with more severe issues.
Mitochondrial disorders	Mitochondrial disorders may be caused by mutations in mitochondrial DNA, in which case they are maternally inherited, or may be caused by mutations in autosomal genes, in which case they are usually autosomal recessively inherited.
	Maternally inherited mitochondrial disorders are generally passed on to all children in the sibship, although the severity of issues may vary from one sibling to another.
Multifactorial disorders	
NTDs are common birth defects with an increased recurrence risk within families	Patients with NTDs have an ∼5% chance of having a child with an NTD.
	Siblings of patients with NTDs, parents, aunts, uncles, etc, also have an increased risk.
	Folate, 4 mg/kg per day, taken 3 mo before conception and through the first trimester, can decrease (but not eliminate) this risk.
	Certain ethnic groups (including people of English and/or Irish, Hispanic, and Chinese descent) have an increased risk of having a child with an NTD and might also consider taking folate prophylactically, even without a family history.
Other	Some disorders are caused by multiple factors including genes that may not be known, teratogens such as alcohol, or nutritional factors such as low folate. Recently available genetic tests including next-generation sequencing panels have helped make specific diagnoses in patients with rare disorders.

COL1A1, collagen type I alpha 1; COL1A2, collagen type I alpha 2; EDS, Ehlers-Danlos syndrome; FGFR3, fibroblast growth factor receptor 3; FRAXTAS, fragile X-associated tremor/ataxia syndrome; NTD, neural tube defect; OI, osteogenesis imperfecta.

adolescent women, regardless of disability status, report being victims of sexual abuse and/or assault.[56] In a cross-sectional survey of 101 students with disabilities from a large northeastern public university, 22% reported some form of abuse over the last year, and nearly 62% ($n = 63$) had experienced some form of physical or sexual abuse before the age of 17.[57] Of those who were abused in the past year, 40% reported little or no knowledge of abuse-related resources, and only 27% reported the incident.[57] Compared with respondents without disabilities, young women with physical disabilities had a higher odds of being a victim of rape (odds ratio: 1.49; 95% confidence interval: 1.06–2.08).[58] Perpetrators of sexual violence against people with disabilities often know their victims well. Nearly one-third of perpetrators of sexual abuse are family members or acquaintances, and an additional 44% of assailants had a care-provider relationship with their victims.[55]

Children and youth with disabilities are more vulnerable to sexual victimization, likely because of a variety of factors depending on the type of disability, including a decreased ability to resist an attack, a desire to please the other person without a full understanding of the circumstances, dependence on others for aspects of care and decision-making, limited communication skills, and increased tolerance of physical intrusion, among others.[55] For example, some individuals with intellectual disability may lack the decision-making capacity, ability to consent, and skills necessary to develop healthy relationships, which can be associated with sexual exploitation, abuse, or coercion.[59,60] Given the increased risk of sexual abuse, coercion, and assault, the pediatric

provider is encouraged to surveil often, in developmentally appropriate ways, and provide resources when a concern is raised.[2,55,61] As is the case for all children, health care providers are mandated reporters, and reporting should occur to the appropriate authorities[61,62] If the youth with disabilities is 18 years or older, reports should be made to adult protective services. In addition, children with disabilities may have been placed in foster care because of sexual abuse; therefore, the pediatric health care provider is encouraged to screen for a history of sexual violence for this population. Specific AAP policies on sexual abuse, coercion, and assault as they relate to children with disabilities can be found in Table 4.

TYPICAL AND PROBLEM SEXUAL BEHAVIORS

There are a wide range of typical and developmentally appropriate child and adolescent sexual behaviors that provide teachable moments for health care providers and families, especially during early development.[63] For example, when a preschooler undresses in the classroom, an adult can comment, "undressing is what we do privately before taking a bath, not in front of our friends at school." Children with developmental disabilities, including autism spectrum disorder (ASD), may extend the ages of typical sexual exploration. Providers need to consider social, cultural, religious, familial, and medical contexts for typical and problem behaviors. It is important to be able to differentiate signs of expected and/or typical versus atypical, aberrant, or problem sexual behaviors in children with disabilities and provide appropriate education and counseling on the topic.

Typical behaviors in early development, which may be seen in

older children who have developmental disabilities, include general sexual curiosity, masturbation, an interest in peer or sibling genitals, standing or sitting too close, trying to view adult nudity, and sometimes crude mimicking of movements associated with sexual acts. These are separated from uncommon and rarely typical behaviors, regardless of cognitive ability, such as explicit imitation of sexual acts, asking peers or adults to engage in sexual activities, insertion of objects into genitals, activity with children who are more than 4 years apart, and frequent sexual behaviors that are resistant to distraction.[63,64] Atypical behaviors at any age or developmental level include sexual behaviors that result in distress or pain, are associated with physical aggression or coercion, or become persistent and resistant to redirection. Sorting out behaviors that involve sexual offense from those that are problem behaviors and challenging to self or others can help determine the acuity and degree of intervention.[31] Regardless, challenging sexualized behaviors associated with developmental disabilities or acquired disorders such as brain injury require assessment of the reason for the behavior. Families and/or caregivers and the clinicians can work with schools, behavioral analysts, and/or psychologists to obtain a functional behavior assessment and customize behavioral interventions.[31,65]

Problem or inappropriate sexual behaviors, such as public masturbation and nonconsensual groping, are exhibited more commonly in children and adolescents with disabilities, specifically developmental disabilities, and may be the most problematic in those with ASD.[65] Core deficits in social reciprocity, communication, and sensory

TABLE 4 Relevant AAP Policy Statements, Clinical Reports, and Technical Reports

Title	Date of Publication and/or Reaffirmation
Long-Acting Reversible Contraception: Specific Issues for Adolescents	August 2020
Barrier Protection Use by Adolescents During Sexual Activity (Policy Statement); Barrier Protection Use by Adolescents During Sexual Activity (Technical Report)	August 2020
Emerging Issues in Male Adolescent Sexual and Reproductive Health Care	May 2020
Emergency Contraception	December 2019
Unique Needs of Adolescents	December 2019
Supporting the Health Care Transition From Adolescence to Adulthood in the Medical Home	November 2018
Ensuring Comprehensive Care and Support for Transgender and Gender-Diverse Children and Adolescents	October 2018
Counseling in Pediatric Population at Risk for Infertility and/or Sexual Dysfunction	August 2018
Sexual and Reproductive Health Care Services in the Pediatric Setting	November 2017
Shared Decision-making and Children with Disabilities: Pathways to Consensus	June 2017
Care of the Adolescent After an Acute Sexual Assault	March 2017; erratum June 2017
Sexuality Education for Children and Adolescents	August 2016
Menstrual Management for Adolescents with Disabilities	July 2016
Contraception for Adolescents	October 2014
Screening for Nonviral Sexually Transmitted Infections in Adolescents and Young Adults	July 2014
Condom Use by Adolescents	November 2013
The Evaluation of Children in the Primary Care Setting When Sexual Abuse Is Suspected	August 2013; reaffirmed August 2018
Office-Based Care for Lesbian, Gay, Bisexual, Transgender, and Questioning Youth (Policy Statement); Office-Based Care for Lesbian, Gay, Bisexual, Transgender, and Questioning Youth (Technical Report)	July 2013
Standards for Health Information Technology to Ensure Adolescent Privacy	November 2012; reaffirmed December 2018
Male Adolescent Sexual and Reproductive Health Care	December 2011; reaffirmed May 2015
Protecting Children from Sexual Abuse by Health Care Providers	August 2011; reaffirmed January 2020
The Use of Chaperones During the Physical Examination of the Pediatric Patient	May 2011; reaffirmed November 2017
Gynecologic Examination for Adolescents in the Pediatric Office Setting	September 2010; reaffirmed May 2013
The Evaluation of Sexual Behaviors in Children	September 2009; reaffirmed October 2018

processing likely contribute to poor adherence to sociosexual norms, as well a limited understanding of the consequences of sexual behavior. In a recent survey of both parents and youth, 29% of young adults with ASD experienced challenging sexualized behaviors, most commonly masturbation in public.[66] When parents of children and youth with ASD, Down syndrome, and typical development were interviewed, those with ASD had significantly more trouble in multiple domains of sexual functioning, including social behavior, privacy awareness, sex education, sexual behavior, and parental concerns.[67]

Improving sociosexual education can help prevent or minimize many of these behaviors and should begin at a young age.[68] Health care providers, educators, and family members and caregivers can work collaboratively toward extinguishing problem behaviors and use reminders, distractions, or replacement with socially appropriate gestures or places. Specific resources to address problem behaviors can be found in Table 5.

SEXUALITY AND ADOLESCENTS WITH ASD

Adulthood is a highly social construct. Negotiating the transition to adulthood from supervised, structured home and school settings can be challenging for all adolescents, especially for individuals with ASD.[69-71] It is not surprising that the core deficits of ASD, including difficulty with social reciprocity and pragmatic communication, complicate experiences and relationships of youth with ASD, compared with their typical or cognitively delayed peers.[67,72] Although youth and adults with ASD did not significantly differ from their counterparts without ASD in their knowledge of sexual language and interest in sexual experiences,[72,73] more than a dozen studies including direct report by individuals with ASD

TABLE 5 Resources for Problem Behaviors

Problem Behavior	Resources
Excessive or public masturbation	Suggested conversation: "Today, we discussed that masturbation is a normal behavior. Excessive and/or inappropriate masturbation is often difficult to control because it can be a self-reinforcing behavior. We discussed that although inappropriate masturbation, such as public masturbation, may not completely go away, your child can learn to be redirected to perform the behavior in private. The key to approaching this is to ensure that your child both has a personal space and that he or she understands the appropriate place for private behaviors. Recommend using a schedule or timer to set boundaries for these behaviors."
	Specific protocols for minimizing excessive public masturbation include interrupting the behavior, reminding the person of appropriate time and place, redirection, and allowing masturbation in private. Often, working with a behavior therapist who can offer applied behavior analysis is recommended.
	Resources: Kate E. Reynolds books: *Things Tom Likes: A Book About Sexuality and Masturbation for Boys and Young Men with Autism and Related Conditions* (2015) and *Things Ellie Likes: A Book About Sexuality and Masturbation for Girls and Young Women with Autism and Related Conditions* (2015).
Inappropriate interactions (stalking), touching, or romantic gestures	Through the Individualized Education Program, request a functional behavior assessment and a behavior intervention plan for positive supports such as a social skills group, scripting, video modeling and feedback, self-management, and rule governed behaviors.
	Resource: Teaching Moment: Teaching Your Kids Appropriate and Inappropriate Touching (https://www.northshore.org/healthy-you/teaching-your-kids-appropriate-touching/).
Using public restrooms	Resources: Kate E Reynolds books: *Tom Needs to Go: A Book About How to Use Public Toilets Safely for Boys and Young Men with Autism and Related Conditions* (2015) and *Ellie Needs to Go: A Book About How to Use Public Toilets Safely for Girls and Young Women with Autism and Related Conditions* (2015).

indicate lower levels of sexual knowledge (including understanding of privacy norms) decreased social opportunities, and increased social anxiety and vulnerability.[66,74,75] In addition, at a population level, teenagers and young adults with ASD without an intellectual disability have greater diversity in sexual orientation and gender identity, compared with typically developing peers, which they state can be confusing.[76] As understanding of sexual knowledge and health differences between individuals with ASD increases, there are new opportunities to individualize safety and sex education to understand sexual orientation and prevent socially isolating problem sexual behaviors, sexual coercion, and abuse.[74] Typical sex education may not be

sufficient for people with ASD, and specific methods and curricula are necessary to match their needs (Table 1).[77] An enhancement of clinical services and additional research is needed to ensure people with ASD have their informational needs met and are able to achieve a healthy sexuality.[78]

SEXUALITY AND ADOLESCENTS WITH SPINA BIFIDA OR A SPINAL CORD INJURY

Individuals with spina bifida or a spinal cord injury have some amount of lower extremity paralysis and also tend to have a neurogenic bowel and bladder as well as loss of nerve signals to their sex organs. The neurologic consequences of spinal cord injury and spina bifida can alter sexual and reproductive experiences

for people with these conditions, affect confidence and self-esteem, and hinder relationship building.[12,79–81] Although many youth with spina bifida do not understand their reproductive potential, women with spinal cord injury or spina bifida tend to have normal fertility but require high-risk obstetric care before and during their pregnancies.[12,82] Many women with spinal cord injury or spina bifida, when sexually aroused, do not have full vulvar engorgement or vaginal lubrication, making penetration difficult or painful.[83] Some women with these conditions are able to experience orgasms.[82] Men with spina bifida or spinal cord injury tend to have altered fertility.[84] In addition, the performance of sexual intercourse may be hindered by erectile dysfunction, including an inability to achieve or maintain an erection for penetration and retrograde, absent, or incomplete ejaculation.[79,85] For both men and women with these conditions, engaging in sexual activity may be complicated by incontinence from neurogenic bowel or bladder.[86,87] Both men and women may be counseled to catheterize their bladders before and after sexual activity.[83] Men who have retrograde ejaculation often need to flush their bladders after sex to remove semen from the bladder.[88] Sexual education and guidance should be tailored to the individual's needs and should consider the cognitive and physical capabilities of the individual.[86] Many people with spina bifida also commonly have learning disabilities and other cognitive problems.[89] People with spina bifida also need to be counseled about the use of nonlatex condoms because of the risk of latex allergies in this population.

SEXUALITY AND HEALTH CARE TRANSITION

Viewing sexuality as a normative part of adolescence in people with disabilities, including ASD, is conceptually new, compared with long-standing myths of universal asexuality and limited sexual experiences.[72,75] The 2018 AAP clinical report, "Supporting the Health Care Transition From Adolescence to Adulthood in the Medical Home," provides a strong framework for primary care providers to longitudinally promote and integrate healthy sexuality for all youth, both with and without disabilities, from understanding pubertal changes and gender identity to experiencing sexual feelings and understanding sexual orientation to ultimately exploring and developing capacity for intimacy and reproduction.[22] This ongoing longitudinal relationship, similar to that for typically developing youth, includes confidential conversations, appropriate genital examinations, openness to sexual and gender

diversity and individual and family preferences, and, if needed, sensitive reporting of sexual abuse or violence.[90] As opportunities for employment, postsecondary education, and community living increase for a large portion of the population with disabilities, it is imperative to prepare and support them in their sociosexual self-efficacy, safety, and well-being.

THE PEDIATRIC HEALTH CARE PROVIDER'S ROLE

Pediatric health care providers play a crucial and longitudinal role in the development of healthy sexuality of children and youth with disabilities. The unique relationship with the patient and family over time allows the pediatric health care provider to discuss and promote important social and sexual skills at an individualized pace appropriate for each patient.

- Pediatric health care providers can examine and adjust or reinforce their knowledge, beliefs, and attitudes about sexuality and gender identity to ensure their own behavior reflects inclusivity and autonomy of all their patients, especially children and adolescents with disabilities; all people have the right to develop relationships, exercise choice and autonomy, and receive education to promote a healthy sexuality, regardless of sexual orientation or gender identity. Communication that is open and respectful can help develop trust and foster shared decision-making.
- At the earliest ages, including preschoolers, pediatric health care providers are encouraged to discuss appropriate "private" versus "public" behaviors. Pediatric health care providers can help children with disabilities and their families understand boundaries and the concept of body ownership and consent. Explaining "good touch,"

"bad touch," and "necessary touch" can help children frame their understanding of appropriate and inappropriate circumstances and situations. Using anatomically correct language for body parts at young ages helps children to understand their bodies in a positive, healthy way and offers children a way to express healthy sexuality.

- By at least 8 or 9 years of age, pediatric health care providers should begin to discuss puberty and may need to do so sooner if the child is at risk for precocious puberty. Discussing puberty, preparing children and families, and offering additional materials (separate from school curriculum; Table 1) to review in a quiet comfortable place such as the home allows for questions, clarification, and anticipatory guidance for supports in hygiene and normalization of experiences.
- As with all adolescents, pediatric health care providers are encouraged to offer youth with disabilities an opportunity to speak with their provider confidentially during a visit. This allows youth to express their thoughts and experiences and ask questions. This is especially important for youth who are discovering their nonbinary gender identity or nonheterosexual sexual orientation. The pediatric health care provider's office should be a safe place to discuss these issues for all youth, including those with disabilities.
- Pediatric health care providers have opportunities with families and caregivers to introduce topics such as healthy sexual development and exploration while limiting risk of harm. Encouraging coeducational supervised group activities to include individuals with disabilities in typical teenager interactions often is best received by families and caregivers as anticipatory guidance by their trusted

provider. This is also a good time to encourage families and caregivers to be a primary source of sexual education for their children. There are many resources available, including those listed in Table 1. Pediatric health care providers can partner with families and caregivers who may feel uncomfortable addressing sexual health through a shared decision-making process that is culturally responsive and elevates the rights of children with disabilities to gain knowledge and understanding regarding their developing sexuality.

- Pediatric health care providers are the best resource to counsel all youth, including youth with disabilities, regarding the prevention of STIs and unwanted pregnancy as well as the benefits of HPV vaccination.
- Pediatric health care providers can help youth with disabilities procure contraceptives in a confidential manner, with adherence to informed consent rules.
- Pediatric health care providers can screen for STIs or ensure that appropriate referrals are in place (eg, gynecology or urology) for routine screening as part of their role in providing care in a medical home.
- Pediatric health care providers are well suited to provide families with resources to help them address problematic or inappropriate sexual behaviors (Table 5).
- Pediatric health care providers can partner with schools to ensure that children with disabilities have access to a developmentally appropriate sexual education that includes knowledge building around sexual victimization, safer sex practices, consent, and respect through their Individualized Education Programs or as part of the typical curriculum.
- Pediatric health care providers may need to offer education to schools regarding the high risk of sexual victimization for children with disabilities, how best to prevent it, and how to identify it if it occurs.
- Pediatric health care providers are vigilant about the knowledge that children and youth with disabilities are at an increased risk for sexual abuse and assault and can help families understand this risk. Asking about unwanted or coercive interactions and monitoring for emotional disturbance that may indicate sexual abuse or coercion can happen at every visit. If concerns arise, ensuring that proper reporting occurs and follow-up care is delivered is a role pediatric health care providers are trained to provide.

Pediatric health care providers are encouraged to approach sexual education and guidance individually for children and youth with disabilities, taking into account their patient's developmental trajectory and understanding the functional limitations of health conditions that can affect the development of healthy sexuality. Numerous other AAP reports can help inform the pediatric health provider on the topic of sexuality (Table 4). Framing healthy sexuality through a "competence lens" helps providers recognize the strengths and challenges for each individual patient. To be competent at something, an individual must have sufficient knowledge and skills to engage in action. Although there may be barriers to the development of skills needed for healthy sexuality in individuals with disabilities, it is important to prioritize ongoing skill development, compensatory strategies, and opportunities for autonomy and self-actualization.

LEAD AUTHORS

Amy Joy Houtrow, MD, PhD, MPH, FAAP
Ellen Roy Elias, MD, FAAP, FACMG
Beth Ellen Davis, MD, MPH, FAAP

COUNCIL ON CHILDREN WITH DISABILITIES EXECUTIVE COMMITTEE, 2020–2021

Dennis Z. Kuo, MD, MHS, FAAP, Chairperson
Rishi Agrawal, MD, MPH, FAAP
Lynn F. Davidson, MD, FAAP
Kathryn A. Ellerbeck, MD, FAAP
Jessica E.A. Foster, MD, MPH, FAAP
Ellen Fremion, MD, FAAP, FACP
Mary O'Connor Leppert, MD, FAAP
Barbara S. Saunders, DO, FAAP
Christopher Stille, MD, MPH, FAAP
Jilda Vargus-Adams, MD, MSc, FAAP
Larry Yin, MD, MSPH, FAAP

PAST COUNCIL ON CHILDREN WITH DISABILITIES EXECUTIVE COMMITTEE MEMBERS

Kenneth Norwood, Jr, MD, FAAP, Immediate Past Chairperson

LIAISONS

Cara Coleman, JD, MPH – *Family Voices*
Marie Y. Mann, MD, MPH, FAAP – *Maternal and Child Health Bureau*
Edwin Simpser, MD, FAAP – *Section on Home Care*
Jennifer Poon, MD, FAAP – *Section on Developmental and Behavioral Pediatrics*
Marshalyn Yeargin-Allsopp, MD, FAAP – *Centers for Disease Control and Prevention*

STAFF

Alexandra Kuznetsov

ABBREVIATIONS

AAP: American Academy of Pediatrics
ASD: autism spectrum disorder
HPV: human papillomavirus
STI: sexually transmitted infection

DOI: https://doi.org/10.1542/peds.2021-052043

Address correspondence to Amy Houtrow, MD, PhD, MPH, FAAP. E-mail: houtrow@upmc.edu

PEDIATRICS (ISSN Numbers: Print, 0031-4005; Online, 1098-4275).

FINANCIAL DISCLOSURE: The authors have indicated they have no financial relationships relevant to this article to disclose.

FUNDING: No external funding.

POTENTIAL CONFLICT OF INTEREST: The authors have indicated they have no potential conflicts of interest to disclose.

REFERENCES

1. World Health Organization. Defining sexual health. Available at: www.who.int/reproductivehealth/topics/sexual_health/sh_definitions/en/. Accessed September 30, 2020

2. Breuner CC, Mattson G; COMMITTEE ON ADOLESCENCE; COMMITTEE ON PSYCHOSOCIAL ASPECTS OF CHILD AND FAMILY HEALTH. Sexuality education for children and adolescents. *Pediatrics.* 2016;138(2):e20161348

3. Swartzendruber A, Zenilman JM. A national strategy to improve sexual health. *JAMA.* 2010;304(9):1005–1006

4. American College of Obstetricians and Gynecologists. Comprehensive sexuality education. Available at: https://www.acog.org/-/media/project/acog/acogorg/clinical/files/committee-opinion/articles/2016/11/comprehensive-sexuality-education.pdf. Accessed July 15, 2020

5. Lee S, Fenge LA, Collins B. Promoting sexual well-being in social work education and practice. *Soc Work Educ.* 2018;37(3):315–327

6. Marcell AV, Burstein GR; COMMITTEE ON ADOLESCENCE. Sexual and reproductive health care services in the pediatric setting. *Pediatrics.* 2017;140(5):e20200627

7. Child and Adolescent Health Measurement Initiative. Data search results. Available at: www.childhealthdata.org/browse/survey/results?q=4668&r=1. Accessed September 30, 2020

8. Hagerman TK, Houtrow AJ. Variability in prevalence estimates of disability among children in the National Survey of Children's Health. *JAMA Pediatr.* 2021;175(3):307–310

9. Rosenbaum P, Gorter JW. The 'F-words' in childhood disability: I swear this is how we should think! *Child Care Health Dev.* 2012;38(4):457–463

10. DiGiulio G. Sexuality and people living with physical or developmental disabilities: a review of key issues. *Can J Hum Sex.* 2003;12(1):53–68

11. Horner-Johnson W, Moe EL, Stoner RC, et al. Contraceptive knowledge and use among women with intellectual, physical, or sensory disabilities: a systematic review. *Disabil Health J.* 2019;12(2):139–154

12. Sawin KJ, Buran CF, Brei TJ, Fastenau PS. Sexuality issues in adolescents with a chronic neurological condition. *J Perinat Educ.* 2002;11(1):22–34

13. Finlay WM, Rohleder P, Taylor N, Culfear H. 'Understanding' as a practical issue in sexual health education for people with intellectual disabilities: a study using two qualitative methods. *Health Psychol.* 2015;34(4):328–338

14. Schaafsma D, Kok G, Stoffelen JMT, Curfs LMG. People with intellectual disabilities talk about sexuality: implications for the development of sex education. *Sex Disabil.* 2017;35(1):21–38

15. Barnard-Brak L, Schmidt M, Chesnut S, Wei T, Richman D. Predictors of access to sex education for children with intellectual disabilities in public schools. *Intellect Dev Disabil.* 2014;52(2):85–97

16. Swango-Wilson A. Meaningful sex education programs for individuals with intellectual/developmental disabilities. *Sex Disabil.* 2011;29(2):113–118

17. Adams RC, Levy SE; COUNCIL ON CHILDREN WITH DISABILITIES. Shared decision-making and children with disabilities: pathways to consensus. *Pediatrics.* 2017;139(6):e20170956

18. Houtrow A, Jones J, Ghandour R, Strickland B, Newacheck P. Participation of children with special health care needs in school and the community. *Acad Pediatr.* 2012;12(4):326–334

19. Milligan MS, Neufeldt AH. The myth of asexuality: a survey of social and empirical evidence. *Sex Disabil.* 2001;19(2):91–109

20. Hagan JF, Shaw JS, Duncan PM, eds. *Bright Futures: Guidelines for Health Supervision of Infants, Children, and Adolescents.* 4th ed. Elk Grove Village, IL: American Academy of Pediatrics; 2017

21. Center for Parent Information & Resources. Sexuality education for students with disabilities. Available at: https://www.parentcenterhub.org/sexed/. Accessed September 30, 2020

22. White PH, Cooley WC; TRANSITIONS CLINICAL REPORT AUTHORING GROUP; AMERICAN ACADEMY OF PEDIATRICS; AMERICAN ACADEMY OF FAMILY PHYSICIANS; AMERICAN COLLEGE OF PHYSICIANS. Supporting the health care transition from adolescence to adulthood in the medical home. *Pediatrics.* 2018;142(5):182–200

23. Rafferty J; COMMITTEE ON PSYCHOSOCIAL ASPECTS OF CHILD AND FAMILY HEALTH; COMMITTEE ON ADOLESCENCE; SECTION ON LESBIAN, GAY, BISEXUAL, AND TRANSGENDER HEALTH AND WELLNESS. Ensuring comprehensive care and support for transgender and gender-diverse children and adolescents. *Pediatrics.* 2018;142(4):e20182162

24. Wolfe PS, Wertalik JL, Domire Monaco S, Gardner S, Ruiz S. Review of sociosexuality curricular content for individuals with developmental disabilities. *Focus Autism Other Dev Disabl.* 2019;34(3):153–162

25. Ailey SH, Marks BA, Crisp C, Hahn JE. Promoting sexuality across the life span for individuals with intellectual

and developmental disabilities. *Nurs Clin North Am.* 2003;38(2):229–252

26. Michaud P-A, Ambresin AE. Consultation for disordered puberty: what do adolescent medicine patients teach us? *Endocr Dev.* 2016;29:240–255

27. American College of Obstetricians and Gynecologists. Committee opinion No. 710: counseling adolescents about contraception. *Obstet Gynecol.* 2017;130(2):e74–e80

28. Cholley F, Trivin C, Sainte-Rose C, Souberbielle JC, Cinalli G, Brauner R. Disorders of growth and puberty in children with non-tumoral hydrocephalus. *J Pediatr Endocrinol Metab.* 2001;14(3):319–327

29. Kaplowitz P, Bloch C; Section on Endocrinology, American Academy of Pediatrics. Evaluation and referral of children with signs of early puberty. *Pediatrics.* 2016;137(1):e20153732

30. Kaplowitz PB, Mehra R. Clinical characteristics of children referred for signs of early puberty before age 3. *J Pediatr Endocrinol Metab.* 2015;28(9–10): 1139–1144

31. McLay L, Carnett A, Tyler-Merrick G, van der Meer L. A systematic review of interventions for inappropriate sexual behavior of children and adolescents with developmental disabilities. *Rev J Autism Dev Disord.* 2015;2(4):357–373

32. Quint EH, O'Brien RF; COMMITTEE ON ADOLESCENCE; North American Society for Pediatric and Adolescent Gynecology. Menstrual management for adolescents with disabilities. *Pediatrics.* 2016;138(1):e20160295

33. Grover SR. Gynaecological issues in adolescents with disability. *J Paediatr Child Health.* 2011;47(9):610–613

34. Tracy J, Grover S, Macgibbon S. Menstrual issues for women with intellectual disability. *Aust Prescr.* 2016;39(2):54–57

35. Quint EH. Menstrual and reproductive issues in adolescents with physical and developmental disabilities. *Obstet Gynecol.* 2014;124(2, pt 1):367–375

36. American College of Obstetricians and Gynecologists' Committee on Adolescent Health Care. Committee opinion No. 668: menstral manipulation for adolescents with physical and developmental disabilities. *Obstet Gynecol.* 2016;128(2):e20–e25

37. Acharya K, Lantos JD. Considering decision-making and sexuality in menstrual suppression of teens and young adults with intellectual disabilities. *AMA J Ethics.* 2016;18(4):365–372

38. Baines S, Emerson E, Robertson J, Hatton C. Sexual activity and sexual health among young adults with and without mild/moderate intellectual disability. *BMC Public Health.* 2018;18(1):667

39. Abells D, Kirkham YA, Ornstein MP. Review of gynecologic and reproductive care for women with developmental disabilities. *Curr Opin Obstet Gynecol.* 2016;28(5):350–358

40. Spiegel T, Pollak Y. Corrigendum: attention deficit/hyperactivity disorder and increased engagement in sexual risk-taking behavior: the role of benefit perception. *Front Psychol.* 2019;10:2152

41. Schoenfelder EN, Kollins SH. Topical review: ADHD and health-risk behaviors: toward prevention and health promotion. *J Pediatr Psychol.* 2016;41(7):735–740

42. LeFevre ML; US Preventive Services Task Force. Behavioral counseling interventions to prevent sexually transmitted infections: U.S. Preventive Services Task Force recommendation statement. *Ann Intern Med.* 2014;161(12):894–901

43. Grubb LK; COMMITTEE ON ADOLESCENCE. Barrier protection use by adolescents during sexual activity. *Pediatrics.* 2020;146(2):e2020007237

44. Menon S; COMMITTEE ON ADOLESCENCE. Long-acting reversible contraception: specific issues for adolescents. *Pediatrics.* 2020;146(2):e2020007252

45. Alderman EM, Breuner CC; COMMITTEE ON ADOLESCENCE. Unique needs of the adolescent. *Pediatrics.* 2019;144(6):e20193150

46. Gavin L, Moskosky S, Carter M, et al; Centers for Disease Control and Prevention (CDC). Providing quality family planning services: recommendations of CDC and the U.S. Office of Population Affairs. *MMWR Recomm Rep.* 2014;63(RR-04):1–54

47. Workowski KA, Bolan GA; Centers for Disease Control and Prevention. Sexually transmitted diseases treatment guidelines, 2015. *MMWR Recomm Rep.* 2015;64(RR-03):1–137

48. Blake DR, Middleman AB. Human papillomavirus vaccine update. *Pediatr Clin North Am.* 2017;64(2):321–329

49. COMMITTEE ON INFECTIOUS DISEASES. Recommended childhood and adolescent immunization schedule: United States, 2020. *Pediatrics.* 2020;145(3):e20193995

50. Centers for Disease Control and Prevention. Recommended child and adolescent immunization schedule for ages 18 years or younger, United States, 2021. Available at: https://www.cdc.gov/vaccines/schedules/hcp/imz/child-adolescent.html#notes. Accessed July 15, 2020

51. American College of Obstetricians and Gynecologists. ACOG committee opinion No. 768 summary: genetic syndromes and gynecologic implications in adolescents. *Obstet Gynecol.* 2019;133(3):598–599

52. Stein Q, Loman R, Zuck T. Genetic counseling in pediatrics. *Pediatr Rev.* 2018;39(7):323–331

53. Bull MJ; Committee on Genetics. Health supervision for children with Down syndrome [published correction appears in *Pediatrics.* 2011;128(6):1212]. *Pediatrics.* 2011;128(2):393–406

54. Smith N, Harrell S. Sexual abuse of children with disabilities: a national snapshot. *Child Law Practice Today.* July 1, 2013. Available at: https://www.americanbar.org/groups/public_interest/child_law/resources/child_law_practiceonline/child_law_practice/vol_32/july-2013/sexual-abuse-of-children-with-disabilities--a-national-snapshot0/. Accessed September 30, 2020

55. Crawford-Jakubiak JE, Alderman EM, Leventhal JM; COMMITTEE ON CHILD ABUSE AND NEGLECT; COMMITTEE ON ADOLESCENCE. Care of the adolescent after an acute sexual assault. [published correction appears in *Pediatrics.* 2017;139(6):e20170958]. *Pediatrics.* 2017;139(3):e20164243

56. Finkelhor D, Shattuck A, Turner HA, Hamby SL. The lifetime prevalence of child sexual abuse and sexual assault assessed in late adolescence. *J Adolesc Health.* 2014;55(3):329–333

57. Findley PA, Plummer SB, McMahon S. Exploring the experiences of abuse of college students with disabilities. *J Interpers Violence.* 2016;31(17):2801–2823

58. Haydon AA, McRee AL, Tucker Halpern C. Unwanted sex among young adults in the United States: the role of physical disability and cognitive performance. *J Interpers Violence*. 2011;26(17):3476–3493

59. McDaniels B, Fleming A. Sexuality education and intellectual disability: time to address the challenge. *Sex Disabil*. 2016;34(2):215–225

60. Murphy GH, O'Callaghan A. Capacity of adults with intellectual disabilities to consent to sexual relationships. *Psychol Med*. 2004;34(7):1347–1357

61. Jenny C, Crawford-Jakubiak JE; Committee on Child Abuse and Neglect; American Academy of Pediatrics. The evaluation of children in the primary care setting when sexual abuse is suspected. *Pediatrics*. 2013;132(2):e558–e567

62. Christian CW; Committee on Child Abuse and Neglect, American Academy of Pediatrics. The evaluation of suspected child physical abuse. *Pediatrics*. 2015;135(5):e1337–e1354

63. Kellogg ND; Committee on Child Abuse and Neglect, American Academy of Pediatrics. Clinical report—the evaluation of sexual behaviors in children. *Pediatrics*. 2009;124(3):992–998

64. Kenny MC, Abreu RL. Training mental health professionals in child sexual abuse: curricular guidelines. *J Child Sex Abuse*. 2015;24(5):572–591

65. Clay CJ, Bloom SE, Lambert JM. Behavioral interventions for inappropriate sexual behavior in individuals with developmental disabilities and acquired brain injury: a review. *Am J Intellect Dev Disabil*. 2018;123(3):254–282

66. Fernandes LC, Gillberg CI, Cederlund M, Hagberg B, Gillberg C, Billstedt E. Aspects of sexuality in adolescents and adults diagnosed with autism spectrum disorders in childhood. *J Autism Dev Disord*. 2016; 46(9):3155–3165

67. Ginevra MC, Nota L, Stokes MA. The differential effects of Autism and Down's syndrome on sexual behavior. *Autism Res*. 2016;9(1):131–140

68. Beddows N, Brooks R. Inappropriate sexual behaviour in adolescents with autism spectrum disorder: what education is

recommended and why. *Early Interv Psychiatry*. 2016;10(4):282–289

69. Bennett AE, Miller JS, Stollon N, Prasad R, Blum NJ. Autism spectrum disorder and transition-aged youth. *Curr Psychiatry Rep*. 2018;20(11):103

70. van Schalkwyk GI, Volkmar FR. Autism spectrum disorders: challenges and opportunities for transition to adulthood. *Child Adolesc Psychiatr Clin N Am*. 2017;26(2):329–339

71. Roux A, Shattuck P, Rast J, Anderson K. *National Autism Indicators Report: Developmental Disability Services and Outcomes in Adulthood*. Philadelphia, PA: Drexel University; 2017

72. Dewinter J, Vermeiren R, Vanwesenbeeck I, Nieuwenhuizen CV. Parental awareness of sexual experience in adolescent boys with autism spectrum disorder. *J Autism Dev Disord*. 2016;46(2):713–719

73. Gilmour L, Schalomon P, Smith V. Sexuality in a community based sample of adults with autism spectrum disorder. *Res Autism Spectr Disord*. 2012;6(1):313–318

74. Hancock GIP, Stokes MA, Mesibov GB. Socio-sexual functioning in autism spectrum disorder: a systematic review and meta-analyses of existing literature. *Autism Res*. 2017;10(11):1823–1833

75. Kellaher DC. Sexual behavior and autism spectrum disorders: an update and discussion. *Curr Psychiatry Rep*. 2015;17(4):562

76. Turner D, Briken P, Schöttle D. Autism-spectrum disorders in adolescence and adulthood: focus on sexuality. *Curr Opin Psychiatry*. 2017;30(6):409–416

77. Hannah LA, Stagg SD. Experiences of sex education and sexual awareness in young adults with autism spectrum disorder. *J Autism Dev Disord*. 2016;46(12):3678–3687

78. Lehan Mackin M, Loew N, Gonzalez A, Tykol H, Christensen T. Parent perceptions of sexual education needs for their children with autism. *J Pediatr Nurs*. 2016;31(6):608–618

79. Gatti C, Del Rossi C, Ferrari A, Casolari E, Casadio G, Scire G. Predictors of successful sexual partnering of adults with

spina bifida. *J Urol*. 2009;182(4 suppl): 1911–1916

80. Lassmann J, Garibay Gonzalez F, Melchionni JB, Pasquariello PS Jr, Snyder HM III. Sexual function in adult patients with spina bifida and its impact on quality of life. *J Urol*. 2007;178(4, pt 2): 1611–1614

81. Lee NG, Andrews E, Rosoklija I, et al. The effect of spinal cord level on sexual function in the spina bifida population. *J Pediatr Urol*. 2015; 11(3):142.e1–142.e6

82. de Vylder A, van Driel MF, Staal AL, Weijmar Schultz WC, Nijman JM. Myelomeningocele and female sexuality: an issue? *Eur Urol*. 2004;46(4):421–426, discussion 426–427

83. Hess MJ, Hough S. Impact of spinal cord injury on sexuality: broad-based clinical practice intervention and practical application. *J Spinal Cord Med*. 2012;35(4):211–218

84. Deng N, Thirumavalavan N, Beilan JA, et al. Sexual dysfunction and infertility in the male spina bifida patient. *Transl Androl Urol*. 2018;7(6):941–949

85. Bong GW, Rovner ES. Sexual health in adult men with spina bifida. *ScientificWorldJournal*. 2007;7:1466–1469

86. Verhoef M, Barf HA, Vroege JA, et al. Sex education, relationships, and sexuality in young adults with spina bifida. *Arch Phys Med Rehabil*. 2005;86(5):979–987

87. Cardenas DD, Topolski TD, White CJ, McLaughlin JF, Walker WO. Sexual functioning in adolescents and young adults with spina bifida. *Arch Phys Med Rehabil*. 2008;89(1):31–35

88. Barazani Y, Stahl PJ, Nagler HM, Stember DS. Management of ejaculatory disorders in infertile men. *Asian J Androl*. 2012;14(4):525–529

89. Fletcher JM, Copeland K, Frederick JA, et al. Spinal lesion level in spina bifida: a source of neural and cognitive heterogeneity. *J Neurosurg*. 2005;102(3 suppl):268–279

90. Grubb LK, Powers M; COMMITTEE ON ADOLESCENCE. Emerging issues in male adolescent sexual and reproductive health care. *Pediatrics*. 2020;145(5):e20200627

CLINICAL REPORT   Guidance for the Clinician in Rendering Pediatric Care

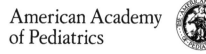

Maltreatment of Children With Disabilities

Lori A. Legano, MD, FAAP,[a] Larry W. Desch, MD, FAAP,[b] Stephen A. Messner, MD, FAAP,[c] Sheila Idzerda, MD, FAAP,[d] Emalee G. Flaherty, MD, FAAP,[e] COUNCIL ON CHILD ABUSE AND NEGLECT, COUNCIL ON CHILDREN WITH DISABILITIES

abstract

Over the past decade, there have been widespread efforts to raise awareness about maltreatment of children. Pediatric providers have received education about factors that make a child more vulnerable to being abused and neglected. The purpose of this clinical report is to ensure that children with disabilities are recognized as a population at increased risk for maltreatment. This report updates the 2007 American Academy of Pediatrics clinical report "Maltreatment of Children With Disabilities." Since 2007, new information has expanded our understanding of the incidence of abuse in this vulnerable population. There is now information about which children with disabilities are at greatest risk for maltreatment because not all disabling conditions confer the same risks of abuse or neglect. This updated report will serve as a resource for pediatricians and others who care for children with disabilities and offers guidance on risks for subpopulations of children with disabilities who are at particularly high risk of abuse and neglect. The report will also discuss ways in which the medical home can aid in early identification and intervene when abuse and neglect are suspected. It will also describe community resources and preventive strategies that may reduce the risk of abuse and neglect.

[a]Department of Pediatrics, Grossman School of Medicine, New York University, New York, New York; [b]Department of Pediatrics, Chicago Medical School, Rosalind Franklin University of Medicine and Science and Advocate Children's Hospital, Oak Lawn, Illinois; [c]Stephanie V. Blank Center for Safe and Healthy Children, Children's Healthcare of Atlanta, Department of Pediatrics, Emory University School of Medicine, Atlanta, Georgia; [d]Billings Clinic, Department of Medicine, University of Washington School of Medicine, Bozeman, Montana; and [e]Department of Pediatrics, Northwestern University Feinberg School of Medicine, Chicago, Illinois

Clinical reports from the American Academy of Pediatrics benefit from expertise and resources of liaisons and internal (AAP) and external reviewers. However, clinical reports from the American Academy of Pediatrics may not reflect the views of the liaisons or the organizations or government agencies that they represent.

The guidance in this report does not indicate an exclusive course of treatment or serve as a standard of medical care. Variations, taking into account individual circumstances, may be appropriate.

All clinical reports from the American Academy of Pediatrics automatically expire 5 years after publication unless reaffirmed, revised, or retired at or before that time.

DOI: https://doi.org/10.1542/peds.2021-050920

Address correspondence to Lori Legano, MD. Email: lori.legano@nyulangone.org

PEDIATRICS (ISSN Numbers: Print, 0031-4005; Online, 1098-4275).

To cite: Legano LA, Desch LW, Messner SA, et al. AAP COUNCIL ON CHILD ABUSE AND NEGLECT, AAP COUNCIL ON CHILDREN WITH DISABILITIES. Maltreatment of Children With Disabilities. *Pediatrics.* 2021;147(5):e2021050920

INTRODUCTION

The maltreatment of children, including those with disabilities, is a critical public health issue. For the purposes of this report, children with disabilities include the full spectrum of children and adolescents with any significant impairment in any area of motor, sensory, social, communicative, cognitive, or emotional functioning. Children and youth with special health care needs is a broader group that shares some of the same risks as children with disabilities. These children have chronic medical issues that may cause impairment and, as a group, require significantly more health care than typically developing children.

Current data on incidence and prevalence of maltreatment in children with disabilities are limited by varying definitions of disability and lack of uniform methods of classifying maltreatment. There is concern that the incidence of child abuse and neglect is underreported in part because many children with disabilities have communication difficulties and cannot directly report problems.[1,2] Nonetheless, children with disabilities and special health care needs are at increased risk of child maltreatment. This report updates the previous clinical report published in 2007, "Assessment of Maltreatment of Children With Disabilities."[1]

The US Children's Bureau reported that an estimated 678 000 children were determined to be victims of abuse or neglect in 2018.[3] Three-fifths (60.8%) of child victims experienced neglect, 10.7% were physically abused, and 7.0% were sexually abused; 15.5% of these children suffered from 2 or more maltreatment types.[3] The 2010 reauthorization of the Child Abuse Prevention and Treatment Act (CAPTA) improved the data collection from states on children with disabilities by mandating that states report the number of children younger than 3 years who are involved in a substantiated case of child maltreatment and are eligible to be referred for early intervention services and the number of children who were actually referred for those services.[4] It did not require collecting information regarding types of disabilities or the number of children with disabilities who are older than 3 years when they enter the child welfare system.[4]

On the basis of national data from 2015, child victims with a disability accounted for 14.1% of all victims of abuse and neglect.[4] In that report, children with the following conditions were considered to have a disability: intellectual disability (ID), severe

emotional disturbance, visual or hearing impairment, learning disability, physical disability, behavior problem, or a few other chronic medical conditions. It was believed that children with such conditions are undercounted because not every child received a clinical diagnostic assessment when child maltreatment was suspected. A recent study of the data from the National Survey of Child and Adolescent Well-Being II, which included children older than 3 years, found that nearly one-half of children investigated by child protective services (CPS) were not typically developing.[5]

Child abuse and neglect is reported in 3% to 10% of the population with disabilities.[6–10] The rate of child abuse and neglect is at least 3 times higher in children with disabilities than in the typically developing population.[11] In a recent study by the Federal Bureau of Justice Statistics, during the period from 2011 to 2015, among all people older than 12 years who had disabilities, people between 12 and 15 years of age had the highest rate of violent victimization.[8]

Using data from the National Child Abuse and Neglect Data System, Kistin et al[12] evaluated the incidence and timing of rereferral to CPS, substantiated maltreatment, determined foster care placement for children who had been reported to CPS and had unsubstantiated neglect, and compared typically developing children and children with disabilities. Children with disabilities were re-referred to CPS more frequently, were found to have been abused more frequently, and were more often subsequently placed in foster care.[12] Once placed in foster care, children with ID were more likely to experience placement instability[13] and were more likely to have adoption disruption and less likely to be reunified with a parent or other family member.[13]

A systematic review of violence against children with disabilities revealed that, overall, children with disabilities are more likely to be victims of violence than their peers without disabilities. However, the authors of that review reported limitations in the literature because of a lack of well-designed research studies, with poor standards of measurement of disability and violence and insufficient exploration about whether violence preceded the disability.[11]

Child maltreatment may result in the development of disabilities, which in turn can precipitate further abuse. Abusive head trauma, for example, is known to cause disabilities in children.[14] The majority of survivors of abusive head trauma have developmental delays, seizures, motor impairments, feeding difficulties, and later behavioral and educational dysfunction, with only 28% having no impairment.[15] Vision loss can result from occipital cortical injury and optic nerve injury.[16] Neglect is associated with short-term and long-term effects on children's cognitive, socioemotional, and behavioral development.[17,18] Neglect that occurs early in life can have more profound effects on development.

Injury from abuse is augmented by the impact it has on the cortisol stress response and consequent physiologic impact. Adverse childhood experiences, including child abuse and neglect, cause physiologic disruptions that can persist into adulthood and lead to lifelong poor physical and mental health.[19] Exposure to traumatic events is associated with significant negative effects on long-term cognitive development, such as IQ scores, language development, and academic achievement.[20] Specifically, witnessing intimate partner violence in early childhood, particularly during the first 2 years of life, is associated with decreased cognitive scores later in childhood.[21]

FACTORS THAT INCREASE THE RISK OF CHILD ABUSE AND NEGLECT

In general, the causes of abuse and neglect of children with disabilities are the same as those for all children; however, several elements may increase the risk of abuse for children with disabilities. Children with chronic illnesses or disabilities sometimes can place higher emotional, physical, economic, and social demands on their families.[22]

The financial stress of raising a child with disabilities is often high, and this contributes significantly to family stress.[23,24] Other studies have found that families of children with disabilities have significantly more out-of-pocket costs for health care expenditures.[24,25] Caregivers may feel more overwhelmed and unable to cope with the care and supervision responsibilities that are required.[25] Lack of respite or other breaks in child care responsibilities for caregivers may contribute to an increased risk of abuse and neglect in children with disabilities. Neglect, the most common form of child maltreatment, is more prevalent in children with disabilities than in children without disabilities.[7] The complex needs of children with disabilities, in both special health care and educational needs, may result in the failure of the child to receive essential medications, therapies, and appropriate educational placement.[24,26]

A substance use disorder in the mother is a risk factor for child maltreatment[27] and may be the cause of the child's disability. Fetal alcohol spectrum disorder (FASD) is a classic example. The use of alcohol or other substances during pregnancy can cause a range of lifelong physical and behavioral disabilities and IDs.[28] Children with FASD often have learning problems and speech and language issues and are typically impulsive, lack focus, and have poor judgment. These problems can be extremely frustrating for any caregiver of a child with FASD. Parents with ongoing substance use disorders may also be less able to handle their children's challenging behaviors and be more punitive to their children.[29]

Parenting a child with disabilities is often challenging. Some children with disabilities may not respond to traditional means of reinforcement, and sometimes their behaviors, such as aggressiveness, noncompliance, and communication problems, can become frustrating, thus increasing caregiver stress.[30] These behavioral challenges can increase the risk of physical abuse by children's caregivers.[26]

Parents of a child with a disability may also overestimate their child's capabilities. In one study from the United States, parents of children with disabilities sometimes held unrealistically high expectations for their children.[9] Unrealistic expectations were also associated with a decreased degree of empathetic awareness of their child's limitations. Parents of children with intellectual or communication problems may sometimes turn to inappropriate physical punishment because of frustration about what they perceive as stubbornness or intentional failure to respond to verbal guidance.[31] Inappropriate expectations and ignorance of challenges a child with a disability might face can be linked to a higher risk for maltreatment. Pediatric providers can intervene by providing reasonable expectations for parents regarding their children with disabilities.[9] Parents need information and support to understand their child's abilities and challenges. They also need knowledge about proper strategies to use that are appropriate for the disability-related problems and the developmental status of their child.[25]

Although the use of aversive procedures and restraints for children who have disabilities has fortunately been diminishing, in part because of legislative changes (eg, modifications of the Individuals with Disabilities Education Act [Pub L No. 108-446 (2004)]), these practices are still sometimes used in homes, schools, programs, nursing homes, group homes, and other institutions.[32] Aversive techniques are procedures that use painful or unpleasant stimuli (such as biting the child, administering a noxious electric stimulus, or applying hot sauce to mucosal surfaces) to modify a behavior, and these techniques are always unacceptable or inappropriate. Restraints are physical measures (such as tie-downs or prolonged seclusion) used to prevent something physical from happening or for punishment. Physical restraints include forced holding, a technique that has been repudiated as being harmful.[33]

State laws are often unclear, contradictory, and varied regarding aversive and restraint techniques and do not always consider the techniques maltreatment.[34] Pediatricians and others can find additional information about the problems occurring from the use of aversive procedures or the use of restraints from the Web site Stop Hurting Kids (http://stophurtingkids.com/resources/). Over the past 20 years, research has demonstrated the effectiveness of alternative measures, commonly called "positive behavioral supports," to change behavior.[9] Pediatricians are encouraged to advocate for this approach. Information about positive behavioral support guidelines is available from a US Department of Education-funded program, the Technical Assistance Center on Positive Behavioral Interventions and Supports, at www.pbis.org, as well as other national and international programs. The American Academy of Child and Adolescent Psychiatry also provides guidance on this subject (https://www.aacap.org).

The presence of multiple caregivers can either increase or decrease the risk of abuse of children with disabilities. Children with disabilities who require multiple caregivers or providers may have contact with numerous individuals, thereby increasing the opportunity for abuse. However, advantages to having a large number of caregivers are that there are more individuals who may detect the injuries or signs of abuse, and the additional assistance may actually decrease the amount of stress placed on the primary caregivers. Risk may be minimized by careful screening and selection of caregivers, sporadic and unscheduled monitoring of care, and recognizing that any child may become a victim of child abuse and neglect.

Children with disabilities may be unintentionally conditioned to comply with authority, which could result in them failing to recognize abusive behaviors as maltreatment.[35] Children with disabilities are often perceived as easy targets because their intellectual limitations may prevent them from being able to discern the experience as abuse and their impaired communication abilities may prevent them from disclosing abuse. Because some forms of therapy may be painful (eg, injections or manipulation as part of physical therapy), a child may not be able to differentiate appropriate pain from inappropriate pain.

ASSOCIATION BETWEEN DISABILITY TYPE AND FORM OF ABUSE

Recent research has evaluated how differences in risk of abuse and neglect correlated with the type and severity of the child's disability. The World Health Organization describes disabilities by the domains of function that are affected (ie, cognition, mobility, self-care, getting along, life activities, and participation).[36] The most severely affected children are at a lower risk of maltreatment than mobile, verbal children who are still delayed, especially those with cognitive disabilities.[37] Children who are nonverbal or hearing impaired are more likely than others to experience neglect or sexual abuse.[4]

In an Australian study, researchers examined the relationship between different types of disabilities (eg, Down syndrome, autism) and the rate of substantiated maltreatment allegations.[10] The authors found that children with ID, mental or behavioral problems, or conduct disorder had an increased risk of an abuse allegation and for a substantiated allegation. In contrast, children with autism had a lower risk than children with Down syndrome, and those with birth defects or cerebral palsy had the same risk as children without disability after adjusting for child, family, and neighborhood risk factors. The type of abuse was not specified.

In another study from South Carolina, researchers examined the relationship between autism spectrum disorder (ASD) and ID and child maltreatment.[38] There were higher odds of reported and substantiated maltreatment among children with ASD only, ASD plus ID, and ID only, compared with a control group after controlling for sociodemographic factors. In a 2018 study from Tennessee, children with ASD had more referrals to a child abuse hotline than those without ASD, although substantiation rates were similar between the 2 groups.[39] In a 2018 study using data from the National Survey of Child and Adolescent Well-Being II data, children with multiple developmental delays were more likely to have recurrence of child abuse reporting.[40]

Physical Abuse

Sullivan and Knutson found that children with a disability were 3.79 times more likely to be physically abused than those without a disability.[41] Helton and Cross[37] also found that there is an association between disability and physical abuse. Rather than comparing children on the basis of diagnosis, they compared children on the basis of their level of functioning. The highest rates of physical abuse were in children with mild cognitive disabilities and no motor disability. Paradoxically, children whose disabilities are less severe are more likely to be the victims of physical abuse. These authors stated,

> "Conceptually, we can hypothesize that children with minor impairment are at greater risk because they have a complicated mix of dysfunctionality and functionality. Their dysfunctionality increases the probability that they will act in a way that elicits a negative reaction from parents, while their functionality increases their parents' expectations of them and increase their ability to take actions that may frustrate their parents."[37]

Harsh discipline, whether physical or verbal, can negatively affect children emotionally. Therefore, it is important to counsel parents of children with and without special needs about methods of discipline specifically as they relate to the developmental level of their child.[42]

Neglect

In their study, Van Horne et al followed the risks of substantiated maltreatment in a cohort of children younger than 2 years with cleft lip and palate, Down syndrome, and spina bifida. In this study, the authors found that, although children with Down syndrome had the same rate of overall substantiated maltreatment as typically developing peers, children with cleft lip and palate and spina bifida had 2 times the rate of maltreatment. However, the risk of medical neglect was significantly greater among all 3 birth defect groups than in the unaffected group of children. The medical complexity of these children may account for the increase in medical neglect.[7] In a follow-up study by Van Horne et al[43] on children aged 2 to 10 years with the same disabilities, children with cleft lip and palate, Down syndrome, and spina bifida all had a higher rate of medical neglect compared with children who were unaffected. In a study by McDonnell et al,[38] children with ASD alone, ASD plus ID, and ID alone were found to be at greater risk of physical neglect. Children with disabilities and unsubstantiated referrals for neglect experienced future maltreatment sooner and more often than other children.[12]

Sexual Abuse

In addition to physical abuse and neglect, children with disabilities are at an increased risk for being sexually abused.[41,44] Caldas and Bensy[44] studied children aged 6 to 17 years in the school setting and examined types of abuse, profiles of the victims of abuse, and profiles of the abusers. They found that children with disabilities are at 3 times the risk of sexual abuse compared with typically developing peers. The children with the greatest risk of abuse were children who had special education classroom supports. One-half of these abused children were victimized by peers, and one-half were victimized by school personnel. In a 2007 study from Israel, researchers found that children with disabilities were more likely to suffer more severe forms of sexual abuse.[45]

Multiple factors have been found to contribute to this increased rate of sexual abuse in children with disabilities, including the increased number of caregivers that children with disabilities encounter and limited access to information and training on personal safety and sexual abuse prevention.[44,46] Parents support education on human sexuality but are uncertain of how this topic should be presented to their child with IDs or communicative or motor disabilities.[47]

It is also important to recognize that health care providers have been implicated in sexual abuse of children with disabilities.[48] Data about the incidence and prevalence of sexual abuse by health care providers are sparse and do not allow a thorough analysis of the incidence of the types of abuse or the types of perpetrators because the terms "health care provider" or "health care worker" encompass many subgroups, including physicians, nurses, and therapists. Given the increased number of health care providers that children with disabilities routinely encounter, it is essential that the prohibition of sexual abuse and exploitation be discussed and taught during the training of all health care providers. The 2011 American Academy of Pediatrics (AAP) policy statement "Protecting Children From Sexual Abuse by Health Care Providers" is an excellent resource to help with this training.[48]

Emotional Abuse

In a study from the United Kingdom, children with conduct disorder, nonconduct psychological disorders, or speech and language difficulties were associated with a higher likelihood of child protection registration for emotional abuse.[49] Children with a psychiatric diagnosis are at higher risk for psychological maltreatment and emotional abuse.[50] In a study from Turkey, children with attention-deficit/hyperactivity disorder (ADHD) were found to have higher rates of emotional abuse than controls.[51] In a retrospective study of adults with and without ADHD, adults with ADHD reported higher rates of emotional abuse experienced as children when compared with adults who did not have ADHD.[52]

PEDIATRICIAN'S ROLE

Pediatricians and other health care providers need to be actively involved in the prevention, identification, and assessment of possible maltreatment of children with disabilities. Recognizing that these children are at a much higher risk is essential. It is important to assess whether immunizations and other well-child care are up to date and to ensure that necessary appointments with specialists or for illness or injuries are kept. Many children with disabilities have a team of professionals (including but not limited to teachers, paraprofessionals, and medical providers) who regularly interact with them and have direct knowledge about the limitations, abilities, and behaviors of that individual child. By working closely with these professionals, the pediatrician can gather additional insight into any concerns about maltreatment and use this information to guide the medical evaluation.

Pediatricians and other health care providers play a key role in evaluating and documenting medical conditions that may or may not predispose children with disabilities to injury. For example, documenting the presence of, or a risk for, osteopenia, is helpful in assessing fractures that may occur later. Self-injurious behaviors, such as headbanging and self-scratching, can elicit a CPS referral.[53] Careful and thorough documentation is often key in making a determination about whether an injury is consistent with abuse or is a result of self-injurious behavior. Health care providers can document abnormal physical examination findings, observed behaviors, and reported behaviors to establish the problem list for children with disabilities. Many electronic health records now have the capability to add digital photographs and "for your information" flags and alerts to the charts that can aid in assessing future injuries or changes in behavior based on preexisting conditions. This documentation is useful for collaboration with in-hospital providers, such as emergency medicine providers, hospitalists, and critical care providers who may also be part of the system of care for children with disabilities who are victims of abuse and neglect.

If abuse or neglect is suspected after a careful assessment, a report must be made to the appropriate CPS agency.[54] Collaboration with a multidisciplinary child abuse team or child abuse pediatrician can provide both technical assistance in the evaluation and guidance with the reporting process. Pediatricians may also need to educate CPS about medical findings to assist with the investigation by CPS. Careful consideration should be given regarding whether the evaluation is best completed in the outpatient versus inpatient setting. There are advantages and disadvantages to both; however, the safety of the child needs to be kept at the forefront in the decision-making process. If there are reports of self-injurious behavior that have not previously been documented or observed by a third party, an inpatient evaluation should be considered to observe the child's behaviors as part of the full medical evaluation.

Appropriate medical treatment can be provided for any identified injuries, infections, or other conditions. Each case of abuse or neglect that is clinically confirmed or strongly suspected requires a multidisciplinary treatment plan. Behavioral health referrals to clinicians experienced with caring for children with disabilities needs to be considered as part of the treatment plan. Evidence-based trauma therapy is available for children with disabilities, although this type of specific therapy may not be available in all communities (https://www.nctsn.org/resources/facts-traumatic-stress-and-children-developmental-disabilities).

Pediatricians are responsible for the transition of care to adult physicians but may continue to manage patients beyond their 18th birthday when they are no longer minors. When patients enter adulthood, abuse concerns are then referred to adult protective services. Pediatricians can familiarize themselves with adult protective services in their state.

Prevention

Support and assistance with parenting skills are often needed by families, and the need is greater for families with children and youth with special health care needs or disabilities. Pediatricians, as trusted family advisors, can acknowledge family needs, provide encouragement, and address parents' physical, social, and mental health needs.[55] They can present disability-specific injury prevention guidelines to help the family minimize injury.[56] The availability of parent support groups, respite care, and home health services should be explored, and referrals may be made when appropriate. Pediatricians can learn about services for parents of children with disabilities, such as respite and medical waiver subsidies and programs specific to each state and how to qualify for such funds.[57] Table 1 lists some resources for families of children with disabilities.

During each health supervision encounter, pediatric providers can address the medical, social, economic, behavioral, and psychological needs of the child and the family. Proactively addressing discipline concerns and encouraging positive parenting are especially needed in this population.[58] The AAP published a report strongly discouraging spanking and providing alternative discipline practices.[42] It is helpful to recognize and support child and family strengths at each encounter.[55] The AAP provides several resources for positive parenting (eg, www.healthychildren.org[59]; *Bright Futures: Guidelines for Health Supervision of Infants, Children, and Adolescents*, Fourth Edition[60]; and Connected Kids[61]). Pediatricians can share other positive parenting resources with families as well, such as the Centers for Disease Control and Prevention's Essentials for Parenting Toddlers and Preschoolers (http://www.cdc.gov/parents/essentials/overview.html).

All children, with or without disabilities, benefit from a medical home consisting of a health care professional who is readily accessible to the family to answer questions, help coordinate care, and discuss concerns.[62] A medical home may incorporate other professionals, including social workers, to help with accessing resources. The medical home can also collaborate with

TABLE 1 Resources for Families of Children With Disabilities

	Resources
Financial	Supplemental Security Income (SSI), Special Supplemental Nutrition Program for Women, Infants, and Children (WIC), Medicaid waiver, therapist fees, Title V maternal and child health services programs for children and youth with special health care needs
Respite or extended care	Respite centers, baby-sitting, after-school programs, emergency respite, residential supports
Specialized medical needs	In-home nursing services, durable medical equipment
Emotional support	Support groups, counseling services for families, family-to-family health information centers
Educational support	IFSPs, IEPs, special education teachers and paraprofessionals
Recreational opportunities	Camps, after-school recreation, sports

IEP, Individualized Education Program; IFSP, Individualized Family Service Plan.

partners from other disciplines, including education, child care, mental health, and faith-based organizations. While working with families of children with disabilities, health care providers can educate and encourage them to work with community agencies that provide the resources and services they need to improve the child's care and the family's coping. Child abuse prevention, including indicators of abuse, can be discussed with parents and caregivers, especially those dealing with children with disabilities, and taking into account the family's language and culture.[55]

Education

In-service training for CPS and adult protective service workers, law enforcement professionals, health care professionals, child care providers, early childhood educators, teachers, and judges is crucial, and protocols are necessary for the identification, reporting, and referral of all cases of suspected child maltreatment in all schools, programs, and institutional settings. Experts in either child maltreatment or childhood disabilities can assist with this educational endeavor. General pediatricians can help local school districts with training in positive behavioral interventions and supports.[32] Education on risk factors for maltreatment of children with disabilities is important.

Pediatricians can be important role models to parents, trainees, and others. Pediatricians and other health care providers who provide care for children with disabilities can avoid using physical restraints during procedures for these children. Often, taking the time to explain procedures in terms appropriate to developmental level or other ways to prepare a child can make restraints unnecessary except in situations when children are dangerous to themselves or others. Even when some types of restraints are needed,

such as to prevent a child from scratching at newly repaired lacerations, such restraints should be as comfortable and as minimal as possible and used for the shortest time feasible. Pediatricians can also be flexible about performing procedures, such as delaying blood draws that are not essential.

Pediatricians may also assist in education about child abuse to peers, residents, medical students, and other health care students. All health care professionals need adequate training to monitor children with disabilities for signs of abuse and neglect and to screen suspected victims of child maltreatment for possible delays or disabilities.[63]

Advocacy

The pediatrician, in providing the medical home and acting as the patient's and family's advocate, may review care that is provided by various agencies and resources. Much of this advocacy effort can be performed by coordinating efforts and ensuring that recommendations are implemented.[57] By providing prevention-based continuity of care, additional patient needs, such as changes in services, can be expediently identified and resolved.

Pediatricians play an important advocacy role in their relationships with various governmental and nongovernmental agencies. AAP chapters can also have an influential role in these arenas. State, educational, social, foster care, financial, and health care systems often function in isolation from each other, with little coordination or communication.[35] Foster children with disabilities and their foster parents, for example, often suffer from lack of adequate support systems.[1] Community involvement can often lead to the development of needed resources, including child care and respite services for families with a child with a special health care

need.[6] Pediatricians can advocate for the caregivers to receive financial support to access services, such as respite. Communication with schools and other systems with which families interact is another avenue to increase the awareness of the needs of children who have disabilities and/ or special health care needs.

As child advocates, pediatricians are in an ideal position to influence public policy by sharing information and giving educational presentations on child maltreatment and the needs of children with disabilities. There can be advocacy for training in recognizing both abuse and findings that mimic abuse for providers of children with disabilities. Pediatricians can advocate for state policies that mandate CPS agencies to gather disability information on child maltreatment cases. Pediatricians can emphasize the devastating costs of child maltreatment to legislators, policy makers, and the public. Pediatricians can advocate for state Medicaid programs to provide prompt automatic Medicaid eligibility at enrollment in foster care, including kinship care. Pediatricians can also advocate for health care not to be disrupted if a child with disabilities is placed into Medicaid managed-care plans that do not have the child's existing specialists in network. Pediatricians can also advocate for proper coverage in both private and public insurance plans. In the case of primary care, there should be a time-limited presumptive authorization extended to a current primary care provider for well visits and timely immunization visits. Pediatricians can advocate that Medicaid programs pay for services necessary for the effective transition of care when there must be a change in specialty providers. Pediatricians can also advocate for screening procedures for potential employees in educational, recreational, and residential settings to help ensure the safety of all children in their care.[32]

SUMMARY

Children with disabilities are a vulnerable population at increased risk of child abuse and neglect and, therefore, merit special attention to reduce this risk. Children with milder forms of disability are at higher risk of abuse and neglect than more profoundly affected children.

Certain types of disabilities are associated with different forms of abuse. Children with behavioral difficulties are at a greater risk for physical abuse. Children who are nonverbal or hearing impaired are more likely to experience neglect or sexual abuse. Children with multiple developmental delays are more at risk for recurrence of child abuse reporting. Conduct disorder, nonconduct psychological disorders, speech and language difficulties, and ADHD are associated with emotional abuse.

Addressing financial struggles, family stress, and the long-term needs of these children can reduce the risk of child abuse and neglect. Pediatricians are a unique resource to children with disabilities through the medical home model and in multidisciplinary teams.

GUIDANCE FOR PEDIATRICIANS

1. Recognize signs and symptoms of child maltreatment in all children and adolescents, including those with disabilities, and understand mandatory, state-specific reporting requirements for child and adult protective services.

2. Use each medical visit as an opportunity to assess family well-being.

3. Understand that families of children with disabilities benefit from assistance in addressing their child's abilities and needs. Provide reasonable expectations for parents regarding their children with disabilities and be prepared to offer concrete suggestions about how to respond to common developmentally based challenges for the child with a disability.

4. Refer families of children with disabilities to available community resources and agencies that provide necessary services designed to aid children with disabilities and their families.

5. Structure discussions about appropriate discipline within well-child visits for the child with a disability. Parents may be uncertain as to how to deal with discipline, especially for children who are verbal but developmentally delayed, so provide guidance on positive parenting. Consider referring these families to specialists with expertise in parenting skills for children with disabilities.

6. Be actively involved with both educational and medical treatment plans developed for children with disabilities and participate in collaborative team approaches.

7. Advocate at the state and local level for system changes that support at-risk children and those with disabilities and their families.

SUGGESTED RESOURCES

A Call to Action: Ending Crimes of Violence against Children and Adults with Disabilities: this report includes recommendations on policy, surveillance systems and data collection, violence prevention, intervention, and research needs. Available at: https://www.aucd.org/docs/annual_mtg_2006/symp_marge2003.pdf.

www.pbis.org: this Web-based resource offers information about programs supporting positive behavioral parenting for families and other caregivers.

Toolkit for medical providers about trauma-informed practice from the National Child Traumatic Stress Network. Available at: http://www.nctsnet.org/trauma-types/pediatric-medical-traumatic-stress-toolkit-for-health-care-providers.

Stop Hurting Kids: this Web site was created by the Alliance to Prevent Restraint, Aversive Interventions, and Seclusion (APRAIS,) a coalition of organizations and advocates who dedicate their time and resources to ending restraint and seclusion abuse in US schools. Available at: http://stophurtingkids.com/resources/.

Hagan JF, Shaw JS, Duncan PM, eds. *Bright Futures: Guidelines for Health Supervision of Infants, Children, and Adolescents.* 4th ed. Elk Grove Village, IL: American Academy of Pediatrics; 2017. Available at: https://brightfutures.aap.org/Pages/default.aspx.

American Academy of Pediatrics. Connected Kids: Safe, Strong, Secure. Available at: https://www.aap.org/en-us/advocacy-and-policy/aap-health-initiatives/Pages/Connected-Kids.aspx.

LEAD AUTHORS

Lori A. Legano, MD, FAAP
Larry W. Desch, MD, FAAP
Stephen A. Messner, MD, FAAP
Sheila Idzerda, MD, FAAP
Emalee G. Flaherty, MD, FAAP

COUNCIL ON CHILD ABUSE AND NEGLECT, 2019–2020

Suzanne B. Haney, MD, FAAP, Chairperson
Andrew P. Sirotnak, MD, FAAP, Immediate Past Chairperson
Amy R. Gavril, MD, MSCI, FAAP
Rebecca Greenlee Girardet, MD, FAAP
Amanda Bird Hoffert Gilmartin, MD, FAAP
Sheila M. Idzerda, MD, FAAP
Antoinette Laskey, MD, MPH, MBA, FAAP
Lori A. Legano, MD, FAAP
Stephen A. Messner, MD, FAAP
Bethany Anne Mohr, MD, FAAP
Shalon Marie Nienow, MD, FAAP
Norell Rosado, MD, FAAP

ABBREVIATIONS

AAP: American Academy of Pediatrics
ADHD: attention-deficit/hyperactivity disorder
ASD: autism spectrum disorder
CPS: child protective services
FASD: fetal alcohol spectrum disorder
ID: intellectual disability

FINANCIAL DISCLOSURE: The authors have indicated they have no financial relationships relevant to this article to disclose.

FUNDING: No external funding.

POTENTIAL CONFLICT OF INTEREST: The authors have indicated they have no potential conflicts of interest to disclose.

REFERENCES

1. Hibbard RA, Desch LW; American Academy of Pediatrics Committee on Child Abuse and Neglect; American Academy of Pediatrics Council on Children With Disabilities. Maltreatment of children with disabilities. *Pediatrics.* 2007;119(5):1018–1025

2. Prkachin KM, Solomon PE, Ross J. Underestimation of pain by health-care providers: towards a model of the process of inferring pain in others. *Can J Nurs Res.* 2007;39(2):88–106

3. US Department of Health and Human Services, Administration for Children and Families, Administration on Children, Youth and Families, Children's Bureau. Child maltreatment 2018. Available at:https://www.acf.hhs.gov/sites/default/files/documents/cb/cm2018.pdf. Accessed July 10, 2020

4. Child Welfare Information Gateway. *The Risk and Prevention of Maltreatment of Children with Disabilities.* Washington,

   DC: US Department of Health and Human Services, Children's Bureau; 2018

5. Helton JJ, Lightfoot E, Fu QJ, Bruhn CM. Prevalence and severity of child impairment in a US sample of child maltreatment investigations. *J Dev Behav Pediatr.* 2019;40(4):285–292

6. Turner HA, Vanderminden J, Finkelhor D, Hamby S, Shattuck A. Disability and victimization in a national sample of children and youth. *Child Maltreat.* 2011;16(4):275–286

7. Van Horne BS, Moffitt KB, Canfield MA, et al. Maltreatment of children under age 2 with specific birth defects: a population-based study. *Pediatrics.* 2015;136(6). Available at: www.pediatrics.org/cgi/content/full/136/6/e1504

8. Harrell E. *Crime Against People With Disabilities, 2009-2015—Statistical Tables.* Washington, DC: Bureau of

   Justice Statistics, US Department of Justice; 2017. Available at: www.bjs.gov/index.cfm?ty=pbdetail&iid=5986. Accessed September 9, 2020

9. Zand DH, Pierce KJ, Nibras S, Maxim R. Parental risk for the maltreatment of developmentally delayed/disabled children. *Clin Pediatr (Phila).* 2015; 54(3):290–292

10. Maclean MJ, Sims S, Bower C, Leonard H, Stanley FJ, O'Donnell M. Maltreatment risk among children with disabilities. *Pediatrics.* 2017;139(4): e20161817

11. Jones L, Bellis MA, Wood S, et al. Prevalence and risk of violence against children with disabilities: a systematic review and meta-analysis of observational studies. *Lancet.* 2012; 380(9845):899–907

12. Kistin CJ, Tompson MC, Cabral HJ, Sege RD, Winter MR, Silverstein M. Subsequent maltreatment in children

with disabilities after an unsubstantiated report for neglect. *JAMA.* 2016;315(1):85–87

13. Slayter E, Springer C. Child welfare-involved youth with intellectual disabilities: pathways into and placements in foster care. *Intellect Dev Disabil.* 2011;49(1):1–13

14. Frasier LD. Abusive head trauma in infants and young children: a unique contributor to developmental disabilities. *Pediatr Clin North Am.* 2008; 55(6):1269–1285, vii

15. Nuño M, Ugiliweneza B, Zepeda V, et al. Long-term impact of abusive head trauma in young children. *Child Abuse Negl.* 2018;85:39–46

16. Levin AV. Retinal hemorrhages: advances in understanding. *Pediatr Clin North Am.* 2009;56(2):333–344

17. Blaisdell KN, Imhof AM, Fisher PA. Early adversity, child neglect, and stress neurobiology: from observations of impact to empirical evaluations of mechanisms. *Int J Dev Neurosci.* 2019; 78:139–146

18. Maguire SA, Williams B, Naughton AM, et al. A systematic review of the emotional, behavioural and cognitive features exhibited by school-aged children experiencing neglect or emotional abuse. *Child Care Health Dev.* 2015;41(5):641–653

19. Shonkoff JP, Garner AS; Committee on Psychosocial Aspects of Child and Family Health; Committee on Early Childhood, Adoption, and Dependent Care; Section on Developmental and Behavioral Pediatrics. The lifelong effects of early childhood adversity and toxic stress. *Pediatrics.* 2012;129(1). Available at: www.pediatrics.org/cgi/content/full/129/1/e232

20. Pechtel P, Pizzagalli DA. Effects of early life stress on cognitive and affective function: an integrated review of human literature. *Psychopharmacology (Berl).* 2011;214(1):55–70

21. Enlow MB, Egeland B, Blood EA, Wright RO, Wright RJ. Interpersonal trauma exposure and cognitive development in children to age 8 years: a longitudinal study. *J Epidemiol Community Health.* 2012;66(11):1005–1010

22. Peer JW, Hillman SB. Stress and resilience for parents of children with intellectual and developmental disabilities: a review of key factors and recommendations for practitioners. *J Policy Pract Intell Disabil.* 2014;11(2): 92–98

23. Witt WP, Litzelman K, Mandic CG, et al. Healthcare-related financial burden among families in the U.S.: the role of childhood activity limitations and income. *J Fam Econ Issues.* 2011;32(2): 308–326

24. Murphy N. Maltreatment of children with disabilities: the breaking point. *J Child Neurol.* 2011;26(8):1054–1056

25. Romley JA, Shah AK, Chung PJ, Elliott MN, Vestal KD, Schuster MA. Family-provided health care for children with special health care needs. *Pediatrics.* 2017;139(1):e20161287

26. Goudie A, Narcisse MR, Hall DE, Kuo DZ. Financial and psychological stressors associated with caring for children with disability. *Fam Syst Health.* 2014; 32(3):280–290

27. Dubowitz H, Kim J, Black MM, Weisbart C, Semiatin J, Magder LS. Identifying children at high risk for a child maltreatment report. *Child Abuse Negl.* 2011;35(2):96–104

28. Centers for Disease Control and Prevention. Fetal alcohol spectrum disorders (FASDs). Available at: https://www.cdc.gov/ncbddd/fasd/index.html. Accessed March 22, 2021

29. Miller BA, Smyth NJ, Mudar PJ. Mothers' alcohol and other drug problems and their punitiveness toward their children. *J Stud Alcohol.* 1999;60(5): 632–642

30. Ouyang L, Fang X, Mercy J, Perou R, Grosse SD. Attention-deficit/hyperactivity disorder symptoms and child maltreatment: a population-based study. *J Pediatr.* 2008;153(6): 851–856

31. Scaramella LV, Leve LD. Clarifying parent-child reciprocities during early childhood: the early childhood coercion model. *Clin Child Fam Psychol Rev.* 2004; 7(2):89–107

32. Turnbull HR, Wilcox BL, Stowe M, Raper C, Hedges LP. Public policy foundations for positive behavioral interventions, strategies, and supports. *J Posit Behav Interv.* 2000;2(4):218–230

33. Mohr WK, Petti TA, Mohr BD. Adverse effects associated with physical restraint. *Can J Psychiatry.* 2003;48(5): 330–337

34. Kutz GD. *Seclusions and Restraints: Selected Cases of Death and Abuse at Public and Private Schools and Treatment Centers.* Washington, DC: US Government Accountability Office; 2009. Available at: https://www.gao.gov/products/GAO-09-719T. Accessed September 9, 2020

35. Sullivan P, Cork PM. *Developmental Disabilities Training Project.* Omaha, NE: Center for Abused Children with Disabilities, Boys Town National Research Hospital, Nebraska Department of Health and Human Services; 1996

36. World Health Organization. International classification of functioning, disability and health. Available at: www.who.int/classifications/icf/en/. Accessed September 9, 2020

37. Helton JJ, Cross TP. The relationship of child functioning to parental physical assault: linear and curvilinear models. *Child Maltreat.* 2011;16(2):126–136

38. McDonnell CG, Boan AD, Bradley CC, Seay KD, Charles JM, Carpenter LA. Child maltreatment in autism spectrum disorder and intellectual disability: results from a population-based sample. *J Child Psychol Psychiatry.* 2019;60(5):576–584

39. Fisher MH, Epstein RA, Urbano RC, Vehorn A, Cull MJ, Warren Z. A population-based examination of maltreatment referrals and substantiation for children with autism spectrum disorder. *Autism.* 2019;23(5): 1335–1340

40. Perrigo JL, Berkovits LD, Cederbaum JA, Williams ME, Hurlburt MS. Child abuse and neglect re-report rates for young children with developmental delays. *Child Abuse Negl.* 2018;83:1–9

41. Sullivan PM, Knutson JF. Maltreatment and disabilities: a population-based epidemiological study. *Child Abuse Negl.* 2000;24(10):1257–1273

42. Sege RD, Siegel BS; Council on Child Abuse and Neglect; Committee on Psychosocial Aspects of Child and Family Health. Effective discipline to

raise healthy children. [published correction appears in *Pediatrics*;143(2): e20183609]. *Pediatrics*. 2018;142(6): e20183112

43. Van Horne BS, Caughy MO, Canfield M, et al. First-time maltreatment in children ages 2-10 with and without specific birth defects: a population-based study. *Child Abuse Negl*. 2018;84: 53–63

44. Caldas SJ, Bensy ML. The sexual maltreatment of students with disabilities in American school settings. *J Child Sex Abuse*. 2014;23(4):345–366

45. Hershkowitz I, Lamb ME, Horowitz D. Victimization of children with disabilities. *Am J Orthopsychiatry*. 2007; 77(4):629–635

46. Servais L. Sexual health care in persons with intellectual disabilities. *Ment Retard Dev Disabil Res Rev*. 2006;12(1): 48–56

47. Eastgate G, Scheermeyer E, van Driel ML, Lennox N. Intellectual disability, sexuality and sexual abuse prevention - a study of family members and support workers. *Aust Fam Physician*. 2012; 41(3):135–139

48. Committee on Child Abuse and Neglect. Protecting children from sexual abuse by health care providers. *Pediatrics*. 2011;128(2):407–426

49. Spencer N, Devereux E, Wallace A, et al. Disabling conditions and registration for child abuse and neglect:

a population-based study. *Pediatrics*. 2005;116(3):609–613

50. Cuevas CA, Finkelhor D, Ormrod R, Turner H. Psychiatric diagnosis as a risk marker for victimization in a national sample of children. *J Interpers Violence*. 2009;24(4):636–652

51. Sari Gokten E, Saday Duman N, Soylu N, Uzun ME. Effects of attention-deficit/ hyperactivity disorder on child abuse and neglect. *Child Abuse Negl*. 2016;62: 1–9

52. Rucklidge JJ, Brown DL, Crawford S, Kaplan BJ. Retrospective reports of childhood trauma in adults with ADHD. *J Atten Disord*. 2006;9(4):631–641

53. Minshawi NF, Hurwitz S, Fodstad JC, Biebl S, Morriss DH, McDougle CJ. The association between self-injurious behaviors and autism spectrum disorders. *Psychol Res Behav Manag*. 2014;7:125–136

54. Kellogg N; American Academy of Pediatrics Committee on Child Abuse and Neglect. The evaluation of sexual abuse in children. *Pediatrics*. 2005; 116(2):506–512

55. Mattson G, Kuo DZ; Committee on Psychosocial Aspects of Child and Family Health; Council on Children With Disabilities. Psychosocial factors in children and youth with special health care needs and their families. *Pediatrics*. 2019;143(1):e20183171

56. Gaebler-Spira D, Thornton LS. Injury prevention for children with

disabilities. *Phys Med Rehabil Clin N Am*. 2002;13(4):891–906

57. Friedman SL, Kalichman MA; Council on Children with Disabilities. Out-of-home placement for children and adolescents with disabilities. *Pediatrics*. 2014; 134(4):836–846

58. Office of Special Education Programs, US Department of Education. Positive behavioral interventions and supports. Available at: https://www.PBIS.org. Accessed October 22, 2018

59. American Academy of Pediatrics. HealthyChildren.org. Available at: www.healthychildren.org/English/Pages/default.aspx. Accessed August 13, 2019

60. Hagan JF, Shaw JS, Duncan PM, eds.. *Bright Futures: Guidelines for Health Supervision of Infants, Children, and Adolescents*, 4th ed. Elk Grove Village, IL: American Academy of Pediatrics; 2017

61. American Academy of Pediatrics. Connected kids: safe, strong, secure. Available at: https://www.aap.org/en-us/advocacy-and-policy/aap-health-initiatives/Pages/Connected-Kids.aspx. Accessed September 9, 2020

62. Medical Home Initiatives for Children With Special Needs Project Advisory Committee. American Academy of Pediatrics. The medical home. *Pediatrics*. 2002;110(1 pt 1):184–186

63. Botash AS, Church CC. Child abuse and disabilities: a medical perspective. *APSAC Advisor*. 1999;12:10–13, 18

CLINICAL REPORT Guidance for the Clinician in Rendering Pediatric Care

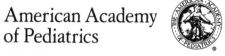

American Academy
of Pediatrics

DEDICATED TO THE HEALTH OF ALL CHILDREN™

Promoting the Participation of Children and Adolescents With Disabilities in Sports, Recreation, and Physical Activity

Paul S. Carbone, MD, FAAP,[a] Peter J. Smith, MD, MA, FAAP,[b] Charron Lewis, MD, FAAP,[c] Claire LeBlanc, MD, FAAP,[d]
COUNCIL ON CHILDREN WITH DISABILITIES, COUNCIL ON SPORTS MEDICINE AND FITNESS

abstract

The benefits of physical activity are likely universal for all children, including children and adolescents with disabilities (CWD). The participation of CWD in physical activity, including adaptive or therapeutic sports and recreation, promotes inclusion, minimizes deconditioning, optimizes physical functioning, improves mental health as well as academic achievement, and enhances overall well-being. Despite these benefits, CWD face barriers to participation and have lower levels of fitness, reduced rates of participation, and a higher prevalence of overweight and obesity compared with typically developing peers. Pediatricians and caregivers may overestimate the risks or overlook the benefits of physical activity in CWD, which further limits participation. Preparticipation evaluations often include assessment of health status, functional capacity, individual activity preferences, availability of appropriate programs, and safety precautions. Given the complexity, the preparticipation evaluation for CWD may not occur in the context of a single office visit but rather over a period of time with input from the child's multidisciplinary team (physicians, coaches, physical education teachers, school nurses, adaptive recreation specialists, physical and occupational therapists, and others). Some CWD may desire to participate in organized sports to experience the challenge of competition, and others may prefer recreational activities for enjoyment. To reach the goal of inclusion in appropriate physical activities for all children with disabilities, child, family, financial, and societal barriers to participation need to be identified and addressed. Health care providers can facilitate participation by encouraging physical activity among CWD and their families during visits. Health care providers can create "physical activity prescriptions" for CWD on the basis of the child's preferred activities, functional status, need for adaptation of the activity and the recreational opportunities available in the community. This clinical report discusses the

[a]Department of Pediatrics, The University of Utah, Salt Lake City, Utah; [b]Section on Developmental and Behavioral Pediatrics, The University of Chicago, Chicago, Illinois; [c]Division of Developmental-Behavioral Pediatrics and Psychology, Rainbow Babies and Children's Hospital, Cleveland, Ohio; and [d]Department of Pediatrics, McGill University, Montreal, Quebec, Canada

All authors participated in conception, design, drafting, and critical revision of the clinical report and approved the final manuscript as submitted.

Clinical reports from the American Academy of Pediatrics benefit from expertise and resources of liaisons and internal (AAP) and external reviewers. However, clinical reports from the American Academy of Pediatrics may not reflect the views of the liaisons or the organizations or government agencies that they represent.

The guidance in this report does not indicate an exclusive course of treatment or serve as a standard of medical care. Variations, taking into account individual circumstances, may be appropriate.

All clinical reports from the American Academy of Pediatrics automatically expire 5 years after publication unless reaffirmed, revised, or retired at or before that time.

DOI: https://doi.org/10.1542/peds.2021-054664

To cite: Carbone PS, Smith PJ, Lewis C, et al.; AAP Council on Children With Disabilities, Council on Sports Medicine and Fitness Promoting the Participation of Children and Adolescents With Disabilities in Sports, Recreation, and Physical Activity. *Pediatrics.* 2021;148(6):e2021054664

importance of participation in sports, recreation, and physical activity for CWD and offers practical suggestions to health care providers.

GLOSSARY OF TERMS

- Children and youth with special health care needs (CYSHCN) are "children who have or are at increased risk for a chronic physical, developmental, behavioral or emotional condition and who also require health and related services of a type or amount beyond that required by children generally."[1] In the United States, 19% of children have a special health care need.[2] CYSHCN are a diverse group of children, ranging from children with chronic conditions, to those with medical complexity, to children with cognitive, behavioral, or emotional conditions. The term CYSHCN includes children with disabilities (CWD) and children with medical complexity, whom are described below and shown in Fig 1.

- CWD are defined under the Individuals with Disabilities Education Act (IDEA) as children with intellectual disabilities, hearing impairments (including deafness), speech or language impairments, visual impairments (including blindness), serious emotional disturbance, orthopedic impairments, autism spectrum disorder, traumatic brain injury, other health impairments, or specific learning disabilities and who, by reason thereof, need special education and related services.[3] Although not part of the IDEA definition, the World Health Organization International Classification of Functioning, Disability and Health (ICF) framework provides an important alternative framework for disability because of its emphasis on body function, pursuit of meaningful activities, and community participation as primary determinates of the health of individuals rather than emphasis on any particular diagnosis or deficit (Fig 2).[4]

- Children with medical complexity have multiple significant chronic health problems resulting in functional limitations, high health care service needs, and often the need for or use of medical technology.[5] An example of a child with medical complexity is one with a genetic syndrome with an associated congenital heart defect, difficulty swallowing, cerebral palsy, and a urologic condition. This child would typically require the care of a primary care physician; multiple pediatric medical subspecialists or pediatric surgical specialists, home nurses, and rehabilitative and habilitative therapists; community-based services; extensive pharmaceutical therapies; special attention to his or her nutritional needs and growth; and durable medical equipment to maintain health, maximize development, and promote function.

- Participation, defined by the ICF, is the nature and extent of a person's involvement in desired activities, such as recreation, leisure activities, and community life. The ICF also emphasizes the interconnection of contextual factors, environmental and personal, that can have profound influences on participation. For example, finding out what recreational activities are enjoyable and fun for CWD (personal factors) and supporting families (environmental factors) can foster increased community participation and bolster overall health.[6,7]

- Physical activity refers to any body movement produced by skeletal muscles that requires energy expenditure.[8]

- Exercise is planned, structured, and repetitive physical activity that aims to improve or maintain one or more component of physical fitness.[8] Exercise may be subdivided into aerobic (cardiovascular endurance), flexibility (increase muscle and joint range of motion), anaerobic (resistance training), and high-impact weight-bearing exercise (that promotes bone health).[8]

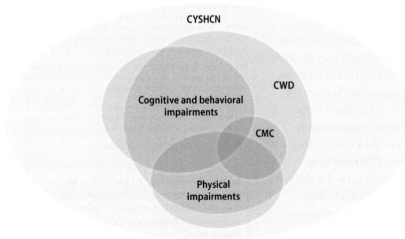

FIGURE 1 Diverse subgroups within CYSHCN. CMC, children with medical complexity.

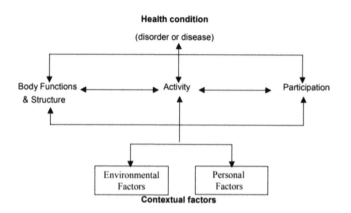

FIGURE 2 The World Health Organization International Classification of Functioning, Disability and Health. Reprinted with permission from World Health Organization. *Towards a Common Language for Functioning, Disability and Health.* Geneva, Switzerland: World Health Organization; 2002:9.

- PAVS, physical activity vital sign.
- AAI, atlantoaxial instability.

INTRODUCTION

International efforts to promote the well-being of CWD through participation in exercise, sports, recreation, and physical activities began with the first competitive sporting event for individuals with disabilities in 1948, followed by the first Paralympics competition in 1960. Special Olympics was established in 1968 and is now the largest recreational program for children and adults with intellectual disabilities, with 5.5 million athletes in 1930 countries.[9] Despite the success of these programs, opportunities for CWD to participate in physical activity, exercise, or competitive sports remain limited, and they are less likely to participate compared with their peers without disabilities.[10-12] In the absence of such opportunities and the encouragement to participate, many CWD engage in more sedentary and solitary activities, leading to a higher prevalence of overweight and obesity, lower levels of cardiorespiratory fitness, and increasing social isolation.[13-19] Taking part in physical activity through recreation and sport provides CWD the opportunity to achieve better physical and mental health, develop skills and competencies, express creativity, form friendships, and improve quality of life.[20-23] Thus, the American Academy of Pediatrics *Bright Futures: Guidelines for Health Supervision of Infants, Children, and Adolescents, Fourth Edition*, includes promotion of physical activity as a key health promotion theme and includes recommendations for health care providers to help CYSHCN and their families identify appropriate and enjoyable activities and implement adaptations based on need and ability.[24]

This clinical report discusses the importance of physical activity for CWD, reviews potential barriers to inclusion, and offers practical solutions for clinicians to facilitate participation. Of note, the terms CYSHCN, CWD, and children with medical complexity are overlapping (Fig 1). This clinical report focuses on the needs of CWD, but many of the comments and recommendations apply also to the larger group of CYSHCN. However, not all points or problems apply equally to the diverse subgroups of CWD. For example, some recommendations may apply more to children with physical impairments or children with cognitive or behavioral impairments. Furthermore, the subgroups within CWD are also overlapping and can shift over time, such as the case in which a child with primary motor impairments as a young child might be more impacted by cognitive or behavioral impairments as an adolescent (Fig 1). Regardless of the subgroup, CYSHCN and all children with different abilities are at risk for being "left out," which can adversely affect wellness, community integration, and full actualization of their individuality. Although it is hoped that children with and without disabilities engage in physical activity together, there will be times when CWD and their families opt for adaptive programs that are focused specifically on their needs. It must also be noted that there is a heterogeneity of adaptive recreation and sports programs, varying both by the type of primary impairment they are focused on and by the competitive levels of the programs. For example, Paralympians are high-performance competitive athletes who generally self-identify as primarily having physical or visual impairments, whereas Special Olympians are often individuals with intellectual and developmental disabilities who compete in many different sports at various competitive levels.[9,25] There are also sports programs for people with hearing impairments, with the most elite being the Deaflympics.[26] Although adaptive recreation programs have existed for more than 50 years, recently there has been accelerated growth in the number of programs, especially those with a primary purpose of fostering physical activity in a noncompetitive, fun environment. Whatever the activity or the level of competition, health care providers can engage in shared decision-making with CWD and their families with the goal of pursuing appropriate opportunities for physical activity.[27]

BENEFITS OF PARTICIPATION IN PHYSICAL ACTIVITIES

The benefits of physical activity are likely universal for all children, including those with disabilities. CWD are underrepresented in exercise intervention research, resulting in a limited understanding of how research involving children without disabilities can be translated into guidance for physical activity programs for CWD. The limited research conducted to date points to at least short-term benefits for CWD, such as improvements in aerobic capacity, muscular strength, physical and cognitive function, body weight and composition, social skills, relationships, and psychological well-being.[28–30] Although many studies of exercise interventions for children with physical disabilities have small sample sizes and lack randomization, they support safe participation and improvements in fitness and well-being.[31] Several studies rated from moderate- to high-quality show that children and youth with physical disabilities who participate in physical activity programs improve their locomotor performance and skills, object control, social skills, peer interactions, and self-confidence.[29] One randomized trial of an 8-month weight-bearing physical activity program for children with cerebral palsy showed improvements in bone mineral density.[32] In some CWD, exercise interventions may even be able to slow disease progression. For example, in 2 randomized trials of assisted bicycle and upper extremity training, functional motor deterioration slowed in boys with Duchenne muscular dystrophy.[33,34] Ambulatory children with spina bifida can also increase their walking speed and cardiorespiratory fitness with treadmill training programs.[35] Thus, *Bright Futures: Guidelines for Health Supervision of Infants, Children, and Adolescents, Fourth Edition*, includes recommendations for health care providers to help CYSHCN and their families identify appropriate and enjoyable physical activities and implement adaptations on the basis of their needs and abilities.

Physical activity also has benefits for children with primarily cognitive and behavioral disabilities. Children with autism spectrum disorder (hereafter referred to as autism), who are more likely to be diagnosed with overweight or obesity, have this risk attenuated with regular physical activity and sports participation.[36] Short periods of walking or running before educational sessions also help children with autism increase the proportion of correct academic responses and work tasks completed in school settings.[37,38] Other exercise interventions for children with autism, such as horseback riding, martial arts, swimming, yoga, or dance, can result in better social responsiveness and decreased irritability, stereotypical behavior, and hyperactivity.[39–43] Although stimulant medication is the mainstay in addressing core symptoms for children with attention-deficit/hyperactivity disorder, aerobic exercise offers a safe and widely beneficial adjunct in decreasing hyperactivity and improving attention and executive function.[44] Youth with intellectual disability who are overweight or obese benefit from participating in an integrative training program, with improved cardiorespiratory fitness, balance, muscle strength, and endurance as well as lower BMI.[45] Adolescents and adults with Down syndrome who receive individualized progressive resistance training over 10 weeks have increased muscular strength and become more physically active.[46]

Beyond the physiologic benefits, regular physical activity, recreation, and sports participation are associated with both psychosocial well-being and quality of life of CWD as well as with improving academic achievements.[21] For example, participants in Special Olympics show heightened self-esteem, perceived physical competence, and peer acceptance when compared with nonparticipants.[47] Physically active individuals with cerebral palsy experience higher quality of life and happiness compared with those who are less active.[20] Children with autism who have higher levels of participation in organized activities, including sports, have better social-emotional adjustment as well as reduced loneliness and depression.[48,49] Children with muscular dystrophies who participate in physical activities, such as swimming, benefit by cultivation of friendships, increased self-confidence, and enjoyment.[50] Children with hearing impairment who participated in a 3-month ice skating program were found by their parents to have improvements in self-esteem, behavior, and sleep quality.[51]

Despite the physical, behavioral, cognitive, and psychosocial benefits of physical activity for CWD, the incorporation of physical activity is often prioritized below other interventions in treatment planning.[49] Yet, as the above examples illustrate, inclusion of physical activity into treatment plans allows CWD real-world and enjoyable opportunities to work on motor, communication, and social skill goals identified in traditional therapies, such as physical, speech, and occupational therapy.

BARRIERS TO PARTICIPATION

Despite the potential benefits, CWD participate in sports, recreation, and physical activity less than children without disabilities, and they experience barriers to participation that go beyond the functional limitations associated with their disabilities (Table 1).[52–57] Without

TABLE 1 Benefits, Barriers, and Considerations for Participation in Sports by CWD

Benefits of participation
    Improved wellness
    Increased community integration
    Improved muscle strength
    Improved fundamental movement skills
    Enhanced psychosocial well-being
    Increased cardiorespiratory fitness
    Decreased morbidity (ie, pressure ulcers, infections, overweight and obesity, etc)
    Improved bone health
    Improved motor coordination
    Improved attention and focus
    Decreased maladaptive behaviors
Barriers to participation
    False belief: no programs for this population
    False belief: participation is unsafe or too risky
    False belief: rules of sports too hard to learn or cannot be adapted to accommodate CWD
    Low physical literacy
    Lack of transportation to and from activities
    Lack of needed supervision or expertise
    Extra cost and time commitment
Facilitators to participation
    Preparticipation evaluations to maximize safety with appropriate accommodations
    Organized sports that are focused on fun over competition
    Clinicians, physical education teachers, and coaches who create physical activity prescriptions
      and recognize individual needs
    Adaptations such as longer rest periods, lower coach to athlete ratios, copious positive
      feedback, and close monitoring for symptoms of fatigue or injury

Reproduced with permission from: American Academy of Pediatrics. Athletes with a disability. In: Bernhardt DT, Roberts WO, eds. *PPE: Preparticipation Physical Evaluation*. 5th ed. Itasca, IL: American Academy of Pediatrics; 2019:185

addressing barriers to physical activity, CWD often fill leisure time with sedentary screen-based activities.[18,58] Frequently identified barriers to participation of CWD in sports and physical activity are the child's functional limitations, negative self-perceptions, high cost, lack of accessible facilities, lack of nearby facilities or programs, and lack of providers with adaptive recreation expertise.[10,59-62] In addition, many individuals with disabilities are still, to a large extent, socially segregated and experience negative societal stereotypes and low performance expectations, providing them with limited opportunities for participation in group-based physical activities.[57,60,63] Some CWD may be discouraged to participate by an implicit societal bias that favors competitiveness and winning over participation for the sake of fun, enjoyment, and inclusion. When CWD do attempt to participate in sports, they are also more likely to be bullied by their peers[64,65]; this is especially true for CWD with obesity, who may experience additional weight-bias stigmatization. Primary care providers who have longitudinal and trusting relationships with CWD and their families can be positive role models and use nonjudgmental language and motivational interviewing to identify short-term goals and strategies related to eating and physical activity.[66] With negative experiences and lack of opportunities, support, or encouragement, some CWD may become disinterested or discouraged to participate. Older children and adolescents with disabilities may lose self-confidence to participate as skill gaps between them and their typically developing peers widen and sports become more competitive. Through required physical education services of a child's Individualized Education Program (IEP), schools can develop goals to address deficits in fundamental movement skills to foster physical literacy. However, most CWD take general physical education classes, and although physical education teachers may make accommodations for some, budget constraints and lack of training are cited as barriers to participation.[67,68] Pediatricians, other professionals, and parents may also overestimate the risk of injury during physical activity, although involvement in sports has been shown to be reasonably safe for CWD; one recent study found a lower risk of injury in CWD after controlling for personal and environmental factors.[60,69-71] Nevertheless, parents of CWD are justified in desiring high-quality, accessible, and safe adaptive recreation programs, yet they report marked variation in recreational activity availability, long waiting lists for adaptive programs, absence of suitable transport to these facilities, a reduced number of skilled instructors to run these programs, and poor advertisement of programs in the community.[60,61] Likewise, pediatricians may be unaware of adaptive recreation opportunities within the community or of the family's interest in pursuing these opportunities.[72]

Overall, misconceptions and attitudinal barriers at the level of the individual, family, and community need to be addressed to integrate children of all abilities into recreational and physical activities. Pediatricians can help families and children balance the benefits of participation with the potential risks, recognizing that historically, being "too safe" and assuming that CWD "can't do that," has been a persistent barrier to participation.

FACILITATORS TO PARTICIPATION

The combined efforts of well-informed health care providers, parents, educators, coaches, and others are needed to ensure and promote the participation of all children in sports, recreation, and physical activity (Table 1). Health care providers can facilitate participation by asking about current levels of activity and using tools, such as a physical activity vital sign (PAVS) in the electronic health record, to start the conversation about physical activity during visits.[23] The PAVS consists of 2 screening questions that are used to assess how many days per week the individual engages in physical activity that is moderate (causes the child or youth to sweat a little and breathe harder, such as bike riding or playground activities) to vigorous (causes the child or youth to sweat and be out of breath, such as running or swimming) and how many minutes this level of physical activity is maintained. Use of the PAVS has been associated with a greater likelihood of physician exercise counseling and improved metabolic outcomes in adults.[73] Clinicians can then create "physical activity prescriptions" for CWD with goals for participation and referrals to specific programs or resources that are based on baseline physical activity, preferred activities, functional limitations that may require adaptation of the activity and preparticipatory planning, and the evidence base of the physical activity regarding risks and benefits.[23] Providers can explore the child and family's beliefs and attitudes about physical activity through motivational interviewing and arrive at a treatment plan through shared decision-making (Appendix 1).[27,74] Lastly, by their own commitment to physical activity, health care providers can serve as role models for CWD and their families. For example, pediatricians with self-reported higher levels of fitness are more likely to discuss physical activity during health supervision visits.[75]

To facilitate participation, providers can refer CWD to specialized adaptive programs staffed by recreational, physical, or occupational therapists that create a safe and fun recreational environment while allowing coordination with the primary care provider if medical concerns occur.[76] Specifically, health care providers and care coordinators within practices can partner with local adaptive recreational programs that address traditional barriers to participation (time, cost, transportation) and share this information with families. For example, many city and county parks and recreation departments offer low-cost adaptive recreation opportunities for CWD, and some adaptive recreational programs offer scholarships and provide transportation to and from activities. Therapists and coaches at specialized adaptive recreation programs facilitate participation for CWD by having lower participant to coach or instructor ratios (fewer than 4 participants for each coach), using positive feedback, and individualizing activities to the preferences of each participant.[77]

Lastly, providers can work with local and state public health agencies to promote physical activity to create and strengthen recreational programs for CWD. The Title V Maternal and Child Health Services Block Grant Program has a National Performance Measure on physical activity, with only 25% of CYSHCN with more complex health needs meeting the measure of being physically active at least 60 minutes per day.[78] At the federal level, the Centers for Disease Control and Prevention funds and supports 2 national centers on disability: Special Olympics and the National Center on Health, Physical Activity and Disability. These centers identify and expand physical activity programs, provide training for professionals, and provide data to establish best practices.[79]

Parents, caregivers, and peers are important facilitators of physical activity for CWD. Parents who believe in the benefits of physical activity report higher levels of activity in their CWD.[70] In one study, CWD whose parents were physically active at least 3 hours per week were 4.2 times as likely to be physically active compared with those whose parents were less active.[80] Therefore, an important message from pediatric health care providers to parents of CWD is to prioritize their own physical activity and to include CWD in family recreational activities.[81] Additionally, CWD are too often left behind regarding organized sports participation despite the clear benefit of participation for CWD. Parents can advocate for and support organized sports that encourage inclusion and focus on fun instead of winning, such as Special Olympics, because these are important influencers of sustained participation by CWD.[65] In addition, peer-mediated interventions to facilitate play skills and foster inclusion and acceptance of CWD by modeling behaviors can be an effective counterbalance to the barrier of systematic exclusion that has (in the past) resulted in opportunities for bullying behaviors.[82,83]

The American Heart Association has called for schools to play a central role in ensuring all students participate in enough physical activity to develop healthy lifestyles.[84] With only 24% of CWD engaging in 60 minutes of physical activity daily, schools can help a greater proportion reach this level of activity.[85] The Centers for Disease Control and Prevention recommends that a substantial percentage of students' overall physical activity should be obtained through school physical education. The right of CWD to participate in physical activity and sports in school is rooted in several federal laws. The

IDEA mandates free, appropriate public education in the least restrictive environment, and Section 504 of the Rehabilitation Act of 1973 requires that no individual shall be excluded because of disability in programs that receive federal funds.[86] Physical education is a federally mandated component of special education services, including the promotion of physical fitness, fundamental movement skills, and skills in individual and group games and sports.[67] However, many school districts allow exemption from physical education requirements for students with cognitive and other disabilities.[87] Physical education curricula for CWD can promote enjoyment of movement and skill development that can be incorporated before, during, and after school hours.[88] Pediatric providers and parents can partner with the educational team to include physical activity goals in progress metrics within a child's IEP to facilitate participation in physical activity at school.[86] Physical activity can be accurately measured for CWD through subjective and objective measures.[89] Adaptive physical education teachers can address physical activity goals by modifying recreational programs to accommodate the motor skills, muscle strength, and fitness of each child. Strategies physical education teachers use to accommodate CWD may include simplified instruction, additional skill modeling, peer teaching, equipment modification, and coordinating activities with a special education teacher.[68] Beyond physical education, the Comprehensive School Physical Activity Program developed by the Centers for Disease Control and Prevention and the Society of Health and Physical Educators, is a framework to capture all opportunities for school-based physical activity for CWD.[90] School nurses can coordinate with pediatricians in developing and implementing health care plans that promote safe participation in physical activity.[91] School-based physical activity programs, such as recess or physical education, that are focused on fun and enjoyment are strongly associated with daily physical activity in CWD.[88]

PREPARTICIPATION CONSIDERATIONS

It is important that all CWD participate in activity-related recreational programs while minimizing risks of illness or injury. Well-designed programs can target fundamental movement skills (throwing, catching, kicking, jumping, running, hopping, balance), flexibility, cardiorespiratory endurance, and muscular strength while maximizing enjoyment and safety. Rather than being excluded from sports participation, all children can be empowered to take part with a can-do attitude, enjoying the dignity of taking acceptable risk during participation just as individuals without disabilities are allowed to do. It is also important to involve parents and caregivers early and often in discussions of the importance of participation in sports, recreation, and physical activity for CWD.

A first step toward regular physical activity of all children, including CWD, is achieving physical literacy, which is the "the ability, confidence, and desire to be physically active for life."[92] For children with typical development, fundamental movement skills emerge in early childhood after the attainment of gross and fine motor milestones in infancy. Later in childhood, provided the child has opportunities to engage regularly in active play and physical activity throughout the day, additional competences are gained in coordination, balance, running, kicking, throwing, and catching.[23] The attainment of these fundamental movement skills influences physical literacy, is a strong predictor of future physical activity levels of children, and is linked to improvement in cardiovascular fitness scores and BMI.[93] Thus, CWD who have decreased gross motor function or other developmental delays may lack fundamental movement skills, may have low physical literacy, and are subsequently at risk for developing a low preference for physical activity during childhood and later in life.[23,94] Physical literacy assessments by health care providers are essential to allow early identification of any deficits.[95] Physical literacy assessments for all children begin in early childhood and encompass surveillance and screening for motor delay and exploring the child and family's knowledge, motivation, and feelings related to physical activity and movement.[23,96,97] Figure 3 provides an adaptation of the ICF framework for pediatricians to use in assessing physical literacy and promoting physical activity in CWD.[7] For CWD who have motor delays, referrals to exercise-related specialists (physical therapist, physical medicine and rehabilitation physician, recreation therapist, sports medicine physician) for structured programming may help to maximize the child's potential in developing fundamental movement skills, which in turn may foster confidence and desire to participate in sports and recreation.[98,99] Furthermore, young CWD can be given the same opportunities as other children to participate in free play and recess to develop fundamental movement skills and to foster the notion that physical activity is fun.[100,101] One such program to include students with autism with typically developing peers during recess activities led to improvements in peer engagement.[102]

How Much Physical Activity to Recommend?

All children, including CWD, are encouraged to strive to follow

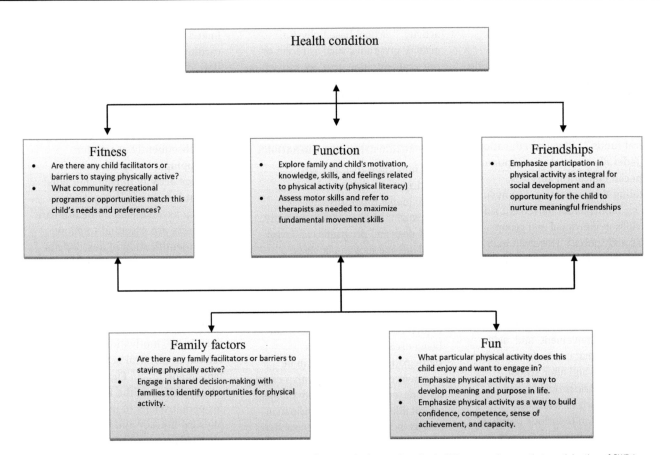

FIGURE 3 Adaptation of the International Classification of Function as a framework of assessing physical literacy and promoting participation of CWD in sports, recreation, and physical activity.[7] Adapted from World Health Organization. *Towards a Common Language for Functioning, Disability and Health.* Geneva, Switzerland: World Health Organization; 2002:9.

guidelines established by the 2018 Physical Activity Guidelines Advisory Committee, which recommends that children and adolescents (6–17 years) take part in at least 60 minutes of moderate to vigorous physical activity daily as well as in bone and muscle strengthening activities at least 3 days a week.[103] Parents of infants are encouraged to keep them active several times a day through interactive floor-based play, and parents of preschool-aged children (3–5 years) are encouraged to have their children accumulate at least 3 hours of light- to moderate-intensity activity throughout the day to develop movement skills.[23,104–106] For CWD, some modifications may be required to the frequency, intensity, and/or duration of physical activity. Goals need to be realistic, with an emphasis on encouraging children and families to do whatever they can through a gradual exploration of increases in time, intensity, and duration.[104] By asking CWD and their families about usual weekly duration and intensity of physical activity, health care providers can adapt physical activity guidelines to accommodate for neuromuscular deficits and cardiorespiratory profiles associated with specific conditions.

The Preparticipation Evaluation: Special Concerns for CWD

Families of CWD will sometimes schedule mandatory preparticipation physical evaluations or recommended health supervision visits. In either case, these visits allow opportunities for families and providers to discuss medical and psychosocial issues that are relevant for participation in physical activity.

The concepts of self-determination and shared decision-making have emerged as important themes in the care of CWD.[27] Discussions with children and families may start with a query about the child's current level of physical activity and the importance the family and child place on being physically active. Families of CWD may experience high levels of day-to-day stress and may consider time for physical activity a lower priority. Using behavioral techniques, such as motivational interviewing, providers can explore the family's beliefs and develop achievable physical activity goals. Once the wishes of the child and family are known, conditions that may interfere with participation or predispose the child to injury can be collaboratively discussed between the child, family, provider, and other treatment team members.

The child's current health status and functional ability, demands of the sport (including level of competition), and whether the sport can be modified with protective or adaptive equipment to allow for safer participation are important considerations. Given the complexity, the preparticipation evaluation for CWD may not occur in the context of a single office visit but rather over a period of time with the assistance of care coordination from the primary care medical home to obtain input from the child's multidisciplinary team, which may include subspecialists such as physical medicine and rehabilitation or sports medicine physicians; school nurses, coaches, and physical education teachers; and recreation, physical, and occupational therapists. Ideally, members of the multidisciplinary team can periodically reassess CWD to update treatment plans, including recommendations about sport participation, adaptations, and any restrictions deemed necessary.

The goal of the preparticipation evaluation is to review the desired activities of the child and family and the current state of disability-specific and co-occurring conditions to provide an appropriate menu of activities and potential accommodations or precautions that may be needed. Tables 2 and 3 show elements of a preparticipation history and physical examination that can be used for CWD. For example, children with physical disabilities, such as cerebral palsy, may have decreased flexibility with joint contractures, muscle strength imbalances, and lack of motor control, coordination, and equilibrium, which may increase the risk of lower extremity overuse injuries, strains, and sprains. If a child with cerebral palsy wishes to play baseball and there are limitations in skills (catching, throwing, and using a bat), it may be advisable to consider ways to adapt

the sport or the child's participation to prevent injury to the athlete or other participants.[107] Children with neurologic conditions who use wheelchairs for ambulation are at higher risk of upper extremity overuse injuries, peripheral nerve entrapment (eg, carpal tunnel syndrome), and pressure sores affecting the sacrum and ischial tuberosities.[108] The preparticipation evaluation presents an opportunity to screen for skin ulcerations and, when present, initiate appropriate treatment before sports participation.[109,110] Inspecting the adaptive or medical equipment used by CWD participating in sport so that braces are appropriately fitted and sports wheelchairs are in proper working order promotes optimum performance and injury prevention. Families can be encouraged to bring all equipment used during physical activity to the preparticipation visit so that these assessments can be conducted. If needed, referrals to exercise-related subspecialists (physical therapist, physical medicine and rehabilitation physician, recreation therapist, sports medicine physician) can be made for equipment adjustments or other equipment concerns.

The preparticipation evaluation also allows for the provision of anticipatory guidance that promotes safe participation for children with physical disabilities. For example, athletes with spinal cord pathology above the sixth thoracic level may develop autonomic dysreflexia, which is excessive and uncontrolled sympathetic nervous system output. This condition, which can be life-threatening, may be triggered by bladder infections, sunburns, and other stimuli or may be self-induced by an act such as occluding a bladder catheter in an attempt to improve sport performance (also known as "boosting"). Autonomic dysreflexia may present with symptoms and signs such as

headache, high blood pressure, or bradycardia, and these symptoms prompt immediate removal of the precipitating factor and prompt medical care.[107] Children with spinal cord injuries and cerebral palsy are also at risk for abnormal thermoregulation and exertional heat illness resulting from impaired sweating and control of peripheral blood flow as well the use of certain medications (such as those with anticholinergic properties).[107,111] As is the current practice for most adaptive and therapeutic sports organizations, coaches can modify the activity as needed, provide frequent breaks of appropriate duration, have ready access to fluids, and use appropriate clothing and equipment, which can mitigate this risk.[107,111,112]

Children with developmental disabilities also benefit from preparticipation planning and anticipatory guidance. For example, children with autism may have apraxia and motor coordination deficits, increasing the risk for injuries.[113] This risk can be managed by adaptations to the activity or the equipment or with additional neuromotor training to develop kinesthetic awareness.[114] Children with intellectual disability may have lower muscle strength, balance, flexibility, and endurance and may benefit from exercise that is of lower intensity as well as preparatory conditioning, such as resistance training, to reduce the risk of injury.[108] Children with Down syndrome are at slight increased risk of symptomatic atlantoaxial instability (AAI). Neurologic manifestations of AAI with cervical cord myelopathy include significant neck pain, radicular pain, weakness, spasticity or change in tone, gait difficulties, hyperreflexia, and change in bowel or bladder function or other signs or symptoms of myelopathy. In the

TABLE 2 Elements of a History During Preparticipation Evaluation for CWD

History	Comments
Is there a history of seizures?	Children with uncontrolled seizures or implantable devises (eg, ventriculoperitoneal shunt, vagal nerve stimulator) may benefit from consultation with a neurologist or neurosurgeon, respectively, to assist with medical eligibility. Although there is no universal exclusion for participation in contact sports for children with epilepsy, some families may choose to avoid sports in which seizure activity would pose risk to self or others (eg, archery, riflery, weightlifting, and sports that involve heights). There are considerations related to prevention of drowning in children with epilepsy who swim.[118] In addition, some antiepilepsy drugs can impair normal sweating.
Is there a history or concern for hearing or vision loss?	Boxing and full-contact martial arts are not recommended for functionally one-eyed athletes.[119] Visually asymptomatic CWD are encouraged to have a vision screening based on the *Bright Futures* periodicity table. Those with ocular signs or symptoms are recommended to have a complete examination by a pediatric ophthalmologist.[120]
Is there a history or concern for cardiopulmonary disease?	Children with stage 2 hypertension are recommended to refrain from high-static sports (weightlifting, gymnastics). Children with congenital heart disease, structural heart disease, and dysrhythmias are encouraged to have consultation with a cardiologist.[119]
Is there history of symptomatic AAI?	Children with symptomatic AAI may report or demonstrate fatigue, gait abnormalities, neck pain, limited neck range of motion, changes in coordination, spasticity, hyperreflexia, clonus, or extensor-plantar reflex. Parents can be advised that participation in contact sports, such as football, soccer, and gymnastics, places children at risk for spinal cord injury.[115]
Is there a history of heat stroke or heat exhaustion?	Thermoregulation in children with spinal cord injuries can be impaired because of skeletal muscle paralysis (impaired shivering and reduced ability to produce heat) and a loss of autonomic nervous system control (impaired sweating and vasodilation to dissipate heat). Athletes who have a history of heat illness are more at risk to develop the condition again.
Is there a history of fractures or dislocations?	Ligamentous laxity and joint hypermobility are more common in some disabilities, such as Down syndrome and Ehlers-Danlos syndrome. Children with obesity, those with osteogenesis imperfecta, and athletes in wheelchairs may have reduced bone mineral density with increased fracture risk.
Are there adaptive devices used during sports participation?	Health care providers are encouraged to be aware of the child's need for adaptive equipment. Athletes using wheelchairs are at increased risk for shoulder and wrist injuries and upper extremity peripheral nerve entrapment syndrome.
Is there a need for bladder catheterization?	Athletes with spinal cord injuries or other neurologic conditions may have neurogenic bladder and need an indwelling catheter or require intermittent catheterization.
Is there a history of pressure sores or ulcers?	Children who use wheelchairs are prone to pressure ulcers over the sacrum and ischial tuberosities.
What medications is the child taking?	Medications used for pain and bladder dysfunction can interfere with the normal sweating response; medications that alter QT intervals also may require special assessments.
Is there a history of autonomic dysreflexia?	Autonomic dysreflexia is acute onset of excessive, unregulated sympathetic output that can occur in children with spinal cord injuries at or above the sixth thoracic spinal cord level. This condition may occur spontaneously or may be self-induced (boosting) in an attempt to improve performance.[121]

Adapted from American Academy of Pediatrics. Athletes with a disability. In: Bernhardt DT, Roberts WO, eds. *PPE: Preparticipation Physical Evaluation*. 5th ed. Itasca, IL: American Academy of Pediatrics; 2019:182–183.

absence of myelopathic signs and symptoms during the preparticipation evaluation, routine radiographic evaluation of the cervical spine is not recommended.

Children and youth with Down syndrome can be encouraged to participate in activities they enjoy, although contact sports, such as football, soccer, and gymnastics, may place them at increased risk of spinal cord injury.[115]

As the above examples illustrate, for each child and youth with a

TABLE 3 Elements of a Physical Examination During Preparticipation Evaluation for CWD

Physical Examination Components	Items to Screen
Ocular	Decreased visual acuity
	Ocular health
	Strabismus
	Abnormalities in ocular appearance
Cardiovascular	Cardiovascular heart disease
	Hypertension
Neurologic	Peripheral neuropathies
	Inadequate motor control
	Inadequate coordination and balance
	Clonus
	Impaired hand-eye coordination
	Sensory dysfunction
	AAI
	Hyperreflexia
	Ataxia
	Muscle weakness
	Spasticity
	Upper motor neuron and posterior column signs and symptoms
Dermatologic	Abrasions
	Lacerations
	Blisters
	Pressure ulcers
	Rashes
Musculoskeletal	Limited neck range of motion
	AAI
	Torticollis
	Decreased flexibility, often with contractures; decreased strength; and muscle strength imbalance
	Wrist and elbow extensor tendinitis in athletes using wheelchairs
	Rotator cuff tendinitis and impingement in athletes using wheelchairs
	Pelvic dysfunction caused by lower extremity prosthetic device causing unequal leg lengths

Reproduced with permission from: American Academy of Pediatrics. Athletes with a disability. In: Bernhardt DT, Roberts WO, eds. *PPE: Preparticipation Physical Evaluation*. 5th ed. Itasca, IL: American Academy of Pediatrics; 2019:185

disability, pediatricians can review condition-specific information, current medications, and other individualized aspects of the history to offer recommendations that promote safe participation. Concerns or questions that arise during the preparticipation visit can be addressed through consultation with a sports medicine or physical medicine and rehabilitation physician, who can provide additional guidance. Although a comprehensive review of preparticipation considerations is beyond the scope of this report, health care providers are encouraged to refer to the publication *PPE: Preparticipation Physical Evaluation, Fifth Edition*, which has a chapter titled "Athletes with Disability." A supplemental history form for athletes with a disability and a Special Olympics medical form are available for download at https://www.aap.org/en-us/advocacy-and-policy/aap-health-initiatives/Pages/PPE.aspx or in Supplemental Fig 4.[116]

RECOMMENDATIONS

Pediatricians can promote participation of children and adolescents with disabilities in sports, recreation, and physical activity in the following ways:

1. Assess motor development, physical literacy, and physical activity levels at all health supervision visits with CWD.

   a. Adding a PAVS to visits can help start conversations about physical activity with CWD and their families.

Communicate the physical, beha-vioral, cognitive, and social-emotional benefits of participation in sports, recreation, and physical activity to CWD and their caregivers (Table 1).

   a. Promotion of physical activity is a *Bright Futures* key health promotion theme to be aware of in each stage of child development.[24]

Health care providers can make a difference when they agree to "take the pledge" to talk to their patients about physical activity (https://www.nchpad.org/pledge/doctalk). Encourage parents to be physically active and encourage inclusion of CWD in family recreational activities. Recognize, identify, and address barriers to participation at the individual, family, community, and societal levels to increase the opportunities for CWD to be physically active (Table 1).

   a. Refer CWD to local adaptive and therapeutic recreation programs that decrease the barriers to participation. If there is limited access to local programs, home-based programs with adapted exercises and movements can be recommended. Free-to-access videos are available through the National Center on Health, Physical Activity and Disability (https://www.nchpad.org/Videos).

Pediatricians can partner with families, schools, and community organizations in advocating for safe, affordable, accessible, and inclusive recreational programs for CWD to reduce disparities in participation in physical activity;

Encourage participation by discu-ssing physical activity goals with CWD and their families and partnering with interdisciplinary team members to develop physical activity prescriptions that can be incorporated within an after-visit summary within the electronic medical record. If a handwritten paper note is preferred, a free physical activity prescription pad is available through the Americans with Disabilities Fund at http://foundationforpmr.org/old/physicians/diagnostic-population/rx-for-exercise-pediatrics-new/.

  a. Participation in recreation, sports, and physical activity has inherent risk for all. Rather than exclusion from sports participation, pediatricians can encourage CWD to adopt a can-do attitude, enjoying the dignity of taking acceptable risk during participation just as individuals without disabilities are allowed to do.

While striving to meet the 2018 Physical Activity Guidelines Advisory Committee recommendations for physical activity, some CWD will require modifications to the frequency, intensity, and/or duration of physical activity. Realistic goals can be based on gradual increases in baseline duration and intensity of physical activity.

Perform preparticipation evaluations for CWD, in collaboration with the child, family, pediatric specialists, and therapists, leading to opportunities to participate in sports and recreational activities with appropriate adaptation to minimize risk of injury (Tables 2 and 3).

  a. Encourage families to bring ada-ptive equipment used during physical activity to visits to assess need for adjustments or referrals.

PPE: Preparticipation Physical Evaluation, Fifth Edition, serves as a resource for medical providers to keep athletes safe and healthy while participating in sports and includes condition-specific preparticipation considerations for athletes with disabilities.

The use of a preparticipation form can promote the documentation of relevant medical issues that can be shared with therapeutic recreation programs, schools, and coaches (Supplemental Fig 4; https://www.aap.org/en-us/advocacy-and-policy/aap-health-initiatives/Pages/PPE.aspx). Partner with children, parents, and educational teams to include physical activity goals and modifications in a student's IEP and advocate for school-based physical activity programs for CWD.

Be aware of and actively refer to local school and community-based organizations that offer appropriate physical activity programs and sports for CWD.

  a. Local and state disability organizations, such as family-to-family health information centers and Family Voices, may have up-to-date lists of adaptive recreation programs (https://familyvoices.org/).

Web sites of national organizations, such as Special Olympics, the National Center on Health, Physical Activity and Disability, and Move United, can provide information on local activities (see Resources for Health Care Providers and Families).

Advocate at the local, state, and national levels for policies that that promote inclusion of CWD in sports, recreation, and physical activity and for surveillance systems that include CWD to track participation and access.[117]

SUMMARY AND CONCLUSIONS

Participation in free play, sports, recreational programs, and physical activity improves health, well-being, and quality of life for CWD and their families. Although more research is needed to confirm specific outcomes and benefits, particularly among individuals with higher levels of disability, clinicians should not hesitate to promote physical activity for CWD. Well-informed decisions regarding each child's participation are made through consideration of individual activity preferences, overall health status, motor skills, balance, muscle strength, bone strength, fitness level, and the availability of adaptive programs. Child, family, and societal barriers to participation continue to exist and need to be directly identified and addressed through advocacy at the local, state, and federal levels. Pediatric health care providers are urged to promote healthy, active living for CWD through physical activity, exercise, recreation, and organized sport by creating specific physical activity prescriptions suited to the child's interests and ability. The benefits are substantial not only for the children who participate but also for communities that welcome them.

RESOURCES FOR HEALTH CARE PROVIDERS AND FAMILIES

- National centers on health promotion for people with disabilities: National Center on Health, Physical Activity and Disability (http://www.nchpad.org) and Special Olympics (https://www.specialolympics.org);
- Paralympics (https://www.paralympic.org);
- US Association of Blind Athletes (usaba.org);
- Miracle League (http://www.themiracleleague.net);
- Move United (https://www.moveunited.org);
- Achilles International (achillesinternational.org);
- National Wheelchair Basketball Association (nwba.org);
- Easter Seals (http://www.easterseals.com/our-programs/camping-recreation/recreation-and-sports.html);

- *PPE: Preparticipation Physical Evaluation, Fifth Edition* (https://www.aap.org/en-us/advocacy-and-policy/aap-health-initiatives/Pages/PPE.aspx);
- America the Beautiful access pass for federal recreation sites (https://www.nps.gov/planyourvisit/passes.htm); and
- Medical Home Portal, Recreational Activities page (https://www.medicalhomeportal.org/living-with-child/other-needs/recreation-activities).

APPENDIX: SAMPLE PROCESSES IN CREATING PHYSICAL ACTIVITY PRESCRIPTIONS FOR CWD

Example 1

During a health supervision visit for a 10-year-old girl with autism spectrum disorder, the clinician notes her BMI is greater than the 95th percentile. On the PAVS, the mother reports 1 day of physical activity per week for 20 minutes. When asked, the child indicates she likes playing basketball, but her mother reports that previous attempts at several team sports, including basketball, have been negative experiences. Her mother explains that the skills required, the pace of play, and the increasingly competitive aspect of the team exceeded her capability, resulting in her becoming discouraged and quitting. She has since become more involved in sedentary activities, such as video games and television viewing. Through a previous collaboration with the state parent-to-parent network, the care coordinator for the practice maintains a list of local adaptive recreational programs. The clinician informs the family of a low-cost adaptive basketball program for CWD offered by the nearby parks and recreation department. Through motivational interviewing, the child and parent agree to walk the family dog to the park 3 times per week, where she can practice basketball in addition to the twice weekly basketball activities offered through the adaptive recreation program. Her after-visit summary includes a physical activity prescription with the contact information for the program and the goals of basketball 3 times per week and walking to the park 3 times per week. At follow-up in 3 months, the child proudly shows the clinician the team photograph of her adaptive basketball team. Her PAVS has improved to 4 days of activity per week for 40 minutes. Her mother reports meeting families of other CWD through the program, which has resulted in friendships and the child wanting to enroll in other sports offered.

Example 2

A 12-year-old boy with hemiplegic cerebral palsy, intellectual disability, and attention-deficit/hyperactivity disorder is seen in follow-up. Despite taking stimulant medication, he continues to display impulsive and oppositional behaviors, especially at home. He is tripping and falling and complaining of more pain, leading to less physical activity. He previously had an ankle foot orthosis but stopped wearing it after excessive skin irritation and pain. His PAVS filled out by his mother shows 2 days of activity per week for 30 minutes. His examination shows increased right upper and lower extremity tone and hyperreflexia. His right hamstrings and gastrocnemius muscles are tight, and his right ankle does not dorsiflex past 0°. Through motivational interviewing, he expresses a desire to participate in martial arts, which his mother states he initially enjoyed before quitting because of pain. His after-visit summary includes a physical activity prescription for martial arts after consultation for further preparticipation planning with several specialists. He is referred for a physical medicine and rehabilitation consultation with the request for assistance in preparticipation planning for martial arts. In the physical medicine and rehabilitation clinic, his spasticity is treated with intramuscular botulinum toxin injections, and he is fitted with a new ankle foot orthosis. He is referred to physical therapy and has weekly sessions to address goals of improving core strength, balance, and lower extremity flexibility and to refine and reinforce his home exercise program. He visits with his primary care pediatrician regularly, often bringing the latest color belt that he has earned in karate. His mother feels that the stimulant medication, his home exercise program, and martial arts have helped with attention, focus, and quality of life.

LEAD AUTHORS

Paul S. Carbone, MD, FAAP
Peter J. Smith, MD, MA, FAAP
Charron Lewis, MD, FAAP
Claire LeBlanc, MD, FAAP

COUNCIL ON CHILDREN WITH DISABILITIES EXECUTIVE COMMITTEE, 2021–2022

Garey Noritz, MD, FAAP, Chairperson
Rishi Agrawal, MD, MPH, FAAP
Kathryn A. Ellerbeck, MD, MPH, FAAP
Jessica E.A. Foster, MD, MPH, FAAP
Ellen Fremion, MD, FAAP, FACP
Sheryl Frierson, MD, MEd, FAAP
Mary O'Connor Leppert, MD, FAAP
Barbara S. Saunders, DO, FAAP
Christopher Stille, MD, MPH, FAAP
Jilda Vargus-Adams, MD, MSc, FAAP
Katharine Zuckerman, MD, MPH, FAAP

PAST COUNCIL ON CHILDREN WITH DISABILITIES EXECUTIVE COMMITTEE MEMBERS

Lynn Davidson, MD, FAAP
Kenneth Norwood Jr, MD, FAAP
Larry Yin, MD, MSPH, FAAP
Dennis Z. Kuo, MD, MHS, FAAP, Immediate Past Chairperson

LIAISONS

Allysa Ware, MSW – *Family Voices*
Marie Mann, MD, MPH, FAAP – *Maternal and Child Health Bureau*
Edwin Simpser, MD, FAAP – *Section on Home Care*
Jennifer Poon, MD, FAAP – *Section on Developmental and Behavioral Pediatrics*
Marshalyn Yeargin-Allsopp, MD, FAAP – *Centers for Disease Control and Prevention*

STAFF

Alexandra Kuznetsov

COUNCIL ON SPORTS MEDICINE AND FITNESS EXECUTIVE COMMITTEE 2019–2020

M. Alison Brooks, MD, FAAP, Chairperson

Susannah M. Briskin, MD, FAAP
Greg Canty, MD, FAAP
Rebecca L. Carl, MD, MS, FAAP
Alex B. Diamond, DO, MPH, FAAP
William Hennrikus, MD, FAAP
Kelsey Logan, MD, MPH, FAAP
Andrew R. Peterson, MD, MSPH, FAAP
Francisco Jose Silva, MD, FAAP
Paul R. Stricker, MD, FAAP
Kevin D. Walter, MD, FAAP

PAST COUNCIL ON SPORTS MEDICINE AND FITNESS EXECUTIVE COMMITTEE MEMBERS

Blaise A. Nemeth, MD, MS, FAAP
Cynthia R. LaBella, MD, FAAP,
Immediate Past Chairperson

CONSULTANT

Avery D. Faigenbaum, EdD, FACSM

LIAISONS

Donald W. Bagnall – *National Athletic Trainers' Association*

PAST LIAISONS

Claire LeBlanc, MD, FAAP – *Canadian Paediatric Society*

STAFF

Anjie Emanuel, MPH

Address correspondence to Paul S. Carbone, MD, FAAP. Email: paul.carbone@hsc.utah.edu

PEDIATRICS (ISSN Numbers: Print, 0031-4005; Online, 1098-4275).

Copyright © 2021 by the American Academy of Pediatrics

FINANCIAL DISCLOSURE: Dr Smith has disclosed his spouse has an employee relationship with Walgreens; Drs Carbone, Lewis, and LeBlanc have indicated they have no financial relationships relevant to this article to disclose.

FUNDING: No external funding.

POTENTIAL CONFLICT OF INTEREST: The authors have indicated they have no potential conflicts of interest to disclose.

REFERENCES

1. McPherson M, Arango P, Fox H, et al. A new definition of children with special health care needs. *Pediatrics.* 1998;102(1 pt 1):137–140

2. Health Resources & Services Administration. Children and youth with special health care needs. Available at: https://mchb.hrsa.gov/maternal-child-health-topics/children-and-youth-special-health-needs. Accessed April 14, 2019

3. US Department of Education. Individuals with Disabilities Education Act. Available at: https://sites.ed.gov/idea/. Accessed April 14, 2019

4. World Health Organization. *Towards a Common Language for Functioning, Disability and Health.* Geneva, Switzerland: World Health Organization; 2002

5. Cohen E, Kuo DZ, Agrawal R, et al. Children with medical complexity: an emerging population for clinical and research initiatives. *Pediatrics.* 2011;127(3):529–538

6. World Health Organization. International Classification of Functioning,

Disability and Health (ICF). Available at: https://www.who.int/classifications/icf/en/. Accessed April 15, 2019

7. Rosenbaum P, Gorter JW. The 'F-words' in childhood disability: I swear this is how we should think! *Child Care Health Dev.* 2012;38(4):457–463

8. World Health Organization. Physical activity. Available at: https://www.who.int/dietphysicalactivity/pa/en/. Accessed April 15, 2019

9. Special Olympics. Available at: www.specialolympics.org. Accessed April 20, 2019

10. Rimmer JH, Padalabalanarayanan S, Malone LA, Mehta T. Fitness facilities still lack accessibility for people with disabilities. *Disabil Health J.* 2017;10(2):214–221

11. Woodmansee C, Hahne A, Imms C, Shields N. Comparing participation in physical recreation activities between children with disability and children with typical development: a secondary analysis of matched

data. *Res Dev Disabil.* 2016;49–50:268–276

12. Li C, Haegele JA, Wu L. Comparing physical activity and sedentary behavior levels between deaf and hearing adolescents. *Disabil Health J.* 2019;12(3):514–518

13. Bandini L, Danielson M, Esposito LE, et al. Obesity in children with developmental and/or physical disabilities. *Disabil Health J.* 2015;8(3):309–316

14. Oppewal A, Hilgenkamp TI, van Wijck R, Evenhuis HM. Cardiorespiratory fitness in individuals with intellectual disabilities–a review. *Res Dev Disabil.* 2013;34(10):3301–3316

15. Wouters M, Evenhuis HM, Hilgenkamp TI. Systematic review of field-based physical fitness tests for children and adolescents with intellectual disabilities. *Res Dev Disabil.* 2017;61:77–94

16. Centers for Disease Control and Prevention. Overweight and obesity among people with disabilities. Available at: https://www.cdc.gov/ncbddd/

disabilityandhealth/documents/ obesityfactsheet2010.pdf. Accessed April 15, 2019

17. Neter JE, Schokker DF, de Jong E, Renders CM, Seidell JC, Visscher TL. The prevalence of overweight and obesity and its determinants in children with and without disabilities. *J Pediatr.* 2011;158(5):735–739

18. Must A, Phillips S, Curtin C, Bandini LG. Barriers to physical activity in children with autism spectrum disorders: relationship to physical activity and screen time. *J Phys Act Health.* 2015;12(4): 529–534

19. Jones RA, Downing K, Rinehart NJ, et al. Physical activity, sedentary behavior and their correlates in children with autism spectrum disorder: a systematic review. *PLoS One.* 2017;12(2):e0172482

20. Maher CA, Toohey M, Ferguson M. Physical activity predicts quality of life and happiness in children and adolescents with cerebral palsy. *Disabil Rehabil.* 2016;38(9):865–869

21. Te Velde SJ, Lankhorst K, Zwinkels M, Verschuren O, Takken T, de Groot J; HAYS study group. Associations of sport participation with self-perception, exercise self-efficacy and quality of life among children and adolescents with a physical disability or chronic disease-a cross-sectional study. *Sports Med Open.* 2018;4(1):38

22. Nyquist A, Jahnsen RB, Moser T, Ullenhag A. The coolest I know - a qualitative study exploring the participation experiences of children with disabilities in an adapted physical activities program. *Disabil Rehabil.* 2020;42(17):2501–2509

23. Lobelo F, Muth ND, Hanson S, Nemeth BA; Council on Sports Medicine and Fitness; Section on Obesity. Physical activity assessment and counseling in pediatric clinical settings. *Pediatrics.* 2020;145(3):e20193992

24. Bright Futures. Promoting physical activity. Available at: https:// brightfutures.aap.org/Bright% 20Futures%20Documents/ BF4_PhysicalActivity.pdf. Accessed November 1, 2020

25. International Paralympic Committee. Available at: https://www.paralympic. org/. Accessed November 5, 2020

26. Deaflympics. Available at: https://www. deaflympics.com/. Accessed November 5, 2020

27. Adams RC, Levy SE; Council on Children with Disabilities. Shared decision-making and children with disabilities: pathways to consensus. *Pediatrics.* 2017;139(6):e20170956

28. Lai B, Lee E, Wagatsuma M, et al. Research trends and recommendations for physical activity interventions among children and youth with disabilities: a review of reviews. *Adapt Phys Activ Q.* 2020;37(2):211–234

29. Arbour-Nicitopoulos KP, Grassmann V, Orr K, McPherson AC, Faulkner GE, Wright FV. A scoping review of inclusive out-of-school time physical activity programs for children and youth with physical disabilities. *Adapt Phys Activ Q.* 2018;35(1):111–138

30. Lai B, Lee E, Kim Y, et al. Leisure-time physical activity interventions for children and adults with cerebral palsy: a scoping review. *Dev Med Child Neurol.* 2021;63(2):162–171

31. O'Brien TD, Noyes J, Spencer LH, Kubis HP, Hastings RP, Whitaker R. Systematic review of physical activity and exercise interventions to improve health, fitness and well-being of children and young people who use wheelchairs. *BMJ Open Sport Exerc Med.* 2016;2(1): e000109

32. Chad KE, Bailey DA, McKay HA, Zello GA, Snyder RE. The effect of a weight-bearing physical activity program on bone mineral content and estimated volumetric density in children with spastic cerebral palsy. *J Pediatr.* 1999;135(1): 115–117

33. Alemdaroğlu I, Karaduman A, Yilmaz OT, Topaloğlu H. Different types of upper extremity exercise training in Duchenne muscular dystrophy: effects on functional performance, strength, endurance, and ambulation. *Muscle Nerve.* 2015;51(5):697–705

34. Jansen M, van Alfen N, Geurts AC, de Groot IJ. Assisted bicycle training delays functional deterioration in boys with Duchenne muscular dystrophy: the randomized controlled trial "no use is disuse". *Neurorehabil Neural Repair.* 2013;27(9):816–827

35. de Groot JF, Takken T, van Brussel M, et al. Randomized controlled study of home-based treadmill training for ambulatory children with spina bifida. *Neurorehabil Neural Repair.* 2011; 25(7):597–606

36. McCoy SM, Jakicic JM, Gibbs BB. Comparison of obesity, physical activity, and sedentary behaviors between adolescents with autism spectrum disorders and without. *J Autism Dev Disord.* 2016;46(7):2317–2326

37. Oriel KN, George CL, Peckus R, Semon A. The effects of aerobic exercise on academic engagement in young children with autism spectrum disorder. *Pediatr Phys Ther.* 2011;23(2):187–193

38. Rosenthal-Malek A, Mitchell S. Brief report: the effects of exercise on the self-stimulatory behaviors and positive responding of adolescents with autism. *J Autism Dev Disord.* 1997;27(2):193–202

39. Gabriels RL, Agnew JA, Holt KD, et al. Pilot study measuring the effects of therapeutic horseback riding on school-age children and adolescents with autism spectrum disorders. *Res Autism Spectr Disord.* 2012;6(2): 578–588

40. Rosenblatt LE, Gorantla S, Torres JA, et al. Relaxation response-based yoga improves functioning in young children with autism: a pilot study. *J Altern Complement Med.* 2011;17(11): 1029–1035

41. Bahrami F, Movahedi A, Marandi SM, Abedi A. Kata techniques training consistently decreases stereotypy in children with autism spectrum disorder. *Res Dev Disabil.* 2012;33(4):1183–1193

42. Pan CY. Effects of water exercise swimming program on aquatic skills and social behaviors in children with autism spectrum disorders. *Autism.* 2010;14(1):9–28

43. McDaniel Peters BC, Wood W. Autism and equine-assisted interventions: a systematic mapping review. *J Autism Dev Disord.* 2017;47(10):3220–3242

44. Cerrillo-Urbina AJ, García-Hermoso A, Sánchez-López M, Pardo-Guijarro MJ, Santos Gómez JL, Martínez-Vizcaíno V. The effects of physical exercise in children with attention deficit hyperactivity disorder: a systematic review and

meta-analysis of randomized control trials. *Child Care Health Dev.* 2015;41(6):779–788

45. Wu WL, Yang YF, Chu IH, Hsu HT, Tsai FH, Liang JM. Effectiveness of a cross-circuit exercise training program in improving the fitness of overweight or obese adolescents with intellectual disability enrolled in special education schools. *Res Dev Disabil.* 2017;60:83–95

46. Shields N, Taylor NF, Wee E, Wollersheim D, O'Shea SD, Fernhall B. A community-based strength training programme increases muscle strength and physical activity in young people with Down syndrome: a randomised controlled trial. *Res Dev Disabil.* 2013;34(12):4385–4394

47. Tint A, Thomson K, Weiss JA. A systematic literature review of the physical and psychosocial correlates of Special Olympics participation among individuals with intellectual disability. *J Intellect Disabil Res.* 2017;61(4):301–324

48. Bohnert A, Lieb R, Arola N. More than leisure: organized activity participation and socio-emotional adjustment among adolescents with autism spectrum disorder. *J Autism Dev Disord.* 2019;49(7):2637–2652

49. Spratt E, Mercer MA, Grimes A, et al. Translating benefits of exercise on depression for youth with autism spectrum disorder and neurodevelopmental disorders. *J Psychol Psychiatr.* 2018;2:109

50. de Valle KL, Davidson ZE, Kennedy RA, Ryan MM, Carroll KM. Physical activity and the use of standard and complementary therapies in Duchenne and Becker muscular dystrophies. *J Pediatr Rehabil Med.* 2016;9(1):55–63

51. Dursun OB, Erhan SE, Ibiş EO, et al. The effect of ice skating on psychological well-being and sleep quality of children with visual or hearing impairment. *Disabil Rehabil.* 2015;37(9):783–789

52. Carlon SL, Taylor NF, Dodd KJ, Shields N. Differences in habitual physical activity levels of young people with cerebral palsy and their typically developing peers: a systematic review. *Disabil Rehabil.* 2013;35(8):647–655

53. Buffart LM, van der Ploeg HP, Bauman AE, et al. Sports participation in adolescents and young adults with myelomeningocele and its role in total physical activity behaviour and fitness. *J Rehabil Med.* 2008;40(9):702–708

54. Bandini LG, Gleason J, Curtin C, et al. Comparison of physical activity between children with autism spectrum disorders and typically developing children. *Autism.* 2013;17(1):44–54

55. Phillips AC, Holland AJ. Assessment of objectively measured physical activity levels in individuals with intellectual disabilities with and without Down's syndrome. *PLoS One.* 2011;6(12):e28618

56. Hinckson EA, Curtis A. Measuring physical activity in children and youth living with intellectual disabilities: a systematic review. *Res Dev Disabil.* 2013;34(1):72–86

57. Bedell G, Coster W, Law M, et al. Community participation, supports, and barriers of school-age children with and without disabilities. *Arch Phys Med Rehabil.* 2013;94(2):315–323

58. Wilson PB, Haegele JA, Zhu X. Mobility status as a predictor of obesity, physical activity, and screen time use among children aged 5-11 years in the United States. *J Pediatr.* 2016;176:23–29.e1

59. Shields N, Synnot A. Perceived barriers and facilitators to participation in physical activity for children with disability: a qualitative study. *BMC Pediatr.* 2016;16:9

60. Shields N, Synnot AJ, Barr M. Perceived barriers and facilitators to physical activity for children with disability: a systematic review. *Br J Sports Med.* 2012;46(14):989–997

61. Wiart L, Darrah J, Kelly M, Legg D. Community fitness programs: what is available for children and youth with motor disabilities and what do parents want? *Phys Occup Ther Pediatr.* 2015;35(1):73–87

62. Martin Ginis KA, Ma JK, Latimer-Cheung AE, Rimmer JH. A systematic review of review articles addressing factors related to physical activity participation among children and adults with physical disabilities. *Health Psychol Rev.* 2016;10(4):478–494

63. Wright A, Roberts R, Bowman G, Crettenden A. Barriers and facilitators to physical activity participation for children with physical disability: comparing and contrasting the views of children, young people, and their clinicians. *Disabil Rehabil.* 2019;41(13):1499–1507

64. Stirling AE, Bridges EJ, Cruz EL, Mountjoy ML; Canadian Academy of Sport and Exercise Medicine. Canadian Academy of Sport and Exercise Medicine position paper: abuse, harassment, and bullying in sport. *Clin J Sport Med.* 2011;21(5):385–391

65. Logan K, Cuff S; Council on Sports Medicine and Fitness. Organized sports for children, preadolescents, and adolescents. *Pediatrics.* 2019;143(6):e20190997

66. Curtin C, Hyman SL, Boas DD, et al. Weight management in primary care for children with autism: expert recommendations. *Pediatrics.* 2020;145(suppl 1):S126–S139

67. Wrightslaw. Physical education for students with disabilities. Available at: https://www.wrightslaw.com/info/pe.index.htm. Accessed May 28, 2019

68. US Government Accountability Office. *Students With Disabilities: More Information and Guidance Could Improve Opportunities in Physical Education and Athletics.* Washington, DC: US Government Accountability Office; 2010

69. Ng KW, Tynjälä J, Rintala P, Kokko S, Kannas L. Do adolescents with long-term illnesses and disabilities have increased risks of sports related injuries? *Inj Epidemiol.* 2017;4(1):13

70. Pitchford EA, Siebert E, Hamm J, Yun J. Parental perceptions of physical activity benefits for youth with developmental disabilities. *Am J Intellect Dev Disabil.* 2016;121(1):25–32

71. Courtney-Long EA, Stevens AC, Carroll DD, Griffin-Blake S, Omura JD, Carlson SA. Primary care providers' level of preparedness for recommending physical activity to adults with disabilities. *Prev Chronic Dis.* 2017;14:E114

72. Jaarsma EA, Dijkstra PU, de Blécourt AC, Geertzen JH, Dekker R. Barriers and facilitators of sports in children with physical disabilities: a mixed-method study. *Disabil Rehabil.* 2015;37(18):1617–1623; quiz 1624–1625

73. Grant RW, Schmittdiel JA, Neugebauer RS, Uratsu CS, Sternfeld B. Exercise as a vital sign: a quasi-experimental

analysis of a health system intervention to collect patient-reported exercise levels. *J Gen Intern Med.* 2014; 29(2):341–348

74. Daniels SR, Hassink SG; Committee on Nutrition. The role of the pediatrician in primary prevention of obesity. *Pediatrics.* 2015;136(1). Available at: www.pediatrics. org/cgi/content/full/136/1/e275

75. Binns HJ, Mueller MM, Ariza AJ. Healthy and fit for prevention: the influence of clinician health and fitness on promotion of healthy lifestyles during health supervision visits. *Clin Pediatr (Phila).* 2007;46(9):780–786

76. American Therapeutic Recreation Association. About recreational therapy. Available at: https://www.atra-online. com/page/AboutRecTherapy. Accessed June 12, 2019

77. Rosso EGF. Brief report: coaching adolescents with autism spectrum disorder in a school-based multi-sport program. *J Autism Dev Disord.* 2016;46(7):2526–2531

78. Data Resource Center for Child & Adolescent Health. National Survey of Children's Health interactive data query (2016–present). Available at: https:// www.childhealthdata.org/browse/ survey. Accessed November 11, 2020

79. Centers for Disease Control and Prevention. National programs on health promotion for people with disabilities. Available at: https://www.cdc.gov/ ncbddd/disabilityandhealth/ national-programs.html. Accessed November 6, 2020

80. Yazdani S, Yee CT, Chung PJ. Factors predicting physical activity among children with special needs. *Prev Chronic Dis.* 2013;10:E119

81. National Park Service. Entrance passes. Available at: https://www.nps. gov/planyourvisit/passes.htm. Accessed June 12, 2019

82. Kent C, Cordier R, Joosten A, Wilkes-Gillan S, Bundy A. Can I learn to play? Randomized control trial to assess effectiveness of a peer-mediated intervention to improve play in children with autism spectrum disorder. *J Autism Dev Disord.* 2021;51(6): 1823–1838

83. Klavina A, Block ME. The effect of peer tutoring on interaction behaviors in

inclusive physical education. *Adapt Phys Activ Q.* 2008;25(2):132–158

84. Pate RR, Davis MG, Robinson TN, Stone EJ, McKenzie TL, Young JC; American Heart Association Council on Nutrition, Physical Activity, and Metabolism (Physical Activity Committee); Council on Cardiovascular Disease in the Young; Council on Cardiovascular Nursing. Promoting physical activity in children and youth: a leadership role for schools: a scientific statement from the American Heart Association Council on Nutrition, Physical Activity, and Metabolism (Physical Activity Committee) in collaboration with the Councils on Cardiovascular Disease in the Young and Cardiovascular Nursing. *Circulation.* 2006;114(11): 1214–1224

85. Child and Adolescent Health Measurement Initiative. 2017–18 National Survey of Children's Health (NSCH) combined data set. www.childhealthdata.org. Accessed April 28, 2020

86. Lipkin PH, Okamoto J; Council on Children With Disabilities; Council on School Health. The Individuals With Disabilities Education Act (IDEA) for children with special educational needs. *Pediatrics.* 2015;136(6). Available at: www.pediatrics.org/cgi/content/full/ 136/6/e1650

87. Centers for Disease Control and Prevention. Results from the school health policies and practices study 2014. 2015. Available at: https://www.cdc.gov/ healthyyouth/data/shpps/pdf/ SHPPS-508-final_101315.pdf. Accessed January 6, 2020

88. Jin J, Yun J, Agiovlasitis S. Impact of enjoyment on physical activity and health among children with disabilities in schools. *Disabil Health J.* 2018;11(1): 14–19

89. Yun J, Beamer J. Promoting physical activity in adapted physical education. *J Phys Educ Recreat Dance.* 2018;89(4): 7–13

90. Society of Health and Physical Educators. CSPAP Comprehensive School Physical Activity Program. Available at: https://www.shapeamerica.org/cspap/ what.aspx. Accessed January 6, 2021

91. Council on School Health. Role of the school nurse in providing school

health services. *Pediatrics.* 2016; 137(6):e20160852

92. Aspen Institute Project Play. Sport for All Play for Life. Available at: www. aspenprojectplay.org. Accessed October 21, 2021

93. Jaakkola T, Yli-Piipari S, Huotari P, Watt A, Liukkonen J. Fundamental movement skills and physical fitness as predictors of physical activity: a 6-year follow-up study. *Scand J Med Sci Sports.* 2016;26(1):74–81

94. Kantomaa MT, Purtsi J, Taanila AM, et al. Suspected motor problems and low preference for active play in childhood are associated with physical inactivity and low fitness in adolescence. *PLoS One.* 2011;6(1):e14554

95. Bopp T, Stellefson M, Weatherall B, Spratt S. Promoting physical literacy for disadvantaged youth living with chronic disease. *Am J Health Educ.* 2019;50(3):153–158

96. Noritz GH, Murphy NA; Neuromotor Screening Expert Panel. Motor delays: early identification and evaluation. *Pediatrics.* 2013;131(6). Available at: www.pediatrics.org/cgi/content/full/ 131/6/e2016

97. Cairney J, Clark HJ, James ME, Mitchell D, Dudley DA, Kriellaars D. The preschool physical literacy assessment tool: testing a new physical literacy tool for the early years. *Front Pediatr.* 2018;6:138

98. Farhat F, Masmoudi K, Hsairi I, et al. The effects of 8 weeks of motor skill training on cardiorespiratory fitness and endurance performance in children with developmental coordination disorder. *Appl Physiol Nutr Metab.* 2015;40(12):1269–1278

99. Houtrow A, Murphy N; Council on Children With Disabilities. Prescribing physical, occupational, and speech therapy services for children with disabilities. *Pediatrics.* 2019;143(4):e20190285

100. Yogman M, Garner A, Hutchinson J, Hirsh-Pasek K, Golinkoff RM; Committee on Psychological Aspects of Child and Family Health; Council on Communications and Media. The power of play: a pediatric role in enhancing development in young children. *Pediatrics.* 2018;142(3):e20182058

101. Murray R, Ramstetter C; Council on School Health, American Academy of

Pediatrics. The crucial role of recess in school. *Pediatrics*. 2013;131(1):183–188

102. Kretzmann M, Shih W, Kasari C. Improving peer engagement of children with autism on the school playground: a randomized controlled trial. *Behav Ther*. 2015;46(1):20–28

103. US Department of Health and Human Services. 2018 Physical Activity Guidelines Advisory Committee scientific report. 2018. Available at: https://health.gov/sites/default/files/2019-09/PAG_Advisory_Committee_Report.pdf. Accessed March 15, 2021

104. US Department of Health and Human Services. *Physical Activity Guidelines for Americans*. Washington, DC: US Department of Health and Human Services; 2018

105. Tremblay MS, Leblanc AG, Carson V, et al; Canadian Society for Exercise Physiology. Canadian physical activity guidelines for the early years (aged 0-4 years). *Appl Physiol Nutr Metab*. 2012;37(2):345–369

106. Lipnowski S, Leblanc CM; Canadian Paediatric Society, Healthy Active Living and Sports Medicine Committee. Healthy active living: physical activity guidelines for children and adolescents. *Paediatr Child Health*. 2012;17(4):209–212

107. Klenck C, Gebke K. Practical management: common medical problems in disabled athletes. *Clin J Sport Med*. 2007;17(1):55–60

108. Patel DR, Greydanus DE. Sport participation by physically and cognitively

challenged young athletes. *Pediatr Clin North Am*. 2010;57(3):795–817

109. Fullerton HD, Borckardt JJ, Alfano AP. Shoulder pain: a comparison of wheelchair athletes and nonathletic wheelchair users. *Med Sci Sports Exerc*. 2003;35(12):1958–1961

110. Dec KL, Sparrow KJ, McKeag DB. The physically-challenged athlete: medical issues and assessment. *Sports Med*. 2000;29(4):245–258

111. Simon LM, Ward DC. Preparing for events for physically challenged athletes. *Curr Sports Med Rep*. 2014;13(3):163–168

112. Bergeron MF, Devore C, Rice SG; Council on Sports Medicine and Fitness and Council on School Health, American Academy of Pediatrics. Policy statement—climatic heat stress and exercising children and adolescents. *Pediatrics*. 2011;128(3). Available at: www.pediatrics.org/cgi/content/full/128/3/e741

113. Ramirez M, Yang J, Bourque L, et al. Sports injuries to high school athletes with disabilities. *Pediatrics*. 2009;123(2):690–696

114. Srinivasan SM, Pescatello LS, Bhat AN. Current perspectives on physical activity and exercise recommendations for children and adolescents with autism spectrum disorders. *Phys Ther*. 2014;94(6):875–889

115. Bull MJ; Committee on Genetics. Health supervision for children with Down syndrome. *Pediatrics*. 2011;128(2):393–406

116. Bernhardt DT, Roberts WO, eds. *PPE: Preparticipation Physical Evaluation*. 5th ed. Itasca, IL: American Academy of Pediatrics; 2019

117. US Department of Health and Human Services. The national youth sports strategy. 2019. Available at: https://health.gov/sites/default/files/2019-10/National_Youth_Sports_Strategy.pdf. Accessed March 16, 2021

118. Denny SA, Quan L, Gilchrist J, et al; Council on Injury, Violence, and Poison Prevention. Prevention of drowning. *Pediatrics*. 2019;143(5):e20190850

119. Rice SG; American Academy of Pediatrics Council on Sports Medicine and Fitness. Medical conditions affecting sports participation. *Pediatrics*. 2008;121(4):841–848

120. Donahue S, Nixon C; Section on Opthamology, American Academy of Pediatrics; Committee on Practice and Ambulatory Medicine, American Academy of Pediatrics; American Academy of Ophthalmology; American Association for Pediatric Ophthalmology and Strabismus; American Association of Certified Orthoptists. Visual system assessment in infants, children, and young adults by pediatricians. *Pediatrics*. 2016;137(1):28–30

121. International Paralympic Committee. Position statement on autonomic dysreflexia and boosting. In: *International Paralympic Committee Handbook*. Bonn, Germany: International Paralympic Committee; 2016

POLICY STATEMENT   Organizational Principles to Guide and Define the Child Health
Care System and/or Improve the Health of all Children

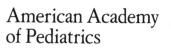

American Academy
of Pediatrics

DEDICATED TO THE HEALTH OF ALL CHILDREN®

Children With Intellectual and Developmental Disabilities as Organ Transplantation Recipients

Mindy B. Statter, MD, MBE,[a] Garey Noritz, MD,[b] COMMITTEE ON BIOETHICS, COUNCIL ON CHILDREN WITH DISABILITIES

abstract

The demand for transplantable solid organs far exceeds the supply of deceased donor organs. Patient selection criteria are determined by individual transplant programs; given the scarcity of solid organs for transplant, allocation to those most likely to benefit takes into consideration both medical and psychosocial factors. Children with intellectual and developmental disabilities have historically been excluded as potential recipients of organ transplants. When a transplant is likely to provide significant health benefits, denying a transplant to otherwise eligible children with disabilities may constitute illegal and unjustified discrimination. Children with intellectual and developmental disabilities should not be excluded from the potential pool of recipients and should be referred for evaluation as recipients of solid organ transplants.

[a]Division of Pediatric Surgery, Department of Surgery, Children's Hospital at Montefiore, Bronx, New York; and [b]Department of Pediatrics and Center for Pediatric Bioethics, The Ohio State University and Nationwide Children's Hospital, Columbus, Ohio

Policy statements from the American Academy of Pediatrics benefit from expertise and resources of liaisons and internal (AAP) and external reviewers. However, policy statements from the American Academy of Pediatrics may not reflect the views of the liaisons or the organizations or government agencies that they represent.

The guidance in this statement does not indicate an exclusive course of treatment or serve as a standard of medical care. Variations, taking into account individual circumstances, may be appropriate.

All policy statements from the American Academy of Pediatrics automatically expire 5 years after publication unless reaffirmed, revised, or retired at or before that time.

DOI: https://doi.org/10.1542/peds.2020-0625

Address correspondence to Mindy B. Statter, MD, MBE. E-mail: mstatter@montefiore.org

PEDIATRICS (ISSN Numbers: Print, 0031-4005; Online, 1098-4275).

FINANCIAL DISCLOSURE: The authors have indicated they have no financial relationships relevant to this article to disclose.

To cite: Statter MB, Noritz G, AAP COMMITTEE ON BIOETHICS, COUNCIL ON CHILDREN WITH DISABILITIES. Children With Intellectual and Developmental Disabilities as Organ Transplantation Recipients. *Pediatrics.* 2020; 145(5):e20200625

INTRODUCTION

The American Academy of Pediatrics policy statement "Pediatric Organ Donation and Transplantation" published in 2010 provides recommendations to promote awareness for increased organ donation and the role of organ donation as an integral part of end-of-life care but does not discuss recipient candidacy and eligibility.[1] The demand for transplantable solid organs far exceeds the supply of deceased donor organs. Patient selection criteria are determined by individual transplant programs. Given the scarcity of solid organs for transplant, organs are allocated to those most likely to experience maximal benefit, taking into consideration both medical and psychosocial factors. Historically, patients with intellectual and developmental disabilities (IDDs) have often been excluded as potential recipients of organ transplants. The issue of intellectual disability (ID) in donors is not in the scope of this statement.

IDD is defined as "a group of developmental conditions characterized by significant impairment of cognitive functions, which are associated with limitations of learning, adaptive behaviour and skills."[2] Patients with an

CLINICAL REPORT   Guidance for the Clinician in Rendering Pediatric Care

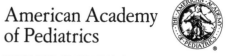

American Academy
of Pediatrics

DEDICATED TO THE HEALTH OF ALL CHILDREN™

Prescribing Physical, Occupational, and Speech Therapy Services for Children With Disabilities

Amy Houtrow, MD, PhD, MPH, FAAP, FAAPMR,[a] Nancy Murphy, MD, FAAP, FAAPMR,[b] COUNCIL ON CHILDREN WITH DISABILITIES

Clinical Report – Reaffirmed With Reference & Data Updates

This clinical report was reaffirmed in July 2023 with reference and data updates. New or updated references and datapoints are indicated in bold typeface. No other changes have been made to the text or content. The AAP would like to acknowledge Amy Houtrow, MD, PhD, MPH, FAAP, and Jilda Vargus-Adams, MD, MSc, FAAP, for these updates.

Pediatric health care providers are frequently responsible for prescribing physical, occupational, and speech therapies and monitoring therapeutic progress for children with temporary or permanent disabilities in their practices. This clinical report will provide pediatricians and other pediatric health care providers with information about how best to manage the therapeutic needs of their patients in the medical home by reviewing the International Classification of Functioning, Disability and Health; describing the general goals of habilitative and rehabilitative therapies; delineating the types, locations, and benefits of therapy services; and detailing how to write a therapy prescription and include therapists in the medical home neighborhood.

abstract

[a]Department of Physical Medicine and Rehabilitation and Pediatrics, University of Pittsburgh, Pittsburgh, Pennsylvania; and [b]Division of Pediatric Physical Medicine and Rehabilitation, Department of Pediatrics, University of Utah, Salt Lake City, Utah

Drs Houtrow and Murphy were each responsible for all aspects of conceptualizing, writing, editing, and preparing the document for publication; and both authors approved the final manuscript as submitted.

Clinical reports from the American Academy of Pediatrics benefit from expertise and resources of liaisons and internal (AAP) and external reviewers. However, clinical reports from the American Academy of Pediatrics may not reflect the views of the liaisons or the organizations or government agencies that they represent.

The guidance in this report does not indicate an exclusive course of treatment or serve as a standard of medical care. Variations, taking into account individual circumstances, may be appropriate.

All clinical reports from the American Academy of Pediatrics automatically expire 5 years after publication unless reaffirmed, revised, or retired at or before that time.

DOI: https://doi.org/10.1542/peds.2019-0285

Address correspondence to Amy J. Houtrow, MD, PhD, MPH, FAAP, FAAPMR. E-mail: houtrow@upmc.edu

PEDIATRICS (ISSN Numbers: Print, 0031-4005; Online, 1098-4275).

To cite: Houtrow A, Murphy N, AAP COUNCIL ON CHILDREN WITH DISABILITIES. Prescribing Physical, Occupational, and Speech Therapy Services for Children With Disabilities. *Pediatrics.* 2019;143(4):e20190285

Pediatricians and other pediatric health care providers have a vitally important role of linking children and youth with disabilities in their family-centered primary care medical homes with appropriate community-based services.[1] Pediatric providers are often asked (frequently by families) or recognize the need to prescribe habilitative and rehabilitative therapies (physical, occupational, and speech and language) for infants, children, and youth with disabilities in their clinical practices. Many general pediatric providers describe inadequate training to appropriately prescribe therapy in the various settings in which they may be available to children with disabilities.[2–5] This clinical report will review (1) the framework of the International Classification of Functioning, Disability and Health (ICF) for understanding the interaction between health conditions and personal and environmental factors that result

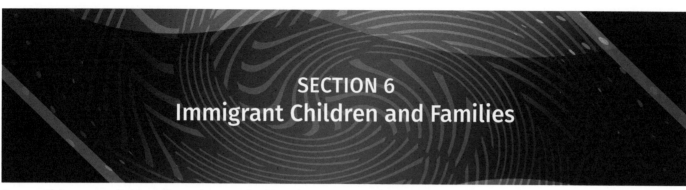

SECTION 6
Immigrant Children and Families

Some articles are available online only; scan the QR code to access online content.

POLICY STATEMENT Organizational Principles to Guide and Define the Child Health Care System and/or Improve the Health of all Children

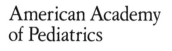

American Academy of Pediatrics

DEDICATED TO THE HEALTH OF ALL CHILDREN™

Providing Care for Children in Immigrant Families

Julie M. Linton, MD, FAAP,[a,b] Andrea Green, MDCM, FAAP,[c] COUNCIL ON COMMUNITY PEDIATRICS

abstract

Children in immigrant families (CIF), who represent 1 in 4 children in the United States, represent a growing and ever more diverse US demographic that pediatric medical providers nationwide will increasingly encounter in clinical care. Immigrant children are those born outside the United States to non–US citizen parents, and CIF are defined as those who are either foreign born or have at least 1 parent who is foreign born. Some families immigrate for economic or educational reasons, and others come fleeing persecution and seeking safe haven. Some US-born children with a foreign-born parent may share vulnerabilities with children who themselves are foreign born, particularly regarding access to care and other social determinants of health. Therefore, the larger umbrella term of CIF is used in this statement. CIF, like all children, have diverse experiences that interact with their biopsychosocial development. CIF may face inequities that can threaten their health and well-being, and CIF also offer strengths and embody resilience that can surpass challenges experienced before and during integration. This policy statement describes the evolving population of CIF in the United States, briefly introduces core competencies to enhance care within a framework of cultural humility and safety, and discusses barriers and opportunities at the practice and systems levels. Practice-level recommendations describe how pediatricians can promote health equity for CIF through careful attention to core competencies in clinical care, thoughtful community engagement, and system-level support. Advocacy and policy recommendations offer ways pediatricians can advocate for policies that promote health equity for CIF.

[a]Departments of Pediatrics and Public Health, School of Medicine Greenville, University of South Carolina, Greenville, South Carolina; [b]Department of Pediatrics, School of Medicine, Wake Forest University, Winston-Salem, North Carolina; and [c]Larner College of Medicine, The University of Vermont, Burlington, Vermont

Drs Linton and Green drafted, reviewed, and revised the manuscript; and both authors approved the final manuscript as submitted.

This document is copyrighted and is property of the American Academy of Pediatrics and its Board of Directors. All authors have filed conflict of interest statements with the American Academy of Pediatrics. Any conflicts have been resolved through a process approved by the Board of Directors. The American Academy of Pediatrics has neither solicited nor accepted any commercial involvement in the development of the content of this publication.

Policy statements from the American Academy of Pediatrics benefit from expertise and resources of liaisons and internal (AAP) and external reviewers. However, policy statements from the American Academy of Pediatrics may not reflect the views of the liaisons or the organizations or government agencies that they represent.

The guidance in this statement does not indicate an exclusive course of treatment or serve as a standard of medical care. Variations, taking into account individual circumstances, may be appropriate.

All policy statements from the American Academy of Pediatrics automatically expire 5 years after publication unless reaffirmed, revised, or retired at or before that time.

DOI: https://doi.org/10.1542/peds.2019-2077

Address correspondence to Julie M. Linton, MD, FAAP. E-mail: Julie.linton@prismahealth.org

PEDIATRICS (ISSN Numbers: Print, 0031-4005; Online, 1098-4275).

FINANCIAL DISCLOSURE: The authors have indicated they have no financial relationships relevant to this article to disclose.

FUNDING: No external funding.

To cite: Linton JM, Green A, AAP COUNCIL ON COMMUNITY PEDIATRICS. Providing Care for Children in Immigrant Families. *Pediatrics.* 2019;144(3):e20192077

DEMOGRAPHICS

Health care of children in immigrant families (CIF) in the United States has received increasing attention over the past decade, in part because of increasing migration of children caused by conflicts globally, greater diversity among migrant populations, and divisive sociopolitical discussion regarding immigration policy. Definitions regarding immigrant children vary, but for the purposes of this policy statement, immigrant

children are those born outside the
United States to non–US citizen
parents. The term CIF includes both
those who are foreign born and those
who are born in the United States and
have at least 1 parent who was
foreign born. In 2015, 43 million
people, representing 13% of the
US population, were immigrants,
approaching the historic high of
14.8% in 1890.[1,2] Currently, 3% of US
children are foreign born, and 25% of
US children live in immigrant
families.[3,4] It is projected that by
2065, 18% of the US population will
be foreign born and an additional
18% will be US-born children of
immigrants.[2] Immigrant children and
CIF reside in all 50 states (Figs 1
and 2).

Children immigrate to the United
States with or without their parents
for diverse and complex reasons,
including, but not limited to,
economic needs, educational pursuits,
international adoption, human
trafficking, or escape from
threatening conditions in pursuit of
safe haven. Immigrants may arrive

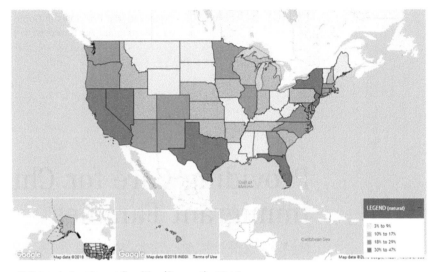

Children In Immigrant Families (Percent) - 2016

National KIDS COUNT
KIDS COUNT Data Center, datacenter.kidscount.org
A project of the Annie E. Casey Foundation

FIGURE 2
CIF, 2016. Reprinted with permission from The Annie E. Casey Foundation, KIDS COUNT Data Center,
https://datacenter.kidscount.org.

with temporary visas (eg, work visa,
student visa, tourist visa, J-1
classification), have or obtain
permanent permission to remain in
the United States (eg, lawful
permanent residents [LPRs] or "green
card" holders), come with
refugee status, seek legal protection
on arrival to the United States,
or remain without legal status
(Table 1). Refugees, who obtain legal
status before arrival, and asylees,
who can obtain legal status after
arrival in the United States, must have
a well-founded fear of persecution
based on race, religion, nationality,
sexual/gender orientation, political
opinion, or membership in
a particular social group.[5] LPRs and
refugees can apply for citizenship
after 5 years of living in the United
States.[6] In addition to asylum, other
forms of protection (eg, special
immigrant juvenile status, T
nonimmigrant status, and U
nonimmigrant status) may also be
available to particular children and
families seeking safe haven in the
United States.[7] If parents or children
do not qualify for a legal form of
protection, they may choose to
remain in the United States
without legal status. Specifically,
approximately 11.1 million
individuals in the United States lack
current legal status,[8] and 5.1 million
US children live with at least 1

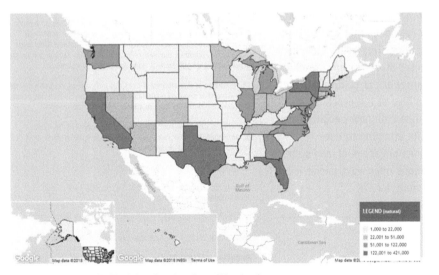

Child Population By Nativity: Foreign-Born (Number) -
2017

National KIDS COUNT
KIDS COUNT Data Center, datacenter.kidscount.org
A project of the Annie E. Casey Foundation

FIGURE 1
Population of immigrant children in the United States, 2017. Reprinted with permission from The
Annie E. Casey Foundation, KIDS COUNT Data Center, https://datacenter.kidscount.org.

TABLE 1 Definitions

Term	Description
Children in immigrant families (CIF)	Children who are foreign born and those who are born in the United States and have at least 1 parent who was foreign born
Immigrant children	Children born outside the United States
Lawful permanent residents (LPR)	Immigrants with permission to live and work permanently in the United States
Refugee	Children or adults who fled persecution in their home countries and legally entered the United States after being screened and approved by US agencies abroad
Asylum	Status that can be granted to people already in the United States who have a well-founded fear of persecution by or permitted by their government on the basis of 1 of 5 grounds and who satisfy the requirements for refugee status
T nonimmigrant status ("T visa")	Victims of severe forms of trafficking who can demonstrate that they would suffer extreme hardship involving unusual or severe harm if removed from the United States
U nonimmigrant status ("U visa")	Victims of certain serious crimes who have cooperated with law enforcement in the investigation or prosecution of the crime
Special immigrant juvenile status (SIJS)	Noncitizen minors who were abused, neglected, or abandoned by 1 or both parents
Temporary protected status (TPS)	Status granted to individuals physically present in the United States who are from countries designated by the Secretary of the US Department of Homeland Security as unsafe to accept their return
J-1 classification (exchange visitors)	Status granted to those who intend to participate in an approved program for the purposes of teaching, instructing or lecturing, studying, observing, conducting research, consulting, demonstrating special skills, receiving training, or receiving graduate medical education or training
Deferred Action for Childhood Arrivals (DACA)	Temporary relief from deportation with strict criteria based on age of arrival to United States, whether the individual is in school or working, and whether the individual has no criminal offenses or threats
Deferred Action for Parents of Americans and Lawful Permanent Residents	Temporary relief from deportation for parents of children who are US citizens or have LPR that was never implemented

immigrant parent without legal status.[9]

In 2016, half of the 22.5 million refugees worldwide were 18 years or younger, and less than 1% are resettled annually.[10] Ongoing humanitarian needs are acutely exacerbated by global migration crises, exemplified by the displacement of nearly 12 million Syrians by the end of 2015.[10] The number of refugees entering the United States is set annually by Congress and the president and historically has fluctuated on the basis of sociopolitical events. All 50 states, with the exception of Wyoming, have refugee resettlement programs.[11]

Migration to the United States varies on the basis of global poverty, armed conflict, and exceedingly complex sociopolitical circumstances. Despite these complexities, the United Nations Convention on the Rights of the Child, endorsed by the American Academy of Pediatrics (AAP) but not ratified by the US government, is an

internationally recognized legal framework for the protection of children's basic rights, regardless of the reasons children migrate.[12,13] The AAP policy statement "The Effects of Armed Conflict on Children" delineates the impact of armed conflict on children and the role of child health professionals in a global response.[14]

Responses to migration, and especially migration of children, are equally varied and complicated.[15] For instance, increasing arrivals of unaccompanied children and family units from Guatemala, Honduras, El Salvador, and Mexico at the southern US border beginning in 2014 triggered a series of governmental responses, including escalating detention of immigrant children, described in detail in the AAP policy statement "Detention of Immigrant Children."[7,16] Additionally, the Deferred Action for Childhood Arrivals (DACA) program was developed to allow young adults who had arrived in the United States as

children without legal status but had grown up in the United States to apply for deportation relief and work permits.[15] A related program, Deferred Action for Parents of Americans and Lawful Permanent Residents (DAPA), would have offered similar protections for parents without legal status who have US-born children, but it was halted in federal courts and was subsequently rescinded by presidential executive order before it could be implemented.[15,17] In 2017, the president signed new executive orders focused on heightened immigration enforcement, increased border security, and limits to the US refugee program. Furthermore, changes to temporary protected status (TPS), granted to individuals physically present in the United States who are from countries designated by the secretary of the US Department of Homeland Security as unsafe to accept their return, have created uncertainty for the nearly 320 000 TPS beneficiaries and their families.[18]

In addition to changes in the numbers and demographics of immigrants and the legal protections afforded them, family immigration status represents an important and often-neglected social determinant of health. The immigration status of children and their parents relates directly to their subsequent access to and use of health care, perceived health status, and health outcomes.[7,19-26] Family immigration status is intertwined with other social determinants of health, including poverty,[27] food insecurity,[28,29] housing instability,[30,31] discrimination,[32,33] and health literacy.[34-37]

RESILIENCE AND INTEGRATION

Despite the challenges that immigrant children and families often face, many offer tremendous assets and demonstrate remarkable resilience. On first arrival in the United States, immigrant children may be healthier than native-born peers, a phenomenon often described as "the immigrant paradox" or "the healthy immigrant effect."[27,33] A strengths-based approach to immigrant child health celebrates assets of immigrant families and populations, buffers marginalization, and supports integration. Understanding cultural assets, such as ethnic-racial identity and cultural values, may offer opportunities to build resilience among immigrant children.[38-40] Furthermore, recognizing assets facilitates productive dialogue that supports immigrant families not as threats but as valuable resources to our society.[40]

CULTURAL HUMILITY AND SAFETY

When caring for CIF, health care providers must recognize the role culture plays in understanding illness without reflexively assuming that challenges are always attributable to cultural differences.[41-45] Because culture is dynamic, cultural competency is never fully realized,[46]

but rather serves as a developmental process.[47] Providers bring personal cultural biases, as well as biases of biomedicine, that can implicitly or explicitly affect the provision of care.[48,49] Cultural humility is the concept of openness and respect for differences.[50-52] Cultural safety reflects the recognition of the power differences and inequities in health and the clinical encounter that result from social, historical, economic, and political circumstances.[53-55] By recognizing ourselves and others as cultural beings, by building trust through respect and awareness of power differentials and cultural beliefs, and by developing and implementing communication skills that facilitate mutual understanding, health care providers work to minimize disparities and promote equity in a health encounter.

Culturally sensitive systems of health care, ones that value cultural humility and safety, emerge when patients and families are engaged with 3 core values: curiosity, empathy, and respect.[56] Some immigrants bring with them a system of healing that, like biomedicine practiced in the United States, claims to be curative, includes interventions that can be applied by an expert practitioner, and offers a body of theory regarding disease causation, classification, and treatment.[57] With acculturation, these individuals may or may not modify their healing system to incorporate biomedical concepts. Culturally sensitive care systems have the flexibility to support health literacy, to recognize values of community and family that may supersede individual rights, to engage spirituality and respect traditions, and to include diverse perspectives in implementation and evaluation. The reciprocity of culturally sensitive health care offers us a wider lens that reduces health inequities and strengthens the practice of healing through multicultural medicine and

medical practice that acknowledges nonallopathic traditions.[58,59]

CARE OF CIF: CORE COMPETENCIES

Immigrant children benefit from increased access and communication offered in a patient- and family-centered medical home with an identified primary care provider in which care "is respectful of and responsive to individual patient preferences, needs, and values."[60-64] The medical home, infused with cultural humility and safety, supports continuous, comprehensive, and compassionate care and increases collaboration with community supports, including schools, places of worship, legal agencies, and extracurricular activities. Interpreters are an essential part of the medical team to support health literacy, improve access, and ensure quality medical care.[65,66] However, disparities in access to care for CIF, and especially for those with special health care needs, have persisted.[24,25,67-72] Immigrant families, particularly those with children with special health care needs, often benefit from intensive supports in negotiating a complex medical system, special education system, and network of community resources. Pediatric providers can play a lead role for the medical home team in implementing and educating on core competencies that are meant to build health equity for CIF. Core resources for the provision of care for CIF include, but are not limited to, the AAP Immigrant Child Health Toolkit[44] and the Centers for Disease Control and Prevention Refugee Health Guidelines.[73]

Cross-cultural Approach

Rather than learning generalities of a given culture, a practical framework can guide the clinical approach.[74,75] A classic patient-based model recommends assessing for core cross-cultural issues, exploring the meaning of the illness, determining the social context, and engaging in negotiation around treatment plans.[76] Core cross-cultural issues include styles of communication, trust, family dynamics, traditions and spirituality, and sexual and gender considerations.[75] Kleinman and Benson's[45] 7 questions for cultural assessment are helpful to explore patient's perspectives; most crucially, this includes what matters most to the patient and family within the context of illness and treatment (Table 2). The efficacy of treatment may need to be understood "within the scope of cultural beliefs and not that of the scientific evidence."[77,78] Therefore, there may be need for cross-cultural negotiation facilitated through tools like "LEARN" (listen, explain, acknowledge, recommend, negotiate).[57,79]

Knowledge and skills can be developed regarding cross-cultural patient care, migration health issues, and unique vulnerabilities and strengths of immigrant families. Although all children and families are unique, origin-country profiles may be helpful to provide generalized information about immigrant groups.[80–82]

Migration Health Issues

Care of immigrant children requires knowledge of unique health issues in the child's country of origin and country or countries of refuge before arrival as well as an understanding of

TABLE 2 Questions to Elicit the Patient Explanatory Model

Questions
1. What do you call this problem?
2. What do you believe is the cause of this problem?
3. What course do you expect it to take? How serious is it?
4. What do you think this problem does inside your body?
5. How does it affect your body and your mind?
6. What do you most fear about this condition?
7. What do you most fear about the treatment?

Copyright 2006 Kleinman and Benson.[45] Reprinted under the terms of the Creative Commons Attribution License.

the challenges of resettlement and acculturation once within the United States. When taking a medical history, it is therefore necessary to elicit details of migration[73] as well as the child's birth; medical, immunization, developmental, social, and family history; and exposure to trauma and violence.[73,83] Past medical and immunization records may require translation as well as awareness and management of different global immunization schedules.[84,85] CIF often return to their families' countries of origin to visit relatives, and providers need to be familiar with travel risks, prophylactic medications, and unique vaccine needs.[86]

Communicable Disease

When screening for and treating infectious diseases, a public health approach is advantageous.[44,87] For refugees, some screenings may have been performed in another country, and presumptive treatments may have been provided through the International Organization for Migration.[88] Depending on the migration history, immigrant children may need screening on arrival in the United States for infectious diseases (eg, tuberculosis; malaria; Chagas disease; intestinal parasites such as helminths, schistosomiasis, and strongyloides; chronic hepatitis B; HIV; syphilis; and other vertically and horizontally transmitted sexual infections).[44,87–94] Comprehensive reproductive and mental health services are warranted for immigrant children with a history of sexual activity, trafficking, exploitation, or victimization.

Oral Health

The global burden of oral diseases is high.[95] Caries risk varies depending on previous country of residence.[96,97] Differences in oral health may reflect cultural practices and norms related to weaning and brushing, dietary changes, and limited oral health literacy.[98–101] Access to dental

services and education on oral health is essential for immigrant children.[102]

Noncommunicable Disease

The incidence of noncommunicable diseases globally has grown.[103–105] Rates of asthma, obesity, autism,[106–110] depression, anxiety, and posttraumatic stress disorder (PTSD) may be similar or disproportionately increased in immigrant children.[71,111–114] In addition, newly arrived immigrant children may present with diseases not yet diagnosed or further progressed. Examples include genetic conditions related to consanguinity. Furthermore, newborn screening for hearing loss, hypothyroidism, metabolic diseases, or hemoglobinopathies may not have been performed.[94,115] Vision problems and elevated blood lead concentrations are also common and must be considered.[94,116–120]

Nutrition and Growth

During assessment of nutrition and growth on entry into medical care, immigrant children may be recognized as wasted, having underweight, having overweight, or stunted.[97,121–124] Health care providers will need to be familiar with global diets, dietary restrictions, and vitamin and nutrient sources.[124–126] Anemia, thalassemia, glucose-6-phosphate dehydrogenase deficiency, and micronutrient deficiencies (including iron, vitamin D, and vitamin B_{12}) may exist.[97,127–129] Families can be screened for food insecurity and connected to relevant resources.[126,130,131]

Developmental and Educational Considerations

Age-appropriate developmental and behavioral screening is possible with the use of validated multilingual screening tools, such as the Ages and Stages Questionnaire[132] and the Survey of Well-being of Young Children,[133] and with historical assessment of milestones.[134,135] Care must be taken to recognize cultural bias and experiential differences in skill development.[136–139] Screening needs to be sensitive to cultural differences in parenting[140,141] and disparities in reading or sharing books with children,[142] but referral should not be delayed if screening results are concerning.[143] Age-appropriate vision and hearing screening is essential.[144] Providers' encouragement of a language-rich environment in the parent's primary language recognizes the strengths of bilingualism.[145–150]

One in 10 students from kindergarten to 12th grade in the United States is an English-language learner.[151] Dual-language learners, defined as children younger than 8 years with at least 1 parent who speaks another language in the home other than English, make up one-third of young children in the United States currently. Dual-language learners are less likely to be enrolled in high-quality early child care and preschools compared with peers, potentially limiting kindergarten readiness.[152,153]

All children are entitled to free public education and specialized educational services regardless of immigration status.[154] Immigrant children may face particular academic challenges.[155,156] Before arrival to the United States, some children may have had no opportunity for formal schooling or may have faced protracted educational interruptions. Students with interrupted or no schooling may lack strong literacy skills, age-appropriate content knowledge, and socioemotional skills; in addition, they may need to learn the English language.[157] Learning may also be affected by traumatic brain injury, cerebral malaria, malnutrition, personal trauma, in utero exposures (eg, alcohol),[94] and toxic exposures (eg, lead).[116–120] Testing for developmental and learning challenges in the school setting may result in overrepresentation of students with limited English proficiency (LEP) in

special education.[158–161] Through collaboration with parents and schools, pediatricians can facilitate thoughtful consideration of learning difficulties in the setting of LEP. Supplemental anticipatory guidance may include recognition of family strengths and differences in parent-child relationships, child-rearing practices and discipline, dietary preferences, safety risks and use of car restraints and safe sleep practices, and acculturation.[162–168]

Mental Health

Many immigrant children and youth may have had disruptions to the basic experiences that allow for healthy development.[169] Immigrant children and their families may experience trauma before migration, during their journey, on arrival at our borders, and while integrating into American communities[170–176] and, as a result of their increased risk, require "health and related services of a type or amount beyond that required by children generally."[177] Trauma may include personal history of physical or sexual abuse, witnessing interpersonal violence, human trafficking, actual or threatened separation from parents, or exposure to armed conflict.[173,174,176,178] Traumatized children with traumatized parents (or, in some cases, without their parents) may be at risk for toxic stress or prolonged serious stress in the absence of buffering relationships.[179] In addition to intergenerational transfer of mental health problems, core stressors include trauma, acculturation, isolation, and resettlement.[172] In particular, acculturation includes stressors that families experience as they navigate between the culture of their country of origin and the culture in their new country.[172]

On arrival, many refugee and unaccompanied children have high levels of anxiety, depression, and PTSD.[174,180–186] Compared with US-

origin youth, refugee youth have higher rates of community violence exposure, dissociative symptoms, traumatic grief, somatization, and phobic disorder.[187] Unaccompanied minors have even higher levels of PTSD compared with accompanied immigrants,[188] which may be further heightened if they are seeking asylum.[189] Immigration-related trauma history may be shared over time as a trusting relationship develops with the physician.[190] Some CIF who were born in the United States may face difficulty with emotional and behavioral problems relating to identity formation.[191] Initial and ongoing screening for mental and behavioral health problems with multiple cross-culturally validated tools (eg, the Ages and Stages Questionnaire-Social Emotional, the Survey of Well-being of Young Children, the Strengths and Difficulty Questionnaire, the Refugee Health Screener 15, and the Child Behavior Checklist) facilitates recognition of distress and concerns.[44,132,133,192–195]

By understanding the interplay of biological, social, environmental, and psychological risk and protective factors, emotional disorders can be modulated on population, community, and individual levels.[196] Protective factors and sources of resilience observed in immigrants include having a positive outlook, having strong coping skills, having positive parental coping strategies, connection to prosocial organizations such as places of worship and athletics, and cultural pride reinforcement.[32,197–200] Resilience is fostered through strong family relationships and community support.[201] Bicultural identity, a strong attachment to one's culture of origin in addition to a sense of belonging within the culture of residence, promotes resilience.[140,202]

Because of the shame and stigma associated with mental health problems, families may be reluctant to seek treatment.[203] Providers can increase access and minimize stigma by integrating culturally tailored mental health services into the medical home, in the school setting, and through engagement with community mental health resources,[78,175,204] including home visitation.[205] Community-wide strategies that foster belonging, reduce discrimination, and provide social supports can facilitate healing and reduce stigma.

Traditional Health Care and Cultural Practices

Traditional healing and cultural practices, common among some immigrant populations, warrant awareness by health care providers.[206] Patients may not disclose use of herbal and traditional treatments unless directly asked.[42,207] Some immigrant families use traditional forms of protection for vulnerable infants, such as prayer, amulets, kohl, or myrrh. Other immigrant families use traditional practices to treat illness (eg, cupping, coining, and uvulectomy), and stigmata of these traditional treatments may be observed on examination and may be misinterpreted as abuse.[208,209]

Female genital cutting or mutilation (FGC/M) is still practiced in some communities in Africa, in the Middle East, and in parts of Asia despite increased efforts to educate on risks.[210,211] Performing FGC/M is against the law in the United States and has been defined as torture by the United Nations, but foreign-born girls may have experienced this before entry into the United States.[210,212] Resources exist regarding the types of FGC/M, complications that can result, recommended documentation in the medical record, and strategies to sensitively discuss this with families.[213,214] In 2013, the United States passed the Transport for Female Genital Mutilation Act, which prohibits knowingly transporting

a girl out of the United States for the purpose of "vacation cutting."[215] The need to screen for FGC/M further underscores the importance of examining the external genitalia of children at all preventive visits in addition to sensitively counseling families regarding the laws and other concerns regarding FGM/C.

PRACTICE-LEVEL BARRIERS AND POTENTIAL OPPORTUNITIES

Communication challenges between families with LEP and health care providers must be addressed to provide high-quality care. Fifty-four percent of CIF have resident parents who have difficulty speaking English.[3] Parental LEP is associated with worse health care access and quality for children.[216-220] National Standards for Culturally and Linguistically Appropriate Services in Health Care were issued by the US Department of Health and Human Services, in accordance with Title VI of the Civil Rights Act. Culturally and Linguistically Appropriate Services in Health Care Standards describe the federal expectation that health care organizations receiving federal funding must provide meaningful access to verbal and written-language services for patients with LEP.[221,222] Interpreters are an integral part of the medical home team for CIF and hold the same confidentiality standards as the physician.[67,68] Most state insurance programs and private insurers do not offer reimbursement for language services. Although teaching health care providers when and how to work with interpreters can improve care, few providers receive such training.[223,224] For these and other reasons, some providers inappropriately use family members as ad hoc interpreters.[225] However, family members, friends, and especially children are not acceptable substitutes for trained interpreters.[226,227] Trained medical interpreters, via phone or tablet or in-person, facilitate mutual

understanding and a high quality of communication.[228,229] Use of trained interpreters maintains confidentiality, reduces errors and cost, and increases the quality of health care delivery.[227,228,230-232] Interpretation requires that extra time be allotted to health care encounters. Qualified bicultural and bilingual staff can receive medical interpreter training if expected to perform as interpreters, and bilingual providers can ideally demonstrate dual-language proficiency before engaging with families in their preferred language without an interpreter.[233-235] Access can be further improved by the use of multilingual signage, screening tools, handouts, and other key documents (eg, consent forms and hospital discharge summaries) that are prepared by qualified translators.

Although some immigrant families integrate without hardship, many CIF face inequities resulting from complex determinants, including poverty, immigration status, insurance status, education, and discrimination on the basis of race and/or ethnicity.[32,33] For some, fear regarding family immigration status threatens children's health, development, and access to care.[22,32,236-238] For others, growing up in 2-parent families and having environmental stimulation at home, particularly for those with low socioeconomic status, may be protective.[33,239] Screening for social determinants of health can trigger referrals to community-based supports.[240] The hallmarks of the medical home, comprehensive care and enhanced care coordination, are important supports for immigrant families. Integrated mental health, nutrition, social work, and patient navigation services allow for ease of access and for reduction in stigma and barriers. Community health workers who are members of immigrant communities have been effective in reducing disparity and improving health outcomes.[241-246]

Interagency partnerships with the local health department, home-visiting programs, community mental health providers, schools, and immigrant service organizations facilitate access to medical homes and cross-sector communication. "Warm hand-offs," or in-person transfer of care between health care team members with patients and families present, can help to ensure linkage between providers and relevant resources.[247]

SYSTEMS-LEVEL BARRIERS AND POTENTIAL OPPORTUNITIES

Health literacy challenges experienced by CIF include not only language comprehension but also the myriad of system barriers in the health care network. Limited health literacy can complicate enrollment in public benefits for CIF. Immigrant children are specifically less likely to have a medical home[67,68] and health insurance, resulting in delayed or foregone care.[248] Most immigrant children with legal status are eligible for health coverage. A majority of states have opted to allow lawfully residing immigrant children to receive Medicaid and/or Children's Health Insurance Program coverage using federal Medicaid and Children's Health Insurance Program funds without a 5-year waiting period, an option given to states by the Children's Health Insurance Program Reauthorization Act of 2009; however, 17 states have not taken the Children's Health Insurance Program Reauthorization Act of 2009 option.[249-253] Only a minority of states offer health coverage to children regardless of immigration status.[252,253] Additionally, immigrant children without legal status, including DACA youth, are excluded from eligibility for most federal programs, including health insurance, although some states have included and/or are considering inclusion of DACA youth (or, more broadly, other noncitizen children) as eligible for

programs such as in-state tuition or professional licensing.[254,255] Opportunities to mitigate these literacy, access, and health insurance enrollment challenges include system-wide use and funding of interpreters and multilingual tools and use of community health workers and patient navigators to reduce barriers through facilitation, education, and advocacy.[43,58,59,256,257] For CIF without health coverage, federally qualified health centers, public health departments, free clinics, and charity care systems may offer access to consistent care. Home-visiting programs can support immigrant parents and parents with LEP who may be isolated and unable to access public services[152,258]; attention to cultural safety is particularly critical when engaging in home-based services. Quality after-school programming, with support of school social work, can also facilitate integration and build resilience for CIF.[259,260]

IMMIGRATION AND RELATED LEGAL ISSUES

Federal immigration policies can adversely affect immigrant health coverage, access, and outcomes. Immigration status of children and/or their parents continues to affect access to services and public benefits, despite some improvement.[33,261,262] Increased fears about the use of public programs and immigration status has deterred immigrants from accessing programs regardless of eligibility.[263-265] In addition, immigration enforcement activities that occur at or near sensitive locations, such as hospitals, may prevent families from accessing needed medical care.[264] Sensitive locations include medical treatment and health care facilities, places of worship, and schools, and US Immigration and Customs Enforcement actions, including apprehension, interviews, searches, or surveillance, should not occur at

these locations.[266,267] Fear of immigration enforcement or discrimination may exacerbate transportation barriers and worsen perceived access to care.[23,237,268-271] Discrimination relating to immigration may intersect with religion (eg, Muslim immigrants) and race in complex ways.[264,272-274] Discrimination and immigration enforcement policies may also create fear and uncertainty, which threaten the mental health of immigrant children[275] and their families.[19,236,264,276] Families living on the US-Mexico border face particular risk of mistreatment and victimization.[277] Policies that offer protection from deportation, such as DACA, may confer large mental health benefits for youth and for the children of parenting youth.[278,279]

Immigrant children who have been detained and are in immigration proceedings face almost universal traumatic histories and ongoing stress, including actual or threatened separation from their parents at the border.[7] Immigrant children, including unaccompanied children, are not guaranteed a right to legal counsel, and as such, roughly 50% of children arriving in the United States have no one to represent them in immigration court.[280] Lack of guaranteed legal representation for immigrant children and families at risk for deportation is further complicated by funding restrictions; specifically, medical-legal partnerships receiving federal funding that operate under Legal Services Corporation guidelines cannot accept most cases related to immigration.[281] Many nongovernmental efforts have sought to address lack of legal representation for children, but opportunities remain to better provide immigration-specific legal support for immigrant families,[282,283] including novel medical-legal partnerships with different funding streams that do not exclude people without legal status and offer representation in immigration court. In addition, traumatized immigrant children can benefit from system-level supports for integration of mental health and social work supports into schools, the medical home, and protected community settings.[284]

Evidence-based programs can systematically build resilience among CIF by supporting integration into US culture while preserving home cultural heritage. Although specific evidence regarding CIF is limited, home-visiting programs offer opportunities to celebrate unique strengths and mitigate stress in a natural environment.[258,285] Programs that support literacy and encourage play, such as Reach Out and Read, can reinforce parent-child relationships, build parenting skills, support development, and prepare children for academic success.[150,286,287] For children experiencing parental reunification after prolonged separation, mental health services and educational support are particularly critical.[238] Given the strong role of communities in many cultures, community-based interventions may be particularly effective for immigrant families.

Opportunities to investigate strategies, mitigate barriers, and optimize health and well-being for CIF include research, medical education, and community engagement, including community-based participatory research and health education. Research used to examine acculturative stress and resilience of immigrant children over time is limited. Among CIF, diversity within and between racial and ethnic groups (eg, Hispanic, Asian, African, and Caribbean) and between CIF of varying socioeconomic statuses is also understudied and underappreciated.[288] Medical education has become increasingly responsive to health disparities for immigrants and to the opportunities for experiential broadening of global

health. By implementing core competencies in the care of immigrant populations, trainees can learn to support a culture of health equity for CIF. Pediatricians can support families within and beyond the medical home through efforts supported by cross-sector community collaboration, including fields such as education and law, innovative research, and thoughtful advocacy, to inspire progressive policy.[171,180,289] Grants that are focused on minority and underserved pediatric populations have the potential to mitigate inequities for immigrant children.[171]

SUMMARY AND RECOMMENDATIONS

With ever-increasing levels of migration worldwide, the population of CIF residing in the United States grows. The following practice- and policy-level recommendations offer guidance for pediatricians caring for CIF. Although it is aspirational to fully implement all recommendations in all situations, most are achievable by intentionally enacting practice- and systems-based changes over time.

Practice-Level Recommendations

1. All pediatricians are encouraged to recognize their inherent biases and work to improve their skills in cultural humility and effective communication through professional development.

2. CIF benefit from comprehensive, coordinated, continuous, and culturally and linguistically effective care in a quality medical home with an identified primary care provider.

3. Co-located or integrated mental health, social work, patient navigation, and legal services are recommended to improve access and minimize barriers.

4. Trained medical interpreters, via phone or tablet or in-person, are recommended to facilitate mutual understanding and a high quality

of communication. Family members, friends, and especially children are not recommended for interpretation. Materials may be translated into the patient's preferred language by qualified translators whenever possible. Consideration should be given for the extended time needed for interpretation during medical encounters.

5. It is recommended that pediatricians and staff receive training on working effectively with language services and that bilingual providers and staff demonstrate dual-language competency before interacting with patients and families without medical interpreters.

6. Pediatricians and pediatric trainees are encouraged to engage in professional development activities that include specific competencies (including immigrant health; global health, including the global burden of disease; integrative medicine; and travel medicine) and to incorporate these competencies into the evaluation and care of CIF.

7. Pediatricians caring for CIF are urged to apply a trauma-informed lens, with sensitivity to and screening for multigenerational trauma. Mental health professionals adept at treating immigrants can be integrated into the medical home or identified in the community.

8. Screening for social determinants of health, including risks and protective factors, is recommended.

9. Assessment of development, learning, and behavior is warranted for all immigrant children, regardless of age. Pediatricians can support dual language as an asset and as part of cultural pride reinforcement.

Advocacy and Policy Recommendations

1. The AAP endorses the United Nations Convention on the Rights of the Child and the principles included in this document as a legal framework for the protection of children's basic rights.

2. All US federal government, private, and community-based organizations involved with immigrant children should adopt policies that protect and prioritize their health, well-being, and safety and should consider children's best interests in all decisions by government and private actors.

3. Interagency collaboration is recommended between service providers (eg, medical, mental health, public health, legal, education, social work, and ethnic-community based) to enhance care, prevent marginalization of immigrant families, and build resilience among immigrant communities.

4. Health coverage should be provided for all children regardless of immigration status. Neither immigrant children with legal status nor their parents should be subject to a 5-year waiting period for health coverage or other federal benefits.

5. Private and public insurance payers should pay for qualified medical interpretation and translation services. Given the increased cost-effectiveness and quality of care provided with medical interpretation, payers should recognize and reimburse for the increased time needed during a medical encounter when using an interpreter.

6. Both the separation of children from their parents and the detention of children with parents as a tool of law enforcement are inhumane, counterproductive, and threatening to short- and long-term health. Immigration authorities should not separate children from their parents nor place children in detention.

7. Immigration enforcement activities should not occur at or near sensitive locations such as hospitals, health care facilities, schools (including child care and Head Start), places of worship, and other sensitive locations. Pediatricians have the right to report and protest any such enforcement. Medical records should be protected from immigration enforcement actions. Health systems can develop protocols to minimize fear and enhance trust for those seeking health care.

8. Children in immigration proceedings should have access to legal representation at no cost to the child. Medical-legal partnerships that include immigration representation (eg, Terra Firma[290]) and efforts to increase legal representation (eg, KIND,[291] the Young Center for Immigrant Children's Rights,[292] RAICES[293]) should be supported practically and financially at local, state, and federal levels.

9. Immigration policy that prioritizes children and families by ensuring access to health care and educational and economic supports, by keeping families together, and by protecting vulnerable unaccompanied children is of fundamental importance for comprehensive immigration reform. Humanitarian protection (eg, refugee resettlement and protection for victims of trafficking and asylum seekers) supports trauma-informed care of children and is an essential component of immigration policy.

10. All children with LEP merit early, intensive, and longitudinal educational support with culturally responsive teaching. Literacy skills are necessary for health literacy, an essential health need.

11. Enhanced funding is recommended to support research regarding immigrant child health, including, but not limited to, health outcomes; screening tools for development, mental health, and social determinants of health that are culturally and linguistically sensitive; developmental and/or learning difficulties in children whose home language is not English; and reduction of barriers to health access and equity.

12. Medical education can facilitate education of trainees and health care professionals through implementation of core competencies in the care of immigrant populations and through advocacy curricula that incorporate special populations, including CIF.

13. AAP chapters can work with state governments to adopt policies that protect and prioritize immigrant children's health, well-being, and safety.

CONCLUSIONS

CIF represent a growing, diverse demographic in the United States. Pediatricians play an essential role in addressing vulnerabilities, minimizing barriers to care, and supporting optimal short- and long-term health and well-being of CIF within the medical home and in communities across the nation.

With compassionate, respectful, and progressive policy, CIF can achieve their full potential for health and well-being.

LEAD AUTHORS

Julie M. Linton, MD, FAAP
Andrea Green, MD, FAAP

COUNCIL ON COMMUNITY PEDIATRICS EXECUTIVE COMMITTEE, 2017–2018

Lance A. Chilton, MD, FAAP, Chairperson
James H. Duffee, MD, MPH, FAAP, Vice-Chairperson
Kimberley J. Dilley, MD, MPH, FAAP
Andrea Green, MD, FAAP

J. Raul Gutierrez, MD, MPH, FAAP
Virginia A. Keane, MD, FAAP
Scott D. Krugman, MD, MS, FAAP
Julie M. Linton, MD, FAAP
Carla D. McKelvey, MD, MPH, FAAP
Jacqueline L. Nelson, MD, FAAP

LIAISONS

Gerri L. Mattson, MD, MPH, FAAP – *Chairperson, Public Health Special Interest Group*
Kathleen Rooney-Otero, MD, MPH – *Section on Pediatric Trainees*
Donene Feist – *Family Voices North Dakota*

STAFF

Dana Bennett-Tejes, MA, MNM
Jean Davis, MPP
Tamar Magarik Haro

ACKNOWLEDGMENT

We thank Jennifer Nagda, JD (Young Center for Immigrant Children's Rights).

ABBREVIATIONS

AAP: American Academy of Pediatrics
CIF: children in immigrant families
DACA: Deferred Action for Childhood Arrivals
FGC/M: female genital cutting or mutilation
LEP: limited English proficiency
LPR: lawful permanent resident
PTSD: posttraumatic stress disorder
TPS: temporary protected status

POTENTIAL CONFLICT OF INTEREST: The authors have indicated they have no potential conflicts of interest to disclose.

REFERENCES

1. Migration Policy Institute. Immigrant profiles and demographics. US data. Available at: https://www.migrationpolicy.org/topics/us-data. Accessed July 26, 2019

2. Pew Research Center. *Modern immigration wave brings 59 million to US, driving population growth and change through 2065: views of immigration's impact on US society mixed.* 2015. Available at: www.pewhispanic.org/2015/09/28/modern-immigration-wave-brings-59-million-to-u-s-driving-population-growth-and-change-through-2065/. Accessed August 30, 2018

3. The Annie E. Casey Foundation; Kids Count Data Center. Children in immigrant families in the United States. Available at: https://datacenter.kidscount.org/data/tables/115-children-in-immigrant-families?loc=1&loct=1#detailed/1/any/false/871,870,573,869,36,868,867,133,38,35/any/445,446. Accessed July 26, 2019

4. Urban Institute. Children of immigrants data tool. Available at: http://webapp.urban.org/charts/datatool/pages.cfm. Accessed August 30, 2018

5. United Nations Office of the High Commissioner for Refugees. Convention and protocol relating to the status of refugees. 2010. Available at: www.unhcr.org/en-us/protection/basic/3b66c2aa10/convention-protocol-relating-status-refugees.html. Accessed August 30, 2018

6. The National Child Traumatic Stress Network. Bridging refugee youth and children's services. Refugee 101. Available at: https://www.nctsn.org/resources/bridging-refugee-youth-and-childrens-services-refugee-101. Accessed August 30, 2018

7. Linton JM, Griffin M, Shapiro AJ; Council on Community Pediatrics. Detention of immigrant children. *Pediatrics.* 2017;139(5): e20170483

8. Passel JS, Cohn D. Overall number of US unauthorized immigrants holds steady since 2009. 2016. Available at: www.pewhispanic.org/2016/09/20/overall-number-of-u-s-unauthorized-immigrants-holds-steady-since-2009/. Accessed December 27, 2017

9. Capps R, Fix M, Zong J. A profile of U.S. children with unauthorized immigrant parents. Available at: https://www.migrationpolicy.org/research/profile-us-children-unauthorized-immigrant-parents. Accessed December 27, 2017

10. United Nations Office of the High Commissioner for Refugees. *Global Trends: Forced Displacement in 2015.* Geneva, Switzerland: United Nations Office of the High Commissioner for Refugees; 2016

11. Administration for Children and Families. Office of refugee resettlement. 2017. Available at: https://www.acf.hhs.gov/orr. Accessed June 12, 2017

12. Haggerty RJ. The convention on the rights of the child: it's time for the United States to ratify. *Pediatrics.* 1994; 94(5):746–747

13. United Nations General Assembly. Convention on the rights of the child. 1989. Available at: www.ohchr.org/Documents/ProfessionalInterest/crc.pdf. Accessed April 8, 2016

14. Shenoda S, Kadir A, Pitterman S, Goldhagen J; Section on International Child Health. The effects of armed conflict on children. *Pediatrics.* 2018; 142(6):e20182585

15. Cohn D. *How U.S. Immigration Laws and Rules Have Changed through History.* Washington, DC: Pew Research Center; 2015. Available at: www.pewresearch.

org/fact-tank/2015/09/30/how-u-s-immigration-laws-and-rules-have-changed-through-history/. Accessed June 16, 2017

16. US Customs and Border Protection. United States border patrol southwest family unit subject and unaccompanied alien children apprehensions fiscal year 2016. Available at: https://www.cbp.gov/newsroom/stats/southwest-border-unaccompanied-children/fy-2016. Accessed December 26, 2016

17. US Department of Homeland Security. Frequently asked questions: rescission of memorandum providing for Deferred Action for Parents of Americans and Lawful Permanent Residents ("DAPA"). 2017. Available at: https://www.dhs.gov/news/2017/06/15/frequently-asked-questions-rescission-memorandum-providing-deferred-action-parents. Accessed June 15, 2017

18. Cohn D, Passel JS, Bialik K. Many Immigrants With Temporary Protected Status Face Uncertain Future in U.S. 2017. Available at: www.pewresearch.org/fact-tank/2017/11/08/more-than-100000-haitian-and-central-american-immigrants-face-decision-on-their-status-in-the-u-s/. Accessed December 27, 2017

19. Martinez O, Wu E, Sandfort T, et al. Evaluating the impact of immigration policies on health status among undocumented immigrants: a systematic review [published correction appears in *J Immigr Minor Health*. 2016;18(1):288]. *J Immigr Minor Health*. 2015;17(3):947–970

20. Novak NL, Geronimus AT, Martinez-Cardoso AM. Change in birth outcomes among infants born to Latina mothers after a major immigration raid. *Int J Epidemiol*. 2017;46(3):839–849

21. Hardy LJ, Getrich CM, Quezada JC, Guay A, Michalowski RJ, Henley E. A call for further research on the impact of state-level immigration policies on public health. *Am J Public Health*. 2012;102(7):1250–1254

22. Vargas ED, Ybarra VD. U.S. citizen children of undocumented parents: the link between state immigration policy and the health of Latino children. *J Immigr Minor Health*. 2017;19(4):913–920

23. Lopez WD, Kruger DJ, Delva J, et al. Health implications of an immigration raid: findings from a Latino community in the midwestern United States. *J Immigr Minor Health*. 2017;19(3):702–708

24. Yun K, Fuentes-Afflick E, Curry LA, Krumholz HM, Desai MM. Parental immigration status is associated with children's health care utilization: findings from the 2003 new immigrant survey of US legal permanent residents. *Matern Child Health J*. 2013;17(10):1913–1921

25. Javier JR, Huffman LC, Mendoza FS, Wise PH. Children with special health care needs: how immigrant status is related to health care access, health care utilization, and health status. *Matern Child Health J*. 2010;14(4):567–579

26. Siddiqi A, Zuberi D, Nguyen QC. The role of health insurance in explaining immigrant versus non-immigrant disparities in access to health care: comparing the United States to Canada. *Soc Sci Med*. 2009;69(10):1452–1459

27. Child Trends. Immigrant children. 2017. Available at: https://www.childtrends.org/indicators/immigrant-children. Accessed August 27, 2018

28. Chilton M, Black MM, Berkowitz C, et al. Food insecurity and risk of poor health among US-born children of immigrants. *Am J Public Health*. 2009;99(3):556–562

29. Walsemann KM, Ro A, Gee GC. Trends in food insecurity among California residents from 2001 to 2011: inequities at the intersection of immigration status and ethnicity. *Prev Med*. 2017;105(1):142–148

30. Koball H, Capps R, Perrera K, et al. *Health and Social Service Needs of US-Citizen Children With Detained or Deported Immigrant Parents*. Washington, DC: Urban Institute, Migration Policy Institute; 2015, Available at: https://www.urban.org/research/publication/health-and-social-service-needs-us-citizen-children-detained-or-deported-immigrant-parents/view/full_report. Accessed December 27, 2017

31. Hooper K, Zong J, Capps R, Fix M. *Young Children of Refugees in the United States: Integration Successes and Challenges*. Washington, DC: Migration Policy Institute; 2016, Available at: https://www.migrationpolicy.org/research/young-children-refugees-united-states-integration-successes-and-challenges. Accessed August 27, 2018

32. Brown CS. *The Educational, Psychological, and Social Impact of Discrimination on the Immigrant Child*. Washington, DC: Migration Policy Institute; 2015, Available at: https://www.migrationpolicy.org/research/educational-psychological-and-social-impact-discrimination-immigrant-child. Accessed August 27, 2018

33. Singh GK, Rodriguez-Lainz A, Kogan MD. Immigrant health inequalities in the United States: use of eight major national data systems. *ScientificWorldJournal*. 2013;2013:512313

34. Braveman P, Barclay C. Health disparities beginning in childhood: a life-course perspective. *Pediatrics*. 2009;124(suppl 3):S163–S175

35. Braveman P, Egerter S, Williams DR. The social determinants of health: coming of age. *Annu Rev Public Health*. 2011;32:381–398

36. Simich L. Health literacy and immigrant populations. Public Health Agency of Canada and Metropolis Canada, Ottawa, Canada. 2009. Available at: http://www.metropolis.net/pdfs/health_literacy_policy_brief_jun15_e.pdf. Accessed August 27, 2018

37. Lee HY, Rhee TG, Kim NK, Ahluwalia JS. Health literacy as a social determinant of health in Asian American immigrants: findings from a population-based survey in California. *J Gen Intern Med*. 2015;30(8):1118–1124

38. Rivas-Drake D, Stein GL. Multicultural developmental experiences: implications for resilience in transitional age youth. *Child Adolesc Psychiatr Clin N Am*. 2017;26(2):271–281

39. US Department of Health and Human Services, Office of Minority Health. *National Standards for Culturally and Linguistically Appropriate Services in Health Care*. Washington, DC: US Department of Health and Human Services; 2001

40. Baran M, Kendall-Taylor N, Lindland E, O'Neil M, Haydon A. Getting to "we":

mapping the gaps between expert and public understandings of immigration and immigration reform. Available at: www.frameworksinstitute.org/assets/files/Immigration/immigration_mtg.pdf. Accessed December 28, 2017

41. Kodjo C. Cultural competence in clinician communication. *Pediatr Rev.* 2009;30(2):57–63; quiz 64

42. Brach C, Fraser I. Can cultural competency reduce racial and ethnic health disparities? A review and conceptual model. *Med Care Res Rev.* 2000;57(suppl 1):181–217

43. Committee on Pediatric Workforce. Enhancing pediatric workforce diversity and providing culturally effective pediatric care: implications for practice, education, and policy making. *Pediatrics.* 2013;132(4). Available at: www.pediatrics.org/cgi/content/full/132/4/e1105

44. American Academy of Pediatrics. Immigrant Child Health Toolkit. 2015. Available at: https://www.aap.org/en-us/advocacy-and-policy/aap-health-initiatives/Immigrant-Child-Health-Toolkit/Pages/Immigrant-Child-Health-Toolkit.aspx. Accessed October 29, 2018

45. Kleinman A, Benson P. Anthropology in the clinic: the problem of cultural competency and how to fix it. *PLoS Med.* 2006;3(10):e294

46. Kirmayer LJ. Rethinking cultural competence. *Transcult Psychiatry.* 2012; 49(2):149–164

47. Cross T, Bazron BJ, Dennis KW, Isaacs MR. *Towards a Culturally Competent System of Care: A Monograph on Effective Services for Minority Children Who Are Severely Emotionally Disturbed.* Washington, DC: Georgetown University Child Development Center, CASSP Technical Assistance Center; 1989

48. Project Implicit. About us. Available at: https://implicit.harvard.edu/implicit/aboutus.html. Accessed September 17, 2018

49. Blair IV, Steiner JF, Fairclough DL, et al. Clinicians' implicit ethnic/racial bias and perceptions of care among Black and Latino patients. *Ann Fam Med.* 2013; 11(1):43–52

50. Tervalon M, Murray-García J. Cultural humility versus cultural competence: a critical distinction in defining physician training outcomes in multicultural education. *J Health Care Poor Underserved.* 1998;9(2):117–125

51. Hook JN, Davis DE, Owen J, Worthington EL, Utsey SO. Cultural humility: measuring openness to culturally diverse clients. *J Couns Psychol.* 2013; 60(3):353–366

52. Yeager KA, Bauer-Wu S. Cultural humility: essential foundation for clinical researchers. *Appl Nurs Res.* 2013;26(4):251–256

53. Papps E, Ramsden I. Cultural safety in nursing: the New Zealand experience. *Int J Qual Health Care.* 1996;8(5): 491–497

54. Darroch F, Giles A, Sanderson P, et al. The United States does CAIR about cultural safety: examining cultural safety within indigenous health contexts in Canada and the United States. *J Transcult Nurs.* 2017;28(3): 269–277

55. Bozorgzad P, Negarandeh R, Raiesifar A, Poortaghi S. Cultural safety: an evolutionary concept analysis. *Holist Nurs Pract.* 2016;30(1):33–38

56. Green AR, Betancourt JR, Carillo JE. Cultural competence: a patient-based approach to caring for immigrants. In: Walker PF, Barnett ED, eds. *Immigrant Medicine.* 1st ed. Philadelphia, PA: Elsevier Health Sciences; 2007:83–97

57. Culhane-Pera KA, Borkan JM. Multicultural medicine. In: Walker PF, Barnett ED, eds. *Immigrant Medicine.* 1st ed. Philadelphia, PA: Elsevier Health Sciences; 2007:69–82

58. McPhail-Bell K, Bond C, Brough M, Fredericks B. 'We don't tell people what to do': ethical practice and Indigenous health promotion. *Health Promot J Austr.* 2015;26(3):195–199

59. Swota AH, Hester DM. Ethics for the pediatrician: providing culturally effective health care. *Pediatr Rev.* 2011; 32(3):e39–e43

60. American Academy of Pediatrics. National center for patient/family-centered medical home. Available at: https://medicalhomeinfo.aap.org/Pages/default.aspx. Accessed October 29, 2018

61. Medical Home Initiatives for Children With Special Needs Project Advisory Committee; American Academy of Pediatrics. The medical home. *Pediatrics.* 2002;110(1, pt 1):184–186

62. Barry MJ, Edgman-Levitan S. Shared decision making–pinnacle of patient-centered care. *N Engl J Med.* 2012; 366(9):780–781

63. Bennett AC, Rankin KM, Rosenberg D. Does a medical home mediate racial disparities in unmet healthcare needs among children with special healthcare needs? *Matern Child Health J.* 2012; 16(suppl 2):330–338

64. Okumura MJ, Van Cleave J, Gnanasekaran S, Houtrow A. Understanding factors associated with work loss for families caring for CSHCN. *Pediatrics.* 2009;124(suppl 4): S392–S398

65. Hsieh E, Ju H, Kong H. Dimensions of trust: the tensions and challenges in provider–interpreter trust. *Qual Health Res.* 2010;20(2):170–181

66. Hsieh E, Kramer EM. Medical interpreters as tools: dangers and challenges in the utilitarian approach to interpreters' roles and functions. *Patient Educ Couns.* 2012;89(1):158–162

67. Raphael JL, Guadagnolo BA, Beal AC, Giardino AP. Racial and ethnic disparities in indicators of a primary care medical home for children. *Acad Pediatr.* 2009;9(4):221–227

68. Kan K, Choi H, Davis M. Immigrant families, children with special health care needs, and the medical home. *Pediatrics.* 2016;137(1):e20153221

69. Mendoza FS. Health disparities and children in immigrant families: a research agenda. *Pediatrics.* 2009; 124(suppl 3):S187–S195

70. Yu SM, Huang ZJ, Kogan MD. State-level health care access and use among children in US immigrant families. *Am J Public Health.* 2008;98(11):1996–2003

71. Javier JR, Wise PH, Mendoza FS. The relationship of immigrant status with access, utilization, and health status for children with asthma. *Ambul Pediatr.* 2007;7(6):421–430

72. Health Resources and Services Administration Maternal and Child Health. Children with special health

care needs. Available at: https://mchb.hrsa.gov/maternal-child-health-topics/children-and-youth-special-health-needs. Accessed January 9, 2018

73. Centers for Disease Control and Prevention. Domestic examination for newly arrived refugees: guidelines and discussion of the history and physical examination. Available at: https://www.cdc.gov/immigrantrefugeehealth/guidelines/domestic/guidelines-history-physical.html. Accessed August 14, 2018

74. Betancourt JR. Cultural competence and medical education: many names, many perspectives, one goal. *Acad Med.* 2006;81(6):499–501

75. Epner DE, Baile WF. Patient-centered care: the key to cultural competence. *Ann Oncol.* 2012;23(suppl 3):33–42

76. Carrillo JE, Green AR, Betancourt JR. Cross-cultural primary care: a patient-based approach. *Ann Intern Med.* 1999;130(10):829–834

77. Kleinman A, Eisenberg L, Good B. Culture, illness, and care: clinical lessons from anthropologic and cross-cultural research. *Ann Intern Med.* 1978;88(2):251–258

78. Roldán-Chicano MT, Fernández-Rufete J, Hueso-Montoro C, García-López MDM, Rodríguez-Tello J, Flores-Bienert MD. Culture-bound syndromes in migratory contexts: the case of Bolivian immigrants. *Rev Lat Am Enfermagem.* 2017;25:e2915

79. Berlin EA, Fowkes WC Jr. A teaching framework for cross-cultural health care. Application in family practice. *West J Med.* 1983;139(6):934–938

80. Centers for Disease Control and Prevention. Refugee health profiles. Available at: https://www.cdc.gov/immigrantrefugeehealth/profiles/index.html. Accessed August 14, 2018

81. Cultural Orientation Resource Center. Refugee backgrounders. Available at: www.culturalorientation.net/learning/backgrounders. Accessed August 14, 2018

82. EthnoMed. Clinical topics. Available at: https://ethnomed.org/clinical. Accessed August 14, 2018

83. Centers for Disease Control and Prevention. Immigrant and refugee health. Available at: https://www.cdc.gov/immigrantrefugeehealth/index.html. Accessed August 14, 2018

84. Centers for Disease Control and Prevention. Catch-up immunization schedule for persons aged 4 months-18 years who start late or who are more than 1 month behind—United States. 2019. Available at: https://www.cdc.gov/vaccines/schedules/hcp/imz/catchup.html. Accessed July 26, 2019

85. World Health Organization. WHO Vaccine-preventable diseases monitoring system. 2019 Global Summary. Available at: https://apps.who.int/immunization_monitoring/globalsummary. Accessed July 29, 2019

86. Centers for Disease Control and Prevention. Travelers' health. Available at: https://wwwnc.cdc.gov/travel/destinations/list/. Accessed August 24, 2018

87. Centers for Disease Control and Prevention. Refugee health guidelines: guidelines for pre-departure and post-arrival medical screening and treatment of U.S.-bound refugees. Available at: https://www.cdc.gov/immigrantrefugeehealth/guidelines/refugee-guidelines.html. Accessed July 26, 2019

88. Centers for Disease Control and Prevention. Guidelines for overseas presumptive treatment of strongyloidiasis, schistosomiasis, and soil-transmitted helminth infections. 2018. Available at: https://www.cdc.gov/immigrantrefugeehealth/guidelines/overseas/intestinal-parasites-overseas.html. Accessed August 14, 2018

89. Seery T, Boswell H, Lara A. Caring for refugee children. *Pediatr Rev.* 2015;36(8):323–338

90. Haber BA, Block JM, Jonas MM, et al; Hepatitis B Foundation. Recommendations for screening, monitoring, and referral of pediatric chronic hepatitis B. *Pediatrics.* 2009;124(5). Available at: www.pediatrics.org/cgi/content/full/124/5/e1007

91. Ciaccia KA, John RM. Unaccompanied immigrant minors: where to begin. *J Pediatr Health Care.* 2016;30(3):231–240

92. Muennig P, Pallin D, Sell RL, Chan MS. The cost effectiveness of strategies for the treatment of intestinal parasites in immigrants. *N Engl J Med.* 1999;340(10):773–779

93. Centers for Disease Control and Prevention. Domestic intestinal parasite guidelines. Available at: https://www.cdc.gov/immigrantrefugeehealth/guidelines/domestic/intestinal-parasites-domestic.html. Accessed July 17, 2017

94. Jones VF, Schulte EE; Council on Foster Care, Adoption, and Kinship Care. Comprehensive health evaluation of the newly adopted child. *Pediatrics.* 2019;143(5):e20190657

95. Petersen PE, Bourgeois D, Ogawa H, Estupinan-Day S, Ndiaye C. The global burden of oral diseases and risks to oral health. *Bull World Health Organ.* 2005;83(9):661–669

96. Cote S, Geltman P, Nunn M, Lituri K, Henshaw M, Garcia RI. Dental caries of refugee children compared with US children. *Pediatrics.* 2004;114(6). Available at: www.pediatrics.org/cgi/content/full/114/6/e733

97. Shah AY, Suchdev PS, Mitchell T, et al. Nutritional status of refugee children entering DeKalb County, Georgia. *J Immigr Minor Health.* 2014;16(5):959–967

98. Finnegan DA, Rainchuso L, Jenkins S, Kierce E, Rothman A. Immigrant caregivers of young children: oral health beliefs, attitudes, and early childhood caries knowledge. *J Community Health.* 2016;41(2):250–257

99. Davidson N, Skull S, Calache H, Murray SS, Chalmers J. Holes a plenty: oral health status a major issue for newly arrived refugees in Australia. *Aust Dent J.* 2006;51(4):306–311

100. Butani Y, Weintraub JA, Barker JC. Oral health-related cultural beliefs for four racial/ethnic groups: assessment of the literature. *BMC Oral Health.* 2008;8:26

101. Riggs E, Gibbs L, Kilpatrick N, et al. Breaking down the barriers: a qualitative study to understand child oral health in refugee and migrant communities in Australia. *Ethn Health.* 2015;20(3):241–257

102. Nicol P, Al-Hanbali A, King N, Slack-Smith L, Cherian S. Informing a culturally appropriate approach to oral health and dental care for pre-school refugee

children: a community participatory study. *BMC Oral Health.* 2014;14:69

103. Beaglehole R, Horton R. Chronic diseases: global action must match global evidence. *Lancet.* 2010;376(9753): 1619–1621

104. United Nations General Assembly. Political declaration of the high-level meeting of the General Assembly on the prevention and control of non-communicable diseases. Available at: www.who.int/nmh/events/un_ncd_summit2011/political_declaration_en.pdf. Accessed August 14, 2018

105. World Health Organization. Noncommunicable diseases and mental health. Global status report on noncommunicable diseases 2014. 2014. Available at: www.who.int/nmh/publications/ncd-status-report-2014/en/. Accessed August 14, 2018

106. Pondé MP, Rousseau C. Immigrant children with autism spectrum disorder: the relationship between the perspective of the professionals and the parents' point of view. *J Can Acad Child Adolesc Psychiatry.* 2013;22(2): 131–138

107. Lin SC, Yu SM, Harwood RL. Autism spectrum disorders and developmental disabilities in children from immigrant families in the United States. *Pediatrics.* 2012;130(suppl 2):S191–S197

108. Becerra TA, von Ehrenstein OS, Heck JE, et al. Autism spectrum disorders and race, ethnicity, and nativity: a population-based study. *Pediatrics.* 2014;134(1). Available at: www.pediatrics.org/cgi/content/full/134/1/e63

109. Croen LA, Grether JK, Selvin S. Descriptive epidemiology of autism in a California population: who is at risk? *J Autism Dev Disord.* 2002;32(3): 217–224

110. Schieve LA, Boulet SL, Blumberg SJ, et al. Association between parental nativity and autism spectrum disorder among US-born non-Hispanic white and Hispanic children, 2007 National Survey of Children's Health. *Disabil Health J.* 2012;5(1):18–25

111. Akbulut-Yuksel M, Kugler AD. Intergenerational persistence of health: do immigrants get healthier as they remain in the U.S. for more generations? *Econ Hum Biol.* 2016;23: 136–148

112. Bischoff A, Schneider M, Denhaerynck K, Battegay E. Health and ill health of asylum seekers in Switzerland: an epidemiological study. *Eur J Public Health.* 2009;19(1):59–64

113. Perreira KM, Ornelas IJ. The physical and psychological well-being of immigrant children. *Future Child.* 2011; 21(1):195–218

114. Centers for Disease Control and Prevention. Non-communicable diseases (NCDs). Central American refugee health profile. Available at: https://www.cdc.gov/immigrantrefugeehealth/profiles/central-american/health-information/chronic-disease/index.html. Accessed August 14, 2018

115. Hamdoun E, Karachunski P, Nathan B, et al. Case report: the specter of untreated congenital hypothyroidism in immigrant families. *Pediatrics.* 2016; 137(5):e20153418

116. Minnesota Department of Health. Lead poisoning prevention programs biennial report to the Minnesota legislature 2019. Available at: https://www.health.state.mn.us/communities/environment/lead/docs/reports/bienniallegrept.pdf. Accessed July 29, 2019

117. Centers for Disease Control and Prevention. Managing elevated blood lead levels among children: recommendations from the Advisory Committee on Childhood Lead Poisoning Prevention. Available at: https://www.cdc.gov/nceh/lead/casemanagement/casemanage_main.htm. Accessed August 30, 2018

118. Centers for Disease Control and Prevention (CDC). Elevated blood lead levels in refugee children—New Hampshire, 2003-2004 [published correction appears in *MMWR Morb Mortal Wkly Rep.* 2005;54(3):76]. *MMWR Morb Mortal Wkly Rep.* 2005;54(2): 42–46

119. Geltman PL, Brown MJ, Cochran J. Lead poisoning among refugee children resettled in Massachusetts, 1995 to 1999. *Pediatrics.* 2001;108(1):158–162

120. Centers for Disease Control and Prevention. Screening for lead during the domestic medical examination for newly arrived refugees. 2013. Available at: www.cdc.gov/immigrantrefugeehealth/guidelines/lead-guidelines.html. Accessed July 16, 2017

121. Yun K, Matheson J, Payton C, et al. Health profiles of newly arrived refugee children in the United States, 2006-2012. *Am J Public Health.* 2016;106(1):128–135

122. Dawson-Hahn EE, Pak-Gorstein S, Hoopes AJ, Matheson J. Comparison of the nutritional status of overseas refugee children with low income children in Washington state. *PLoS One.* 2016;11(1):e0147854

123. Dawson-Hahn E, Pak-Gorstein S, Matheson J, et al. Growth trajectories of refugee and nonrefugee children in the United States. *Pediatrics.* 2016; 138(6):e20160953

124. Centers for Disease Control and Prevention. Guidelines for evaluation of the nutritional status and growth in refugee children during the domestic medical screening examination. 2012. Available at: https://www.cdc.gov/immigrantrefugeehealth/pdf/nutrition-growth.pdf. Accessed August 14, 2018

125. Oldways. Inspiring good health through cultural food traditions. Available at: https://oldwayspt.org. Accessed July 6, 2017

126. Centers for Disease Control and Prevention. Guidelines for evaluation of the nutritional status and growth in refugee children during the domestic medical screening examination. 2013. Available at: www.cdc.gov/immigrantrefugeehealth/guidelines/domestic/nutrition-growth.html. Accessed July 6, 2017

127. Centers for Disease Control and Prevention (CDC). Vitamin B12 deficiency in resettled Bhutanese refugees—United States, 2008-2011. *MMWR Morb Mortal Wkly Rep.* 2011; 60(11):343–346

128. Hintzpeter B, Scheidt-Nave C, Müller MJ, Schenk L, Mensink GB. Higher prevalence of vitamin D deficiency is associated with immigrant background among children and adolescents in Germany. *J Nutr.* 2008;138(8):1482–1490

129. Penrose K, Hunter Adams J, Nguyen T, Cochran J, Geltman PL. Vitamin D

deficiency among newly resettled refugees in Massachusetts. *J Immigr Minor Health*. 2012;14(6):941–948

130. Council on Community Pediatrics; Committee on Nutrition. Promoting food security for all children. *Pediatrics*. 2015;136(5). Available at: www. pediatrics.org/cgi/content/full/136/5/ e1431

131. Food Research and Action Center. Addressing food insecurity: a toolkit for pediatricians. Available at: http://frac. org/aaptoolkit. Accessed August 14, 2018

132. Ages and Stages Questionnaires. Social-emotional health: look to ASQ:SE-2 for truly accurate screening. 2018. Available at: http://agesandstages.com/ products-services/asqse-2/. Accessed August 14, 2018

133. Floating Hospital for Children at Tufts Medical Center. The survey of well-being of young children. Available at: https:// www.floatinghospital.org/The-Survey-of-Wellbeing-of-Young-Children/Overview. aspx. Accessed August 14, 2018

134. Kroening AL, Moore JA, Welch TR, Halterman JS, Hyman SL. Developmental screening of refugees: a qualitative study. *Pediatrics*. 2016; 138(3):e20160234

135. Martin-Herz SP, Kemper T, Brownstein M, McLaughlin JF. Developmental screening with recent immigrant and refugee children: a preliminary report. 2012. Available at: http://ethnomed.org/ clinical/pediatrics/developmental-screening-with-recent-immigrant-and-refugee-children. Accessed August 14, 2018

136. Rogoff B. *The Cultural Nature of Human Development*. New York, NY: Oxford University Press; 2003

137. Cowden JD, Kreisler K. Development in children of immigrant families. *Pediatr Clin North Am*. 2016;63(5):775–793

138. Pachter LM, Dworkin PH. Maternal expectations about normal child development in 4 cultural groups. *Arch Pediatr Adolesc Med*. 1997;151(11): 1144–1150

139. Stein MT, Flores G, Graham EA, Magana L, Willies-Jacobo L, Gulbronson M. Cultural and linguistic determinants in the diagnosis and management of

developmental delay in a 4-year-old. *Pediatrics*. 2004;114(suppl 6):1442–1447

140. Johnson L, Radesky J, Zuckerman B. Cross-cultural parenting: reflections on autonomy and interdependence. *Pediatrics*. 2013;131(4):631–633

141. deVries MW, deVries MR. Cultural relativity of toilet training readiness: a perspective from East Africa. *Pediatrics*. 1977;60(2):170–177

142. Festa N, Loftus PD, Cullen MR, Mendoza FS. Disparities in early exposure to book sharing within immigrant families. *Pediatrics*. 2014;134(1). Available at: www.pediatrics.org/cgi/ content/full/134/1/e162

143. Toppelberg CO, Collins BA. Language, culture, and adaptation in immigrant children. *Child Adolesc Psychiatr Clin N Am*. 2010;19(4):697–717

144. Hagan JF Jr, Shaw JS, Duncan PM, eds. *Bright Futures: Guidelines for Health Supervision of Infants, Children, and Adolescents*. 4th ed. Elk Grove Village, IL: American Academy of Pediatrics; 2017

145. Adesope OO, Lavin T, Thompson T, Ungerleider C. A systematic review and meta-analysis on the cognitive correlates of bilingualism. *Rev Educ Res*. 2010;80(2):207–245

146. Feliciano C. The benefits of biculturalism: exposure to immigrant culture and dropping out of school among Asian and Latino youths. *Soc Sci Q*. 2001;82(4):865–879

147. Zhou M. Growing up American: the challenge confronting immigrant children and children of immigrants. *Annu Rev Sociol*. 1997;23(1):63–95

148. Engel de Abreu PM, Cruz-Santos A, Tourinho CJ, Martin R, Bialystok E. Bilingualism enriches the poor: enhanced cognitive control in low-income minority children. *Psychol Sci*. 2012;23(11):1364–1371

149. Bialystok E. Reshaping the mind: the benefits of bilingualism. *Can J Exp Psychol*. 2011;65(4):229–235

150. High PC, Klass P; Council on Early Childhood. Literacy promotion: an essential component of primary care pediatric practice. *Pediatrics*. 2014; 134(2):404–409

151. Education Commission of the States. English language learners. The

progress of education reform. 2013. Available at: https://www.rwjf.org/en/ library/research/2011/11/caring-across-communities–.html. Accessed July 26, 2019

152. Park M, O'Toole A, Katsiaficas C. *Dual Language Learners: A National Demographic and Policy Profile*. Washington, DC: Migration Policy Institute; 2017

153. Morland L, Ives N, McNeely C, Allen C. Providing a head start: improving access to early childhood education for refugees. Migration Policy Institute. 2016. Available at: https://www. migrationpolicy.org/research/ providing-head-start-improving-access-early-childhood-education-refugees. Accessed August 30, 2018

154. Plyler v Doe, 457 US 202 (1982)

155. Graham HR, Minhas RS, Paxton G. Learning problems in children of refugee background: a systematic review. *Pediatrics*. 2016;137(6): e20153994

156. Walker SP, Wachs TD, Gardner JM, et al; International Child Development Steering Group. Child development: risk factors for adverse outcomes in developing countries. *Lancet*. 2007; 369(9556):145–157

157. DeCapua A. Reaching students with limited or interrupted formal education through culturally responsive teaching. *Lang Linguist Compass*. 2016;10(5): 225–237

158. Macswan J, Rolstad K. How language proficiency tests mislead us about ability: implications for English language learner placement in special education. *Teach Coll Rec (1970)*. 2006; 108(11):2304–2328

159. Wagner RK, Francis DJ, Morris RD. Identifying English language learners with learning disabilities: key challenges and possible approaches. *Learn Disabil Res Pract*. 2005;20(1): 6–15

160. McCardle P, Mele-McCarthy J, Cutting L, Leos K, D'Emilio T. Learning disabilities in English language learners: identifying the issues. *Learn Disabil Res Pract*. 2005;20(1):1–5

161. Figueroa RA, Newsome P. The diagnosis of LD in English learners: is it

nondiscriminatory? *J Learn Disabil.* 2006;39(3):206–214

162. Lara M, Gamboa C, Kahramanian MI, Morales LS, Bautista DE. Acculturation and Latino health in the United States: a review of the literature and its sociopolitical context. *Annu Rev Public Health.* 2005;26:367–397

163. Bornstein MH, Cote LR, eds. *Acculturation and Parent–Child Relationships: Measurement and Development.* Mahwah, NJ: Lawrence Erlbaum Associates, Inc; 2006

164. Antecol H, Bedard K. Unhealthy assimilation: why do immigrants converge to American health status levels? *Demography.* 2006;43(2): 337–360

165. Zamboanga BL, Schwartz SJ, Jarvis LH, Van Tyne K. Acculturation and substance use among Hispanic early adolescents: investigating the mediating roles of acculturative stress and self-esteem. *J Prim Prev.* 2009; 30(3–4):315–333

166. Myers R, Chou CP, Sussman S, Baezconde-Garbanati L, Pachon H, Valente TW. Acculturation and substance use: social influence as a mediator among Hispanic alternative high school youth. *J Health Soc Behav.* 2009;50(2):164–179

167. Ho J, Birman D. Acculturation gaps in Vietnamese immigrant families: impact on family relationships. *Int J Intercult Relat.* 2010;34(1):22–23

168. Birman D, Taylor-Ritzler T. Acculturation and psychological distress among adolescent immigrants from the former Soviet Union: exploring the mediating effect of family relationships. *Cultur Divers Ethnic Minor Psychol.* 2007;13(4): 337–346

169. Refugee Health Technical Assistance Center. Youth and mental health. Available at: http://refugeehealthta.org/physical-mental-health/mental-health/youth-and-mental-health/. Accessed August 30, 2018

170. The National Child Traumatic Stress Network. Learning center for child and adolescent trauma. Refugee Services Toolkit (RST). 2012. Available at: https://www.nctsn.org/resources/refugee-services-core-stressor-assessment-tool. Accessed July 26, 2019

171. Sawyer CB, Márquez J. Senseless violence against Central American unaccompanied minors: historical background and call for help. *J Psychol.* 2017;151(1):69–75

172. The National Child Traumatic Stress Network. Refugee trauma. 2017. Available at: http://nctsn.org/trauma-types/refugee-trauma/learn-about-refugee-core-stressors. Accessed August 14, 2017

173. United Nations Office of the High Commissioner for Refugees. Children on the run. Available at: www.unhcr.org/en-us/about-us/background/56fc266f4/children-on-the-run-full-report.html. Accessed August 30, 2018

174. Cleary SD, Snead R, Dietz-Chavez D, Rivera I, Edberg MC. Immigrant trauma and mental health outcomes among Latino youth. *J Immigr Minor Health.* 2018;20(5):1053–1059

175. Isakson BL, Legerski JP, Layne CM. Adapting and implementing evidence-based interventions for trauma-exposed refugee youth and families. *J Contemp Psychother.* 2015;45(4): 245–253

176. Greenbaum J, Bodrick N; Committee on Child Abuse and Neglect; Section on International Child Health. Global human trafficking and child victimization. *Pediatrics.* 2017;140(6): e20173138

177. McPherson M, Arango P, Fox H, et al. A new definition of children with special health care needs. *Pediatrics.* 1998; 102(1, pt 1):137–140

178. Dreby J. U.S. immigration policy and family separation: the consequences for children's well-being. *Soc Sci Med.* 2015;132:245–251

179. Garner AS, Shonkoff JP; Committee on Psychosocial Aspects of Child and Family Health; Committee on Early Childhood, Adoption, and Dependent Care; Section on Developmental and Behavioral Pediatrics. Early childhood adversity, toxic stress, and the role of the pediatrician: translating developmental science into lifelong health. *Pediatrics.* 2012;129(1). Available at: www.pediatrics.org/cgi/content/full/129/1/e224

180. Lustig SL, Kia-Keating M, Knight WG, et al. Review of child and adolescent

refugee mental health. *J Am Acad Child Adolesc Psychiatry.* 2004;43(1):24–36

181. Savin D, Seymour DJ, Littleford LN, Bettridge J, Giese A. Findings from mental health screening of newly arrived refugees in Colorado. *Public Health Rep.* 2005;120(3):224–229

182. Allwood MA, Bell-Dolan D, Husain SA. Children's trauma and adjustment reactions to violent and nonviolent war experiences. *J Am Acad Child Adolesc Psychiatry.* 2002;41(4):450–457

183. Jaycox LH, Stein BD, Kataoka SH, et al. Violence exposure, posttraumatic stress disorder, and depressive symptoms among recent immigrant schoolchildren. *J Am Acad Child Adolesc Psychiatry.* 2002;41(9): 1104–1110

184. Fazel M, Wheeler J, Danesh J. Prevalence of serious mental disorder in 7000 refugees resettled in western countries: a systematic review. *Lancet.* 2005;365(9467):1309–1314

185. Weine SM, Vojvoda D, Becker DF, et al. PTSD symptoms in Bosnian refugees 1 year after resettlement in the United States. *Am J Psychiatry.* 1998;155(4): 562–564

186. Sack WH, Clarke GN, Seeley J. Multiple forms of stress in Cambodian adolescent refugees. *Child Dev.* 1996; 67(1):107–116

187. Betancourt TS, Newnham EA, Birman D, Lee R, Ellis BH, Layne CM. Comparing trauma exposure, mental health needs, and service utilization across clinical samples of refugee, immigrant, and U.S.-origin children. *J Trauma Stress.* 2017;30(3):209–218

188. Hodes M, Jagdev D, Chandra N, Cunniff A. Risk and resilience for psychological distress amongst unaccompanied asylum seeking adolescents. *J Child Psychol Psychiatry.* 2008;49(7):723–732

189. Jakobsen M, Meyer DeMott MA, Wentzel-Larsen T, Heir T. The impact of the asylum process on mental health: a longitudinal study of unaccompanied refugee minors in Norway. *BMJ Open.* 2017;7(6):e015157

190. Majumder P, O'Reilly M, Karim K, Vostanis P. 'This doctor, I not trust him, I'm not safe': the perceptions of mental health and services by unaccompanied

refugee adolescents. *Int J Soc Psychiatry*. 2015;61(2):129–136

191. Belhadj Kouider E, Koglin U, Petermann F. Emotional and behavioral problems in migrant children and adolescents in American countries: a systematic review. *J Immigr Minor Health*. 2015; 17(4):1240–1258

192. Youthinmind. SDQ: Information for researchers and professionals about the Strengths & Difficulties Questionnaires. Available at: www. sdqinfo.com. Accessed September 17, 2018

193. Refugee Health Technical Assistance Center. Refugee Health Screener-15 (RHS-15) packet. Available at: http:// refugeehealthta.org/2012/07/31/ refugee-health-screener-15-rhs-15- packet/. Accessed August 30, 2018

194. Achenbach System of Empirically Based Assessment. Multicultural applications. Available at: https://aseba.org/ multicultural-applications/. Accessed July 29, 2019

195. Fazel M, Betancourt TS. Preventive mental health interventions for refugee children and adolescents in high- income settings. *Lancet Child Adolesc Health*. 2018;2(2):121–132

196. Institute of Medicine. *Preventing Mental, Emotional, and Behavioral Disorders Among Young People: Progress and Possibilities*. Washington, DC: The National Academies Press; 2009

197. Carlson BE, Cacciatore J, Klimek B. A risk and resilience perspective on unaccompanied refugee minors. *Soc Work*. 2012;57(3):259–269

198. Eide K, Hjern A. Unaccompanied refugee children–vulnerability and agency. *Acta Paediatr*. 2013;102(7):666–668

199. Timshel I, Montgomery E, Dalgaard NT. A systematic review of risk and protective factors associated with family related violence in refugee families. *Child Abuse Negl*. 2017;70:315–330

200. Anderson AT, Jackson A, Jones L, Kennedy DP, Wells K, Chung PJ. Minority parents' perspectives on racial socialization and school readiness in the early childhood period. *Acad Pediatr*. 2015;15(4):405–411

201. Ellis BH, Hulland EN, Miller AB, Bixby CB, Cardozo BL, Betancourt TS. Mental

health risks and resilience among Somali and Bhutanese refugee parents. 2016. Available at: https://www. migrationpolicy.org/research/mental- health-risks-and-resilience-among- somali-and-bhutanese-refugee-parents. Accessed August 30, 2018

202. Rothe EM, Tzuang D, Pumariega AJ. Acculturation, development, and adaptation. *Child Adolesc Psychiatr Clin N Am*. 2010;19(4):681–696

203. Geltman PL, Augustyn M, Barnett ED, Klass PE, Groves BM. War trauma experience and behavioral screening of Bosnian refugee children resettled in Massachusetts. *J Dev Behav Pediatr*. 2000;21(4):255–261

204. Caballero TM, DeCamp LR, Platt RE, et al. Addressing the mental health needs of Latino children in immigrant families. *Clin Pediatr (Phila)*. 2017;56(7): 648–658

205. De Milto L. National program executive summary report—caring across communities: addressing mental health needs of diverse children and youth. Available at: https://www.rwjf.org/en/ library/research/2011/11/caring- across-communities–.html. Accessed July 26, 2019

206. Al-Rawi SN, Fetters MD. Traditional Arabic & Islamic medicine: a conceptual model for clinicians and researchers. *Glob J Health Sci*. 2012; 4(3):164–169

207. Pachter LM. Culture and clinical care. Folk illness beliefs and behaviors and their implications for health care delivery. *JAMA*. 1994;271(9):690–694

208. Risser AL, Mazur LJ. Use of folk remedies in a Hispanic population. *Arch Pediatr Adolesc Med*. 1995;149(9): 978–981

209. EthnoMed. Ethnic medicine information from Harborview Medical Center. Available at: https://depts.washington. edu/ethnomed/HMCproject/ hmcproject_talk_0302/F_EthnoMed% 20Home%20Page.htm. Accessed August 30, 2018

210. World Health Organization. *Eliminating Female Genital Mutilation. An Interagency Statement*. Geneva, Switzerland: World Health Organization; 2008. Available at: www.un.org/ womenwatch/daw/csw/csw52/

statements_missions/Interagency_ Statement_on_Eliminating_FGM.pdf. Accessed August 30, 2018

211. United Nations Children's Fund. Female genital mutilation/cutting: a statistical overview and exploration of the dynamics of change. 2013. Available at: https://www.unicef.org/publications/ index_69875.html. Accessed August 30, 2018

212. Refugee Legal Aid Information for Lawyers Representing Refugees Globally Rights in Exile Programme. United States. Available at: www. refugeelegalaidinformation.org/united- states-america-fgm. Accessed August 30, 2018

213. Hearst AA, Molnar AM. Female genital cutting: an evidence-based approach to clinical management for the primary care physician. *Mayo Clin Proc*. 2013; 88(6):618–629

214. Vissandjée B, Denetto S, Migliardi P, Proctor J. Female genital cutting (FGC) and the ethics of care: community engagement and cultural sensitivity at the interface of migration experiences. *BMC Int Health Hum Rights*. 2014;14:13

215. National Defense Authorization Act for Fiscal Year 2013, HR 4310, 112th Cong, 2nd Sess (2012). Available at: https:// www.gpo.gov/fdsys/pkg/BILLS-112hr431 0enr/pdf/BILLS-112hr4310enr.pdf. Accessed August 30, 2018

216. Eneriz-Wiemer M, Sanders LM, Barr DA, Mendoza FS. Parental limited English proficiency and health outcomes for children with special health care needs: a systematic review. *Acad Pediatr*. 2014; 14(2):128–136

217. Arthur KC, Mangione-Smith R, Meischke H, et al. Impact of English proficiency on care experiences in a pediatric emergency department. *Acad Pediatr*. 2015;15(2):218–224

218. Jimenez N, Jackson DL, Zhou C, Ayala NC, Ebel BE. Postoperative pain management in children, parental English proficiency, and access to interpretation. *Hosp Pediatr*. 2014;4(1): 23–30

219. Levas MN, Cowden JD, Dowd MD. Effects of the limited English proficiency of parents on hospital length of stay and home health care referral for their home health care-eligible children with

infections. *Arch Pediatr Adolesc Med.* 2011;165(9):831–836

220. Gallagher RA, Porter S, Monuteaux MC, Stack AM. Unscheduled return visits to the emergency department: the impact of language. *Pediatr Emerg Care.* 2013; 29(5):579–583

221. Title VI of the Civil Rights Act of 1964, 42 USC §2000d-1–2000d-7 (2009). Available at: http://uscode.house.gov/view.xhtml? path=%2Fprelim%40title42% 2Fchapter21&req=granuleid%3AUSC-prelim-title42-chapter21&f=&fq= &num=0&hl=false&edition=prelim. Accessed November 15, 2018

222. Office of the Surgeon General; Center for Mental Health Services; National Institute of Mental Health. *Mental Health: Culture, Race, and Ethnicity: A Supplement to Mental Health: A Report of the Surgeon General.* Rockville, MD: Substance Abuse and Mental Health Services Administration; 2001. Available at: https://www.ncbi. nlm.nih.gov/books/NBK44243/. Accessed August 30, 2018

223. Flores G, Torres S, Holmes LJ, Salas-Lopez D, Youdelman MK, Tomany-Korman SC. Access to hospital interpreter services for limited English proficient patients in New Jersey: a statewide evaluation. *J Health Care Poor Underserved.* 2008;19(2):391–415

224. Jacobs EA, Diamond LC, Stevak L. The importance of teaching clinicians when and how to work with interpreters. *Patient Educ Couns.* 2010; 78(2):149–153

225. DeCamp LR, Kuo DZ, Flores G, O'Connor K, Minkovitz CS. Changes in language services use by US pediatricians. *Pediatrics.* 2013;132(2). Available at: www.pediatrics.org/cgi/content/ full/132/2/e396

226. Flores G, Laws MB, Mayo SJ, et al. Errors in medical interpretation and their potential clinical consequences in pediatric encounters. *Pediatrics.* 2003; 111(1):6–14

227. Flores G, Abreu M, Barone CP, Bachur R, Lin H. Errors of medical interpretation and their potential clinical consequences: a comparison of professional versus ad hoc versus no interpreters. *Ann Emerg Med.* 2012; 60(5):545–553

228. Juckett G, Unger K. Appropriate use of medical interpreters. *Am Fam Physician.* 2014;90(7):476–480

229. Hsieh E. Not just "getting by": factors influencing providers' choice of interpreters. *J Gen Intern Med.* 2015; 30(1):75–82

230. Jacobs EA, Shepard DS, Suaya JA, Stone EL. Overcoming language barriers in health care: costs and benefits of interpreter services. *Am J Public Health.* 2004;94(5):866–869

231. Johnstone MJ, Kanitsaki O. Culture, language, and patient safety: making the link. *Int J Qual Health Care.* 2006; 18(5):383–388

232. Flores G. The impact of medical interpreter services on the quality of health care: a systematic review. *Med Care Res Rev.* 2005;62(3):255–299

233. Moreno MR, Otero-Sabogal R, Newman J. Assessing dual-role staff-interpreter linguistic competency in an integrated healthcare system. *J Gen Intern Med.* 2007;22(suppl 2):331–335

234. Tang G, Lanza O, Rodriguez FM, Chang A. The Kaiser Permanente Clinician Cultural and Linguistic Assessment Initiative: research and development in patient-provider language concordance. *Am J Public Health.* 2011;101(2):205–208

235. Lion KC, Thompson DA, Cowden JD, et al. Impact of language proficiency testing on provider use of Spanish for clinical care. *Pediatrics.* 2012;130(1). Available at: www.pediatrics.org/cgi/content/ full/130/1/e80

236. Dreby J. The burden of deportation on children in Mexican immigrant families. *J Marriage Fam.* 2012;74(4):829–845

237. Rhodes SD, Mann L, Simán FM, et al. The impact of local immigration enforcement policies on the health of immigrant Hispanics/Latinos in the United States. *Am J Public Health.* 2015; 105(2):329–337

238. Suárez-Orozco C, Todorova IL, Louie J. Making up for lost time: the experience of separation and reunification among immigrant families. *Fam Process.* 2002; 41(4):625–643

239. Crosnoe R, Leventhal T, Wirth RJ, Pierce KM, Pianta RC; NICHD Early Child Care Research Network. Family socioeconomic status and consistent

environmental stimulation in early childhood. *Child Dev.* 2010;81(3): 972–987

240. Council on Community Pediatrics. Poverty and child health in the United States. *Pediatrics.* 2016;137(4): e20160339

241. Singh P, Chokshi DA. Community health workers—a local solution to a global problem. *N Engl J Med.* 2013;369(10): 894–896

242. Postma J, Karr C, Kieckhefer G. Community health workers and environmental interventions for children with asthma: a systematic review. *J Asthma.* 2009;46(6):564–576

243. Coker TR, Chacon S, Elliott MN, et al. A parent coach model for well-child care among low-income children: a randomized controlled trial. *Pediatrics.* 2016;137(3):e20153013

244. Enard KR, Ganelin DM. Reducing preventable emergency department utilization and costs by using community health workers as patient navigators. *J Healthc Manag.* 2013; 58(6):412–427; discussion 428

245. Pati S, Ladowski KL, Wong AT, Huang J, Yang J. An enriched medical home intervention using community health workers improves adherence to immunization schedules. *Vaccine.* 2015; 33(46):6257–6263

246. Anugu M, Braksmajer A, Huang J, Yang J, Ladowski KL, Pati S. Enriched medical home intervention using community health worker home visitation and ED use. *Pediatrics.* 2017;139(5):e20161849

247. Agency for Healthcare Research and Quality. Design guide for implementing warm handoffs. 2017. Available at: https://www.ahrq.gov/sites/default/ files/wysiwyg/professionals/quality-patient-safety/patient-family-engagement/pfeprimarycare/ warmhandoff-designguide.pdf. Accessed August 30, 2018

248. Blewett LA, Johnson PJ, Mach AL. Immigrant children's access to health care: differences by global region of birth. *J Health Care Poor Underserved.* 2010;21(suppl 2):13–31

249. National Immigration Law Center. Overview of immigrant eligibility for federal programs. 2015. Available at: https://www.nilc.org/issues/economic-

support/overview-immeligfedprograms/. Accessed August 30, 2018

250. National Immigration Law Center. Table: medical assistance programs for immigrants in various states. 2018. Available at: https://www.nilc.org/wp-content/uploads/2015/11/med-services-for-imms-in-states.pdf. Accessed November 14, 2018

251. Georgetown University Health Policy Institute Center for Children and Families. Health coverage for lawfully residing children. 2018. Available at: https://ccf.georgetown.edu/wp-content/uploads/2018/05/ichia_fact_sheet.pdf. Accessed August 30, 2018

252. Brooks T, Wagnerman K, Artiga S, Cornachione E, Ubri P. Medicaid and CHIP eligibility, enrollment, renewal, and cost sharing policies as of January 2017: findings from a 50-state survey. 2017. Available at: https://www.kff.org/medicaid/report/medicaid-and-chip-eligibility-enrollment-renewal-and-cost-sharing-policies-as-of-january-2017-findings-from-a-50-state-survey/. Accessed August 30, 2018

253. National Immigration Law Center. Health care coverage maps. 2018. Available at: https://www.nilc.org/issues/health-care/healthcoveragemaps/. Accessed July 26, 2019

254. Flores SM. State dream acts: the effect of in-state resident tuition polices and undocumented Latino students. *Rev High Ed.* 2010;33(2):239–283

255. New American Economy. Removing barriers: expanding in-state tuition for Dreamers in South Carolina. 2019. Available at: https://www.newamericaneconomy.org/wp-content/uploads/2019/04/SC_InState_Tuition.pdf. Accessed April 4, 2019

256. Mirza M, Luna R, Mathews B, et al. Barriers to healthcare access among refugees with disabilities and chronic health conditions resettled in the US Midwest. *J Immigr Minor Health.* 2014;16(4):733–742

257. National Immigration Law Center. Know your rights: Is it safe to apply for health insurance or seek health care? Available at: https://www.nilc.org/issues/health-care/health-insurance-and-care-rights/. Accessed July 26, 2019

258. Duffee JH, Mendelsohn AL, Kuo AA, Legano LA, Earls MF; Council on Community Pediatrics; Council on Early Childhood; Committee on Child Abuse and Neglect. Early childhood home visiting. *Pediatrics.* 2017;140(3): e20172150

259. Greenberg JP. Determinants of after-school programming for school-age immigrant children. *Child Sch.* 2013; 35(2):101–111

260. Greenberg JP. Significance of after-school programming for immigrant children during middle childhood: opportunities for school social work. *Soc Work.* 2014;59(3):243–251

261. Jarlenski M, Baller J, Borrero S, Bennett WL. Trends in disparities in low-income children's health insurance coverage and access to care by family immigration status. *Acad Pediatr.* 2016; 16(2):208–215

262. Avila RM, Bramlett MD. Language and immigrant status effects on disparities in Hispanic children's health status and access to health care. *Matern Child Health J.* 2013;17(3):415–423

263. Artiga S. Immigration reform and access to health coverage: key issues to consider. 2013. Available at: https://www.kff.org/uninsured/issue-brief/immigration-reform-and-access-to-health-coverage-key-issues-to-consider/. Accessed July 29, 2019

264. Artiga S, Ubri P. *Living in an immigrant family in America: How fear and toxic stress are affecting daily life, well-being, and health.* 2017. Available at: https://www.kff.org/disparities-policy/issue-brief/living-in-an-immigrant-family-in-america-how-fear-and-toxic-stress-are-affecting-daily-life-well-being-health.* Accessed August 30, 2018

265. Artiga S, Garfield R, Damico A. Estimated impacts of the proposed public charge rule on immigrants and Medicaid. 2018. Available at: https://www.cmhnetwork.org/wp-content/uploads/2018/10/Issue-Brief-Estimated-Impacts-of-the-Proposed-Public-Charge-Rule-on-Immigrants-and-Medicaid.pdf. Accessed July 30, 2019

266. US Immigration and Customs Enforcement. FAQ on sensitive locations and courthouse arrests. 2018. Available at: https://www.ice.gov/ero/enforcement/sensitive-loc. Accessed April 3, 2019

267. National Immigration Law Center. Health care providers and immigration enforcement: know your rights, know your patients' rights. Available at: https://www.nilc.org/issues/immigration-enforcement/healthcare-provider-and-patients-rights-imm-enf/. Accessed April 5, 2019

268. Mann L, Simán FM, Downs M, et al. Reducing the impact of immigration enforcement policies to ensure the health of North Carolinians: statewide community-level recommendations. *N C Med J.* 2016;77(4):240–246

269. Hacker K, Chu J, Leung C, et al. The impact of Immigration and Customs Enforcement on immigrant health: perceptions of immigrants in Everett, Massachusetts, USA. *Soc Sci Med.* 2011; 73(4):586–594

270. Montealegre JR, Selwyn BJ. Healthcare coverage and use among undocumented Central American immigrant women in Houston, Texas. *J Immigr Minor Health.* 2014;16(2): 204–210

271. Raymond-Flesch M, Siemons R, Pourat N, Jacobs K, Brindis CD. "There is no help out there and if there is, it's really hard to find": a qualitative study of the health concerns and health care access of Latino "DREAMers". *J Adolesc Health.* 2014;55(3):323–328

272. Giuliani C, Tagliabue S, Regalia C. Psychological well-being, multiple identities, and discrimination among first and second generation immigrant Muslims. *Eur J Psychol.* 2018;14(1): 66–87

273. Suleman S, Garber J, Rutkow L. Xenophobia as a determinant of health: an integrative review. *J Public Health Policy.* 2018;39(4):407–423

274. Budhwani H, Hearld KR, Chavez-Yenter D. Depression in racial and ethnic minorities: the impact of nativity and discrimination. *J Racial Ethn Health Disparities.* 2015;2(1):34–42

275. Davis AN, Carlo G, Schwartz SJ, et al. The longitudinal associations between discrimination, depressive symptoms, and prosocial behaviors in U.S. Latino/a recent immigrant adolescents. *J Youth Adolesc.* 2016;45(3):457–470

276. Gulbas LE, Zayas LH, Yoon H, Szlyk H, Aguilar-Gaxiola S, Natera G. Deportation experiences and depression among U.S. citizen-children with undocumented Mexican parents. *Child Care Health Dev.* 2016;42(2):220–230

277. Sabo S, Shaw S, Ingram M, et al. Everyday violence, structural racism and mistreatment at the US-Mexico border. *Soc Sci Med.* 2014;109:66–74

278. Venkataramani AS, Shah SJ, O'Brien R, Kawachi I, Tsai AC. Health consequences of the US Deferred Action for Childhood Arrivals (DACA) immigration programme: a quasi-experimental study [published correction appears in *Lancet Public Health.* 2017;2(5):e213]. *Lancet Public Health.* 2017;2(4): e175–e181

279. Hainmueller J, Lawrence D, Martén L, et al. Protecting unauthorized immigrant mothers improves their children's mental health. *Science.* 2017; 357(6355):1041–1044

280. Kids in Need of Defense. *No Child Should Appear in Immigration Court Alone.* Washington, DC: Kids in Need of Defense; 2018. Available at: https:// supportkind.org/wp-content/uploads/2 018/01/General-KIND-Fact-Sheet_ January-2018.pdf. Accessed August 30, 2018

281. Houseman AW. Civil legal aid in the United States: an update for 2013. 2013. www.clasp.org/resources-and-publications/publication-1/CIVIL-LEGAL-AID-IN-THE-UNITED-STATES-3.pdf. Accessed August 30, 2018

282. Kids in Need of Defense. *Improving the Protection and Fair Treatment of Unaccompanied Children.* Washington, DC: Kids in Need of Defense; 2016. Available at: https://supportkind.org/ wp-content/uploads/2016/09/KIND-Protection-and-Fair-Treatment-Report_ September-2016-FINAL.pdf. Accessed August 30, 2018

283. National Immigrant Justice Center. *Justice for Unaccompanied Immigrant Children: An Advocacy Best Practices Manual for Legal Service Providers.* Chicago, IL: National Immigrant Justice Center; 2016. Available at: https://www. americanbar.org/content/dam/aba/ administrative/probono_public_ service/ls_pb_uac_doc_uic_best_ practices_4_27_16.pdf. Accessed August 30, 2018

284. Portes A, Rivas A. The adaptation of migrant children. *Future Child.* 2011; 21(1):219–246

285. Avellar S, Paulsell D, Sama-Miller E, Del Grosso P, Akers L, Kleinman R. *Home Visiting Evidence of Effectiveness Review: Executive Summary.* Washington, DC: Office of Planning, Research, and Evaluation, Administration for Children and Families, US Department of Health and Human Services; 2016, Available at: https://homvee.acf.hhs.gov/HomVEE-Executive-Summary-2016_Compliant. pdf. Accessed August 30, 2018

286. Yogman M, Garner A, Hutchinson J, Hirsh-Pasek K, Golinkoff RM; Committee on Psychosocial Aspects of Child and Family Health; Council on Communications and Media. The power of play: a pediatric role in enhancing development in young children. *Pediatrics.* 2018;142(3):e20182058

287. Weisleder A, Cates CB, Dreyer BP, et al. Promotion of positive parenting and prevention of socioemotional disparities. *Pediatrics.* 2016;137(2): e20153239

288. Katigbak C, Foley M, Robert L, Hutchinson MK. Experiences and lessons learned in using community-based participatory research to recruit Asian American immigrant research participants. *J Nurs Scholarsh.* 2016; 48(2):210–218

289. Huemer J, Karnik NS, Voelkl-Kernstock S, et al. Mental health issues in unaccompanied refugee minors. *Child Adolesc Psychiatry Ment Health.* 2009; 3(1):13

290. Terra Firma. Supporting Resilience for Immigrant Children. Available at: http:// www.terrafirma.nyc. Accessed July 30, 2019

291. Kids in Need of Defense. Legal services. Available at: Available at: https:// supportkind.org/our-work/legal-services-2/. Accessed July 30, 2019

292. Young Center for Immigrant Children's Rights. The Goal. Available at: https:// www.theyoungcenter.org/big-picture. Accessed July 30, 2019

293. RAICES. Services. Available at: https:// www.raicestexas.org/services/. Accessed July 30, 2019

POLICY STATEMENT Organizational Principles to Guide and Define the Child Health Care System and/or Improve the Health of all Children

American Academy of Pediatrics

DEDICATED TO THE HEALTH OF ALL CHILDREN™

This Policy Statement was reaffirmed November 2022.

Detention of Immigrant Children

Julie M. Linton, MD, FAAP,[a] Marsha Griffin, MD, FAAP,[b] Alan J. Shapiro, MD, FAAP,[c] COUNCIL ON COMMUNITY PEDIATRICS

abstract

Immigrant children seeking safe haven in the United States, whether arriving unaccompanied or in family units, face a complicated evaluation and legal process from the point of arrival through permanent resettlement in communities. The conditions in which children are detained and the support services that are available to them are of great concern to pediatricians and other advocates for children. In accordance with internationally accepted rights of the child, immigrant and refugee children should be treated with dignity and respect and should not be exposed to conditions that may harm or traumatize them. The Department of Homeland Security facilities do not meet the basic standards for the care of children in residential settings. The recommendations in this statement call for limited exposure of any child to current Department of Homeland Security facilities (ie, Customs and Border Protection and Immigration and Customs Enforcement facilities) and for longitudinal evaluation of the health consequences of detention of immigrant children in the United States. From the moment children are in the custody of the United States, they deserve health care that meets guideline-based standards, treatment that mitigates harm or traumatization, and services that support their health and well-being. This policy statement also provides specific recommendations regarding postrelease services once a child is released into communities across the country, including a coordinated system that facilitates access to a medical home and consistent access to education, child care, interpretation services, and legal services.

[a]Department of Pediatrics, Wake Forest School of Medicine, Winston-Salem, North Carolina; [b]Department of Pediatrics, University of Texas Rio Grande Valley School of Medicine, Harlingen, Texas; and [c]Department of Pediatrics, Albert Einstein College of Medicine, Children's Hospital at Montefiore, Bronx, New York

Drs Linton, Griffin, and Shapiro collectively drafted, critically revised, and reviewed this policy.

DOI: 10.1542/peds.2017-0483

Address correspondence to Julie M. Linton, MD, FAAP. E-mail: jlinton@wakehealth.edu

PEDIATRICS (ISSN Numbers: Print, 0031-4005; Online, 1098-4275).

Copyright © 2017 by the American Academy of Pediatrics

FINANCIAL DISCLOSURE: The authors have indicated they have no financial relationships relevant to this article to disclose.

FUNDING: No external funding.

To cite: Linton JM, Griffin M, Shapiro AJ, AAP COUNCIL ON COMMUNITY PEDIATRICS. Detention of Immigrant Children. Pediatrics. 2017;139(5):e20170483

INTRODUCTION

Communities nationwide have become homes to immigrant and refugee children who have fled countries across the globe.[1] However, in the dramatic increase in arrivals that began in 2014 and continues at the time of writing this policy statement, more than 95% of undocumented children have emigrated from Guatemala, Honduras, and El Salvador (the Northern Triangle countries of Central America), with much smaller numbers from Mexico and other countries. Most of these undocumented children cross into the United States through the southern border.[2] Unprecedented violence, abject poverty, and lack of state protection

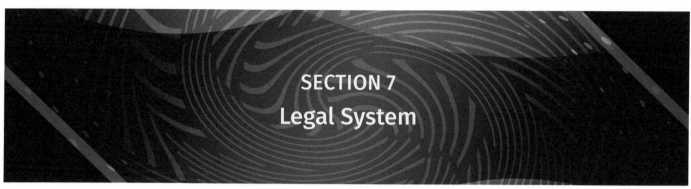

SECTION 7
Legal System

Some articles are available online only; scan the QR code to access online content.

POLICY STATEMENT Organizational Principles to Guide and Define the Child Health Care System and/or Improve the Health of all Children

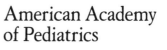

American Academy of Pediatrics

DEDICATED TO THE HEALTH OF ALL CHILDREN®

Advocacy and Collaborative Health Care for Justice-Involved Youth

Mikah C. Owen, MD, MPH, FAAP,[a] Stephenie B. Wallace, MD, MSPH, FAAP,[b] COMMITTEE ON ADOLESCENCE

abstract

Children and adolescents who become involved with the justice system often do so with complex medical, mental health, developmental, social, and legal needs. Most have been exposed to childhood trauma or adversity, which both contribute to their involvement with the justice system and negatively impact their health and well-being. Whether youth are held in confinement or in their home communities, pediatricians play a critical role in promoting the health and well-being of justice-involved youth. Having a working knowledge of the juvenile justice system and common issues facing justice-involved youth may help pediatricians enhance their clinical care and advocacy efforts. This policy statement is a revision of the 2011 policy "Health Care for Youth in the Juvenile Justice System." It provides an overview of the juvenile justice system, describes racial bias and overrepresentation of youth of color in the justice system, reviews the health and mental health status of justice-involved youth, and identifies advocacy opportunities for juvenile justice reform.

[a]Department of Pediatrics, School of Medicine, University of California, Davis, Sacramento, California; and [b]Division of Adolescent Medicine, Department of Pediatrics, School of Medicine, The University of Alabama at Birmingham, Birmingham, Alabama

Policy statements from the American Academy of Pediatrics benefit from expertise and resources of liaisons and internal (AAP) and external reviewers. However, policy statements from the American Academy of Pediatrics may not reflect the views of the liaisons or the organizations or government agencies that they represent.

Drs Owen and Wallace wrote the initial draft, contributed subsequent revisions, and approved the final manuscript as submitted.

The guidance in this statement does not indicate an exclusive course of treatment or serve as a standard of medical care. Variations, taking into account individual circumstances, may be appropriate.

All policy statements from the American Academy of Pediatrics automatically expire 5 years after publication unless reaffirmed, revised, or retired at or before that time.

DOI: https://doi.org/10.1542/peds.2020-1755

Address correspondence to Mikah C. Owen, MD, MPH, FAAP. E-mail: mcowen@ucdavis.edu

PEDIATRICS (ISSN Numbers: Print, 0031-4005; Online, 1098-4275).

FINANCIAL DISCLOSURE: The authors have indicated they have no financial relationships relevant to this article to disclose.

FUNDING: No external funding.

To cite: Owen MC, Wallace SB, AAP COMMITTEE ON ADOLESCENCE. Advocacy and Collaborative Health Care for Justice-Involved Youth. *Pediatrics.* 2020;146(1):e20201755

INTRODUCTION

In 2017, approximately 809 700 persons under the age of 18 were arrested in the United States,[1] a number that has steadily declined from the peak of nearly 2.7 million in 1996.[2] Decreases in juvenile arrests coincide with concomitant decreases in the number of confined youth. In 2017, approximately 202 900 delinquency cases involved detention,[3] a 50% decrease from the peak of 405 700 in 2005.[3] Whether detained pending the resolution of their legal case or committed to a correctional facility by a judge, most youth quickly return to their home communities. In 2017, the median time in placement was 68 days (23 days for detained youth versus 114 days for committed youth).[4] Thus, pediatricians, whether practicing in juvenile correctional facilities or in communities, may have the opportunity to care for youth involved in the justice system.

Despite improving trends in juvenile arrests and confinement, justice-involved youth continue to experience significant barriers to reaching their full potential. Barriers such as racial and ethnic bias, exposure to adverse childhood experiences (ACEs), and unmet physical and mental health needs continue to interfere with the optimal health and development of youth involved with the justice system. Ideally, contact with the juvenile justice system would serve as an opportunity to improve the health and developmental trajectory of youth by identifying precipitants to involvement with the justice system and implementing services to address the young person's needs. Unfortunately, for many youth, involvement with the justice system serves as nothing more than another traumatic experience. Pediatricians, as trusted child advocates, are uniquely positioned to identify and respond to the needs of justice-involved youth and their families. Whether through the provision of clinical care, participation in advocacy activities aimed at reforming the juvenile justice system, or by addressing the root causes of juvenile delinquency, pediatricians have a critical role in improving outcomes for youth involved with the justice system.

OVERVIEW OF THE JUVENILE JUSTICE SYSTEM

In the United States, most children and adolescents suspected of committing a crime are typically placed under the jurisdiction of the juvenile justice system, which is separate from the criminal (adult) justice system. Although each state, and the District of Columbia, have a unique juvenile justice system with different structures and processes, the way a delinquency case progresses through the juvenile justice system is similar among most jurisdictions.[5,6] Law enforcement and non–law enforcement sources (parents, victims, schools) may refer youth under the age of 18 to the juvenile justice system. At the time of arrest, law enforcement agencies may refer the youth for further processing

within the juvenile justice system or divert the case to an alternative program outside the system, known as diversion. At or around the time of arrest, adolescents may be held in facilities pending the resolution of their case (detention). If the legal agency refers a case to juvenile court, an intake officer reviews the case and decides whether to dismiss the case, handle the case informally, or proceed to formal processing in juvenile court (petition). Formal cases in juvenile court proceed to an adjudicatory hearing (trial) in which a judge may find a young person not guilty or adjudicated delinquent (guilty). In the case of adjudication, the case progresses to a disposition hearing (sentencing) in which a juvenile court judge orders the disposition (sanctions). Juvenile court judges have a wide range of disposition options, starting with less severe options such as community service and counseling, progressing to more severe options such as intensive probation or residential placement. Residential placement is the out-of-home placement of adjudicated delinquent youth and may include group homes, residential treatment facilities, and long-term secure facilities.

Not all minors accused of breaking the law progress through the juvenile justice system. The maximum age of juvenile court jurisdiction varies between states: 45 states have a maximum age of 17 and 5 states have a maximum age of 16.[7] Additionally, all states have transfer laws that remove youth from the jurisdiction of juvenile court and place them in the jurisdiction of criminal (adult) court in certain circumstances. Transfer laws and processes vary by state and are discussed in the section of this statement on juvenile transfer laws.

States and local jurisdictions mostly administer juvenile justice systems; however, the federal government has established guidelines for minimum

protections of youth involved with the justice system. The Juvenile Justice Delinquency and Prevention Act (JJDPA), first enacted in 1974[8] and reauthorized by the Juvenile Justice Reform Act of 2018,[9] maintains 4 core protections for youth involved with the justice system:

- deinstitutionalization of status offenders: juveniles who have committed an offense that would not be a crime if committed by an adult (eg, curfew violation or running away) and juveniles who are not charged with any crimes may not be placed in secure detention facilities;
- removal from adult jail: with a few exceptions, juveniles should not be held in adult jails or lockups (this provision was strengthened in 2018, and states have 3 years to comply);
- sight and sound separation: juveniles held in adult facilities should be separated from incarcerated adults by both sight and sound; and
- racial and ethnic disparities: states must implement policy, practice, and system improvement strategies to identify and reduce racial and ethnic disparities among youth who come into contact with the juvenile justice system.

States that do not comply with these core protections are not eligible to receive federal grant funding provided through the JJDPA.

YOUTH INVOLVED WITH THE JUSTICE SYSTEM

Racial and Ethnic Disparities

Despite decreases in youth arrest and confinement rates, there remain significant racial and ethnic disparities throughout the juvenile justice system. As seen in Table 1, racial and ethnic disparities exist at virtually every decision point in the juvenile justice system.

TABLE 1 Racial and/or Ethnic Disparities in the Juvenile Justice System (All Data From 2018, Unless Otherwise Specified)

	White	African American	Hispanic	AIAN	AHPI
US population <18 y,[10] %	50	14	26	1	5
Juvenile arrest relative rate (RR)[11,a]	—	2.6	Not reported[b]	1.3	0.3
Cases referred to juvenile court RR[12]	—	2.9	0.9	1.2	0.2
Cases diverted RR[12]	—	0.6	0.8	0.8	1.0
Cases detained RR[12]	—	1.4	1.5	1.3	1.2
Cases adjudicated delinquent RR[12]	—	0.9	1.1	1.1	1.0
Adjudicated cases resulting in secure confinement RR[12]	—	1.4	1.4	1.2	0.9
Cases judicially waived to criminal court[12]	—	1.6	1.0	0.9	0.9
Juvenile residential placement RR[13]	—	4.6	1.4	2.8	0.2
Decrease juveniles in residential placement 2006–2015,[14] %	54	46	45	51	65
Decline in juvenile court delinquency cases 2005–2015,[15] %	53	44	38	40	57

AIAN, American Indian or Alaskan native; AHPI, Asian American, Hawaiian, or Pacific Islander; —, not applicable.

[a] Relative rates relative to white youth.

[b] Not all agencies provide ethnicity data; thus, arrest rates for Hispanic juveniles are not reported.

Empirical explanations for racial and ethnic disparities within the justice system are commonly grouped into 2 broad conceptual frameworks: differential treatment and differential offending.[16–18] The differential treatment hypothesis[16–18] attributes racial and ethnic disparities to "inequities—intended or unintended —in justice system practices."[18] Multiple studies have demonstrated racial bias against youth of color at all decision points in the juvenile justice system (arrest, referral to court, diversion, detention, petition, adjudication, probation, secure confinement, and transfer to criminal court).[16,19] Authors of a 2018 review article[19] examined official processing of youth of color at various juvenile justice decision points from January 2001 to December 2014. The authors of that review found that 79% of studies showed that status as a person of color had some disadvantaging effect for youth processed in the juvenile justice system. The negative impact of race was especially prominent at earlier decision points in the juvenile justice system (eg, arrest, referral to court, and preadjudication detention). Conversely, the differential offending hypothesis attributes racial and ethnic disparities within the juvenile

justice system to "differences in the incidence, seriousness, and persistence of engagement in delinquent and criminal behavior."[18] The differential offending hypothesis does not ascribe differences in delinquent behavior to biological or genetic differences between races or ethnicities. Instead, the hypothesis posits youth of color are more likely to experience a variety of risk factors for delinquency (poverty, low-performing schools, harsh discipline practices in schools, increased police presence in communities, exposure to violence, incarcerated parents, toxic stress, etc) and thus more likely to commit certain types of crimes.[17] Much of the research supporting this hypothesis relies on the use of official records such as arrest rates, confinement rates, and/or conviction rates. Citing empirical data from official records, which are influenced by inequities in justice system practices (eg, overpolicing of historically disenfranchised neighborhoods, racial profiling, disparate sentencing of youth of color, differential treatment in the plea-bargaining process, implicit and/or explicit bias against youth of color), may overestimate the differences in delinquent and/or criminal behaviors between racial

and ethnic groups and perpetuate bias within the literature. Furthermore, more research is needed to identify how social factors more commonly experienced by youth of color mediate racial and/or ethnic disparities in the juvenile justice system.

Although helpful as conceptual frameworks, the differential treatment and differential offending hypotheses represent an oversimplification of the causes of racial and ethnic disparities within the juvenile justice system. Racial and ethnic disparities within the juvenile justice system exist within the broader context of disparities in child health and well-being. Collectively, the sources of these disparities are rooted in inequities in the social and environmental determinants of health (eg, poverty, racism) and the failure of public policies to adequately address them. Key policy statements from the American Academy of Pediatrics (AAP), "The Impact of Racism on Child and Adolescent Health,"[20] "Poverty and Child Health in the United States"[21] and "Health Equity and Children's Rights"[22] provide insight on how these inequities impact the health and development of children and adolescents and how pediatricians can respond to mitigate their impact.

Children and Adolescents Exposed to ACEs

Research has established the significant impact of childhood trauma, adversity, or ACEs on the health and well-being of children and adolescents.[23] Multiple studies have documented high prevalence rates of childhood trauma among justice-involved youth, with many studies finding that over 90% of youth in the justice system have experienced at least one form of childhood trauma.[24–26] The National Child Traumatic Stress Network found justice-involved youth experience an average of 5 different forms of childhood trauma.[27] Sixty-two percent of youth in the National Center for Child Traumatic Stress study experienced trauma within the first 5 years of life; Table 2 identifies the different types of trauma justice-involved youth experienced in this study.

Aware of the high prevalence of trauma and cognizant that incarceration itself represents a traumatic experience, advocates have called for the implementation of trauma-informed policies, procedures, and standards across the spectrum of juvenile justice settings. In 2015, the National Child Traumatic Stress Network published the *Essential Elements of a Trauma-Informed Juvenile Justice System*,[28] a guide that educates programs working with justice-involved youth to recognize and respond to the needs of youth who have experienced trauma. A 2012 report by the US Department of Justice provides recommendations on how to incorporate trauma-informed care practices throughout the spectrum of the juvenile justice system.[29] Recommendations include the following:

- make trauma-informed screening, assessment, and care the standard in juvenile justice services;

- abandon juvenile justice correctional practices that traumatize children;

- provide juvenile justice services appropriate to children's ethnocultural background;

- provide care and services to address the special circumstances and needs of girls in the juvenile justice system;

- provide care and services to address the special circumstances and needs of lesbian, gay, bisexual, transgender, and queer and/or questioning (LGBTQ) youth in the juvenile justice system;

- develop and implement policies in every school system that aim to keep children in school rather than policies that lead to suspension and expulsion;

- guarantee that all violence-exposed children accused of a crime have legal representation;

- help, do not punish, child victims of sex trafficking; and

- whenever possible, prosecute young offenders in the juvenile justice system.

For justice-involved youth receiving care in the community, the AAP Resilience Project (https://www.aap.org/en-us/advocacy-and-policy/aap-health-initiatives/resilience/Pages/Resilience-Project.aspx) is a great resource to educate pediatricians to

incorporate trauma-informed care into their practice.

Female Youth

Because of larger relative declines in the arrest rates of male youth, the proportion of justice-involved girls and young women has increased.[30] Recent data reveal that female youth accounted for 29% of youth arrests[31] and 15% of youth residential placement.[32]

Available literature suggests that in comparison with male youth, justice-involved female youth experience higher rates of trauma exposure, sexual and physical abuse victimization, and mental illness[25] and are more likely to have been involved with the child welfare system.[33]

In 2015, the Office of Juvenile Justice and Delinquency Prevention issued policy guidance aimed at improving system and programmatic responses for justice-involved female youth.[34] Key recommendations from the report include the following:

- prohibition of placement of minor sex trafficking victims in the juvenile justice system;

- development of alternatives to detention and incarceration for female youth; and

- competency of all programs and services to serve girls and young women in, or at risk of entering, the juvenile justice system.

LGBTQ Youth

Studies report LGBTQ youth compose 13% to 15% of youth in the juvenile justice system,[35-37] but this may be an underestimate because many jurisdictions do not collect information on sexual orientation or gender identity, and youth may not disclose this information because of fear of mistreatment.[35] Most research on LGBTQ youth in the juvenile justice system is focused on sexual orientation and does not include data on transgender or gender-diverse

TABLE 2 Prevalence of Trauma Types Among Justice-Involved Youth[27]

Trauma Type	Percentage of Youth	
	Male	Female
Traumatic loss or bereavement	59	65
Domestic violence	51	56
Impaired caregiver	48	57
Emotional abuse	46	54
Community violence	41	30
Neglect	31	30
Physical maltreatment and/or abuse	39	41
Physical assault	27	24
School violence	23	23
Serious injury or unintentional injury	20	19
Sexual maltreatment and/or abuse	16	32
Sexual assault and/or rape	9	39

youth. Like youth from historically disenfranchised racial and/or ethnic groups, LGBTQ youth experience more risk factors for involvement with the juvenile justice system and differential treatment within the system. LGBTQ youth experience higher rates of physical and sexual violence, familial rejection, bullying, mental health problems, and other risk factors that increase the likelihood of system involvement.[36,37] Literature suggests LGBTQ youth face bias and maltreatment across the spectrum of juvenile justice settings. One study found that LGBTQ and gender-diverse youth were more likely to be detained for truancy, warrants, probation violations, running away, and child sex trafficking.[38] Another study found LGBTQ youth reported youth-on-youth sexual victimization at a rate of nearly 7 times that of heterosexual youth (10.3% vs 1.5%).[39] Multiple reports have found LGBTQ youth in detention facilities experience increased rates of emotional abuse, physical abuse, and time in isolation.[36,37,40] The Prison Rape Elimination Act of the Juvenile Facility Standards of 2003[41] includes provisions to keep LGBTQ youth safe in detention facilities and include, but are not limited to, the following:

- staff must receive training on how to communicate effectively with LGBTQ and gender-nonconforming youth;

- facilities are required to ascertain whether youth are (or are perceived to be) lesbian, bisexual, gay, and/or transgender or gender nonconforming;

- the use of isolation and/or solitary confinement is limited; and

- case-by-case housing decisions are required for transgender and intersex adolescents.

Although the Prison Rape Elimination Act standards provide basic protections for detained LGBTQ youth, they do not set comprehensive standards that promote the overall well-being of confined LGBTQ youth. The Annie E. Casey Foundation[37] and The Equity Project provide best practices and guidance for the development and implementation of more comprehensive standards.[42]

Medical Care for Transgender Youth

Medical care for transgender youth in confinement, including access to hormone therapy, is variable. In a 2015 article, authors analyzed state statutes and department of corrections policies regarding medical services and treatment of transgender inmates and found that 13 states allow for the initiation of hormone treatment and 21 states allow for the continuation of hormone treatment; the authors were unable to identify relevant policies or statues in 10 states.[43] The 2015 National Commission on Correctional Health Care (NCCHC) position statement "Transgender, Transsexual, and Gender Nonconforming Health Care in Correctional Settings"[44] makes recommendations for the health management of transgender patients held in confinement. Recommendations include the following:

- health staff should manage transgender patients in a manner that respects their biomedical and psychosocial needs;

- the management of medical or surgical transgender care should follow accepted standards developed by professionals with expertise in transgender health;

- there should be no blanket administrative or other policies that restrict specific medical treatments; and

- transgender patients who received hormone therapy with or without a prescription before incarceration should have therapy continued without interruption.

Youth Involved With the Child Welfare System

Youth with current or past involvement with the child welfare system, often referred to as crossover or dual-status youth, are overrepresented in the juvenile justice system. Although national data are lacking and estimates vary by jurisdiction, studies reveal the prevalence of dual-status youth in the juvenile justice system commonly exceeds 50%.[45,46] When compared with youth who are not involved in both systems, dual-status youth are younger at the time of first arrest, detained more often, and have more significant mental health and educational needs.[33] The JJDPA requires states to establish polices and systems to incorporate child welfare records into juvenile justice records to establish and implement treatment plans of justice-involved youth.

MEDICAL AND MENTAL HEALTH CARE FOR CONFINED YOUTH

Confined youth have a constitutional right to adequate medical and mental health care[47,48]; however, because of the lack of clearly defined federal standards and differences in state laws regarding the provision of health care for confined youth, on-site medical and mental health care services vary widely between jurisdictions and correctional facilities.[49] States, counties, or private contractors may provide health care services for confined youth.[50] Federal law prohibits the use of Medicaid funds for inmates of a public institution,[50] and local governments (states, counties, cities) are responsible for funding health care services for confined youth.

In addition to state laws governing the provision of health care for confined youth, detention facilities may seek voluntary accreditation from the NCCHC. The NCCHC published "Standards for Health

Services in Juvenile Detention and Confinement Facilities" and provides accreditation for health services in juvenile detention facilities.[51] The AAP, American Academy of Child and Adolescent Psychiatry (AACAP), American College of Obstetricians and Gynecologists (ACOG), and the American Public Health Association support the NCCHC standards, which address 9 general areas: health care services and support, patient care and treatment, special needs and services, governance and administration, safety, personnel and training, health records, health promotion, and medical legal issues.[51] The NCCHC recommends physical, mental, and oral health screenings after admission, a comprehensive health assessment within 7 days of admission, and appropriate follow-up care. Although NCCHC accreditation is voluntary, it is important for providers in confinement facilities to be aware of these standards and juvenile correctional facilities to adopt and comply with the standards.

The 2011 AAP policy statement "Health Care for Youth in the Juvenile Justice System"[52] provided a detailed overview of the physical and mental health needs of confined youth and the provision of health care services for youth in correctional facilities. Since the 2011 policy statement, there have been few additional nationally representative studies on the health status of justice-involved youth published. The Survey of Youth in Residential Placement (SYRP) of 2010[53] remains the most comprehensive nationally representative examination of the health needs of confined youth. The SYRP found 69% of confined youth reported an unmet health care need, including injury, problems with vision or hearing, dental needs, or "other illness." The SYRP did not inquire about specific illnesses or injuries. Common health concerns for these youth include traumatic injuries, oral health needs, sexually transmitted

infections (STIs), and reproductive health needs.[53,54]

Few studies have been used to examine chronic illness in incarcerated youth, and incarcerated youth may have difficulty accessing care before confinement.[52] Quality coordinated care within the justice and medical systems can identify and manage chronic illnesses during confinement. The NCCHC recommends that systems identify and enroll youth with chronic illnesses in a chronic disease management plan.[51]

Reproductive and/or Sexual Health

The 1991 NCCHC study[55] remains the only nationally representative sample evaluating the history of sexual activity and contraceptive use among confined youth. Confined youth reported higher rates of sexual activity, increased likelihood of 4 or more lifetime sexual partners, and lower rates of contraception or condom use during their most recent sexual intercourse. Multiple smaller studies have revealed similar results,[56-59] and these behaviors place justice-involved youth at risk for unintended pregnancy as well as STIs and HIV infections. It is important for adolescents to receive counseling on safe sex practices, which include barrier methods, hormonal contraception, long-acting reversible contraception, and emergency contraception, and receive timely and appropriate reproductive health care during confinement. Reproductive health care includes assessment of youth's self-reported sexual behaviors and practices, STI and HIV testing and treatment, trauma counseling, necessary emergency contraception, and counseling on all other forms of contraception as recommended by the AAP.[60] The NCCHC recommends evaluating all youth assigned female sex at birth for pregnancy risk after admission. Early pregnancy identification allows youth to

consider options regarding their pregnancy and parenthood.

The 2010 SYRP revealed 13% of confined male and 5% of female youth were expecting children.[53] ACOG recommends incarcerated pregnant adolescents receive the same pregnancy care (pregnancy counseling, prenatal and perinatal care, and abortion services) as nonincarcerated adolescents.[61] A unique challenge for pregnant incarcerated women and adolescents is the use of mechanical restraints, commonly known as shackling. ACOG[62] notes that shackling interferes with the ability of the health care clinician to assess and evaluate the health of the woman and fetus and may put the health of both at risk (increased risk of falls, increased risk of venous thrombosis due to limited mobility, interference with normal labor and delivery, and interference with mother-child bonding).[61] ACOG, the American Medical Association, and many other professional organizations have called for prohibiting, or severely restricting, the use of shackles to restrain pregnant women.[62] The Juvenile Justice Reform Act of 2018 prohibits the use of restraints on pregnant women and adolescents during labor, delivery, and postpartum recovery unless there is an immediate threat of harm to self or others (states have 2 years to phase out the use of restraints).[9]

Infections

It is important for health care clinicians to give special attention to screening, immunization, and treatment of specific infections among justice-involved youth.

Tuberculosis

The NCCHC recommends screening all youth for tuberculosis after entry into the justice system unless the local health department determines the community's prevalence does not warrant screening.[51] The 2018 AAP

Red Book: 2018 Report of the Committee on Infectious Diseases outlines methods for assessing risk and screening youth for exposure.[63] The Centers for Disease Control and Prevention also provides recommendations for prevention and control of tuberculosis in detention facilities.[64]

STIs and/or HIV

Data from the Center for Disease Control and Prevention's *Sexually Transmitted Disease Surveillance 2011*[65] found confined youth have elevated rates of STIs (Table 3).

Although HIV prevalence data for confined youth are not available, the same risk factors for STIs place them at risk for HIV infection. In 2017, youth aged 13 to 24 made up 21% of all new HIV diagnoses in the United States.[66]

Routine screening, education (including safe sex practices; abstinence; and barrier, hormonal, long-acting reversible contraception; and emergency contraception), and treatment of STIs and/or HIV among confined youth may decrease the overall disease burden and improve sexual and relationship health. The NCCHC recommends STI testing (chlamydia, gonorrhea, HIV, and syphilis, of which there is significant prevalence) be offered to all youth within 48 hours of arrival.[51]

Immunizations

There is a lack of nationally representative data regarding the immunization status of confined youth, but facility-level data suggest they have significantly lower immunization coverage rates. In a study of one juvenile detention facility in California, authors found only 3% of adolescents had received all recommended immunizations before their first detention.[67] Barriers to full immunization coverage among justice-involved youth may include poor access to health care and lack of a medical home before confinement.[67]

Although immunization requirements for confined youth vary between jurisdictions, confinement may be an opportunity for justice-involved youth to receive immunizations. Studies have revealed that detention and/or secure placement of youth may be associated with higher immunization coverage rates.[67,68] Implementing routine immunization policies in juvenile detention facilities may increase immunization coverage for confined youth. Use of state immunization registries can help determine necessary immunizations.

Mental Health Disorders

Although estimates vary, the prevalence of mental health disorders among justice-involved youth commonly ranges from 50% to 80%.[69-73] Common mental health disorders include depressive disorders, anxiety disorders, disruptive behavior, attention-deficit/hyperactivity disorder, posttraumatic stress disorder, and substance use disorders.[69]

The variable data on the prevalence of mental health disorders among juvenile justice-involved youth are indicative of the limitations of the studies in the literature (use of nonstandardized measures, different diagnostic tools, measurement at different levels of the juvenile justice system, and data specific to individual facility or state). Furthermore, the high prevalence of mental health disorders is interconnected with the high prevalence of trauma and ACEs found in this population.[74,75] Most justice-involved youth experience trauma and polyvictimization from a young age. These experiences, and resulting toxic stress response, may result in maladaptive behaviors such as increased stress reactivity, impulsivity, hyperarousal, and decreased ability to self-regulate.[76] Youth who have experienced multiple traumatic events are at increased risk of delinquency, contact with law enforcement, involvement with the juvenile justice system, school suspension and dropout, volatile relationships, and substance use.[77] Polyvictimized youth are also more likely to receive diagnoses of externalizing disorders such as conduct disorders, oppositional defiant disorder, and antisocial behaviors.[72,78] There is increasing recognition that for many youth, these diagnoses may be rooted in complex trauma and polyvictimization.[79,80]

Substance Use

As illustrated in Table 4, the prevalence of substance use in confined youth exceeds that of the general adolescent population. However, it is important to consider that for many justice-involved youth, substance use may be the instigating factor of their arrest or confinement.

Recognizing the high prevalence of mental health disorders and substance use among justice-involved youth and the lack of appropriate care in many juvenile facilities, many jurisdictions have implemented programs (ie, mental health courts, substance abuse courts) aimed at providing community-based alternatives to detention for those with mental health and/or substance use disorders.[33] Several diversion programs are effective at decreasing recidivism and/or improving

TABLE 3 STI Rates Among Adolescents Aged 12–18 Years in Juvenile Correction Facilities, 2011 (Last Year Data From Juvenile Correctional Facilities Were Included)

Disease	Overall Positivity, %	
	Female	Male
Chlamydia	15.7	7.4
Gonorrhea	4.4	1.2

TABLE 4 Prevalence of Substance Use Among Confined Youth and the General Adolescent Population

Substance	Lifetime Prevalence Among Confined Youth,[53,a] %	Lifetime Prevalence at Grade 12, General Population, 2018,[81,b] %
Alcohol	74	59
Marijuana or hashish	84	44
Cocaine/crack	30	4/1.5
Ecstasy	26	4
Methamphetamine	22	0.7
Acid/LSD	19	5
Heroin	7	0.8
Any illegal drug (excluding marijuana)	50	19

LSD, lysergic acid diethylamide.

[a] Self-reported data from the SYRP, a nationally representative sample of 7073 youth in custody in 2003.

[b] Self-reported data from the Monitoring the Future National Survey on Drug Use.

behavioral health outcomes in justice-involved youth[82]; however, there is significant variability in the design and implementation of these programs, leading to limitations in studying their collective impact.[82] Further studies to identify eligible youth and effective diversion services and programs may improve outcomes in justice-involved youth.

Screening and Assessment for Mental Health and Substance Use Disorders

NCCHC standards recommend screening all confined youth for current or past mental illness and legal and illegal drug use at the time of arrival to the facility.[51] A 2014 survey[83] of juvenile facilities across the United States found 88% of facilities screened all or some youth for substance use and 99% of facilities reported screening all or some youth for mental health needs. Generally, mental health screening involves nonclinical staff using a standardized screening tool.

On-site Psychiatric Care and Psychotropic Medications

The decision to initiate or change medical treatment of psychiatric disorders in confined youth is challenging. The AACAP published recommendations for mental health assessment and treatment of youth in the correctional system.[84] The AACAP recommends psychotropic

medications only be used as part of an individually developed comprehensive treatment plan. To ensure treatment can proceed in a safe and supervised fashion, AACAP guidance recommends determining the youth's legal disposition and placement before initiating or changing medication regimens.[85]

National data are lacking on the use of psychotropic medications for justice-involved youth; however, state- and facility-level data suggest these youth receive psychotropic medications at a higher rate than the general adolescent population. In an analysis of juvenile facilities in 55 California counties, authors found the average proportion of youth receiving psychoactive medication was 17%.[86] In a study of 668 youth in 3 detention facilities in 1 state, authors found that 10% had psychotropic medication dispensed within 1 month of intake.[87] In comparison, from 2005 to 2010, 6% of adolescents reported use of psychotropic medication within the past month.[88]

Suicide and Suicidality

Studies consistently demonstrate justice-involved youth are at increased risk for suicidal thoughts and behaviors. In a longitudinal study of 1829 youth detained at 1 facility over a 3-year period, authors found 36% had ever felt like life was hopeless, 10% had thought about

killing themselves in the past 6 months, and 11% had attempted suicide in the past.[89] In a 2015 literature review, authors found that 19% to 32% of justice-involved youth had suicidal ideations in the past year and 12% to 16% had attempted suicide in the past year.[90]

The 2014 Juvenile Residential Facility Census (JRFC) found that suicide was the most common cause of death for youth in residential placement.[83] From 2000 to 2014, there was an average of 7 suicides per year in juvenile detention facilities across the United States.

The JRFC report found that 93% of reporting facilities screened some or all youth for suicide risk. Available studies indicate facilities with annual suicide prevention training and suicide risk screening shortly after admission reported lower suicide rates.[91,92] Only one-fifth of facilities had the 7 key components deemed necessary for suicide prevention.[91,93] These components include written protocols, intake screening, suicide prevention training, safe housing, observation, mortality review, and cardiopulmonary resuscitation and certification.

Informed Consent and the Right to Refuse Care

According to NCCHC standards, "all examinations, treatments, and procedures are governed by informed consent practices for juvenile care that are applicable in the jurisdiction. A juvenile may refuse specific health evaluations and treatments in accordance with the laws in the jurisdiction."[51] NCCHC standards also state that youth may not be punished for refusing medical or mental health treatment.[51]

Continuity of Care

It is ideal for justice-involved youth to receive comprehensive and coordinated physical and mental health care during confinement and in their communities. Barriers to such care include lack of preventive care in the community, lack of an established medical home, and disruptions in Medicaid or Children's Health Insurance Program coverage. Federal law prohibits the use of Medicaid funds for inmates of a public institution.[94] As a result, many jurisdictions terminate Medicaid eligibility at the time of entry into secure detention facilities.[94] In 2018, Congress passed legislation prohibiting states from terminating Medicaid eligibility for incarcerated juveniles.[95] States may suspend Medicaid coverage during incarceration, but before release, they must conduct a redetermination of eligibility and restore coverage, if eligible. States remain prohibited from using Medicaid to cover incarcerated juveniles.

Identifying and connecting youth with a medical home before release may have long-term benefits to their overall health and well-being. Winkelman et al[96] showed that youth with any justice involvement (detained, paroled, probation, or arrest) were more likely to have an emergency department (ED) visit in the last year compared with youth not involved with the justice system. Similarly, justice-involved youth are more likely to be hospitalized than their peers, and their use of the ED and inpatient services, as measured in person-years, is significantly higher than that of youth not involved with the justice system.[96] Use of the ED and increased hospitalization days by justice-involved youth may contribute to increased health care costs and represents an opportunity to improve the continuity of care for these youth once they return to their communities. It is ideal for these youth to be connected to medical homes and pediatricians who are prepared to address their needs.

Continuity of care starts at the time of admission to the facility. If the youth already has a primary care provider (PCP), it is crucial for the medical staff to contact the PCP to verify previous diagnoses and treatment(s).[97] For cases in which the youth does not have a PCP, medical staff can provide resources to establish primary care. Providing summaries of medical care for the PCP, appropriate subspecialists, or mental health specialists at the time of release to the community is also important. Additionally, detention facilities and jurisdictions can establish policies and procedures that ensure eligible uninsured youth are enrolled in Medicaid or the Children's Health Insurance Program before release from detention and have access to health care coverage as they reenter their home communities.[98,99]

DEVELOPMENTALLY APPROPRIATE CONFINEMENT FACILITIES

Conditions of Confinement

Youth may be confined in a variety of confinement facilities (short-term detention facilities, long-term secure facilities, camps, residential treatment facilities, etc); however, most are confined in locked facilities, many of which resemble adult jails and prisons in form and function (restricted by gates, fences and locked doors, regular use of restraints such as handcuffs and shackles, locking youth in their room for sleep and/or punishment, use of punitive discipline strategies, etc). For youth with a history of trauma, confinement in such facilities may exacerbate symptomatology related to trauma.[100] The trauma of confinement extends beyond the physical environment. Since 2000, systemic abuses of confined youth have been documented in 29 states.[101] Thirty-eight percent of confined youth fear being physically attacked, 50% report detention staff applies punishments without cause, and 33% report the use of unnecessary force.[101] In 2017, the National Council of Juvenile and Family Court Judges passed

a resolution urging states to establish independent monitoring systems (independent bodies responsible for receiving and investigating complaints) for confined youth, with a special focus on the use of isolation, use of mechanical restraints, use of force, access to programming, levels of violence, and access to families.[102] Several jurisdictions have implemented independent monitoring systems for confined youth.[103] The Annie E. Casey Foundation's Juvenile Detention Alternatives Initiative provides guidance and technical assistance for jurisdictions interested in monitoring and improving conditions of confinement.[104]

Isolation and Solitary Confinement

Solitary confinement is "the involuntary placement of a youth alone in a cell, room, or other area for any reason other than as a temporary response to behavior that threatens immediate harm to the youth or others."[105] While in isolation, youth may be denied access to educational material, detention facility programming, recreational activities, and contact with family.[106]

Nationally representative data suggest the use of isolation and solitary confinement is common in juvenile detention facilities. The JRFC found 47% of juvenile detention centers reported locking youth in a room for 4 or more hours within the previous month.[83] The SYRP found 35% of youth reported being held in isolation or solitary confinement.[53] Of those held in isolation, 55% reported being held for more than 24 hours.[53] These reports may understate the use of juvenile isolation and solitary confinement because they do not include youth in adult facilities.

The negative effects of solitary confinement on adults are well documented and may include anxiety, depression, impaired memory, hallucinations, suicidal thoughts, anger, psychosis, paranoia, heart palpitations, headaches, abdominal pain, and insomnia.[107] The 2009 "Juvenile Suicide in Confinement: A National Survey" highlights this vulnerability.[108] In this report, the authors examined 110 juvenile suicides occurring between 1995 and 1999 and found 62% of suicide victims had a history of room confinement, and 51% were on room confinement status at the time of their death.

In 2016, the US Department of Justice issued guiding principles on the use of isolation and solitary confinement and recommended against the use of isolation and solitary confinement in juveniles, stating, "In very rare situations, a juvenile may be separated from others as a temporary response to behavior that poses a serious and immediate risk of physical harm to any person. Even in such cases, the placement should be brief, designed as a 'cool down' period, and done only in consultation with a mental health professional."[109] In 2018, Congress passed legislation prohibiting the use of room confinement (except as a temporary response for juveniles who pose a serious and immediate risk to themselves or others) for youth in federal facilities.[110] There are few juveniles in federal detention centers, and nonfederal detention centers are not obligated to adhere to these principles.

Many states have passed legislation aimed at restricting or eliminating juvenile isolation. A 2016 analysis by the Lowenstein Center for the Public Interest found that 29 states or jurisdictions prohibit the use of punitive solitary confinement in juvenile detention facilities, 15 states impose time limits on the use of punitive solitary confinement, and 7 states place no limits to the use of solitary confinement.[111] In 2016, the AAP endorsed the United Nations position and the AACAP policy statement on solitary confinement of juvenile offenders and opposed the use of solitary confinement for juveniles in correctional facilities.

Many organizations have developed tools to reduce the use of isolation in juvenile confinement. The Council of Juvenile Correctional Administrators published a tool kit[112] outlining steps to reduce the use of isolation and recommendations to use alternative behavior management options and responses. These options may include cognitive behavioral therapy, dialectical behavior therapy, collaborative problem solving and trauma-informed care, and de-escalation training for juvenile correctional employees, workers, and/or officers.

Educational Needs

Youth involved with the justice system often present with significant educational challenges. The SYRP[53] found that 24% of youth reported they were not enrolled in school at the time they entered custody, 61% had been expelled or suspended, and 48% reported being below the level expected for their age. Learning disabilities are more common among youth in custody, with reported rates as high as 30%.[53]

Despite increased educational need, available data suggest confined youth receive inadequate educational support. A 2016 report from the US Department of Education Office for Civil Rights[113] found the number of hours and days of educational programming varies widely between facilities, teachers working in confinement facilities are more likely to be absent, and confinement facilities are less likely to offer essential math and science courses. The US Department of Education and Department of Justice developed guiding principles for the provision of high-quality education in juvenile justice secure settings.[114]

In multiple studies, authors have documented that youth with intellectual and developmental disabilities are overrepresented in the juvenile justice system. Although there is variance between sites, the estimated national average prevalence of intellectual and developmental disabilities in confined youth is 33%.[115] Confined youth with intellectual and developmental disabilities have the same rights under the Individuals with Disabilities Education Act as nonconfined youth and are entitled to individualized education programs and special education services.[115] The National Center on Criminal Justice and Disability provides recommendations for preventing involvement of adolescents with intellectual and developmental disabilities in the justice system and improving the delivery of special education services for confined youth.[116]

JUVENILE JUSTICE REFORM AND OPPORTUNITIES FOR ADVOCACY

Community-Based Interventions and Alternatives to Youth Confinement

Over the last 2 decades, advances in social, developmental, and neurologic sciences have transformed our understanding of health and well-being across the life course. It is recognized that trauma, adversity, and ACEs are associated with a maladaptive stress response, changes in brain architecture, and poor physical, mental, and behavioral health outcomes.[23,26] Advances in neuroscience and neuroimaging have demonstrated numerous structural and functional changes in the brain occur during the period of adolescence.[117] These changes may be associated with impulsive, risk-taking, and reward-seeking behaviors that may make adolescents more likely to interact with the justice system.

This evolving knowledge has contributed to the development and implementation of community-based alternatives to incarceration that are more appropriate for the unique developmental needs of justice-involved youth. Numerous reports have highlighted shortcomings associated with the incarceration of juveniles in the United States. The Annie E. Casey Foundation's *No Place For Kids: The Case for Reducing Juvenile Incarceration* argues that juvenile incarceration is dangerous (documented cases of physical and sexual abuse), ineffective (does not decrease involvement in delinquent behaviors), unnecessary (only 26% of youth confined in residential facilities committed a violent offense), obsolete (community-based alternatives have been demonstrated to reduce recidivism), wasteful (in 2008, an estimated $5 billion was spent on juvenile incarceration), and inadequate (deficient in mental health treatment, substance use treatment, educational programming, and transitional support and often retraumatizes youth).[118]

Many jurisdictions responded to these concerns by implementing reforms (diversion programs, mentor programs, implementation of the Juvenile Detention Alternatives Initiative, etc)[118,119] aimed at reducing the rate of juvenile incarceration and improving outcomes for justice-involved youth. The Juvenile Detention Alternatives Initiative is one available resource and tool that provides training and technical assistance to jurisdictions interested in reforming their juvenile justice systems. Examples of community-based alternatives to detention and secure confinement include day and evening reporting centers (providing youth with supervision and programming during the day and/or evening), electronic monitoring, home- or community-based detention, and intensive family treatment models such as multisystemic therapy, functional

family therapy, and multidimensional foster care.[118,119]

The Office of Juvenile Justice and Delinquency Prevention[120] advocates for a comprehensive strategy of supporting the adolescent's family and engaging core institutions, such as schools, businesses, and religious organizations, to help develop mature and responsible youth. The strategy of delinquency prevention is the most effective approach while recognizing the need for graduated sanctions to protect the community. The best prevention involves targeting risk factors for delinquency, such as ACEs, childhood trauma, drugs and firearms in the community, family conflict, abuse and neglect, poor commitment to school, and negative peer influences, while focusing on protective factors such as a resilient individual temperament; close relationships with family, teachers, other adults, and peers; and promoting school success and avoidance of drugs and crime.[17,29,118–120]

Overall, there is growing evidence that for many youth, community-based alternatives to incarceration are more effective options than confinement.[118,119] This evidence and overall reductions in youth crime have contributed to significant decreases in the rate of juvenile confinement in the United States.

Juvenile Transfer Laws

Juvenile transfer laws govern the relocation of juvenile cases to adult court. Current juvenile transfer laws were created largely as a result of state legislative actions during the 1980s and 1990s, triggered by a rise in youth crime and intense media focus on juvenile crime during that period.[121] States responded by enacting legislation that automatically placed juveniles in the jurisdiction of the adult court for certain offenses or gave prosecutors discretion to place juveniles in adult court. Although juvenile crime rates have steadily

decreased since the mid-1990s, many of the juvenile transfer laws of this era remain in effect.[121]

Although legislators enacted these laws as a deterrent to juvenile crime, evidence suggests that juvenile transfer laws have little or no effect on general juvenile crime rates.[122] Additionally, compared with youth in the juvenile court system, recidivism rates were higher for juveniles with cases in adult criminal court. Recidivism rates were higher particularly for violent offenders.[122] Proposed explanations for increased recidivism rates among youth tried in criminal court include the stigma of having a felony criminal record, less focus on rehabilitation in the adult criminal justice system, and sense of resentment among youth tried and punished as adults.[122]

Currently, all states have transfer laws that allow juvenile offenders to be prosecuted in adult court. The 4 types of transfer laws[7] are as follows:

- statutory exclusion: specific crimes are automatically transferred to adult court;
- judicially controlled transfer: all juvenile cases begin in juvenile court and must be transferred to adult court by the juvenile court;
- prosecutorial discretion: also known as "direct file," prosecutors may choose to file in adult or juvenile court; and
- once an adult, always an adult: once a juvenile has been prosecuted in adult court, all future cases go to adult court.

Juveniles prosecuted in adult court may be confined in adult detention facilities. Juveniles in adult prisons report learning more criminal behavior from adult inmates, fear of victimization, and being least likely to say they would not reoffend. Juveniles in adult facilities, compared with those in juvenile facilities, have an eightfold increase in suicide, fivefold increase in being sexually assaulted, and twofold increase in likelihood of being attacked with a weapon by other inmates or beaten by staff.[123]

Reform efforts have focused on changing the ways in which juveniles may be transferred to adult court. Advocates argue that statutory exclusion and prosecutorial discretion may limit the juvenile court's ability to provide the most appropriate sanctions for youth. There is also concern that prosecutors may use the threat of adult sanctions to coerce youth to accept plea bargains to avoid longer sentences. Several states have successfully enacted legislation limiting the transfer of juveniles to adult court.[123] For example, in 2012, Colorado enacted legislation limiting juvenile transfer to adult court, allowing for judicial review for all juvenile cases and adding juvenile sentencing provisions to convictions in adult court. In the 5 years after this legislation, Colorado saw a 78% reduction in direct file cases and a 99% reduction in adult jailing of juveniles.[124]

Life Without Parole and Death Penalty

Over the last 15 years, the US Supreme Court issued several decisions limiting extreme sentences for juvenile offenders declaring unconstitutional capital punishment of individuals who committed crimes as a juvenile (under age 18)[125] and abolishing mandatory life without parole sentences for crimes committed as a juvenile; however, it is still permissible to impose life without parole sentences for juveniles after judicial consideration of individual case circumstances.[126] The United States is the only country in the world that sentences juveniles to life without the possibility of parole.[127] Extensive advocacy efforts, including litigation, media campaigns, and legislative advocacy are underway with goals of abolishing

juvenile sentences of life without parole in the United States.[128]

Minimum Age of Juvenile Court Jurisdiction

The minimum age of juvenile court jurisdiction is the youngest age at which a child may be referred to a juvenile court for a delinquent act. At the time this policy was written, only 21 states had a minimum age standard, varying from 6 to 11 years of age.[129] In 2017, approximately 29 779 children younger than 12 years were referred to juvenile court, and 3375 were held in detention.[130] Article 40 of the United Nations Convention on the Rights of the Child decrees governments establish "a minimum age below which children shall be presumed not to have the capacity to infringe the penal law"[131] and specified that this age be no younger than 12 years.[132] Many advocates have called for the establishment of state and/or federal laws that set the minimum age of criminal responsibility at no younger than 12 years.[133]

Fines and Fees in the Juvenile Justice System

Juvenile courts throughout the country regularly impose costs that may include court costs, fees for a public defender, probation supervision fees, child support to the state, cost of Global Positioning System monitoring, cost for participation in diversion programs, health care costs, and fines.[134] Low socioeconomic status is a well-established risk factor for involvement with the juvenile justice system, and imposition of such costs may place an undue burden on justice-involved youth and their families.[17] Furthermore, inability or failure to pay these costs may lead to significant consequences for justice-involved youth, including civil judgment, extension of probation, violation of probation, incarceration, suspension of driver's license,

ineligibility for expungement, and imposition of additional fees.[135]

Access to Legal Representation

Children and adolescents accused of crimes have a constitutional right to legal counsel regardless of their ability to pay.[136] However, youth may encounter many barriers to obtaining adequate legal representation. An analysis by the National Juvenile Defender Center[137] found the following:

- only 11 states have a presumption that youth are automatically eligible for an attorney irrespective of financial status;
- no states guarantee lawyers for youth during interrogation; and
- 43 states allow youth to waive their right to a lawyer without first consulting a lawyer.

Youth without adequate access to legal representation throughout their involvement in the justice system may not fully understand their rights and may be influenced to make decisions that are not in their best interest. Recommendations made by the National Juvenile Defender Center[137] include making all youth eligible for a publicly funded juvenile defender, appointing youth a lawyer before interrogation and well in advance of the first court hearing, and prohibiting waiver of counsel until youth have the chance to consult with a lawyer.

Empowerment of Justice-Involved Youth

Decades of research have been conducted on risk factors for juvenile delinquency, protective factors, and outcomes for justice-involved youth; however, until recently, the voices of justice-involved youth have been largely absent from juvenile justice research and policy.[138] Justice-involved youth are the experts of their lived experience and have unique insight into the strengths and weaknesses of the juvenile justice system. Justice-involved youth have demonstrated that when given the opportunity, they can provide both insight into the root causes of juvenile delinquency and offer recommendations for improvement of the juvenile justice system.[138,139]

RECOMMENDATIONS

The following recommendations are provided for caring and advocating for justice-involved youth and their families.

Delivery of Care

- Confined youth should receive the same level and standards of medical, oral, mental health, and substance use care as nonconfined youth accessing care in their communities. Pediatricians should ensure that confidential health care is practiced in accordance with state and local laws, even in correction health clinics.

- All juvenile correctional facilities should adopt and comply with the NCCHC's "Standards for Health Services in Juvenile Detention and Confinement Facilities."

- Facilities should provide youth who are confined for more than 1 week comprehensive preventive services, including a comprehensive history and physical examination; mental health and substance use screening; dental screening; vision screening; pregnancy screening with options counseling; the full range of contraception, including emergency contraception; vaccines; STI and/or HIV testing; adequate pregnancy care; and management of chronic health conditions. Care should be affirming and appropriate for all youth, including those who identify as LGBTQ.

- Consistent with NCCHC recommendations, transgender youth who received hormone therapy before incarceration should have therapy continued without interruption, absent urgent medical reasons to cease treatment.

- All juvenile facilities should implement a comprehensive suicide prevention program that includes ongoing suicide risk assessment.

- Whenever possible, the pediatrician from the medical home should be notified when an adolescent is admitted and discharged from a detention facility. In cases in which confined youth do not have a pediatrician, efforts should be made to establish care in a medical home.

- Strict limits should be placed on the use of restraints for pregnant and hospitalized adolescents.

- Incarcerated youth should maintain eligibility for their existing health insurance benefits. If insurance eligibility is terminated or suspended during confinement, it should be reinstated before release. Eligible uninsured youth should be enrolled in Medicaid while incarcerated.

- Legislation repealing the Medicaid inmate exclusion policy should be supported, thus allowing Medicaid coverage for incarcerated children and adolescents.

Developmentally Appropriate Confinement Facilities

- Children and adolescents should be detained or incarcerated only in facilities with developmentally appropriate programs with staff who are trained to deal with their unique mental health, social, educational, recreational, and supervisory needs and should not be detained in adult facilities.

- Detention facilities and juvenile justice systems should implement a trauma-informed approach that responds to the needs of justice-involved youth and their families.

- Consistent with recommendations of the US Department of Education and Department of Justice, education in confinement facilities should be provided in "a safe, healthy facility-wide climate that prioritizes education, provides the conditions for learning, and encourages the necessary behavioral and social support services that address the individual needs of all youths, including those with disabilities and English learners."[114]

- Use of isolation and solitary confinement for children and adolescents should be prohibited.

- Because of documented cases of systemic and recurring maltreatment of confined youth, jurisdictions should establish independent oversight entities for youth confinement facilities.

- Confinement facilities should recognize and respond to the unique needs of justice-involved female youth, LGBTQ youth, and youth with chronic medical, mental health, and developmental needs.

Advocacy and Juvenile Justice Reform

Many opportunities exist for pediatricians to advocate for juvenile justice reform. Pediatricians can work with the AAP chapter in their state, justice-involved youth and their families, the juvenile justice sections of their state judiciary and bar, state and local governmental officials, detention facilities, and community organizations serving justice-involved youth. Although key issues may vary between jurisdictions, priority targets for juvenile justice reform may include the following recommendations:

- Incarceration of adolescents is a last resort and only for offenders who have committed serious crimes and cannot be safely placed in a community-based program.

- Support research and advocacy efforts aimed at eliminating racial and ethnic disparities within the justice system. Research and advocacy efforts should include an examination of racial and/or ethnic bias throughout the justice system and focus on delinquency prevention by mitigating the impact of interpersonal and structural racism.

- Support legislation that establishes a minimum age of (at least) 12 years for criminal responsibility under which a person may not be charged with a crime.

- Support legislation abolishing sentencing of adolescents to life without the possibility of parole.

- Support legislation reducing and/or eliminating the imposition of fees and fines for justice-involved youth and their families.

- Support legislation ensuring all justice-involved youth receive adequate and timely legal representation.

- Advocate for adolescents to be prosecuted in the juvenile justice system. Transfer to the adult court should occur only after judicial review. A youth's mental health status and exposure to trauma, adversity, and ACEs should be considered as mitigating factors.

- Advocate for research to identify risk factors for involvement with the justice system, protective factors, outcomes for incarcerated youth, and effectiveness of community-based alternatives to incarceration and use resulting data to make evidence-based juvenile justice policy reforms.

- Engage justice-involved youth and families as advocates for juvenile delinquency prevention and juvenile justice reform.

LEAD AUTHORS

Mikah C. Owen, MD, MPH, FAAP
Stephenie B. Wallace, MD, MSPH, FAAP

COMMITTEE ON ADOLESCENCE, 2019–2020

Elizabeth M. Alderman, MD, FAAP, FSAHM, Chairperson
Richard Chung, MD, FAAP
Laura K. Grubb, MD, MPH, FAAP
Janet Lee, MD, FAAP
Makia E. Powers, MD, MPH, FAAP
Maria H. Rahmandar, MD, FAAP
Krishna K. Upadhya, MD, FAAP
Stephenie B. Wallace, MD, MSPH, FAAP

FORMER COMMITTEE MEMBER

Cora C. Breuner, MD, MPH, FAAP, Immediate Past Chairperson

LIAISONS

Liwei L. Hua, MD, PhD – *American Academy of Child and Adolescent Psychiatry*
Ellie Vyver, MD – *Canadian Paediatric Society*
Geri Hewitt, MD – *American College of Obstetricians and Gynecologists*

Seema Menon, MD – *North American Society of Pediatric and Adolescent Gynecology*
Lauren B. Zapata, PhD, MSPH – *Centers for Disease Control and Prevention*

STAFF

Karen Smith
James Baumberger, MPP

ABBREVIATIONS

AACAP: American Academy of Child and Adolescent Psychiatry
AAP: American Academy of Pediatrics
ACE: adverse childhood experience
ACOG: American College of Obstetricians and Gynecologists
ED: emergency department
JJDPA: Juvenile Justice Delinquency and Prevention Act
JRFC: Juvenile Residential Facility Census
LGBTQ: lesbian, gay, bisexual, transgender, and queer and/or questioning
NCCHC: National Commission on Correctional Health Care
PCP: primary care provider
STI: sexually transmitted infection
SYRP: Survey of Youth in Residential Placement

POTENTIAL CONFLICT OF INTEREST: The authors have indicated they have no potential conflicts of interest to disclose.

REFERENCES

1. US Department of Justice; Office of Justice Programs; Office of Juvenile Justice and Delinquency Prevention. Law enforcement & juvenile crime. Juvenile arrests: estimated number of juvenile arrests, 2017. Available at: https://www.ojjdp.gov/ojstatbb/crime/qa05101.asp?qaDate=2017. Accessed December 18, 2019

2. US Department of Justice; Office of Justice Programs; Office of Juvenile Justice and Delinquency Prevention. Law enforcement & juvenile crime. Trends in the number of arrests by age group for all offenses. Available at: https://www.ojjdp.gov/ojstatbb/crime/ucr_trend.asp?table_in=1. Accessed December 18, 2019

3. US Department of Justice; Office of Justice Programs; Office of Juvenile Justice and Delinquency Prevention. Detained delinquency cases, 1985–2017. Available at: https://www.ojjdp.gov/ojstatbb/court/qa06301.asp?qaDate=2018&text=yes. Accessed May 20, 2020

4. US Department of Justice; Office of Justice Programs; Office of Juvenile Justice and Delinquency Prevention. Juveniles in corrections. Time in placement: median days in placement since admission, by placement status, 1997-2017. Available at: https://www.ojjdp.gov/ojstatbb/corrections/qa08405.asp?qaDate=2017. Accessed December 18, 2019

5. US Department of Justice; Office of Justice Programs; Office of Juvenile Justice and Delinquency Prevention. Juvenile justice system structure & process. Case flow diagram. Available at: https://www.ojjdp.gov/ojstatbb/structure_process/case.html. Accessed December 18, 2019

6. National Center for Juvenile Justice; Office of Juvenile Justice and Delinquency Prevention. Juvenile offenders and victims: 2014 national report. 2014. Available at: https://www.ojjdp.gov/ojstatbb/nr2014/downloads/NR2014.pdf. Accessed December 18, 2019

7. National Conference of State Legislatures. Juvenile age of jurisdiction and transfer to adult court laws. Available at: www.ncsl.org/research/civil-and-criminal-justice/juvenile-age-of-jurisdiction-and-transfer-to-adult-court-laws.aspx. Accessed December 18, 2019

8. National Research Council; Division of Behavioral and Social Sciences and Education; Committee on Law and Justice; Committee on a Prioritized Plan to Implement a Developmental Approach in Juvenile Justice Reform. *Implementing Juvenile Justice Reform: The Federal Role.* Washington, DC: National Academies Press; 2014

9. Juvenile Justice Reform Act of 2018, HR 6964, 115th Cong (2017–2018). Publ L No. 115-385. Available at: https://www.congress.gov/115/bills/hr6964/BILLS-115hr6964enr.pdf. Accessed December 18, 2019

10. Federal Interagency Forum on Child and Family Statistics. POP3 race and Hispanic origin composition: percentage of U.S. children ages 0–17 by race and Hispanic origin, 1980–2018 and projected 2019–2050. Available at: https://www.childstats.gov/americaschildren/tables/pop3.asp. Accessed December 18, 2019

11. US Department of Justice; Office of Justice Programs; Office of Juvenile Justice and Delinquency Prevention. Racial and ethnic fairness: juvenile arrest rates by race, 1980–2018. Available at: https://www.ojjdp.gov/ojstatbb/special_topics/qa11502.asp?qaDate=2018&text=yes . Accessed May 20, 2020

12. US Department of Justice; Office of Justice Programs; Office of Juvenile Justice and Delinquency Prevention. Racial and ethnic fairness: case processing characteristics of delinquency offenses by race, 2018. Available at: https://www.ojjdp.gov/ojstatbb/special_topics/qa11601.asp?qaDate=2018

13. US Department of Justice; Office of Justice Programs; Office of Juvenile Justice and Delinquency Prevention. Racial and ethnic fairness: juvenile residential placement rates by race/ethnicity, 1997–2017. Available at: https://www.ojjdp.gov/ojstatbb/special_topics/qa11801.asp?qaDate=2017&text=yes . Accessed May 20, 2020

14. Hockenberry S. *Juveniles in Residential Placement, 2015.* Washington, DC: Office of Juvenile Justice and Delinquency Prevention, Office of Justice Programs, US Department of Justice; 2018

15. Hockenberry S, Puzzanchera C. *Juvenile Court Statistics 2015.* Pittsburgh, PA: National Center for Juvenile Justice; 2018

16. Developmental Services Group, Inc. *Disproportionate Minority Contact.* Washington, DC: Office of Juvenile Justice and Delinquency Prevention, Office of Justice Programs, US Department of Justice; 2014. Available at: https://www.ojjdp.gov/mpg/litreviews/Disproportionate_Minority_Contact.pdf. Accessed December 18, 2019

17. Committee on Assessing Juvenile Justice Reform; Committee on Law and Justice; Division of Behavioral and Social Sciences and Education; National Research Council. In: Bonnie R, Johnson R, Chemers B, Schuck J, eds. *Reforming Juvenile Justice: A Developmental Approach.* Washington, DC: National Academies Press; 2013

18. Kakade M, Duarte C, Liu X, et al. Adolescent substance use and other illegal behaviors and racial disparities in criminal justice system involvement: findings from a US national survey. *Am J Public Health.* 2012;102(7):1307–1310

19. Spinney E, Cohen M, Feyerherm W, Stephenson R, Yeide M, Shreve T. Disproportionate minority contact in the U.S. juvenile justice system: a review of the DMC literature, 2001–2014, Part 1. *J Crime Justice.* 2018;41(5):596–626

20. Trent M, Dooley D, Dougé J; Section on Adolescent Health; Council on Community Pediatrics; Committee on Adolescence. The impact of racism on child and adolescent health. *Pediatrics.* 2019;144(2):e20191765

21. Council on Community Pediatrics. Poverty and child health in the United States. *Pediatrics.* 2016;137(4): e20160339

22. Council on Community Pediatrics and Committee on Native American Child Health. Policy statement--health equity and children's rights. *Pediatrics.* 2010; 125(4):838–849

23. Garner AS, Shonkoff JP; Committee on Psychosocial Aspects of Child and Family Health; Committee on Early Childhood, Adoption, and Dependent Care; Section on Developmental and Behavioral Pediatrics. Early childhood adversity, toxic stress, and the role of the pediatrician: translating development science into lifelong health. *Pediatrics.* 2012;129(1). Available at: www.pediatrics.org/cgi/content/full/129/1/e224

24. Baglivio M, Epps N, Swartz K, Huq M, Sheer A, Hardt N. The prevalence of adverse childhood experiences (ACE) in the lives of juvenile offenders. *J Juv Justice.* 2014;3(2):1–23

25. Kerig PK, Ford JD. *Trauma Among Girls in the Juvenile Justice System.* Los Angeles, CA: National Child Traumatic Stress Network; 2014. Available at www.nctsn.org/sites/default/files/assets/pdfs/trauma_among_girls_in_the_jj_system_2014.pdf. Accessed December 18, 2019

26. Bucci M, Marques S, Oh D, Harris N. Toxic stress in children and adolescents. *Adv Pediatr.* 2016;63(1): 403–428

27. Dierkhising C, Ko S, Woods-Jaeger B, Briggs E, Lee R, Pynoos R. Trauma histories among justice-involved youth: findings from the National Child Traumatic Stress Network. *Eur J Psychotraumatol.* 2013;4

28. National Child Traumatic Stress Network. *Essential Elements of a Trauma-Informed Juvenile Justice System.* Los Angeles, CA: National Child

Traumatic Stress Network; 2015. Available at: https://www.nctsn.org/sites/default/files/resources//essential_elements_trauma_informed_juvenile_justice_system.pdf. Accessed December 18, 2019

29. US Department of Justice. *Report of the Attorney General's National Task Force on Children Exposed to Violence*. Washington, DC: US Department of Justice; 2012. Available at: https://www.justice.gov/defendingchildhood/cev-rpt-full.pdf. Accessed December 18, 2019

30. Puzzanchera C, Ehreman S; National Center for Juvenile Justice. *Spotlight on Girls in the Juvenile Justice System Snapshot*. Washington, DC: Office of Juvenile Justice and Delinquency Prevention; 2018. Available at: https://www.ojjdp.gov/ojstatbb/snapshots/DataSnapshot_GIRLS2015.pdf. Accessed December 18, 2019

31. US Department of Justice; Office of Justice Programs; Office of Juvenile Justice and Delinquency Prevention. Law enforcement & juvenile crime. Juvenile arrests: demographic characteristics of juvenile arrests, 2017. Available at: https://www.ojjdp.gov/ojstatbb/crime/qa05104.asp?qaDate=2017&text=yes. Accessed January 3, 2020

32. US Department of Justice; Office of Justice Programs; Office of Juvenile Justice and Delinquency Prevention. Juveniles in corrections. Demographics: female proportion of juveniles in residential placement, 2017. Available at: https://www.ojjdp.gov/ojstatbb/corrections/qa08202.asp?qaDate=2017&text=yes. Accessed January 3, 2020

33. The Children's Partnership; Robert F. Kennedy National Resource Center for Juvenile Justice. *Building a Brighter Future for Youth With Dual Status: A Policy Roadmap Forward*. Boston, MA: The Children's Partnership/Robert F. Kennedy National Resource Center for Juvenile Justice; 2018. Available at: https://rfknrcjj.org/wp-content/uploads/2018/11/Building-a-Brighter-Future-For-Youth-with-Dual-Status-A-Policy-Roadmap.pdf. Accessed December 18, 2019

34. US Department of Justice; Office of Justice Programs; Office of Juvenile Justice and Delinquency Prevention.

Policy Guidance: Girls and the Juvenile Justice System. Washington, DC: Office of Juvenile Justice and Delinquency Prevention; 2015

35. Development Services Group, Inc. *LGBTQ Youths in the Juvenile Justice System*. Washington, DC: Office of Juvenile Justice and Delinquency Prevention; 2014. Available at: https://www.ojjdp.gov/mpg/litreviews/LGBTQYouthsintheJuvenileJusticeSystem.pdf. Accessed December 18, 2019

36. Majd K, Marksamer J, Reyes C. *Hidden Injustice: Lesbian, Gay, Bisexual and Transgender Youth in Juvenile Courts*. San Francisco, CA: Legal Services for Children/National Juvenile Defender Center/National Center for Lesbian Rights; 2009. Available at: www.nclrights.org/wp-content/uploads/2014/06/hidden_injustice.pdf. Accessed December 18, 2019

37. Wilber S. *A Guide to Juvenile Detention Reform: Lesbian, Gay, Bisexual and Transgender Youth in the Juvenile Justice System*. Baltimore, MD: Annie E. Casey Foundation; 2015. Available at https://www.aecf.org/m/resourcedoc/AECF-lesbiangaybisexualandtransgenderyouthinjj-2015.pdf. Accessed December 18, 2019

38. Irvine A. 'We've had three of them': addressing the invisibility of lesbian, gay, bisexual and gender non-conforming youths in the juvenile justice system. *Columbia J Gend Law*. 2010;19(3):675–701

39. Beck A, Cantor D. *Sexual Victimization in Juvenile Facilities Reported by Youth, 2012: National Survey of Youth in Custody, 2012*. Washington, DC: Bureau of Justice Statistics, US Department of Justice; 2013

40. Movement Advancement Project; Center for American Progress; Youth First. Unjust: LGBTQ Youth Incarcerated in The Juvenile Justice System. Washington, DC: Center for American Progress; 2017. Available at: https://www.lgbtmap.org/file/lgbtq-incarcerated-youth.pdf. Accessed May 20, 2020

41. US Department of Justice. Prison Rape Elimination Act. 28 CFR §115 (2012). Available at: https://www.prearesourcecenter.org/sites/default/files/content/preafinalstandardstype-

juveniles.pdf. Accessed December 18, 2019

42. Bergen S, Chiu L, Curry T, Gilbert C, Reyes C, Wilber S; The Equity Project. *Toward Equity: A Training Curriculum For Understanding Sexual Orientation, Gender Identity, and Gender Expression, and Developing Competency to serve Lesbian, Gay, Bisexual, and Transgender Youth in the Juvenile Justice System*. Washington, DC: The Equity Project; 2015. Available at: www.equityproject.org/wp-content/uploads/2015/01/Equity_Curriculum_Complete.pdf. Accessed December 18, 2019

43. Routh D, Abess G, Makin D, Stohr M, Hemmens C, Yoo J. Transgender inmates in prisons. *Int J Offender Ther Comp Criminol*. 2017;61(6):645–666

44. National Commission on Correctional Health Care. *Transgender, Transsexual, and Gender Nonconforming Health Care in Correctional Settings*. Chicago, IL: National Commission on Correctional Health Care; 2015. Available at: https://www.ncchc.org/transgender-transsexual-and-gender-nonconforming-health-care. Accessed December 18, 2019

45. Hyland N. *JJGPS StateScan: Dual Status Youth: Data Integration to Support System Integration*. Pittsburgh, PA: National Center for Juvenile Justice; 2016. Available at: www.ncjj.org/pdf/JJGPS%20StateScan/JJGPS_U.S._Dual_Status_Youth_Data_Integration_2016_10.pdf. Accessed December 18, 2019

46. Thomas D; When Systems Collaborate. *How Three Jurisdictions Improved Their Handling of Dual-Status Cases*. Pittsburgh, PA: National Center for Juvenile Justice; 2015

47. Umpierre M. Rights and responsibilities of youth, families, and staff. In: National Institutes of Corrections, ed. *Desktop Guide to Quality Practice for Working With Youth in Confinement*. Washington, DC: National Partnership for Juvenile Services/Office of Juvenile Justice and Delinquency Prevention; 2014. Available at https://info.nicic.gov/dtg/node/11. Accessed December 18, 2019

48. Rold W. Thirty years after *Estell v. Gamble*: a legal retrospective. *J Correct Health Care*. 2008;14(1):11–20

49. Perry R, Morris R. Health care for youth involved with the correctional system. *Prim Care*. 2014;41(3):691–705

50. Acoca L, Stephens J, Van Vleet A. *Health Coverage and Care for Youth in the Juvenile Justice System: The Role of Medicaid and CHIP.* Menlo Park, CA: Kaiser Family Foundation; 2014

51. National Commission on Correctional Health Care. *Standards for Health Services in Juvenile Detention and Confinement Facilities.* Chicago, IL: National Commission on Correctional Health Care; 2015

52. Committee on Adolescence. Health care for youth in the juvenile justice system [published correction appears in *Pediatrics*. 2012;129(3):595]. *Pediatrics*. 2011;128(6):1219–1235

53. Sedlak A, McPherson K. *Survey of Youth in Residential Placement: Youth's Needs and Services.* Rockville, MD: Westat; 2010

54. Barnert E, Perry R, Morris R. Juvenile incarceration and health. *Acad Pediatr*. 2016;16(2):99–109

55. Morris R, Harrison E, Knox G, Tromanhauser E, Marquis D, Watts L. Health risk behavioral survey from 39 juvenile correctional facilities in the United States. *J Adolesc Health*. 1995; 17(6):334–344

56. Donaldson A, Burns J, Bradshaw C, Ellen J, Maehr J. Screening juvenile justice-involved females for sexually transmitted infection: a pilot intervention for urban females in community supervision. *J Correct Health Care*. 2013;19(4):258–268

57. Gray S, Holmes K, Bradford D. Factors associated with pregnancy among incarcerated African American adolescent girls. *J Urban Health*. 2016; 93(4):709–718

58. Grubb L, Beyda R, Eissa M, Benjamins L. A contraception quality improvement initiative with detained young women: counseling, initiation, and utilization. *J Pediatr Adolesc Gynecol*. 2018;31(4): 405–410

59. Danielson C, Walsh K, McCauley J, et al. HIV-related sexual risk behavior among African American adolescent girls. *J Womens Health (Larchmt)*. 2014;23(5): 413–419

60. Committee on Adolescence. Contraception for adolescents. *Pediatrics*. 2014;134(4). Available at: www.pediatrics.org/cgi/content/full/134/4/e1244

61. Committee on Health Care for Underserved Women of American College Obstetricians and Gynecologists. ACOG Committee Opinion No. 511: Health care for pregnant and postpartum incarcerated women and adolescent females. Obstet Gynecol. 2011;118(5):1198-1202. doi:10.1097/AOG.0b013e31823b17e3 (Reaffirmed in 2016)

62. American Medical Association. *An "Act to Prohibit the Shackling of Pregnant Prisoners." Model State Legislation.* Chicago, IL: American Medical Association; 2015. Available at: https://www.ama-assn.org/sites/ama-assn.org/files/corp/media-browser/specialty%20group/arc/shackling-pregnant-prisoners-issue-brief.pdf. Accessed December 18, 2019

63. American Academy of Pediatrics. Tuberculosis. In: Kimberlin D, Brady M, Jackson M, Long S, eds. *Red Book: 2018 Report of the Committee on Infectious Diseases*, 31st ed. Itasca, IL: American Academy of Pediatrics; 2018:829–853

64. Centers for Disease Control and Prevention (CDC); National Center for HIV/AIDS, Viral Hepatitis, STD, and TB Prevention. Prevention and control of tuberculosis in correctional and detention facilities: recommendations from CDC. Endorsed by the Advisory Council for the Elimination of Tuberculosis, the National Commission on Correctional Health Care, and the American Correctional Association. *MMWR Recomm Rep*. 2006;55(RR):1–44

65. Centers for Disease Control and Prevention. *Sexually Transmitted Disease Surveillance 2011.* Atlanta, GA: US Department of Health and Human Services; 2012

66. Centers for Disease Control and Prevention. HIV and youth. Available at: https://www.cdc.gov/hiv/group/age/youth/index.html. Accessed December 18, 2019

67. Gaskin G, Glanz J, Binswanger I, Anoshiravani A. Immunization coverage among juvenile justice detainees. *J Correct Health Care*. 2015;21(3): 265–275

68. Balogun T, Troisi C, Swartz M, Lloyd L, Beyda R. Does juvenile detention impact health? *J Correct Health Care*. 2018; 24(2):137–144

69. Underwood L, Washington A. Mental illness and juvenile offenders. *Int J Environ Res Public Health*. 2016;13(2): 228

70. Shufelt J, Cocozza J. *Youth With Mental Health Disorders in the Juvenile Justice System: Results from a Multi-State Prevalence Study. Research and Program Brief.* New York, NY: National Center for Mental Health and Juvenile Justice; 2006

71. Harzke A, Baillargeon J, Baillargeon G, et al. Prevalence of psychiatric disorders in the Texas juvenile correctional system. *J Correct Health Care*. 2012;18(2):143–157

72. Development Services Group, Inc. *Intersection Between Mental Health and the Juvenile Justice System.* Washington, DC: Office of Juvenile Justice and Delinquency Prevention; 2017. Available at: https://www.ojjdp.gov/mpg/litreviews/Intersection-Mental-Health-Juvenile-Justice.pdf. Accessed December 18, 2019

73. Abram KM, Teplin LA, King DC, et al. *PTSD, Trauma, and Comorbid Psychiatric Disorders in Detained Youth.* Washington, DC: Office of Juvenile Justice and Delinquency Prevention; 2013. Available at: https://www.ojjdp.gov/pubs/239603.pdf. Accessed December 18, 2019

74. Barnert E, Abrams L, Bath E. Solving the high unmet behavioral health treatment needs of adolescents involved in the justice system. *J Adolesc Health*. 2019; 64(6):687–688

75. White L, Aalsma M, Salyers M, et al. Behavioral health service utilization among detained adolescents: a meta-analysis of prevalence and potential moderators. *J Adolesc Health*. 2019; 64(6):700–708

76. Grasso D, Ford J, Briggs-Gowan M. Early life trauma exposure and stress sensitivity in young children. *J Pediatr Psychol*. 2013;38(1):94–103

77. Ford J, Elhai J, Connor D, Frueh B. Poly-victimization and risk of posttraumatic,

depressive, and substance use disorders and involvement in delinquency in a national sample of adolescents. *J Adolesc Health.* 2010; 46(6):545–552

78. National Center for Mental Health and Juvenile Justice. Trauma among youth in the juvenile justice system. 2016. Available at: https://www.ncmhjj.com/wp-content/uploads/2016/09/Trauma-Among-Youth-in-the-Juvenile-Justice-System-for-WEBSITE.pdf. Accessed December 18, 2019

79. Cannon Y, Hsi A. Disrupting the path from childhood trauma to juvenile justice: an upstream health and justice approach. *Fordham Urban Law J.* 2016; 43(3):425–493

80. D'Andrea W, Ford J, Stolbach B, Spinazzola J, van der Kolk B. Understanding interpersonal trauma in children: why we need a developmentally appropriate trauma diagnosis. *Am J Orthopsychiatry.* 2012; 82(2):187–200

81. Johnston L, Miech R, O'Malley P, Bachman J, Schulenberg J, Patrick M. *Monitoring the Future National Survey Results on Drug Use 1975–2018: Overview, Key Findings on Adolescent Drug Use.* Ann Arbor, MI: Institute for Social Research, University of Michigan; 2019

82. Development Services Group, Inc. *Diversion From Formal Juvenile Court Processing.* Washington, DC: Office of Juvenile Justice and Delinquency Prevention; 2017. Available at: https://www.ojjdp.gov/mpg/litreviews/Diversion_Programs.pdf. Accessed December 18, 2019

83. Hockenberry S, Wachter A, Sladky A. *Juvenile Residential Facility Census, 2014: Selected Findings.* Washington, DC: Office of Juvenile Justice and Delinquency Prevention; 2016. Available at: https://ojjdp.ojp.gov/sites/g/files/xyckuh176/files/pubs/250123.pdf. Accessed December 18, 2019

84. American Academy of Child and Adolescent Psychiatry. AACAP position statement on oversight of psychotropic medication use for children in state custody: a best principles guideline. Available at: https://www.aacap.org/App_Themes/AACAP/docs/clinical_practice_center/systems_of_care/Foste

rCare_BestPrinciples_FINAL.pdf. Accessed December 18, 2019

85. Penn J, Thomas C. Practice parameter for the assessment and treatment of youth in juvenile detention and correctional facilities. *J Am Acad Child Adolesc Psychiatry.* 2005;44(10): 1085–1098

86. Cohen E, Pfeifer J, Wallace N. Use of psychiatric medications in juvenile detention facilities and the impact of state placement policy. *J Child Fam Stud.* 2014;23:738–744

87. Lyons C, Wasserman G, Olfson M, McReynolds L, Musabegovic H, Keating J. Psychotropic medication patterns among youth in juvenile justice. *Adm Policy Ment Health.* 2013;40(2):58–68

88. Jonas B, Gu Q, Albertorio-Diaz J. Psychotropic medication use among adolescents: United States, 2005-2010. *NCHS Data Brief.* 2013;(135):1–8

89. Abram KM, Choe JY, Washburn JJ, et al. Suicidal thoughts and behaviors among detained youth. 2014. Available at: https://ojjdp.ojp.gov/sites/g/files/xyckuh176/files/pubs/243891.pdf. Accessed December 18, 2019

90. Stokes M, McCoy K, Abram K, Byck G, Teplin L. Suicidal ideation and behavior in youth in the juvenile justice system: a review of the literature. *J Correct Health Care.* 2015;21(3):222–242

91. US Department of Justice; Office of Juvenile Justice and Delinquency Prevention. *Juvenile Suicide in Confinement: A National Survey.* Washington, DC: Office of Juvenile Justice and Delinquency Prevention; 2009. Available at: www.ncjrs.gov/pdffiles1/ojjdp/213691.pdf. Accessed December 18, 2019

92. Gallagher C, Dobrin A. Facility-level characteristics associated with serious suicide attempts and deaths from suicide in juvenile justice residential facilities. *Suicide Life Threat Behav.* 2006;36(3):363–375

93. Hayes LM. Characteristics of juvenile suicide in confinement. 2009. Available at: www.ncjrs.gov/pdffiles1/ojjdp/214434.pdf. Accessed December 18, 2019

94. Acoca L, Stephens J, Van Vleet A. *Health Coverage and Care for Youth in the Juvenile Justice System: The Role of*

Medicaid and CHIP. Menlo Park, CA: Kaiser Family Foundation; 2014. Available at: https://www.kff.org/medicaid/issue-brief/health-coverage-and-care-for-youth-in-the-juvenile-justice-system-the-role-of-medicaid-and-chip/. Accessed December 18, 2019

95. SUPPORT for Patients and Communities Act, HR 6, 115th Cong (2017–2018). Available at: https://www.congress.gov/bill/115th-congress/house-bill/6. Accessed December 18, 2019

96. Winkelman T, Genao I, Wildeman C, Wang E. Emergency department and hospital use among adolescents with justice system involvement. *Pediatrics.* 2017;140(5):e20171144

97. Beyda R, Balogun T, Trojan N, Eissa M. Medical homes for detained youth. *J Adolesc Health.* 2015;56(2):S16–S17

98. Aalsma M, Anderson V, Schwartz K, et al. Preventive care use among justice-involved and non-justice-involved youth. *Pediatrics.* 2017;140(5): e20171107

99. Zemel S, Mooney K, Justice D, Baudouin K; National Academy for State Health Policy. *Facilitating Access to Health Care Coverage for Juvenile Justice-Involved Youth. Models for Change. Systems Reform in Juvenile Justice.* Washington, DC: National Academy for State Health Policy; 2013. Available at: https://nashp.org/wp-content/uploads/sites/default/files/Facilitating_Access_to_Health_Care_Coverage.pdf. Accessed December 18, 2019

100. Burrell S. *Trauma and the Environment of Care in Juvenile Institutions.* Los Angeles, CA: National Center for Child Traumatic Stress; 2013. Available at https://www.nctsn.org/sites/default/files/resources//trauma_and_environment_of_care_in_juvenile_institutions.pdf. Accessed December 18, 2019

101. Mendel RA. *Maltreatment of Youth in U.S. Juvenile Corrections Facilities: An Update.* Baltimore, MD: The Annie E. Casey Foundation; 2015. Available at https://www.aecf.org/m/resourcedoc/aecf-maltreatmentyouthuscorrections-2015.pdf. Accessed December 18, 2019

102. National Council of Juvenile and Family Court Judges. Resolution regarding the need for independent oversight of youth confinement facilities. 2017. Available at: https://www.ncjfcj.org/wp-

content/uploads/2019/08/regarding-the-need-for-independent-oversight-of-youth-confinement-facilities.pdf. Accessed May 20, 2020

103. Center for Children's Law and Policy. Independent monitoring systems for juvenile facilities. 2012. Available at: www.cclp.org/wp-content/uploads/2016/06/IM.pdf. Accessed December 18, 2019

104. The Annie E. Casey Foundation. Juvenile Detention Alternatives Initiative (JDAI). Available at: https://www.aecf.org/work/juvenile-justice/jdai/. Accessed December 18, 2019

105. Stop Solitary for Kids. Position statement with supporters. Available at: https://www.stopsolitaryforkids.org/wp-content/uploads/2017/03/Position-Statement-with-Supporters-7-6-18.pdf. Accessed December 18, 2019

106. American Civil Liberties Union. *Alone & Afraid: Children Held in Solitary Confinement and Isolation in Juvenile Detention and Correctional Facilities.* New York, NY: American Civil Liberties Union; 2014. Available at: https://www.aclu.org/report/alone-afraid. Accessed December 18, 2019

107. Smith P. The effects of solitary confinement on prison inmates: a brief history and review of the literature. *Crime Justice.* 2006;34(1):441–568

108. Hayes LM. *Juvenile Suicide in Confinement: A National Survey.* Washington, DC: Office of Juvenile Delinquency and Prevention; 2009. Available at: https://www.ncjrs.gov/pdffiles1/ojjdp/213691.pdf. Accessed December 18, 2019

109. US Department of Justice. U.S. Department Justice report and recommendations concerning the use of restrictive housing. 2016. Available at: https://www.justice.gov/archives/dag/file/815551/download. Accessed December 18, 2019

110. First Step Act, S 3649, 115th Cong, 2nd Sess (2017–2018) Available at: https://www.congress.gov/bill/115th-congress/senate-bill/3649/text?q=%7B%22search%22%3A%5B%22S.+3649%22%5D%7D&r=1#toc-iddf565a43-5d49-48a4-9f05-011eb4e57668. Accessed December 18, 2019

111. Kraner NJ, Barrowclough ND, Weiss C, Fisch J; Lowenstein Center for the

Public Interest. 51 – jurisdiction survey of juvenile solitary confinement rules in juvenile justice systems. 2016. Available at: https://www.lowenstein.com/media/2825/51-jurisdiction-survey-of-juvenile-solitary-confinement-rules-72616.pdf. Accessed December 18, 2019

112. Council of Juvenile Correctional Administrators. Council of Juvenile Correctional Administrators Toolkit: reducing the use of isolation. 2015. Available at: http://dcfs.nv.gov/uploadedFiles/dcfsnvgov/content/Programs/JJS/CJCA%20Toolkit%20Reducing%20the%20use%20of%20Isolation.pdf. Accessed December 18, 2019

113. US Department of Education and Office of Civil Rights. Protecting the civil rights of students in the juvenile justice system. 2016. Available at: https://www2.ed.gov/about/offices/list/ocr/docs/2013-14-juvenile-justice.pdf. Accessed December 18, 2019

114. US Department of Education; US Department of Justice. Guiding principles for providing high-quality education in juvenile justice secure care settings. 2014. Available at: https://www2.ed.gov/policy/gen/guid/correctional-education/guiding-principles.pdf. Accessed December 18, 2019

115. Developmental Services Group, Inc. *Youths With Intellectual and Developmental Disabilities in the Juvenile Justice System.* Washington, DC: Office of Juvenile Justice and Delinquency Prevention; 2017. Available at: https://www.ojjdp.gov/mpg/litreviews/Intellectual-Developmental-Disabilities.pdf. Accessed December 18, 2019

116. The Arc National Center on Criminal Justice and Disability. *Violence, Abuse and Bullying Affecting People With Intellectual/Developmental Disabilities: A Call to Action for the Criminal Justice Community.* Washington, DC: The Arc National Center on Criminal Justice and Disability; 2015. Available at: https://thearc.org/wp-content/uploads/forchapters/NCCJD%20White%20Paper%20%231%20Violence%20Abuse%20Bullying_5.pdf. Accessed December 18, 2019

117. Balvin N, Banati P, eds. The adolescent brain: a second window of opportunity - a compendium. 2017. Available at:

https://www.unicef-irc.org/publications/933-the-adolescent-brain-a-second-window-of-opportunity-a-compendium.html. Accessed December 18, 2019

118. Mendel RA. *No Place for Kids: The Case for Reducing Juvenile Incarceration.* Baltimore, MD: The Annie E. Casey Foundation; 2011. Available at https://www.aecf.org/resources/no-place-for-kids-full-report/. Accessed December 18, 2019

119. McCarthy P, Schiraldi V, Shark M. *The Future of Youth Justice: A Community-Based Alternative to the Youth Prison Model.* Washington, DC: US Department of Justice, National Institute of Justice; 2016. Available at: https://www.ncjrs.gov/pdffiles1/nij/250142.pdf. Accessed December 18, 2019

120. US Department of Justice; Office of Juvenile Justice and Delinquency Prevention. *OJJPD Research: Making a Difference for Juveniles.* Washington, DC: Office of Juvenile Justice and Delinquency Prevention; 1999. Available at: www.ncjrs.gov/pdffiles1/177602.pdf. Accessed December 18, 2019

121. Griffin P, Addie S, Adams B, Firestine K. *Trying Juveniles as Adults: An Analysis of State Transfer Laws and Reporting.* Washington, DC: Office of Juvenile Justice and Delinquency Prevention; 2011. Available at: https://www.ncjrs.gov/pdffiles1/ojjdp/232434.pdf. Accessed December 18, 2019

122. Redding R. *Juvenile Transfer Laws: An Effective Deterrent To Delinquency?.* Washington, DC: Office of Juvenile Justice and Delinquency Prevention; 2010. Available at: https://www.ncjrs.gov/pdffiles1/ojjdp/220595.pdf. Accessed December 18, 2019

123. Thomas J. *Raising the Bar: State Trends in Keeping Youth Out of Adult Courts (2015-2017),* 4th ed. Washington, DC: Campaign for Youth Justice; 2017

124. Colorado Juvenile Defender Center. Direct file & transfer to adult court. Available at: http://cjdc.org/wp/juvenile-justice-policy/direct-file/. Accessed December 18, 2019

125. *Roper v Simmons,* 543 US 551 (2005), 112 SW 3d 397, affirmed

126. *Miller v Alabama,* 567 US xxx (2012). Available at: https://www.

supremecourt.gov/opinions/11pdf/10-9646g2i8.pdf. Accessed December 18, 2019

127. Kloepfer A. Denial of hope: sentencing children to life in prison without the possibility of parole. *J Civil Rights Econ Dev.* 2012;26(2):387–413

128. Columbia Law School Human Rights Institute. Challenging juvenile life without parole: how has human rights made a difference. 2014. Available at: https://web.law.columbia.edu/sites/default/files/microsites/human-rights-institute/files/jlwop_case_study_hri_0.pdf. Accessed May 20, 2020

129. National Juvenile Defender Center. Minimum age for delinquency adjudication—multi-jurisdiction survey. 2016. Available at: https://njdc.info/practice-policy-resources/state-profiles/multi-jurisdiction-data/minimum-age-for-delinquency-adjudication-multi-jurisdiction-survey/. Accessed December 18, 2019

130. Sickmund M, Sladky A, Kang W. Easy access to juvenile court statistics: 1985-2018: year of disposition by age at referral Available: https://www.ojjdp.gov/ojstatbb/ezajcs/asp/display.asp. Accessed December 18, 2019

131. United Nations Human Rights Office of the High Commissioner. Convention on the Rights of the Child. Available at: www.ohchr.org/EN/ProfessionalInterest/Pages/CRC.aspx. Accessed December 18, 2019

132. United Nations Committee on the Rights of the Child. United Nations Convention on the Rights of the Child. Available at: www2.ohchr.org/English/bodies/crc/docs/CRC.C.GC.10.pdf. Accessed December 18, 2019

133. Barnert E, Abrams L, Maxson C, et al. Setting a minimum age for juvenile justice jurisdiction in California. *Int J Prison Health.* 2017;13(1):49–56

134. Feierman J, Goldstein N, Haney-Caron E, Columbo JF. Debtors' prison for kids? The high cost of fines and fees in the juvenile justice system. 2016. Available at: https://debtorsprison.jlc.org/documents/JLC-Debtors-Prison.pdf. Accessed December 18, 2019

135. National Juvenile Defender Center. The cost of juvenile probation: a critical look into juvenile supervision fees. Available at: http://njdc.info/wp-content/uploads/2017/08/NJDC_The-Cost-of-Juvenile-Probation.pdf. Accessed December 18, 2019

136. United States Courts. Facts and case summary – in re Gault. Available at: https://www.uscourts.gov/educational-resources/educational-activities/facts-and-case-summary-re-gault. Accessed December 18, 2019

137. National Juvenile Defender Center. Access denied: a national snapshot of states' failure to protect children's right to counsel. 2017. Available at: https://njdc.info/wp-content/uploads/2017/05/Snapshot-Final_single-4.pdf. Accessed December 18, 2019

138. Barnert E, Perry R, Azzi V, et al. Incarcerated youth's perspectives on protective factors and risk factors for juvenile offending: a qualitative analysis. *Am J Public Health.* 2015; 105(7):1365–1371

139. The Pittsburgh Foundation. A qualitative study of youth and the juvenile justice system. A 100 Percent Pittsburgh Pilot Project. Available at: https://pittsburghfoundation.org/sites/default/files/100%20Percent%20Pittsburgh%20–%20Youth%20and%20Juvenile%20Justice%20Report.pdf. Accessed December 18, 2019

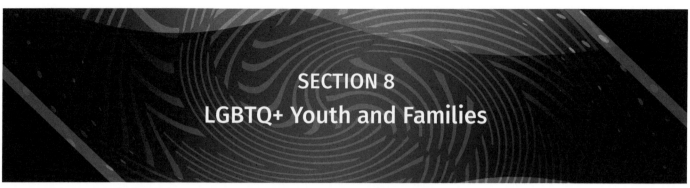

SECTION 8
LGBTQ+ Youth and Families

Some articles are available online only; scan the QR code to access online content.

POLICY STATEMENT Organizational Principles to Guide and Define the Child Health Care System and/or Improve the Health of all Children

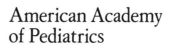

American Academy of Pediatrics

DEDICATED TO THE HEALTH OF ALL CHILDREN™

This Policy Statement was reaffirmed August 2023.

Ensuring Comprehensive Care and Support for Transgender and Gender-Diverse Children and Adolescents

Jason Rafferty, MD, MPH, EdM, FAAP, COMMITTEE ON PSYCHOSOCIAL ASPECTS OF CHILD AND FAMILY HEALTH, COMMITTEE ON ADOLESCENCE, SECTION ON LESBIAN, GAY, BISEXUAL, AND TRANSGENDER HEALTH AND WELLNESS

abstract

As a traditionally underserved population that faces numerous health disparities, youth who identify as transgender and gender diverse (TGD) and their families are increasingly presenting to pediatric providers for education, care, and referrals. The need for more formal training, standardized treatment, and research on safety and medical outcomes often leaves providers feeling ill equipped to support and care for patients that identify as TGD and families. In this policy statement, we review relevant concepts and challenges and provide suggestions for pediatric providers that are focused on promoting the health and positive development of youth that identify as TGD while eliminating discrimination and stigma.

Department of Pediatrics, Hasbro Children's Hospital, Providence, Rhode Island; Thundermist Health Centers, Providence, Rhode Island; and Department of Child Psychiatry, Emma Pendleton Bradley Hospital, East Providence, Rhode Island

Dr Rafferty conceptualized the statement, drafted the initial manuscript, reviewed and revised the manuscript, approved the final manuscript as submitted, and agrees to be accountable for all aspects of the work.

Policy statements from the American Academy of Pediatrics benefit from expertise and resources of liaisons and internal (AAP) and external reviewers. However, policy statements from the American Academy of Pediatrics may not reflect the views of the liaisons or the organizations or government agencies that they represent.

The guidance in this statement does not indicate an exclusive course of treatment or serve as a standard of medical care. Variations, taking into account individual circumstances, may be appropriate.

All policy statements from the American Academy of Pediatrics automatically expire 5 years after publication unless reaffirmed, revised, or retired at or before that time.

INTRODUCTION

In its dedication to the health of all children, the American Academy of Pediatrics (AAP) strives to improve health care access and eliminate disparities for children and teenagers who identify as lesbian, gay, bisexual, transgender, or questioning (LGBTQ) of their sexual or gender identity.[1,2] Despite some advances in public awareness and legal protections, youth who identify as LGBTQ continue to face disparities that stem from multiple sources, including inequitable laws and policies, societal discrimination, and a lack of access to quality health care, including mental health care. Such challenges are often more intense for youth who do not conform to social expectations and norms regarding gender. Pediatric providers are increasingly encountering such youth and their families, who seek medical advice and interventions, yet they may lack the formal training to care for youth that identify as transgender and gender diverse (TGD) and their families.[3]

This policy statement is focused specifically on children and youth that identify as TGD rather than the larger LGBTQ population, providing brief, relevant background on the basis of current available research

To cite: Rafferty J, AAP COMMITTEE ON PSYCHOSOCIAL ASPECTS OF CHILD AND FAMILY HEALTH, AAP COMMITTEE ON ADOLESCENCE, AAP SECTION ON LESBIAN, GAY, BISEXUAL, AND TRANSGENDER HEALTH AND WELLNESS. Ensuring Comprehensive Care and Support for Transgender and Gender-Diverse Children and Adolescents. *Pediatrics.* 2018;142(4): e20182162

TABLE 1 Relevant Terms and Definitions Related to Gender Care

Term	Definition
Sex	An assignment that is made at birth, usually male or female, typically on the basis of external genital anatomy but sometimes on the basis of internal gonads, chromosomes, or hormone levels
Gender identity	A person's deep internal sense of being female, male, a combination of both, somewhere in between, or neither, resulting from a multifaceted interaction of biological traits, environmental factors, self-understanding, and cultural expectations
Gender expression	The external way a person expresses their gender, such as with clothing, hair, mannerisms, activities, or social roles
Gender perception	The way others interpret a person's gender expression
Gender diverse	A term that is used to describe people with gender behaviors, appearances, or identities that are incongruent with those culturally assigned to their birth sex; gender-diverse individuals may refer to themselves with many different terms, such as transgender, nonbinary, genderqueer,[7] gender fluid, gender creative, gender independent, or noncisgender. "Gender diverse" is used to acknowledge and include the vast diversity of gender identities that exists. It replaces the former term, "gender nonconforming," which has a negative and exclusionary connotation.
Transgender	A subset of gender-diverse youth whose gender identity does not match their assigned sex and generally remains persistent, consistent, and insistent over time; the term "transgender" also encompasses many other labels individuals may use to refer to themselves.
Cisgender	A term that is used to describe a person who identifies and expresses a gender that is consistent with the culturally defined norms of the sex they were assigned at birth
Agender	A term that is used to describe a person who does not identify as having a particular gender
Affirmed gender	When a person's true gender identity, or concern about their gender identity, is communicated to and validated from others as authentic
MTF; affirmed female; trans female	Terms that are used to describe individuals who were assigned male sex at birth but who have a gender identity and/or expression that is asserted to be more feminine
FTM; affirmed male; trans male	Terms that are used to describe individuals who were assigned female sex at birth but who have a gender identity and/or expression that is asserted to be more masculine
Gender dysphoria	A clinical symptom that is characterized by a sense of alienation to some or all of the physical characteristics or social roles of one's assigned gender; also, gender dysphoria is the psychiatric diagnosis in the *DSM-5*, which has focus on the distress that stems from the incongruence between one's expressed or experienced (affirmed) gender and the gender assigned at birth.
Gender identity disorder	A psychiatric diagnosis defined previously in the *DSM-IV* (changed to "gender dysphoria" in the *DSM-5*); the primary criteria include a strong, persistent cross-sex identification and significant distress and social impairment. This diagnosis is no longer appropriate for use and may lead to stigma, but the term may be found in older research.
Sexual orientation	A person's sexual identity in relation to the gender(s) to which they are attracted; sexual orientation and gender identity develop separately.

This list is not intended to be all inclusive. The pronouns "they" and "their" are used intentionally to be inclusive rather than the binary pronouns "he" and "she" and "his" and "her." Adapted from Bonifacio HJ, Rosenthal SM. Gender variance and dysphoria in children and adolescents. *Pediatr Clin North Am*. 2015;62(4):1001–1016. Adapted from Vance SR Jr, Ehrensaft D, Rosenthal SM. Psychological and medical care of gender nonconforming youth. *Pediatrics*. 2014;134(6):1184–1192. DSM-5, *Diagnostic and Statistical Manual of Mental Disorders, Fifth Edition*; DSM-IV, *Diagnostic and Statistical Manual of Mental Disorders, Fourth Edition*; FTM, female to male; MTF, male to female.

and expert opinion from clinical and research leaders, which will serve as the basis for recommendations. It is not a comprehensive review of clinical approaches and nuances to pediatric care for children and youth that identify as TGD. Professional understanding of youth that identify as TGD is a rapidly evolving clinical field in which research on appropriate clinical management is limited by insufficient funding.[3,4]

DEFINITIONS

To clarify recommendations and discussions in this policy statement, some definitions are provided. However, brief descriptions of human behavior or identities may not capture nuance in this evolving field.

"Sex," or "natal gender," is a label, generally "male" or "female," that is typically assigned at birth on the basis of genetic and anatomic characteristics, such as genital anatomy, chromosomes, and sex hormone levels. Meanwhile, "gender identity" is one's internal sense of who one is, which results from a multifaceted interaction of biological traits, developmental influences, and environmental conditions. It may be male, female, somewhere in between, a combination of both, or neither (ie, not conforming to a binary conceptualization of gender). Self-recognition of gender identity develops over time, much the same way as a child's physical body does. For some people, gender identity can be fluid, shifting in different contexts. "Gender expression"

refers to the wide array of ways people display their gender through clothing, hair styles, mannerisms, or social roles. Exploring different ways of expressing gender is common for children and may challenge social expectations. The way others interpret this expression is referred to as "gender perception" (Table 1).[5,6]

These labels may or may not be congruent. The term "cisgender" is used if someone identifies and expresses a gender that is consistent with the culturally defined norms of the sex that was assigned at birth. "Gender diverse" is an umbrella term to describe an ever-evolving array of labels that people may apply when their gender identity, expression, or even perception does not conform to the norms and stereotypes others expect of their assigned sex. "Transgender" is usually reserved for a subset of such youth whose gender identity does not match their assigned sex and generally remains persistent, consistent, and insistent over time. These terms are not diagnoses; rather, they are personal and often dynamic ways of describing one's own gender experience.

Gender identity is not synonymous with "sexual orientation," which refers to a person's identity in relation to the gender(s) to which they are sexually and romantically attracted. Gender identity and sexual orientation are distinct but interrelated constructs.[8] Therefore, being transgender does not imply a sexual orientation, and people who identify as transgender still identify as straight, gay, bisexual, etc, on the basis of their attractions. (For more information, *The Gender Book*, found at www.thegenderbook .com , is a resource with illustrations that are used to highlight these core terms and concepts.)

EPIDEMIOLOGY

In population-based surveys, questions related to gender identity are rarely asked, which makes it difficult to assess the size and characteristics of the population that is TGD. In the 2014 Behavioral Risk Factor Surveillance System of the Centers for Disease Control and Prevention, only 19 states elected to include optional questions on gender identity. Extrapolation from these data suggests that the US prevalence of adults who identify as transgender or "gender nonconforming" is 0.6% (1.4 million), ranging from 0.3% in North Dakota to 0.8% in Hawaii.[9] On the basis of these data, it has been estimated that 0.7% of youth ages 13 to 17 years (~150 000) identify as transgender.[10] This number is much higher than previous estimates, which were

extrapolated from individual states or specialty clinics, and is likely an underestimate given the stigma regarding those who openly identify as transgender and the difficulty in defining "transgender" in a way that is inclusive of all gender-diverse identities.[11]

There have been no large-scale prevalence studies among children and adolescents, and there is no evidence that adult statistics reflect young children or adolescents. In the 2014 Behavioral Risk Factor Surveillance System, those 18 to 24 years of age were more likely than older age groups to identify as transgender (0.7%).[9] Children report being aware of gender incongruence at young ages. Children who later identify as TGD report first having recognized their gender as "different" at an average age of 8.5 years; however, they did not disclose such feelings until an average of 10 years later.[12]

MENTAL HEALTH IMPLICATIONS

Adolescents and adults who identify as transgender have high rates of depression, anxiety, eating disorders, self-harm, and suicide.[13–20] Evidence suggests that an identity of TGD has an increased prevalence among individuals with autism spectrum disorder, but this association is not yet well understood.[21,22] In 1 retrospective cohort study of 180 trans youth and matched cisgender peers, 56 youth who identified as transgender reported previous suicidal ideation, and 31 reported a previous suicide attempt, compared with 20 and 11 among matched youth who identified as cisgender, respectively.[13] Some youth who identify as TGD also experience gender dysphoria, which is a specific diagnosis given to those who experience impairment in peer and/or family relationships, school performance, or other aspects of their life as a consequence of the

incongruence between their assigned sex and their gender identity.[23]

There is no evidence that risk for mental illness is inherently attributable to one's identity of TGD. Rather, it is believed to be multifactorial, stemming from an internal conflict between one's appearance and identity, limited availability of mental health services, low access to health care providers with expertise in caring for youth who identify as TGD, discrimination, stigma, and social rejection.[24] This was affirmed by the American Psychological Association in 2008[25] (with practice guidelines released in 2015[8]) and the American Psychiatric Association, which made the following statement in 2012:

Being transgender or gender variant implies no impairment in judgment, stability, reliability, or general social or vocational capabilities; however, these individuals often experience discrimination due to a lack of civil rights protections for their gender identity or expression.... [Such] discrimination and lack of equal civil rights is damaging to the mental health of transgender and gender variant individuals.[26]

Youth who identify as TGD often confront stigma and discrimination, which contribute to feelings of rejection and isolation that can adversely affect physical and emotional well-being. For example, many youth believe that they must hide their gender identity and expression to avoid bullying, harassment, or victimization. Youth who identify as TGD experience disproportionately high rates of homelessness, physical violence (at home and in the community), substance abuse, and high-risk sexual behaviors.[5,6,12,27–31] Among the 3 million HIV testing events that were reported in 2015, the highest percentages of new infections were among women who identified as transgender[32] and were also at particular risk for not knowing their HIV status.[30]

GENDER-AFFIRMATIVE CARE

In a gender-affirmative care model (GACM), pediatric providers offer developmentally appropriate care that is oriented toward understanding and appreciating the youth's gender experience. A strong, nonjudgmental partnership with youth and their families can facilitate exploration of complicated emotions and gender-diverse expressions while allowing questions and concerns to be raised in a supportive environment.[5] In a GACM, the following messages are conveyed:

- transgender identities and diverse gender expressions do not constitute a mental disorder;

- variations in gender identity and expression are normal aspects of human diversity, and binary definitions of gender do not always reflect emerging gender identities;

- gender identity evolves as an interplay of biology, development, socialization, and culture; and

- if a mental health issue exists, it most often stems from stigma and negative experiences rather than being intrinsic to the child.[27,33]

The GACM is best facilitated through the integration of medical, mental health, and social services, including specific resources and supports for parents and families.[24] Providers work together to destigmatize gender variance, promote the child's self-worth, facilitate access to care, educate families, and advocate for safer community spaces where children are free to develop and explore their gender.[5] A specialized gender-affirmative therapist, when available, may be an asset in helping children and their families build skills for dealing with gender-based stigma, address symptoms of anxiety or depression, and reinforce the child's overall resiliency.[34,35] There is a limited but growing body

of evidence that suggests that using an integrated affirmative model results in young people having fewer mental health concerns whether they ultimately identify as transgender.[24,36,37]

In contrast, "conversion" or "reparative" treatment models are used to prevent children and adolescents from identifying as transgender or to dissuade them from exhibiting gender-diverse expressions. The Substance Abuse and Mental Health Services Administration has concluded that any therapeutic intervention with the goal of changing a youth's gender expression or identity is inappropriate.[33] Reparative approaches have been proven to be not only unsuccessful[38] but also deleterious and are considered outside the mainstream of traditional medical practice.[29,39–42] The AAP described reparative approaches as "unfair and deceptive."[43] At the time of this writing,* conversion therapy was banned by executive regulation in New York and by legislative statutes in 9 other states as well as the District of Columbia.[44]

Pediatric providers have an essential role in assessing gender concerns and providing evidence-based information to assist youth and families in medical decision-making. Not doing so can prolong or exacerbate gender dysphoria and contribute to abuse and stigmatization.[35] If a pediatric provider does not feel prepared to address gender concerns when they occur, then referral to a pediatric or mental health provider with more expertise is appropriate. There is little research on communication and efficacy with transfers in care for youth who identify as TGD,

particularly from pediatric to adult providers.

DEVELOPMENTAL CONSIDERATIONS

Acknowledging that the capacity for emerging abstract thinking in childhood is important to conceptualize and reflect on identity, gender-affirmation guidelines are being focused on individually tailored interventions on the basis of the physical and cognitive development of youth who identify as TGD.[45] Accordingly, research substantiates that children who are prepubertal and assert an identity of TGD know their gender as clearly and as consistently as their developmentally equivalent peers who identify as cisgender and benefit from the same level of social acceptance.[46] This developmental approach to gender affirmation is in contrast to the outdated approach in which a child's gender-diverse assertions are held as "possibly true" until an arbitrary age (often after pubertal onset) when they can be considered valid, an approach that authors of the literature have termed "watchful waiting." This outdated approach does not serve the child because critical support is withheld. Watchful waiting is based on binary notions of gender in which gender diversity and fluidity is pathologized; in watchful waiting, it is also assumed that notions of gender identity become fixed at a certain age. The approach is also influenced by a group of early studies with validity concerns, methodologic flaws, and limited follow-up on children who identified as TGD and, by adolescence, did not seek further treatment ("desisters").[45,47] More robust and current research suggests that, rather than focusing on who a child will become, valuing them for who they are, even at a young age, fosters secure attachment and resilience, not only for the child but also for the whole family.[5,45,48,49]

---

* For more information regarding state-specific laws, please contact the AAP Division of State Government Affairs at stgov@ aap.org.

MEDICAL MANAGEMENT

Pediatric primary care providers are in a unique position to routinely inquire about gender development in children and adolescents as part of recommended well-child visits[50] and to be a reliable source of validation, support, and reassurance. They are often the first provider to be aware that a child may not identify as cisgender or that there may be distress related to a gender-diverse identity. The best way to approach gender with patients is to inquire directly and nonjudgmentally about their experience and feelings before applying any labels.[27, 51]

Many medical interventions can be offered to youth who identify as TGD and their families. The decision of whether and when to initiate gender-affirmative treatment is personal and involves careful consideration of risks, benefits, and other factors unique to each patient and family. Many protocols suggest that clinical assessment of youth who identify as TGD is ideally conducted on an ongoing basis in the setting of a collaborative, multidisciplinary approach, which, in addition to the patient and family, may include the pediatric provider, a mental health provider (preferably with expertise in caring for youth who identify as TGD), social and legal supports, and a pediatric endocrinologist or adolescent-medicine gender specialist, if available.[6, 28] There is no prescribed path, sequence, or end point. Providers can make every effort to be aware of the influence of their own biases. The medical options also vary depending on pubertal and developmental progression.

Clinical Setting

In the past year, 1 in 4 adults who identified as transgender avoided a necessary doctor's visit because of fear of being mistreated.[31] All clinical office staff have a role in affirming a patient's gender identity. Making flyers available or displaying posters related to LGBTQ health issues, including information for children who identify as TGD and families, reveals inclusivity and awareness. Generally, patients who identify as TGD feel most comfortable when they have access to a gender-neutral restroom. Diversity training that encompasses sensitivity when caring for youth who identify as TGD and their families can be helpful in educating clinical and administrative staff. A patient-asserted name and pronouns are used by staff and are ideally reflected in the electronic medical record without creating duplicate charts.[52,53] The US Centers for Medicare and Medicaid Services and the National Coordinator for Health Information Technology require all electronic health record systems certified under the Meaningful Use incentive program to have the capacity to confidentially collect information on gender identity.[54,55] Explaining and maintaining confidentiality procedures promotes openness and trust, particularly with youth who identify as LGBTQ.[1] Maintaining a safe clinical space can provide at least 1 consistent, protective refuge for patients and families, allowing authentic gender expression and exploration that builds resiliency.

Pubertal Suppression

Gonadotrophin-releasing hormones have been used to delay puberty since the 1980s for central precocious puberty.[56] These reversible treatments can also be used in adolescents who experience gender dysphoria to prevent development of secondary sex characteristics and provide time up until 16 years of age for the individual and the family to explore gender identity, access psychosocial supports, develop coping skills, and further define appropriate treatment goals. If pubertal suppression treatment is suspended, then endogenous puberty will resume.[20,57,58]

Often, pubertal suppression creates an opportunity to reduce distress that may occur with the development of secondary sexual characteristics and allow for gender-affirming care, including mental health support for the adolescent and the family. It reduces the need for later surgery because physical changes that are otherwise irreversible (protrusion of the Adam's apple, male pattern baldness, voice change, breast growth, etc) are prevented. The available data reveal that pubertal suppression in children who identify as TGD generally leads to improved psychological functioning in adolescence and young adulthood.[20,57–59]

Pubertal suppression is not without risks. Delaying puberty beyond one's peers can also be stressful and can lead to lower self-esteem and increased risk taking.[60] Some experts believe that genital underdevelopment may limit some potential reconstructive options.[61] Research on long-term risks, particularly in terms of bone metabolism[62] and fertility,[63] is currently limited and provides varied results.[57,64,65] Families often look to pediatric providers for help in considering whether pubertal suppression is indicated in the context of their child's overall well-being as gender diverse.

Gender Affirmation

As youth who identify as TGD reflect on and evaluate their gender identity, various interventions may be considered to better align their gender expression with their underlying identity. This process of reflection, acceptance, and, for some, intervention is known as "gender affirmation." It was formerly referred to as "transitioning," but many view the process as an affirmation and acceptance of who they have always been rather than a transition

TABLE 2 The Process of Gender Affirmation May Include ≥1 of the Following Components

Component	Definition	General Age Range[a]	Reversibility[a]
Social affirmation	Adopting gender-affirming hairstyles, clothing, name, gender pronouns, and restrooms and other facilities	Any	Reversible
Puberty blockers	Gonadotropin-releasing hormone analogues, such as leuprolide and histrelin	During puberty (Tanner stage 2–5)[b]	Reversible[c]
Cross-sex hormone therapy	Testosterone (for those who were assigned female at birth and are masculinizing); estrogen plus androgen inhibitor (for those who were assigned male at birth and are feminizing)	Early adolescence onward	Partially reversible (skin texture, muscle mass, and fat deposition); irreversible once developed (testosterone: Adam's apple protrusion, voice changes, and male pattern baldness; estrogen: breast development); unknown reversibility (effect on fertility)
Gender-affirming surgeries	"Top" surgery (to create a male-typical chest shape or enhance breasts); "bottom" surgery (surgery on genitals or reproductive organs); facial feminization and other procedures	Typically adults (adolescents on case-by-case basis[d])	Not reversible
Legal affirmation	Changing gender and name recorded on birth certificate, school records, and other documents	Any	Reversible

[a] Note that the provided age range and reversibility is based on the little data that are currently available.

[b] There is limited benefit to starting gonadotropin-releasing hormone after Tanner stage 5 for pubertal suppression. However, when cross-sex hormones are initiated with a gradually increasing schedule, the initial levels are often not high enough to suppress endogenous sex hormone secretion. Therefore, gonadotropin-releasing hormone may be continued in accordance with the Endocrine Society Guidelines.[68]

[c] The effect of sustained puberty suppression on fertility is unknown. Pubertal suppression can be, and often is indicated to be, followed by cross-sex hormone treatment. However, when cross-sex hormones are initiated without endogenous hormones, then fertility may be decreased.[68]

[d] Eligibility criteria for gender-affirmative surgical interventions among adolescents are not clearly defined between established protocols and practice. When applicable, eligibility is usually determined on a case-by-case basis with the adolescent and the family along with input from medical, mental health, and surgical providers.[68–71]

from 1 gender identity to another. Accordingly, some people who have gone through the process prefer to call themselves "affirmed females, males, etc" (or just "females, males, etc"), rather than using the prefix "trans-." Gender affirmation is also used to acknowledge that some individuals who identify as TGD may feel affirmed in their gender without pursuing medical or surgical interventions.[7,66]

Supportive involvement of parents and family is associated with better mental and physical health outcomes.[67] Gender affirmation among adolescents with gender dysphoria often reduces the emphasis on gender in their lives, allowing them to attend to other developmental tasks, such as academic success, relationship building, and future-oriented planning.[64] Most protocols for gender-affirming interventions incorporate World Professional Association of Transgender

Health[35] and Endocrine Society[68] recommendations and include ≥1 of the following elements (Table 2):

1. Social Affirmation: This is a reversible intervention in which children and adolescents express partially or completely in their asserted gender identity by adapting hairstyle, clothing, pronouns, name, etc. Children who identify as transgender and socially affirm and are supported in their asserted gender show no increase in depression and only minimal (clinically insignificant) increases in anxiety compared with age-matched averages.[48] Social affirmation can be complicated given the wide range of social interactions children have (eg, extended families, peers, school, community, etc). There is little guidance on the best approach (eg, all at once, gradual, creating new social networks, or affirming within existing networks, etc). Pediatric providers

can best support families by anticipating and discussing such complexity proactively, either in their own practice or through enlisting a qualified mental health provider.

2. Legal Affirmation: Elements of a social affirmation, such as a name and gender marker, become official on legal documents, such as birth certificates, passports, identification cards, school documents, etc. The processes for making these changes depend on state laws and may require specific documentation from pediatric providers.

3. Medical Affirmation: This is the process of using cross-sex hormones to allow adolescents who have initiated puberty to develop secondary sex characteristics of the opposite biological sex. Some changes are partially reversible if hormones are stopped, but others become

irreversible once they are fully developed (Table 2).

4. Surgical Affirmation: Surgical approaches may be used to feminize or masculinize features, such as hair distribution, chest, or genitalia, and may include removal of internal organs, such as ovaries or the uterus (affecting fertility). These changes are irreversible. Although current protocols typically reserve surgical interventions for adults,[35,68] they are occasionally pursued during adolescence on a case-by-case basis, considering the necessity and benefit to the adolescent's overall health and often including multidisciplinary input from medical, mental health, and surgical providers as well as from the adolescent and family.[69–71]

For some youth who identify as TGD whose natal gender is female, menstruation, breakthrough bleeding, and dysmenorrhea can lead to significant distress before or during gender affirmation. The American College of Obstetrics and Gynecology suggests that, although limited data are available to outline management, menstruation can be managed without exogenous estrogens by using a progesterone-only pill, a medroxyprogesterone acetate shot, or a progesterone-containing intrauterine or implantable device.[72] If estrogen can be tolerated, oral contraceptives that contain both progesterone and estrogen are more effective at suppressing menses.[73] The Endocrine Society guidelines also suggest that gonadotrophin-releasing hormones can be used for menstrual suppression before the anticipated initiation of testosterone or in combination with testosterone for breakthrough bleeding (enables phenotypic masculinization at a lower dose than if testosterone is used alone).[68] Masculinizing hormones in natal female patients may lead to a cessation of menses,

but unplanned pregnancies have been reported, which emphasizes the need for ongoing contraceptive counseling with youth who identify as TGD.[72]

HEALTH DISPARITIES

In addition to societal challenges, youth who identify as TGD face several barriers within the health care system, especially regarding access to care. In 2015, a focus group of youth who identified as transgender in Seattle, Washington, revealed 4 problematic areas related to health care:

1. safety issues, including the lack of safe clinical environments and fear of discrimination by providers;

2. poor access to physical health services, including testing for sexually transmitted infections;

3. inadequate resources to address mental health concerns; and

4. lack of continuity with providers.[74]

This study reveals the obstacles many youth who identify as TGD face in accessing essential services, including the limited supply of appropriately trained medical and psychological providers, fertility options, and insurance coverage denials for gender-related treatments.[74]

Insurance denials for services related to the care of patients who identify as TGD are a significant barrier. Although the Office for Civil Rights of the US Department of Health and Human Services explicitly stated in 2012 that the nondiscrimination provision in the Patient Protection and Affordable Care Act includes people who identify as gender diverse,[75,76] insurance claims for gender affirmation, particularly among youth who identify as TGD, are frequently denied.[54,77] In 1 study, it was found that approximately 25% of individuals

who identified as transgender were denied insurance coverage because of being transgender.[31] The burden of covering medical expenses that are not covered by insurance can be financially devastating, and even when expenses are covered, families describe high levels of stress in navigating and submitting claims appropriately.[78] In 2012, a large gender center in Boston, Massachusetts, reported that most young patients who identified as transgender and were deemed appropriate candidates for recommended gender care were unable to obtain it because of such denials, which were based on the premise that gender dysphoria was a mental disorder, not a physical one, and that treatment was not medically or surgically necessary.[24] This practice not only contributes to stigma, prolonged gender dysphoria, and poor mental health outcomes,[77] but it may also lead patients to seek nonmedically supervised treatments that are potentially dangerous.[24] Furthermore, insurance denials can reinforce a socioeconomic divide between those who can finance the high costs of uncovered care and those who cannot.[24,77]

The transgender youth group in Seattle likely reflected the larger TGD population when they described how obstacles adversely affect self-esteem and contribute to the perception that they are undervalued by society and the health care system.[74,77] Professional medical associations, including the AAP, are increasingly calling for equity in health care provisions regardless of gender identity or expression.[1,8,23,72] There is a critical need for investments in research on the prevalence, disparities, biological underpinnings, and standards of care relating to gender-diverse populations. Pediatric providers who work with state government and insurance officials can play an essential role in advocating for stronger nondiscrimination policies and improved coverage.

There is a lack of quality research on the experience of youth of color who identify as transgender. One theory suggests that the intersection of racism, transphobia, and sexism may result in the extreme marginalization that is experienced among many women of color who identify as transgender,[79] including rejection from their family and dropping out of school at younger ages (often in the setting of rigid religious beliefs regarding gender),[80] increased levels of violence and body objectification,[81] 3 times the risk of poverty compared with the general population,[31] and the highest prevalence of HIV compared with other risk groups (estimated as high as 56.3% in 1 meta-analysis).[30] One model suggests that pervasive stigma and oppression can be associated with psychological distress (anxiety, depression, and suicide) and adoption of risk behaviors by such youth to obtain a sense of validation toward their complex identities.[79]

FAMILY ACCEPTANCE

Research increasingly suggests that familial acceptance or rejection ultimately has little influence on the gender identity of youth; however, it may profoundly affect young people's ability to openly discuss or disclose concerns about their identity. Suppressing such concerns can affect mental health.[82] Families often find it hard to understand and accept their child's gender-diverse traits because of personal beliefs, social pressure, and stigma.[49,83] Legitimate fears may exist for their child's welfare, safety, and acceptance that pediatric providers need to appreciate and address. Families can be encouraged to communicate their concerns and questions. Unacknowledged concerns can contribute to shame and hesitation in regard to offering support and understanding,[84]

which is essential for the child's self-esteem, social involvement, and overall health as TGD.[48,85–87] Some caution has been expressed that unquestioning acceptance per se may not best serve questioning youth or their families. Instead, psychological evidence suggests that the most benefit comes when family members and youth are supported and encouraged to engage in reflective perspective taking and validate their own and the other's thoughts and feelings despite divergent views.[49,82]

In this regard, suicide attempt rates among 433 adolescents in Ontario who identified as "trans" were 4% among those with strongly supportive parents and as high as 60% among those whose parents were not supportive.[85] Adolescents who identify as transgender and endorse at least 1 supportive person in their life report significantly less distress than those who only experience rejection. In communities with high levels of support, it was found that nonsupportive families tended to increase their support over time, leading to dramatic improvement in mental health outcomes among their children who identified as transgender.[88]

Pediatric providers can create a safe environment for parents and families to better understand and listen to the needs of their children while receiving reassurance and education.[83] It is often appropriate to assist the child in understanding the parents' concerns as well. Despite expectations by some youth with transgender identity for immediate acceptance after "coming out," family members often proceed through a process of becoming more comfortable and understanding of the youth's gender identity, thoughts, and feelings. One model suggests that the process resembles grieving, wherein the family separates from their expectations for their child to embrace a new reality. This process may proceed through stages of shock,

denial, anger, feelings of betrayal, fear, self-discovery, and pride.[89] The amount of time spent in any of these stages and the overall pace varies widely. Many family members also struggle as they are pushed to reflect on their own gender experience and assumptions throughout this process. In some situations, youth who identify as TGD may be at risk for internalizing the difficult emotions that family members may be experiencing. In these cases, individual and group therapy for the family members may be helpful.[49,78]

Family dynamics can be complex, involving disagreement among legal guardians or between guardians and their children, which may affect the ability to obtain consent for any medical management or interventions. Even in states where minors may access care without parental consent for mental health services, contraception, and sexually transmitted infections, parental or guardian consent is required for hormonal and surgical care of patients who identify as TGD.[72,90] Some families may take issue with providers who address gender concerns or offer gender-affirming care. In rare cases, a family may deny access to care that raises concerns about the youth's welfare and safety; in those cases, additional legal or ethical support may be useful to consider. In such rare situations, pediatric providers may want to familiarize themselves with relevant local consent laws and maintain their primary responsibility for the welfare of the child.

SAFE SCHOOLS AND COMMUNITIES

Youth who identify as TGD are becoming more visible because gender-diverse expression is increasingly admissible in the media, on social media, and in schools and communities. Regardless of whether a youth with a gender-diverse identity ultimately identifies as transgender, challenges exist in nearly every social context, from lack of understanding to outright rejection, isolation, discrimination, and victimization. In the US Transgender Survey of nearly 28 000 respondents, it was found that among those who were out as or perceived to be TGD between kindergarten and eighth grade, 54% were verbally harassed, 24% were physically assaulted, and 13% were sexually assaulted; 17% left school because of maltreatment.[31] Education and advocacy from the medical community on the importance of safe schools for youth who identify as TGD can have a significant effect.

At the time of this writing,* only 18 states and the District of Columbia had laws that prohibited discrimination based on gender expression when it comes to employment, housing, public accommodations, and insurance benefits. Over 200 US cities have such legislation. In addition to basic protections, many youth who identify as TGD also have to navigate legal obstacles when it comes to legally changing their name and/or gender marker.[54] In addition to advocating and working with policy makers to promote equal protections for youth who identify as TGD, pediatric providers can play an important role by developing a familiarity with local laws and organizations that provide social work and legal assistance to youth who identify as TGD and their families.

School environments play a significant role in the social and emotional development of children. Every child has a right to feel safe

and respected at school, but for youth who identify as TGD, this can be challenging. Nearly every aspect of school life may present safety concerns and require negotiations regarding their gender expression, including name/pronoun use, use of bathrooms and locker rooms, sports teams, dances and activities, overnight activities, and even peer groups. Conflicts in any of these areas can quickly escalate beyond the school's control to larger debates among the community and even on a national stage.

The formerly known Gay, Lesbian, and Straight Education Network (GLSEN), an advocacy organization for youth who identify as LGBTQ, conducts an annual national survey to measure LGBTQ well-being in US schools. In 2015, students who identified as LGBTQ reported high rates of being discouraged from participation in extracurricular activities. One in 5 students who identified as LGBTQ reported being hindered from forming or participating in a club to support lesbian, gay, bisexual, or transgender students (eg, a gay straight alliance, now often referred to as a genders and sexualities alliance) despite such clubs at schools being associated with decreased reports of negative remarks about sexual orientation or gender expression, increased feelings of safety and connectedness at school, and lower levels of victimization. In addition, >20% of students who identified as LGBTQ reported being blocked from writing about LGBTQ issues in school yearbooks or school newspapers or being prevented or discouraged by coaches and school staff from participating in sports because of their sexual orientation or gender expression.[91]

One strategy to prevent conflict is to proactively support policies and protections that promote inclusion and safety of all students. However, such policies are far from

consistent across districts. In 2015, GLSEN found that 43% of children who identified as LGBTQ reported feeling unsafe at school because of their gender expression, but only 6% reported that their school had official policies to support youth who identified as TGD, and only 11% reported that their school's antibullying policies had specific protections for gender expression.[91] Consequently, more than half of the students who identified as transgender in the study were prevented from using the bathroom, names, or pronouns that aligned with their asserted gender at school. A lack of explicit policies that protected youth who identified as TGD was associated with increased reported victimization, with more than half of students who identified as LGBTQ reporting verbal harassment because of their gender expression. Educators and school administrators play an essential role in advocating for and enforcing such policies. GLSEN found that when students recognized actions to reduce gender-based harassment, both students who identified as transgender and cisgender reported a greater connection to staff and feelings of safety.[91] In another study, schools were open to education regarding gender diversity and were willing to implement policies when they were supported by external agencies, such as medical professionals.[92]

Academic content plays an important role in building a safe school environment as well. The 2015 GLSEN survey revealed that when positive representations of people who identified as LGBTQ were included in the curriculum, students who identified as LGBTQ reported less hostile school environments, less victimization and greater feelings of safety, fewer school absences because of feeling unsafe, greater feelings of connectedness to their school

---

* For more information regarding state-specific laws, please contact the AAP Division of State Government Affairs at stgov@ aap.org.

community, and an increased interest in high school graduation and postsecondary education.[91] At the time of this writing,* 8 states had laws that explicitly forbade teachers from even discussing LGBTQ issues.[54]

MEDICAL EDUCATION

One of the most important ways to promote high-quality health care for youth who identify as TGD and their families is increasing the knowledge base and clinical experience of pediatric providers in providing culturally competent care to such populations, as recommended by the recently released guidelines by the Association of American Medical Colleges.[93] This begins with the medical school curriculum in areas such as human development, sexual health, endocrinology, pediatrics, and psychiatry. In a 2009–2010 survey of US medical schools, it was found that the median number of hours dedicated to LGBTQ health was 5, with one-third of US medical schools reporting no LGBTQ curriculum during the clinical years.[94]

During residency training, there is potential for gender diversity to be emphasized in core rotations, especially in pediatrics, psychiatry, family medicine, and obstetrics and gynecology. Awareness could be promoted through the inclusion of topics relevant to caring for children who identify as TGD in the list of core competencies published by the American Board of Pediatrics, certifying examinations, and relevant study materials. Continuing education and maintenance of certification activities can include topics relevant to TGD populations as well.

---

* For more information regarding state-specific laws, please contact the AAP Division of State Government Affairs at stgov@ aap.org.

RECOMMENDATIONS

The AAP works toward all children and adolescents, regardless of gender identity or expression, receiving care to promote optimal physical, mental, and social well-being. Any discrimination based on gender identity or expression, real or perceived, is damaging to the socioemotional health of children, families, and society. In particular, the AAP recommends the following:

1. that youth who identify as TGD have access to comprehensive, gender-affirming, and developmentally appropriate health care that is provided in a safe and inclusive clinical space;

2. that family-based therapy and support be available to recognize and respond to the emotional and mental health needs of parents, caregivers, and siblings of youth who identify as TGD;

3. that electronic health records, billing systems, patient-centered notification systems, and clinical research be designed to respect the asserted gender identity of each patient while maintaining confidentiality and avoiding duplicate charts;

4. that insurance plans offer coverage for health care that is specific to the needs of youth who identify as TGD, including coverage for medical, psychological, and, when indicated, surgical gender-affirming interventions;

5. that provider education, including medical school, residency, and continuing education, integrate core competencies on the emotional and physical health needs and best practices for the care of youth who identify as TGD and their families;

6. that pediatricians have a role in advocating for, educating, and developing liaison relationships with school districts and other community organizations to promote acceptance and inclusion of all children without fear of harassment, exclusion, or bullying because of gender expression;

7. that pediatricians have a role in advocating for policies and laws that protect youth who identify as TGD from discrimination and violence;

8. that the health care workforce protects diversity by offering equal employment opportunities and workplace protections, regardless of gender identity or expression; and

9. that the medical field and federal government prioritize research that is dedicated to improving the quality of evidence-based care for youth who identify as TGD.

LEAD AUTHOR

Jason Richard Rafferty, MD, MPH, EdM, FAAP

CONTRIBUTOR

Robert Garofalo, MD, FAAP

COMMITTEE ON PSYCHOSOCIAL ASPECTS OF CHILD AND FAMILY HEALTH, 2017–2018

Michael Yogman, MD, FAAP, Chairperson
Rebecca Baum, MD, FAAP
Thresia B. Gambon, MD, FAAP
Arthur Lavin, MD, FAAP
Gerri Mattson, MD, FAAP
Lawrence Sagin Wissow, MD, MPH, FAAP

LIAISONS

Sharon Berry, PhD, LP — *Society of Pediatric Psychology*
Ed Christophersen, PhD, FAAP — *Society of Pediatric Psychology*
Norah Johnson, PhD, RN, CPNP-BC — *National Association of Pediatric Nurse Practitioners*
Amy Starin, PhD, LCSW — *National Association of Social Workers*
Abigail Schlesinger, MD — *American Academy of Child and Adolescent Psychiatry*

STAFF

Karen S. Smith
James Baumberger

ACKNOWLEDGMENTS

We thank Isaac Albanese, MPA, and Jayeson Watts, LICSW, for their thoughtful reviews and contributions.

ABBREVIATIONS

AAP: American Academy of Pediatrics
GACM: gender-affirmative care model
GLSEN: Gay, Lesbian, and Straight Education Network
LGBTQ: lesbian, gay, bisexual, transgender, or questioning
TGD: transgender and gender diverse

DOI: https://doi.org/10.1542/peds.2018-2162

PEDIATRICS (ISSN Numbers: Print, 0031-4005; Online, 1098-4275).

FINANCIAL DISCLOSURE: The author has indicated he has no financial relationships relevant to this article to disclose.

FUNDING: No external funding.

POTENTIAL CONFLICT OF INTEREST: The author has indicated he has no potential conflicts of interest to disclose.

REFERENCES

1. Levine DA; Committee on Adolescence. Office-based care for lesbian, gay, bisexual, transgender, and questioning youth. *Pediatrics.* 2013;132(1). Available at: www.pediatrics.org/cgi/content/full/132/1/e297

2. American Academy of Pediatrics Committee on Adolescence. Homosexuality and adolescence. *Pediatrics.* 1983;72(2):249–250

3. Institute of Medicine; Committee on Lesbian Gay Bisexual, and Transgender Health Issues and Research Gaps and Opportunities. *The Health of Lesbian, Gay, Bisexual, and Transgender People: Building a Foundation for Better Understanding.* Washington, DC: National Academies Press; 2011. Available at: https://www.ncbi.nlm.nih.gov/books/NBK64806. Accessed May 19, 2017

4. Deutsch MB, Radix A, Reisner S. What's in a guideline? Developing collaborative and sound research designs that substantiate best practice recommendations for transgender health care. *AMA J Ethics.* 2016;18(11):1098–1106

5. Bonifacio HJ, Rosenthal SM. Gender variance and dysphoria in children and adolescents. *Pediatr Clin North Am.* 2015;62(4):1001–1016

6. Vance SR Jr, Ehrensaft D, Rosenthal SM. Psychological and medical care of gender nonconforming youth. *Pediatrics.* 2014;134(6):1184–1192

7. Richards C, Bouman WP, Seal L, Barker MJ, Nieder TO, T'Sjoen G. Non-binary or genderqueer genders. *Int Rev Psychiatry.* 2016;28(1):95–102

8. American Psychological Association. Guidelines for psychological practice with transgender and gender nonconforming people. *Am Psychol.* 2015;70(9):832–864

9. Flores AR, Herman JL, Gates GJ, Brown TNT. *How Many Adults Identify as Transgender in the United States.* Los Angeles, CA: The Williams Institute; 2016

10. Herman JL, Flores AR, Brown TNT, Wilson BDM, Conron KJ. *Age of Individuals Who Identify as Transgender in the United States.* Los Angeles, CA: The Williams Institute; 2017

11. Gates GJ. *How Many People are Lesbian, Gay, Bisexual, and Transgender?* Los Angeles, CA: The Williams Institute; 2011

12. Olson J, Schrager SM, Belzer M, Simons LK, Clark LF. Baseline physiologic and psychosocial characteristics of transgender youth seeking care for gender dysphoria. *J Adolesc Health.* 2015;57(4):374–380

13. Reisner SL, Vetters R, Leclerc M, et al. Mental health of transgender youth in care

at an adolescent urban community health center: a matched retrospective cohort study. *J Adolesc Health.* 2015;56(3):274–279

14. Clements-Nolle K, Marx R, Katz M. Attempted suicide among transgender persons: the influence of gender-based discrimination and victimization. *J Homosex.* 2006;51(3):53–69

15. Colizzi M, Costa R, Todarello O. Transsexual patients' psychiatric comorbidity and positive effect of cross-sex hormonal treatment on mental health: results from a longitudinal study. *Psychoneuroendocrinology.* 2014;39:65–73

16. Haas AP, Eliason M, Mays VM, et al. Suicide and suicide risk in lesbian, gay, bisexual, and transgender populations: review and recommendations. *J Homosex.* 2011;58(1):10–51

17. Maguen S, Shipherd JC. Suicide risk among transgender individuals. *Psychol Sex.* 2010;1(1):34–43

18. Connolly MD, Zervos MJ, Barone CJ II, Johnson CC, Joseph CL. The mental health of transgender youth: advances in understanding. *J Adolesc Health.* 2016;59(5):489–495

19. Grossman AH, D'Augelli AR. Transgender youth and life-threatening behaviors. *Suicide Life Threat Behav.* 2007;37(5):527–537

20. Spack NP, Edwards-Leeper L, Feldman HA, et al. Children and adolescents with gender identity disorder referred to a pediatric medical center. *Pediatrics.* 2012;129(3):418–425

21. van Schalkwyk GI, Klingensmith K, Volkmar FR. Gender identity and autism spectrum disorders. *Yale J Biol Med.* 2015;88(1):81–83

22. Jacobs LA, Rachlin K, Erickson-Schroth L, Janssen A. Gender dysphoria and co-occurring autism spectrum disorders: review, case examples, and treatment considerations. *LGBT Health.* 2014;1(4):277–282

23. American Psychiatric Association. *Diagnostic and Statistical Manual of Mental Disorders.* 5th ed. Arlington, VA: American Psychiatric Association; 2013

24. Edwards-Leeper L, Spack NP. Psychological evaluation and medical treatment of transgender youth in an interdisciplinary "Gender Management Service" (GeMS) in a major pediatric center. *J Homosex.* 2012;59(3):321–336

25. Anton BS. Proceedings of the American Psychological Association for the legislative year 2008: minutes of the annual meeting of the Council of Representatives, February 22–24, 2008, Washington, DC, and August 13 and 17, 2008, Boston, MA, and minutes of the February, June, August, and December 2008 meetings of the Board of Directors. *Am Psychol.* 2009;64(5):372–453

26. Drescher J, Haller E; American Psychiatric Association Caucus of Lesbian, Gay and Bisexual Psychiatrists. *Position Statement on Discrimination Against Transgender and Gender Variant Individuals.* Washington, DC: American Psychiatric Association; 2012

27. Hidalgo MA, Ehrensaft D, Tishelman AC, et al. The gender affirmative model: what we know and what we aim to learn. *Hum Dev.* 2013;56(5):285–290

28. Tishelman AC, Kaufman R, Edwards-Leeper L, Mandel FH, Shumer DE, Spack NP. Serving transgender youth: challenges, dilemmas and clinical examples. *Prof Psychol Res Pr.* 2015;46(1):37–45

29. Adelson SL; American Academy of Child and Adolescent Psychiatry (AACAP) Committee on Quality Issues (CQI). Practice parameter on gay, lesbian, or bisexual sexual orientation, gender nonconformity, and gender discordance in children and adolescents. *J Am Acad Child Adolesc Psychiatry.* 2012;51(9):957–974

30. Herbst JH, Jacobs ED, Finlayson TJ, McKleroy VS, Neumann MS, Crepaz N; HIV/AIDS Prevention Research Synthesis Team. Estimating HIV prevalence and risk behaviors of transgender persons in the United States: a systematic review. *AIDS Behav.* 2008;12(1):1–17

31. James SE, Herman JL, Rankin S, Keisling M, Mottet L, Anafi M. *The Report of the 2015 U.S. Transgender Survey.* Washington, DC: National Center for Transgender Equality; 2016

32. Centers for Disease Control and Prevention. *CDC-Funded HIV Testing: United States, Puerto Rico, and the U.S. Virgin Islands.* Atlanta, GA: Centers for Disease Control and Prevention; 2015. Available at: https://www.cdc.gov/hiv/pdf/library/reports/cdc-hiv-funded-testing-us-puerto-rico-2015.pdf. Accessed August 2, 2018

33. Substance Abuse and Mental Health Services Administration. *Ending Conversion Therapy: Supporting and Affirming LGBTQ Youth.* Rockville, MD: Substance Abuse and Mental Health Services Administration; 2015

34. Korell SC, Lorah P. An overview of affirmative psychotherapy and counseling with transgender clients. In: Bieschke KJ, Perez RM, DeBord KA, eds. *Handbook of Counseling and Psychotherapy With Lesbian, Gay, Bisexual, and Transgender Clients.* 2nd ed. Washington, DC: American Psychological Association; 2007:271–288

35. World Professional Association for Transgender Health. *Standards of Care for the Health of Transsexual, Transgender, and Gender Nonconforming People.* 7th ed. Minneapolis, MN: World Professional Association for Transgender Health; 2011. Available at: https://www.wpath.org/publications/soc. Accessed April 15, 2018

36. Menvielle E. A comprehensive program for children with gender variant behaviors and gender identity disorders. *J Homosex.* 2012;59(3):357–368

37. Hill DB, Menvielle E, Sica KM, Johnson A. An affirmative intervention for families with gender variant children: parental ratings of child mental health and gender. *J Sex Marital Ther.* 2010;36(1):6–23

38. Haldeman DC. The practice and ethics of sexual orientation conversion therapy. *J Consult Clin Psychol.* 1994;62(2):221–227

39. Byne W. Regulations restrict practice of conversion therapy. *LGBT Health.* 2016;3(2):97–99

40. Cohen-Kettenis PT, Delemarre-van de Waal HA, Gooren LJ. The treatment of adolescent transsexuals: changing insights. *J Sex Med.* 2008;5(8):1892–1897

41. Bryant K. Making gender identity disorder of childhood: historical lessons for contemporary debates. *Sex Res Soc Policy*. 2006;3(3):23–39

42. World Professional Association for Transgender Health. *WPATH De-Psychopathologisation Statement*. Minneapolis, MN: World Professional Association for Transgender Health; 2010. Available at: https://www.wpath.org/policies. Accessed April 16, 2017

43. American Academy of Pediatrics. AAP support letter conversion therapy ban [letter]. 2015. Available at: https://www.aap.org/en-us/advocacy-and-policy/federal-advocacy/Documents/AAPsupportletterconversiontherapyban.pdf. Accessed August 1, 2018

44. Movement Advancement Project. *LGBT Policy Spotlight: Conversion Therapy Bans*. Boulder, CO: Movement Advancement Project; 2017. Available at: http://www.lgbtmap.org/policy-and-issue-analysis/policy-spotlight-conversion-therapy-bans. Accessed August 6, 2017

45. Ehrensaft D, Giammattei SV, Storck K, Tishelman AC, Keo-Meier C. Prepubertal social gender transitions: what we know; what we can learn—a view from a gender affirmative lens. *Int J Transgend*. 2018;19(2):251–268

46. Olson KR, Key AC, Eaton NR. Gender cognition in transgender children. *Psychol Sci*. 2015;26(4):467–474

47. Olson KR. Prepubescent transgender children: what we do and do not know. *J Am Acad Child Adolesc Psychiatry*. 2016;55(3):155–156.e3

48. Olson KR, Durwood L, DeMeules M, McLaughlin KA. Mental health of transgender children who are supported in their identities. *Pediatrics*. 2016;137(3):e20153223

49. Malpas J. Between pink and blue: a multi-dimensional family approach to gender nonconforming children and their families. *Fam Process*. 2011;50(4):453–470

50. Hagan JF Jr, Shaw JS, Duncan PM, eds. *Bright Futures: Guidelines for Health Supervision of Infants, Children, and Adolescents*. 4th ed. Elk Grove, IL: American Academy of Pediatrics; 2016

51. Minter SP. Supporting transgender children: new legal, social, and medical approaches. *J Homosex*. 2012;59(3):422–433

52. AHIMA Work Group. Improved patient engagement for LGBT populations: addressing factors related to sexual orientation/gender identity for effective health information management. *J AHIMA*. 2017;88(3):34–39

53. Deutsch MB, Green J, Keatley J, Mayer G, Hastings J, Hall AM; World Professional Association for Transgender Health EMR Working Group. Electronic medical records and the transgender patient: recommendations from the World Professional Association for Transgender Health EMR Working Group. *J Am Med Inform Assoc*. 2013;20(4):700–703

54. Dowshen N, Meadows R, Byrnes M, Hawkins L, Eder J, Noonan K. Policy perspective: ensuring comprehensive care and support for gender nonconforming children and adolescents. *Transgend Health*. 2016;1(1):75–85

55. Cahill SR, Baker K, Deutsch MB, Keatley J, Makadon HJ. Inclusion of sexual orientation and gender identity in stage 3 meaningful use guidelines: a huge step forward for LGBT health. *LGBT Health*. 2016;3(2):100–102

56. Mansfield MJ, Beardsworth DE, Loughlin JS, et al. Long-term treatment of central precocious puberty with a long-acting analogue of luteinizing hormone-releasing hormone. Effects on somatic growth and skeletal maturation. *N Engl J Med*. 1983;309(21):1286–1290

57. Olson J, Garofalo R. The peripubertal gender-dysphoric child: puberty suppression and treatment paradigms. *Pediatr Ann*. 2014;43(6):e132–e137

58. de Vries AL, Steensma TD, Doreleijers TA, Cohen-Kettenis PT. Puberty suppression in adolescents with gender identity disorder: a prospective follow-up study. *J Sex Med*. 2011;8(8):2276–2283

59. Wallien MS, Cohen-Kettenis PT. Psychosexual outcome of gender-dysphoric children. *J Am Acad Child Adolesc Psychiatry*. 2008;47(12):1413–1423

60. Waylen A, Wolke D. Sex 'n' drugs 'n' rock 'n' roll: the meaning and social consequences of pubertal timing. *Eur J Endocrinol*. 2004;151(suppl 3):U151–U159

61. de Vries AL, Klink D, Cohen-Kettenis PT. What the primary care pediatrician needs to know about gender incongruence and gender dysphoria in children and adolescents. *Pediatr Clin North Am*. 2016;63(6):1121–1135

62. Vlot MC, Klink DT, den Heijer M, Blankenstein MA, Rotteveel J, Heijboer AC. Effect of pubertal suppression and cross-sex hormone therapy on bone turnover markers and bone mineral apparent density (BMAD) in transgender adolescents. *Bone*. 2017;95:11–19

63. Finlayson C, Johnson EK, Chen D, et al. Proceedings of the working group session on fertility preservation for individuals with gender and sex diversity. *Transgend Health*. 2016;1(1):99–107

64. Kreukels BP, Cohen-Kettenis PT. Puberty suppression in gender identity disorder: the Amsterdam experience. *Nat Rev Endocrinol*. 2011;7(8):466–472

65. Rosenthal SM. Approach to the patient: transgender youth: endocrine considerations. *J Clin Endocrinol Metab*. 2014;99(12):4379–4389

66. Fenway Health. *Glossary of Gender and Transgender Terms*. Boston, MA: Fenway Health; 2010. Available at: http://fenwayhealth.org/documents/the-fenway-institute/handouts/Handout_7-C_Glossary_of_Gender_and_Transgender_Terms__fi.pdf. Accessed August 16, 2017

67. de Vries AL, McGuire JK, Steensma TD, Wagenaar EC, Doreleijers TA, Cohen-Kettenis PT. Young adult psychological outcome after puberty suppression and gender reassignment. *Pediatrics*. 2014;134(4):696–704

68. Hembree WC, Cohen-Kettenis PT, Gooren L, et al. Endocrine treatment of gender-dysphoric/gender-incongruent persons: an endocrine society clinical practice guideline. *J Clin Endocrinol Metab*. 2017;102(11):3869–3903

69. Milrod C, Karasic DH. Age is just a number: WPATH-affiliated surgeons' experiences and attitudes toward

vaginoplasty in transgender females under 18 years of age in the United States. *J Sex Med*. 2017;14(4):624–634

70. Milrod C. How young is too young: ethical concerns in genital surgery of the transgender MTF adolescent. *J Sex Med*. 2014;11(2):338–346

71. Olson-Kennedy J, Warus J, Okonta V, Belzer M, Clark LF. Chest reconstruction and chest dysphoria in transmasculine minors and young adults: comparisons of nonsurgical and postsurgical cohorts. *JAMA Pediatr*. 2018;172(5):431–436

72. Committee on Adolescent Health Care. Committee opinion no. 685: care for transgender adolescents. *Obstet Gynecol*. 2017;129(1):e11–e16

73. Greydanus DE, Patel DR, Rimsza ME. Contraception in the adolescent: an update. *Pediatrics*. 2001;107(3):562–573

74. Gridley SJ, Crouch JM, Evans Y, et al. Youth and caregiver perspectives on barriers to gender-affirming health care for transgender youth. *J Adolesc Health*. 2016;59(3):254–261

75. Sanchez NF, Sanchez JP, Danoff A. Health care utilization, barriers to care, and hormone usage among male-to-female transgender persons in New York City. *Am J Public Health*. 2009;99(4):713–719

76. Transgender Law Center. *Affordable Care Act Fact Sheet*. Oakland, CA: Transgender Law Center; 2016. Available at: https://transgenderlawcenter.org/resources/health/aca-fact-sheet. Accessed August 8, 2016

77. Nahata L, Quinn GP, Caltabellotta NM, Tishelman AC. Mental health concerns and insurance denials among transgender adolescents. *LGBT Health*. 2017;4(3):188–193

78. Grant JM, Mottet LA, Tanis J, Harrison J, Herman JL, Keisling M. *Injustice at Every Turn: A Report of the National Transgender Discrimination Survey*. Washington, DC: National Center for Transgender Equality and National Gay and Lesbian Task Force; 2011 Available at: http://www.thetaskforce.org/static_html/downloads/reports/reports/ntds_full.pdf. Accessed August 6, 2018

79. Sevelius JM. Gender affirmation: a framework for conceptualizing risk behavior among transgender women of color. *Sex Roles*. 2013;68(11–12):675–689

80. Koken JA, Bimbi DS, Parsons JT. Experiences of familial acceptance-rejection among transwomen of color. *J Fam Psychol*. 2009;23(6):853–860

81. Lombardi EL, Wilchins RA, Priesing D, Malouf D. Gender violence: transgender experiences with violence and discrimination. *J Homosex*. 2001;42(1):89–101

82. Wren B. 'I can accept my child is transsexual but if I ever see him in a dress I'll hit him': dilemmas in parenting a transgendered adolescent. *Clin Child Psychol Psychiatry*. 2002;7(3):377–397

83. Riley EA, Sitharthan G, Clemson L, Diamond M. The needs of gender-variant children and their parents: a parent survey. *Int J Sex Health*. 2011;23(3):181–195

84. Whitley CT. Trans-kin undoing and redoing gender: negotiating relational identity among friends and family of transgender persons. *Sociol Perspect*. 2013;56(4):597–621

85. Travers R, Bauer G, Pyne J, Bradley K, Gale L, Papadimitriou M; Trans PULSE; Children's Aid Society of Toronto; Delisle Youth Services. *Impacts of Strong Parental Support for Trans Youth: A Report Prepared for Children's Aid Society of Toronto and Delisle Youth Services*. Toronto, ON: Trans PULSE; 2012. Available at: http://transpulseproject.ca/wp-content/uploads/2012/10/Impacts-of-Strong-Parental-Support-for-Trans-Youth-vFINAL.pdf

86. Ryan C, Russell ST, Huebner D, Diaz R, Sanchez J. Family acceptance in adolescence and the health of LGBT young adults. *J Child Adolesc Psychiatr Nurs*. 2010;23(4):205–213

87. Grossman AH, D'augelli AR, Frank JA. Aspects of psychological resilience among transgender youth. *J LGBT Youth*. 2011;8(2):103–115

88. McConnell EA, Birkett M, Mustanski B. Families matter: social support and mental health trajectories among lesbian, gay, bisexual, and transgender youth. *J Adolesc Health*. 2016;59(6):674–680

89. Ellis KM, Eriksen K. Transsexual and transgenderist experiences and treatment options. *Fam J Alex Va*. 2002;10(3):289–299

90. Lamda Legal. *Transgender Rights Toolkit: A Legal Guide for Trans People and Their Advocates*. New York, NY: Lambda Legal; 2016 Available at: https://www.lambdalegal.org/publications/trans-toolkit. Accessed August 6, 2018

91. Kosciw JG, Greytak EA, Giga NM, Villenas C, Danischewski DJ. *The 2015 National School Climate Survey: The Experiences of Lesbian, Gay, Bisexual, Transgender, and Queer Youth in Our Nation's Schools*. New York, NY: GLSEN; 2016. Available at: https://www.glsen.org/article/2015-national-school-climate-survey. Accessed August 8, 2018

92. McGuire JK, Anderson CR, Toomey RB, Russell ST. School climate for transgender youth: a mixed method investigation of student experiences and school responses. *J Youth Adolesc*. 2010;39(10):1175–1188

93. Association of American Medical Colleges Advisory Committee on Sexual Orientation, Gender Identity, and Sex Development. In: Hollenback AD, Eckstrand KL, Dreger A, eds. *Implementing Curricular and Institutional Climate Changes to Improve Health Care for Individuals Who Are LGBT, Gender Nonconforming, or Born With DSD: A Resource for Medical Educators*. Washington, DC: Association of American Medical Colleges; 2014. Available at: https://members.aamc.org/eweb/upload/Executive LGBT FINAL.pdf. Accessed August 8, 2018

94. Obedin-Maliver J, Goldsmith ES, Stewart L, et al. Lesbian, gay, bisexual, and transgender-related content in undergraduate medical education. *JAMA*. 2011;306(9):971–977

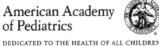

Organizational Principles to Guide and Define the Child
Health Care System and/or Improve the Health of all Children

This Policy Statement was reaffirmed April 2021.

POLICY STATEMENT

Office-Based Care for Lesbian, Gay, Bisexual, Transgender, and Questioning Youth

abstract

The American Academy of Pediatrics issued its last statement on homosexuality and adolescents in 2004. Although most lesbian, gay, bisexual, transgender, and questioning (LGBTQ) youth are quite resilient and emerge from adolescence as healthy adults, the effects of homophobia and heterosexism can contribute to health disparities in mental health with higher rates of depression and suicidal ideation, higher rates of substance abuse, and more sexually transmitted and HIV infections. Pediatricians should have offices that are teen-friendly and welcoming to sexual minority youth. Obtaining a comprehensive, confidential, developmentally appropriate adolescent psychosocial history allows for the discovery of strengths and assets as well as risks. Referrals for mental health or substance abuse may be warranted. Sexually active LGBTQ youth should have sexually transmitted infection/ HIV testing according to recommendations of the Sexually Transmitted Diseases Treatment Guidelines of the Centers for Disease Control and Prevention based on sexual behaviors. With appropriate assistance and care, sexual minority youth should live healthy, productive lives while transitioning through adolescence and young adulthood. *Pediatrics* 2013;132:198–203

INTRODUCTION

The American Academy of Pediatrics issued its first statement on sexual minority teenagers in 1983, with revisions in 1993 and 2004. Since the last report, research areas have rapidly expanded and hundreds of new publications have been produced about lesbian, gay, bisexual, transgender, and questioning (LGBTQ) youth, including an Institute of Medicine publication entitled "The Health of Lesbian, Gay, Bisexual, and Transgender People: Building a Foundation for Better Understanding."[1] Being a member of this group of teenagers is not, in itself, a risk behavior and many sexual minority youth are quite resilient; sexual minority youth should not be considered abnormal. However, the presence of stigma from homophobia and heterosexism often leads to psychological distress, which may be accompanied by an increase in risk behaviors. Health disparities exist in mental health, substance abuse, and sexually transmitted infection (STI)/HIV.

LGBTQ will be used whenever discussing studies and recommendations for all self-identified lesbian, gay, bisexual, transgender, or questioning youth. Many adolescents do not define themselves as a member of a sexual minority group but may have had same gender sexual

COMMITTEE ON ADOLESCENCE

KEY WORDS
sexual orientation, sexual identity, sexual behaviors, adolescents, sexual minority, homosexuality, gay, lesbian, bisexual, transgender

ABBREVIATIONS
CDC—Centers for Disease Control and Prevention
HPV—human papillomavirus
LGBTQ—lesbian, gay, bisexual, transgender, and questioning
MSM—men who have sex with men
STI—sexually transmitted infection
WSW—women who have sex with women

The recommendations in this statement do not indicate an exclusive course of treatment or serve as a standard of medical care. Variations, taking into account individual circumstances, may be appropriate.

All policy statements from the American Academy of Pediatrics automatically expire 5 years after publication unless reaffirmed, revised, or retired at or before that time.

www.pediatrics.org/cgi/doi/10.1542/peds.2013-1282

doi:10.1542/peds.2013-1282

PEDIATRICS (ISSN Numbers: Print, 0031-4005; Online, 1098-4275).

COMPANION PAPER: A companion to this article can be found on page e297, and online at www.pediatrics.org/cgi/doi/10.1542/peds.2013-1283.

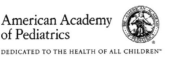

American Academy
of Pediatrics
DEDICATED TO THE HEALTH OF ALL CHILDREN™

This Technical Report was reaffirmed April 2021.

TECHNICAL REPORT

Office-Based Care for Lesbian, Gay, Bisexual, Transgender, and Questioning Youth

David A. Levine, MD, and the COMMITTEE ON ADOLESCENCE

KEY WORDS
sexual orientation, sexual identity, sexual behaviors, adolescents, sexual minority, homosexuality, gay, lesbian, bisexual, transgender

ABBREVIATIONS
CDC—Centers for Disease Control and Prevention
FTM—females transitioning to males
GnRH—gonadotropin-releasing hormone
HPV—human papillomavirus
HSV—herpes simplex virus
IOM—Institute of Medicine
LGBTQ—lesbian, gay, bisexual, transgender, and questioning
MSM—men who have sex with men
MTF—males transitioning to females
STI—sexually transmitted infection
WSW—women who have sex with women
YRBS—Youth Risk Behavior Surveillance

www.pediatrics.org/cgi/doi/10.1542/peds.2013-1283

doi:10.1542/peds.2013-1283

All clinical reports from the American Academy of Pediatrics automatically expire 5 years after publication unless reaffirmed, revised, or retired at or before that time.

(Continued on last page)

abstract

The American Academy of Pediatrics issued its last statement on homosexuality and adolescents in 2004. This technical report reflects the rapidly expanding medical and psychosocial literature about sexual minority youth. Pediatricians should be aware that some youth in their care may have concerns or questions about their sexual orientation or that of siblings, friends, parents, relatives, or others and should provide factual, current, nonjudgmental information in a confidential manner. Although most lesbian, gay, bisexual, transgender, and questioning (LGBTQ) youth are quite resilient and emerge from adolescence as healthy adults, the effects of homophobia and heterosexism can contribute to increased mental health issues for sexual minority youth. LGBTQ and MSM/WSW (men having sex with men and women having sex with women) adolescents, in comparison with heterosexual adolescents, have higher rates of depression and suicidal ideation, higher rates of substance abuse, and more risky sexual behaviors. Obtaining a comprehensive, confidential, developmentally appropriate adolescent psychosocial history allows for the discovery of strengths and assets as well as risks. Pediatricians should have offices that are teen-friendly and welcoming to sexual minority youth. This includes having supportive, engaging office staff members who ensure that there are no barriers to care. For transgender youth, pediatricians should provide the opportunity to acknowledge and affirm their feel-ings of gender dysphoria and desires to transition to the opposite gen-der. Referral of transgender youth to a qualified mental health professional is critical to assist with the dysphoria, to educate them, and to assess their readiness for transition. With appropriate assis-tance and care, sexual minority youth should live healthy, productive lives while transitioning through adolescence and young adulthood. *Pediatrics* 2013;132:e297–e313

INTRODUCTION

The American Academy of Pediatrics issued its first statement on sexual minority teens in 1983, with revisions in 1993 and 2004. Since the last report, research areas have rapidly expanded and hundreds of new publications have been produced about lesbian, gay, bisexual, transgender, and questioning (LGBTQ) youth. In 2011, the Institute of Medicine (IOM) published "The Health of Lesbian, Gay, Bisexual, and Transgender People: Building a Foundation for Better Understanding."[1]

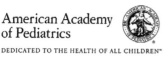

American Academy of Pediatrics
DEDICATED TO THE HEALTH OF ALL CHILDREN®

Organizational Principles to Guide and Define the Child
Health Care System and/or Improve the Health of all Children

This Policy Statement was reaffirmed September 2022.

POLICY STATEMENT

Promoting the Well-Being of Children Whose Parents Are Gay or Lesbian

COMMITTEE ON PSYCHOSOCIAL ASPECTS OF CHILD AND FAMILY HEALTH

KEY WORDS
civil marriage, adoption, foster care, nurturing children, children of gay and lesbian parents, marriage equality

www.pediatrics.org/cgi/doi/10.1542/peds.2013-0376

doi:10.1542/peds.2013-0376

PEDIATRICS (ISSN Numbers: Print, 0031-4005; Online, 1098-4275).

abstract

To promote optimal health and well-being of all children, the American Academy of Pediatrics (AAP) supports access for all children to (1) civil marriage rights for their parents and (2) willing and capable foster and adoptive parents, regardless of the parents' sexual orientation. The AAP has always been an advocate for, and has developed policies to support, the optimal physical, mental, and social health and well-being of all infants, children, adolescents, and young adults. In so doing, the AAP has supported families in all their diversity, because the family has always been the basic social unit in which children develop the supporting and nurturing relationships with adults that they need to thrive. Children may be born to, adopted by, or cared for temporarily by married couples, nonmarried couples, single parents, grandparents, or legal guardians, and any of these may be heterosexual, gay or lesbian, or of another orientation. Children need secure and enduring relationships with committed and nurturing adults to enhance their life experiences for optimal social-emotional and cognitive development. Scientific evidence affirms that children have similar developmental and emotional needs and receive similar parenting whether they are raised by parents of the same or different genders. If a child has 2 living and capable parents who choose to create a permanent bond by way of civil marriage, it is in the best interests of their child(ren) that legal and social institutions allow and support them to do so, irrespective of their sexual orientation. If 2 parents are not available to the child, adoption or foster parenting remain acceptable options to provide a loving home for a child and should be available without regard to the sexual orientation of the parent(s). *Pediatrics* 2013;131:827–830

INTRODUCTION

All children need support and nurturing from stable, healthy, and well-functioning adults to become resilient and effective adults. On the basis of a review of extensive scientific literature, the American Academy of Pediatrics (AAP) affirms that "children's well-being is affected much more by their relationships with their parents, their parents' sense of competence and security, and the presence of social and economic support for the family than by the gender or the sexual orientation of their parents."[1]

American Academy
of Pediatrics

DEDICATED TO THE HEALTH OF ALL CHILDREN™

This Technical Report was reaffirmed September 2022.

TECHNICAL REPORT

Promoting the Well-Being of Children Whose Parents Are Gay or Lesbian

abstract

Extensive data available from more than 30 years of research reveal that children raised by gay and lesbian parents have demonstrated resilience with regard to social, psychological, and sexual health despite economic and legal disparities and social stigma. Many studies have demonstrated that children's well-being is affected much more by their relationships with their parents, their parents' sense of competence and security, and the presence of social and economic support for the family than by the gender or the sexual orientation of their parents. Lack of opportunity for same-gender couples to marry adds to families' stress, which affects the health and welfare of all household members. Because marriage strengthens families and, in so doing, benefits children's development, children should not be deprived of the opportunity for their parents to be married. Paths to parenthood that include assisted reproductive techniques, adop-tion, and foster parenting should focus on competency of the parents rather than their sexual orientation. *Pediatrics* 2013;131: e1374–e1383

Ellen C. Perrin, MD, MA, Benjamin S. Siegel, MD, and the COMMITTEE ON PSYCHOSOCIAL ASPECTS OF CHILD AND FAMILY HEALTH

KEY WORDS
civil marriage, adoption, foster care, nurturing children, gay parents, lesbian parents, health disparities, legal disparities, same sex, same gender, marriage equality

This document is copyrighted and is property of the American Academy of Pediatrics and its Board of Directors. All authors have filed conflict of interest statements with the American Academy of Pediatrics. Any conflicts have been resolved through a process approved by the Board of Directors. The American Academy of Pediatrics has neither solicited nor accepted any commercial involvement in the development of the content of this publication.

The guidance in this report does not indicate an exclusive course of treatment or serve as a standard of medical care. Variations, taking into account individual circumstances, may be appropriate.

All technical reports from the American Academy of Pediatrics automatically expire 5 years after publication unless reaffirmed, revised, or retired at or before that time.

INTRODUCTION

The mission of the American Academy of Pediatrics (AAP) is to promote optimal physical, mental, and social health and well-being for all infants, children, adolescents, and young adults. Historically, the AAP has worked, through its educational, research, advocacy, and policy efforts, to highlight the powerful connection between children's well-being and the functioning of their most enduring source of support and influence —their parents. It is vital that pediatricians understand the unique and complex characteristics of their patients' families and support them to ensure optimal development of children.

All children have the same needs for, and the right to, nurturing, security, and social stability. Children whose parents are gay and lesbian have historically been subjected to laws, social policies, and disapproving attitudes that create social distance and ostracism and challenge the stability of their families as well as their optimal social and psychological development. This technical report provides the scientific rationale, based on the current available evidence, to support the recommendations outlined in the policy statement "Promoting the Well-Being of Children Whose Parents are Gay or Lesbian"[1]: sup-port for marriage equality, including repeal of the federal Defense of

www.pediatrics.org/cgi/doi/10.1542/peds.2013-0377

doi:10.1542/peds.2013-0377

PEDIATRICS (ISSN Numbers: Print, 0031-4005; Online, 1098-4275).

Copyright © 2013 by the American Academy of Pediatrics

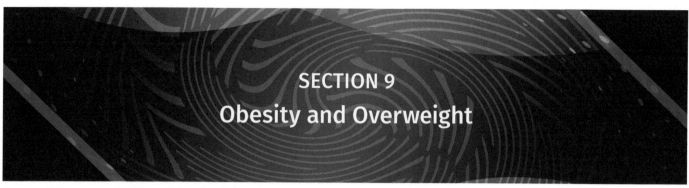

SECTION 9
Obesity and Overweight

Some articles are available online only; scan the QR code to access online content.

CLINICAL PRACTICE GUIDELINE Guidance for the Clinician in Rendering Pediatric Care

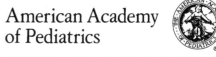

American Academy
of Pediatrics

DEDICATED TO THE HEALTH OF ALL CHILDREN™

Executive Summary: Clinical Practice Guideline for the Evaluation and Treatment of Children and Adolescents With Obesity

Sarah E. Hampl, MD, FAAP,[a] Sandra G. Hassink, MD, FAAP,[b] Asheley C. Skinner, PhD,[c] Sarah C. Armstrong, MD, FAAP,[d] Sarah E. Barlow, MD, MPH, FAAP,[e] Christopher F. Bolling, MD, FAAP,[f] Kimberly C. Avila Edwards, MD, FAAP,[g] Ihuoma Eneli, MD, MS, FAAP,[h] Robin Hamre, MPH,[i] Madeline M. Joseph, MD, FAAP,[j] Doug Lunsford, MEd,[k] Eneida Mendonca, MD, PhD, FAAP,[l] Marc P. Michalsky, MD, MBA, FAAP,[m] Nazrat Mirza, MD, ScD, FAAP,[n] Eduardo R. Ochoa, Jr, MD, FAAP,[o] Mona Sharifi, MD, MPH, FAAP,[p] Amanda E. Staiano, PhD, MPP,[q] Ashley E. Weedn, MD, MPH, FAAP,[r] Susan K. Flinn, MA,[s] Jeanne Lindros, MPH,[t] Kymika Okechukwu, MPA[u]

INTRODUCTION AND APPROACH

Obesity is a common, complex, and often persistent chronic disease associated with serious health and social consequences if not treated.[1] Yet, despite the disease's complexity, treatment of obesity can be successful.[2-4] The current and long-term health of 14.4 million children and adolescents is affected by obesity,[5,6] making it one of the most common pediatric chronic diseases in the United States.[5,7,8]

Obesity has long been stigmatized as a reversible consequence of personal choices but has, in reality, complex genetic, physiologic, socioeconomic, and environmental contributors. An increased understanding of the impact of social determinants of health (SDoHs) on the chronic disease of obesity—along with heightened appreciation of the impact of the chronicity and severity of obesity-related comorbidities—has enabled broader and deeper understanding of the complexity of both obesity risk and treatment.[9,10]

This clinical practice guideline (CPG) aims to inform pediatricians and other pediatric health care providers (PHCPs) about the standard of care for evaluating and treating children with overweight and obesity and related comorbidities. The CPG promotes an approach that considers the child's health status, family system, community context, and resources for treatment to create the best evidence-based treatment plan. The medical home should coordinate the evaluation and treatment of obesity and related conditions; however, the CPG

[a]Children's Mercy Kansas City Center for Children's Healthy Lifestyles & Nutrition, University of Missouri-Kansas City School of Medicine, Kansas City, Missouri; [b]Medical Director, American Academy of Pediatrics, Institute for Healthy Childhood Weight, Wilmington, Delaware; [c]Department of Population Health Sciences, Duke University School of Medicine, Durham, North Carolina; [d]Departments of Pediatrics and Population Health Sciences, Duke Clinical Research Institute, Duke University, Durham, North Carolina; [e]Department of Pediatrics, University of Texas Southwestern Medical Center, Children's Medical Center of Dallas, Dallas, Texas; [f]Department of Pediatrics, University of Cincinnati College of Medicine, Cincinnati, Ohio; [g]Children's Health Policy & Advocacy, Ascension; Department of Pediatrics, Dell Medical School at The University of Texas at Austin, Austin, Texas; [h]Department of Pediatrics, The Ohio State University, Center for Healthy Weight and Nutrition, Nationwide Children's Hospital, Columbus, Ohio; [i]Centers for Disease Control and Prevention, Atlanta, Georgia; [j]Division of Pediatric Emergency Medicine, Department of Emergency Medicine, University of Florida College of Medicine–Jacksonville, University of Florida Health Sciences Center–Jacksonville, Jacksonville, Florida; [k]Family Representative; [l]Departments of Pediatrics and Biostatistics & Health Data Science, Indiana University School of Medicine, Indianapolis, Indiana; [m]Department of Pediatric Surgery, The Ohio State University, College of Medicine, Nationwide Children's Hospital, Columbus, Ohio; [n]Children's National Hospital, George Washington University, Washington, DC; [o]Department of Pediatrics, University of Arkansas for Medical Sciences, Arkansas Children's Hospital, Little Rock, Arkansas;

To cite: Hampl SE, Hassink SG, Skinner AC, et al. Executive Summary: Clinical Practice Guideline for the Evaluation and Treatment of Children and Adolescents With Obesity. *Pediatrics.* 2023;151(2):e2022060641

recommendations are child-centric and not specific to a particular health care setting. The term "pediatricians and other PHCPs" includes pediatric primary and specialty care providers as well as allied health care professionals, all of whom will encounter and may treat children with overweight, obesity, and obesity-related comorbidities.

The CPG is based on a comprehensive evidence review of controlled and comparative effectiveness trials and high-quality longitudinal and epidemiologic studies. The accompanying technical reports (https://doi.org/10.1542/peds.2022-060642 and https://doi.org/10.1542/peds.2022-060643) provide detailed descriptions of the evidence review supporting the CPG's development. Based on this evidence, the CPG contains Key Action Statements (KASs), which represent evidence-based recommendations from randomized controlled and comparative effectiveness trials and high-quality longitudinal and epidemiologic studies. The CPG details an evidence table for each KAS (Table 1) and Appendix 1 in the CPG contains a helpful algorithm to guide care based on these KASs. KASs are supplemented by Consensus Recommendations to provide expert opinion on topics that were not part of the TRs. These Consensus Recommendations are supported by American Academy of Pediatrics (AAP)-endorsed guidelines, clinical guidelines, and/or position statements from professional societies in the field of obesity, and an extensive literature review (see Methodology section of CPG [https://doi.org/10.1542/peds.2022-060640]).

The CPG does not include guidance for overweight and obesity evaluation and treatment of children younger than 2 years of age. Nor does the CPG discuss primary obesity prevention, which will be addressed in a forthcoming AAP policy statement.

Obesity is a Chronic Disease With Complex Contributing Factors

Childhood obesity results from a multifactorial set of socioecological, environmental, and genetic influences that act on children and families (see Epidemiology section of CPG [https://doi.org/10.1542/peds.2022-060640]). The CPG describes risk factors for overweight and obesity, many of which are SDoHs. These SDoHs include factors related to broader policies and systems; institutions and organizations (ie, schools); neighborhoods and communities; and family, socioeconomic, environmental, ecological, genetic, and biological factors[2,3] (see Risk Factors section of CPG [https://doi.org/10.1542/peds.2022-060640]). These risk factors often overlap and/or influence one another and can operate chronically throughout childhood and adolescence, initiating weight gain and escalating degrees of existing obesity. The subcommittee recommends that pediatricians and other PHCPs perform initial and longitudinal assessment of individual, structural, and contextual risk factors to provide individualized and tailored treatment of the child/adolescent with overweight/obesity.

The term "disparities" is commonly used to describe differences in disease prevalence and outcomes in populations, defined by ethnicity, race, gender, and/or age. This word, however, does not acknowledge the causes of these disease prevalence differences, better labeled "inequities," a term that includes structural racism and the lack of "economic, civil-political, cultural, or environmental conditions that are required to generate parity and equality."[4]

This distinction between health disparities and inequities is particularly important when considering obesity because obesity-related risk factors are embedded in the socioecological and environmental fabric of children's lives. There is a danger of stigmatizing children with obesity and their families on the basis of race or ethnicity, age, and/or sex based on the disparities of outcome—without recognizing the systemic challenges that cause and maintain inequities.[11,12] Inequities are often associated with each other[13] and result in disparities in obesity risk and outcomes across the socioecological spectrum. Importantly, they represent neighborhood-, community-, and population-level factors that can be changed.[14] Inequities that promote obesity in childhood can have a longitudinal effect, which leads to disparities in adult health and contributes to adult obesity and other chronic diseases.[15]

Attainment of health equity for children with obesity requires addressing inequities in available resources and systemic barriers to quality health care services.[16] To that end, "practice standards must evolve to support an equity-based practice paradigm," and payment strategies must promote this approach to care.[17]

Individuals with overweight and obesity experience weight stigma and weight-based victimization, teasing, and bullying. This experience contributes to binge eating, social isolation, avoidance of health care services, and decreased physical activity, further complicating the health trajectory.[11,17] It is important for pediatricians and other PHCPs to communicate support and alliance with children, adolescents, and parents/caregivers as they evaluate patients, diagnose obesity and overweight, and guide obesity treatment. Discussions about weight and obesity—even when conducted using nonstigmatizing language and preferred terms—can elicit strong emotional responses, including

TABLE 1 Summary of Key Action Statements and Consensus Recommendations for the Evaluation and Treatment of Children and Adolescents with Overweight and Obesity

KAS	Evidence Quality/Strength	CPG Section
KAS 1. Pediatricians and other PHCPs should measure height and wt, calculate BMI, and assess BMI percentile using age- and sex-specific CDC growth charts or growth charts for children with severe obesity at least annually for all children 2 to 18 y of age to screen for overweight (BMI ≥85th percentile to <95th percentile), obesity (BMI ≥95th percentile), and severe obesity (BMI ≥120% of the 95th percentile for age and sex).	Grade B, Moderate	Diagnosis & Measurement
KAS 2. Pediatricians and other PHCPs should evaluate children 2 to 18 y of age with overweight (BMI ≥85th percentile to <95th percentile) and obesity (BMI ≥95th percentile) for obesity-related comorbidities by using a comprehensive patient history, mental and behavioral health screening, SDoH evaluation, physical examination, and diagnostic studies.	Grade B, Strong	Evaluation
KAS 3. In children 10 y and older, pediatricians and other PHCPs should evaluate for lipid abnormalities, abnormal glucose metabolism, and abnormal liver function in children and adolescents with obesity (BMI ≥95th percentile) and for lipid abnormalities in children and adolescents with overweight (BMI ≥85th percentile to <95th percentile).	Grade B, Strong	Comorbidities
KAS 3.1. In children 10 y and older with overweight (BMI ≥85th percentile to <95th percentile), pediatricians and other PHCPs may evaluate for abnormal glucose metabolism and liver function in the presence of risk factors for T2DM or NAFLD. In children 2 to 9 y of age with obesity (BMI ≥95th percentile), pediatricians and other PHCPs may evaluate for lipid abnormalities.	Grade C, Moderate	Comorbidities
KAS 4. Pediatricians and other PHCPs should treat children and adolescents for overweight (BMI ≥85th percentile to <95th percentile) or obesity (BMI ≥95th percentile) and comorbidities concurrently.	Grade A, Strong	Comorbidities
KAS 5. Pediatricians and other PHCPs should evaluate for dyslipidemia by obtaining a fasting lipid panel in children 10 y and older with overweight (BMI ≥85th percentile to <95th percentile) and obesity (BMI ≥95th percentile) and may evaluate for dyslipidemia in children 2 through 9 y of age with obesity.	Grade B (children ≥10 y with obesity), Strong; Grade C (children 2–9 y), Moderate	Comorbidities
KAS 6. Pediatricians and other PHCPs should evaluate for prediabetes and/or diabetes mellitus with fasting plasma glucose, 2-h plasma glucose after 75-g oral glucose tolerance test (OGTT), or glycosylated hemoglobin (HbA1c).[a]	Grade B, Moderate	Comorbidities
KAS 7. Pediatricians and other PHCPs should evaluate for NAFLD by obtaining an alanine transaminase (ALT) test.[b]	Grade A, Strong	Comorbidities
KAS 8. Pediatricians and other PHCPs should evaluate for hypertension by measuring blood pressure at every visit starting at 3 y of age in children and adolescents with overweight (BMI ≥85 to <95th percentile) and obesity (BMI ≥95th percentile).	Grade C, Moderate	Comorbidities
KAS 9. Pediatricians and other PHCPs should treat overweight (BMI ≥85th percentile to <95th percentile) and obesity (BMI ≥95th percentile) in children and adolescents, following the principles of the medical home and the chronic care model, using a family-centered and nonstigmatizing approach that acknowledges obesity's biologic, social, and structural drivers.	Grade B, Strong	Treatment
KAS 10. Pediatricians and other PHCPs should use motivational interviewing (MI) to engage patients and families in treating overweight (BMI ≥85th percentile to <95th percentile) and obesity (BMI ≥95th percentile).	Grade B, Moderate	Treatment
KAS 11. Pediatricians and other PHCPs should provide or refer children 6 y and older (Grade B) and may provide or refer children 2 through 5 y of age (Grade C) with overweight (BMI ≥85th percentile to <95th percentile) and obesity (BMI ≥95th percentile) to intensive health behavior and lifestyle treatment. Health behavior and lifestyle treatment is more effective with greater contact hours; the most effective treatment includes 26 or more hours of face-to-face, family-based, multicomponent treatment over a 3- to 12-mo period.	Grade B: Ages 6 y and older, Moderate; Grade C: Ages 2–5 y, Moderate	Treatment
KAS 12. Pediatricians and other PHCPs should offer adolescents 12 y and older with obesity (BMI ≥95th percentile) wt loss pharmacotherapy, according to	Grade B	Treatment

TABLE 1 Continued

KAS	Evidence Quality/Strength	CPG Section
medication indications, risks, and benefits, as an adjunct to health behavior and lifestyle treatment.		
KAS 13: Pediatricians and other PHCPs should offer referral for adolescents 13 y and older with severe obesity (BMI ≥120% of the 95th percentile for age and sex) for evaluation for metabolic and bariatric surgery to local or regional comprehensive multidisciplinary pediatric metabolic and bariatric surgery centers.	Grade C	Treatment

Consensus Recommendations	Location
The CPG authors recommend that pediatricians and other pediatric health care providers:	
1. Perform initial and longitudinal assessment of individual, structural, and contextual risk factors to provide individualized and tailored treatment of the child/adolescent with overweight/obesity.	Risk Factors
2. Obtain a sleep history, including symptoms of snoring, daytime somnolence, nocturnal enuresis, morning headaches, and inattention, among children and adolescents with obesity to evaluate for OSA.	Comorbidities
3. Obtain a polysomnogram for children and adolescents with obesity and at least one symptom of disordered breathing.	Comorbidities
4. Evaluate for menstrual irregularities and signs of hyperandrogenism (ie, hirsutism, acne) among female adolescents with obesity to assess risk for PCOS.	Comorbidities
5. Monitor for symptoms of depression in children and adolescents with obesity and conduct annual evaluation for depression for adolescents 12 y and older with a formal self-report tool.	Comorbidities
6. Perform a musculoskeletal review of systems and physical examination (eg, internal hip rotation in growing child, gait) as part of their evaluation for obesity.	Comorbidities
7. Recommend immediate and complete activity restriction, non–wt-bearing with use of crutches, and refer to an orthopedic surgeon for emergent evaluation, if SCFE is suspected. PHCPs may consider sending the child to an emergency department if an orthopedic surgeon is not available.	Comorbidities
8. Maintain a high index of suspicion for IIH with new-onset or progressive headaches in the context of significant wt gain, especially for females.	Comorbidities
9. Deliver the best available intensive treatment to all children with overweight and obesity.	Treatment
10. Build collaborations with other specialists and programs in their communities.	Treatment
11. May offer children ages 8 through 11 y of age with obesity wt loss pharmacotherapy, according to medication indications, risks, and benefits, as an adjunct to health behavior and lifestyle treatment.	Treatment

Implementation Consensus Recommendations	
1: The subcommittee recommends that the AAP and its membership strongly promote supportive payment and public health policies that cover comprehensive obesity prevention, evaluation, and treatment. The medical costs of untreated childhood obesity are well-documented and add urgency to provide payment for treatment. There is a role for AAP policy and advocacy, in partnership with other organizations, to demand more of our government to accelerate progress in prevention and treatment of obesity for all children through policy change within and beyond the health care sector to improve the health and well-being of children. Furthermore, targeted policies are needed to purposefully address the structural racism in our society that drives the alarming and persistent disparities in childhood obesity and obesity-related comorbidities.	Barriers & Implementation Recommendations
2: The subcommittee recommends that public health agencies, community organizations, health care systems, health care providers, and community members partner with each other to expand access to evidence-based pediatric obesity treatment programs and to increase community resources that address social determinants of health in promoting healthy, active lifestyles.	Barriers & Implementation Recommendations
3: The subcommittee recommends that EHR vendors, health systems, and practices implement CDS systems broadly in EHRs to provide prompts and facilitate best practices for managing children and adolescents with obesity.	Barriers & Implementation Recommendations
4: The subcommittee recommends that medical and other health professions schools, training programs, boards, and professional societies improve education and training opportunities related to obesity for both practicing providers and in preprofessional schools and residency/fellowship programs. Such training includes the underlying physiologic basis for wt dysregulation, MI, wt bias, the social and emotional impact of obesity on patients, the need to tailor management to SDoHs that impact wt, and wt-related outcomes and other emerging science.	Barriers & Implementation Recommendations

AAP, American Academy of Pediatrics; BMI, body mass index; CDC, Centers for Disease Control and Prevention; IIH, idiopathic intracranial hypertension; KAS, Key Action Statement; MI, myocardial infarction; NAFLD, pediatric health care provider; OSA, obstructive sleep apnea; PCOS, polycystic ovarian syndrome; PHCP, pediatric health care provider; SCFE, slipped capital femoral epiphysis; SDoH, social determinant of health; T2DM, type 2 diabetes mellitus; wt, weight.

[a] Per KAS 3 and 3.1: Pediatricians and other PHCPs should evaluate children 10 y and older with obesity (BMI ≥95th percentile) for abnormal glucose metabolism and may evaluate children 10 y and older with overweight (BMI ≥85th percentile to <95th percentile) with risk factors for T2DM or NAFLD for abnormal glucose metabolism. (Refer to evidence tables for KAS 3 and 3.1.)

[b] Per KAS 3 and 3.1: Pediatricians and other PHCPs should evaluate children 10 y and older with obesity (BMI ≥95th percentile) for abnormal liver function and may evaluate children 10 y and older with overweight (BMI ≥85th percentile to <95th percentile) with risk factors for T2DM or NAFLD for abnormal liver function. (Refer to evidence tables for KAS 3 and 3.1.)

sadness and anger. Acknowledging and validating these responses, while keeping the focus on the child's health, can help to strengthen the relationship between the pediatrician or other PHCP and patient to support ongoing care.

All services and supports for children and youth with obesity and their families should be implemented and delivered in a linguistically appropriate and accessible manner that recognizes cultural values. The AAP statement on weight bias offers steps to provide supportive and nonbiased behavior, including recognition of the complex genetic and environmental influences on obesity.[17]

Diagnosis and Evaluation

Following comprehensive systematic reviews, the US Preventive Services Task Force issued a Grade B recommendation that pediatricians and other PHCPs screen children and adolescents aged 6 years or older annually for obesity—defined by body mass index (BMI) percentile (**KAS 1**).[18] In clinical practice, BMI is frequently used as both a screening and diagnostic tool for detecting excess body fat because of its ease of use and low cost. BMI is a validated proxy measure of underlying adiposity that is replicable and can track weight status in children and adolescents[19–21] (see Diagnosis/Measurement section of CPG [https://doi.org/10.1542/peds.2022-060640]).

Measuring BMI and assessing weight classification (**KAS 1**) is a screening step that allows the pediatrician or other PHCP to initiate obesity evaluation. Each child with a BMI ≥85th percentile is then evaluated with a comprehensive history, physical examination, and diagnostic studies.

Elements of the history include but are not limited to nutrition, physical activity and sedentary time behaviors, unhealthy weight control practices, sleep patterns, social history (including SDoHs), and mental/behavioral health (**KAS 2**). Specific assessment tools exist for primary care. The purpose of the evaluation is to determine the child's individual health status, including the presence and extent of obesity-related comorbidities, the extent of obesity risk factors present in the child's history and environment, and the resources available to the family to engage in obesity treatment. A timely and comprehensive evaluation is instrumental in tailoring and individualizing care for each patient and family (see Evaluation section of CPG [https://doi.org/10.1542/peds.2022-060640]).

Comorbidities

Children and adolescents with obesity have higher prevalence of comorbidities and a greater risk for obesity during adulthood, morbidity, and premature death (see Comorbidities section of CPG [https://doi.org/10.1542/peds.2022-060640]).[22–25] The risk for obesity-related comorbidities increases with age and severity of obesity and is impacted by a variety of socioecological, environmental, and genetic influences.[26]

Substantial evidence supports concurrent treatment of obesity and related comorbidities to achieve weight loss, avoid further excess weight gain, and improve obesity-related comorbidities (**KAS 4**). Studies report improvement in comorbidities with intensive lifestyle treatment, weight loss medication, and/or metabolic and bariatric surgery.[26–31] BMI reduction in children with obesity can lead to clinically meaningful improvements in obesity-related comorbidities.[31–35]

The CPG provides specific KASs on initial evaluation and diagnostic tests for several common comorbidities: dyslipidemia, type 2 diabetes mellitus (T2DM), nonalcoholic fatty liver disease (NAFLD), and hypertension (**KAS 3, 3.1, 5, 6, 7, 8**). Appendices provide additional information on treatment of these common comorbidities.

The CPG also describes additional comorbidities potentially associated with pediatric obesity, including obstructive sleep apnea, polycystic ovarian syndrome, depression, slipped capital femoral epiphysis, Blount disease, and idiopathic intracranial hypertension (formerly known as pseudotumor cerebri). Consensus Recommendations are provided for addressing these comorbidities; appendices offer a framework for evaluation, reevaluation, and initial management of these comorbidities (see Appendix 3 in the CPG [https://doi.org/10.1542/peds.2022-060640]).

Treatment

Obesity is a chronic disease and should be treated through the medical home with intensive and long-term care strategies, provision of ongoing medical monitoring, and treatment of associated comorbidities and ongoing access to obesity treatment (see Treatment section in CPG [https://doi.org/10.1542/peds.2022-060640]). Comprehensive obesity treatment includes integration and coordination of weight management components and strategies across appropriate disciplines. Comprehensive treatment can include nutrition support, physical activity treatment, behavioral therapy, pharmacotherapy, and metabolic and bariatric surgery.

The CPG recommends that pediatricians and other PHCPs treat overweight and obesity in children and adolescents following the principles of the medical home, and the chronic care model, using a family-centered and nonstigmatizing approach that acknowledges obesity's biologic, social, and structural drivers (**KAS 9**). The chronic care model requires patient-centered care to be delivered with consideration of the child's household and familial influences, access to healthy food and activity spaces, and other SDoHs. Recommendations for obesity treatment should be integrated within existing community and social systems.[36] No evidence exists to exclude children with special health care needs, complex disease, or developmental limitations from the treatment options outlined in the CPG, except where specifically noted (see Treatment Considerations for Children and Youth with Special Health Care Needs section in CPG [https://doi.org/10.1542/peds.2022-060640]).

There is no evidence to support either watchful waiting or unnecessary delay of appropriate treatment of children with obesity. Multiple studies have demonstrated that, although obesity and self-guided dieting place children at high risk for weight fluctuation and disordered eating patterns,[37] participation in structured, supervised weight management programs decreases current and future eating disorder symptoms (including bulimic symptoms, emotional eating, binge eating, and drive for thinness) up to 6 years after treatment.[37–39] The CPG's KASs and Consensus Recommendations share components with effective eating disorder programs, including a focus on increasing healthful food consumption, participation in physical activity for enjoyment and self-care reasons, and improvement in self-esteem and self-concept.

The natural course of obesity across the lifespan is characterized by responses to treatment and relapse when treatment ends[26]; thus, children and adolescents with obesity will need appropriate reassessments of medical and psychological risks and comorbidities and appropriate

modifications to their treatment plan throughout childhood and adolescence into young adulthood (**KAS 9**).[36]

Obesity treatment should be delivered by pediatricians and other PHCPs and their teams in collaboration with (where available) community partners, allied health professionals, pediatric obesity specialists, and metabolic and bariatric surgery teams. The medical home model is the preferred standard of care for children who have chronic conditions; this care coordination should also be accompanied by advocacy for the patient and the family and support for the patient's transition to adult care.

The foundation of all comprehensive obesity treatment is helping the child/adolescent and the family change lifestyle, behavioral, and environmental factors that will allow them to manage their obesity in their individual health and environmental context. Families should be active and core partners in decision-making in all levels of care. Parents/caregivers play a crucial role in obesity treatment through strategies including monitoring, limit-setting, reducing barriers, managing family conflict, and modifying the home environment.[40–43] Medium- to high-intensity parental involvement is associated with weight-related measures of treatment effectiveness.[43] Parents can serve as role models and provide support in obesity treatment. In addition, an enhanced parent–child relationship functions as a mediator in development of healthier behaviors and weight control.[44] Parents themselves and family relationships may also benefit from children's obesity treatment.

Motivational interviewing is a collaborative approach to conversation about change and is a core component of delivering all

levels of comprehensive obesity treatment (**KAS 10**), including engaging patients and families in addressing overweight and obesity, setting goals, and promoting participation in available resources and programs.

Intensive health behavior and lifestyle treatment (IHBLT), although challenging to deliver and not universally available, is the most effective known behavioral treatment of child obesity. The CPG uses "IHBLT" rather than previous terms including "intensive lifestyle/behavioral modification" or "weight management." Pediatricians and other PHCPs should provide or refer children aged 6 years and older—and may provide or refer children 2 through 5 years of age—with overweight and obesity to IHBLT (**KAS 11**). IHBLT is more effective with greater contact hours; the most effective treatments include 26 or more hours of face-to-face, family-based, multicomponent treatment over a 3- to 12-month period. IHBLT should include nutrition, physical activity, and behavioral change support and should be delivered by pediatricians or other PHCPs and their teams in collaboration with pediatric obesity specialists, allied health providers, and community partners.[18]

When an IHBLT program is not available, pediatricians and other PHCPs should provide the most intensive program possible. They can build capacity for obesity treatment by collaborating and connecting families with community resources to support nutrition and address food insecurity (eg, food provision programs), physical activity (eg, local parks, recreation programs), and other SDoHs. Pediatricians and other PHCPs should familiarize themselves with resources and actively collaborate with other specialists and community programs. Registered dietitian nutritionists can complement the care of medical providers and may be the most widely available specialist with whom pediatricians and other PHCPs can provide more intensive, comprehensive obesity treatment. Behavioral health specialists, ideally integrated into primary care, can focus on the process of behavior change, including parenting skills, role modeling, and consistent reinforcement techniques. Exercise specialists can provide counseling and training to engage children and families in noncompetitive, cooperative, and fun activities.[18,26,45]

Pediatricians and other PHCPs should offer adolescents aged 12 years and older with obesity weight loss pharmacotherapy, according to medication indications, risks, and benefits, as an adjunct to health behavior and lifestyle treatment (**KAS 12**). Pharmacotherapy is an adjunct treatment to improve weight loss outcomes. In most studies, pharmacotherapy applies to children with more severe degrees of obesity and/or comorbidities. Pharmacotherapy for obesity treatment, similar to management of ADHD or depression, is most effective when prescribed along with ongoing health behavior and lifestyle treatment.

Pediatricians and other PHCPs should offer referral for adolescents aged 13 years and older with severe obesity for evaluation for metabolic and bariatric surgery to local or regional comprehensive multidisciplinary pediatric metabolic and bariatric surgery centers (**KAS 13**).[46] Although no lower age limit exists to define the safety or effectiveness of surgery among children, there are currently limited data among children younger than age 13 years. Multiple studies support that metabolic and bariatric surgery is safe and effective for adolescents in comprehensive metabolic and bariatric surgery settings that have experience working with youth and their families.

Recommendations for CPG Implementation and Evidence Gaps

Comprehensive obesity treatment requires ongoing evaluation and capacity-building of both practice and community resources. Pediatricians and other PHCPs and families face numerous barriers to promoting healthy and active lifestyles and to supporting obesity treatment among children. The successful implementation of this CPG into routine practice requires careful consideration of barriers and facilitators that can modify implementation, effectiveness, and sustainability. It is anticipated that a pediatrician's or other PHCP's setting, training, and expertise may moderate how elements of the CPG are implemented. Helpful resources can be found in accompanying implementation materials.

The CPG describes changes needed at the policy, community, practice, and provider levels. The CPG offers several Consensus Implementation Recommendations designed to facilitate pediatric obesity treatment. Specifically, the subcommittee recommends that the AAP and its membership should strongly promote supportive payment and public health policies that cover comprehensive multicomponent obesity prevention, evaluation, and treatment, including policy changes within and beyond the health care sector; combat structural racism, which drives disparities and inequities in childhood obesity and obesity-related comorbidities; expand access to evidence-based pediatric obesity treatment

programs and helpful community resources; improve electronic health records to facilitate best practices; and improve education and training opportunities related to obesity (see Implementation Barriers section of CPG [https://doi.org/10.1542/peds.2022-060640]).

Research in the field of pediatric overweight and obesity has progressed in recent years; nonetheless, significant gaps remain. The CPG describes these gaps, which include the need to develop the evidence base on the duration and heterogeneity of treatment effects, to understand how specific treatment components interact, and to conduct epidemiologic and longitudinal studies on specific age ranges, comorbidity prevalence, and optimal age and BMI ranges to begin evaluation and progression of comorbidities (see Evidence Gaps section of CPG [https://doi.org/10.1542/peds.2022-060640]).

CONCLUSION

Obesity in children and adolescents is a chronic, complex, multifactorial, and treatable disease. This CPG recommends early evaluation and treatment at the highest intensity level that is appropriate and available. In addition, understanding the wider determinants of obesity should enable pediatricians and other PHCPs to "raise awareness of the relevance of social and environmental determinants of childhood obesity in their communities."[4] The subcommittee urges pediatricians, other PHCPs, health systems, community partners, payers, and policy makers to work together to advance the equitable and universal provision of evaluation and treatment of children and adolescents with the chronic disease of obesity.

[p]*Department of Pediatrics, Yale School of Medicine, New Haven, Connecticut;* [q]*Louisiana State University Pennington Biomedical Research Center, Baton Rouge, Louisiana;* [r]*Department of Pediatrics, University of Oklahoma Health Sciences Center, Oklahoma City, Oklahoma;* [s]*Medical Writer/Consultant, Washington, DC;* [t]*American Academy of Pediatrics, Itasca, Illinois; and* [u]*American Academy of Pediatrics, Itasca, Illinois*

DOI: https://doi.org/10.1542/peds.2022-060641

Address correspondence to Sarah Hampl, MD. Email: shampl@cmh.edu

PEDIATRICS (ISSN Numbers: Print, 0031-4005; Online, 1098-4275).

FINANCIAL/CONFLICT OF INTEREST DISCLOSURES: An independent review for bias was completed by The American Academy of Pediatrics. Dr Barlow has disclosed a financial relationship with the *Eunice Kennedy Shriver* National Institute of Child Health and Human Development as a co-investigator.

COMPANION PAPER: A companion to this article can be found online at https://doi.org/10.1542/peds.2022-060640.

REFERENCES

1. Centers for Disease Control and Prevention. Childhood obesity causes and consequences. 2021. Available at: https://www.cdc.gov/obesity/childhood/causes.html. Accessed October 4, 2022

2. Karnik S, Kanekar A. Childhood obesity: a global public health crisis. *Int J Prev Med.* 2012;3(1):1–7

3. Pratt CA, Loria CM, Arteaga SS, et al. A systematic review of obesity disparities research. *Am J Prev Med.* 2017;53(1):113–122

4. American Academy of Pediatrics, Council on Community Pediatrics and Committee on Native American Child Health. Policy statement–health equity and children's rights. *Pediatrics.* 2010;125(4):838–849

5. Centers for Disease Control and Prevention. Childhood obesity facts. 2021. Available at: https://www.cdc.gov/obesity/data/childhood.html. Accessed October 4, 2022

6. Fryar CD, Carroll MD, Afful J. Prevalence of overweight, obesity, and severe obesity among children and adolescents aged 2–19 years: United States, 1963–1965 through 2017–2018. NCHS E-Health Stats. 2020. Available at: https://www.cdc.gov/nchs/data/hestat/obesity-child-17-18/obesity-child.htm. Accessed October 4, 2022

7. Hales CM, Fryar CD, Carroll MD, Freedman DS, Ogden CL. Trends in obesity and severe obesity prevalence in US youth and adults by sex and age, 2007-2008 to 2015-2016. *JAMA.* 2018; 319(16):1723–1725

8. Ogden CL, Fryar CD, Martin CB, et al. Trends in obesity prevalence by race and Hispanic origin-1999-2000 to 2017-2018. *JAMA.* 2020;324(12): 1208–1210

9. Medvedyuk S, Ahmednur A, Raphael D. Ideology, obesity and the social determinants of health: a critical analysis of the obesity and health relationship. *Crit Public Health.* 2018;28(5):573–585

10. Centers for Disease Control and Prevention. About Social Determinants of Health (SDOH). 2021. Available at: https://www.cdc.gov/socialdeterminants/about.html. Accessed October 4, 2022

11. Puhl R, Suh Y. Health consequences of weight stigma: implications for obesity prevention and treatment. *Curr Obes Rep.* 2015;4(2):182–190

12. Obesity Canada. Canadian Adult Obesity Clinical Practice Guidelines: Reducing Weight Bias in Obesity Management, Practice and Policy. 2020. Available at: https://obesitycanada.ca/guidelines/weightbias. Accessed October 4, 2022

13. Keating DP, Hertzman C, eds. *Developmental Health and the Wealth of Nations: Social, Biological, and Educational Dynamics.* New York, NY: Guilford Press; 1999

14. Krieger N. A glossary for social epidemiology. *J Epidemiol Community Health.* 2001;55(10):693–700

15. Serdula MK, Ivery D, Coates RJ, Freedman DS, Williamson DF, Byers T. Do obese children become obese adults? A review of the literature. *Prev Med.* 1993;22(2):167–177

16. Whitehead M, Dahlgren G. What can be done about inequalities in health? *Lancet.* 1991;338(8774):1059–1063

17. Pont SJ, Puhl R, Cook SR, Slusser W; American Academy of Pediatrics, Section on Obesity; Obesity Society. Stigma experienced by children and adolescents with obesity. *Pediatrics.* 2017;140(6):e20173034

18. Grossman DC, Bibbins-Domingo K, Curry SJ, et al; US Preventive Services Task Force. Screening for obesity in children and adolescents: US Preventive Services Task Force Recommendation Statement. *JAMA.* 2017;317(23):2417–2426

19. Freedman DS, Sherry B. The validity of BMI as an indicator of body fatness and risk among children. *Pediatrics.* 2009;124(1 Suppl 1):S23–S34

20. Simmonds M, Llewellyn A, Owen CG, Woolacott N. Predicting adult obesity from childhood obesity: a systematic review and meta-analysis. *Obes Rev.* 2016;17(2):95–107

21. Javed A, Jumean M, Murad MH, et al. Diagnostic performance of body mass index to identify obesity as defined by body adiposity in children and adolescents: a systematic review and meta-analysis. *Pediatr Obes.* 2015;10(3):234–244

22. Kelly AS, Barlow SE, Rao G, et al; American Heart Association Atherosclerosis, Hypertension, and Obesity in the Young Committee of the Council on Cardiovascular Disease in the Young, Council on Nutrition, Physical Activity and Metabolism, and Council on Clinical Cardiology. Severe obesity in children and adolescents: identification, associated health risks, and treatment

approaches: a scientific statement from the American Heart Association. *Circulation.* 2013;128(15):1689–1712

23. Baker JL, Olsen LW, Sørensen TI. Childhood body-mass index and the risk of coronary heart disease in adulthood. *N Engl J Med.* 2007;357(23):2329–2337

24. Ward ZJ, Long MW, Resch SC, Giles CM, Cradock AL, Gortmaker SL. Simulation of growth trajectories of childhood obesity into adulthood. *N Engl J Med.* 2017;377(22):2145–2153

25. Skinner AC, Perrin EM, Moss LA, Skelton JA. Cardiometabolic risks and severity of obesity in children and young adults. *N Engl J Med.* 2015;373(14):1307–1317

26. Skinner AC, Staiano A, Armstrong S, et al. Appraisal of clinical care practices for child obesity prevention and treatment to inform quality improvement. Part II: comorbidities. *Pediatrics.* 2023;151(2):e2022060643

27. Inge TH, Coley RY, Bazzano LA, et al; PCORnet Bariatric Study Collaborative. Comparative effectiveness of bariatric procedures among adolescents: the PCORnet bariatric study. *Surg Obes Relat Dis.* 2018;14(9):1374–1386

28. Rajjo T, Almasri J, Al Nofal A, et al. The association of weight loss and cardiometabolic outcomes in obese children: systematic review and meta-regression. *J Clin Endocrinol Metab.* 2017;102(3): 758–762

29. Ryder JR, Xu P, Inge TH, et al. Thirty-year risk of cardiovascular disease events in adolescents with severe obesity. *Obesity (Silver Spring).* 2020;28(3):616–623

30. Savoye M, Shaw M, Dziura J, et al. Effects of a weight management program on body composition and metabolic parameters in overweight children: a randomized controlled trial. *JAMA.* 2007;297(24):2697–2704

31. Andersen IG, Holm JC, Homøe P. Obstructive sleep apnea in children and adolescents with and without obesity. *Eur Arch Otorhinolaryngol.* 2019; 276(3):871–878

32. Hadjiyannakis S, Ibrahim Q, Li J, et al. Obesity class versus the Edmonton Obesity Staging System for Pediatrics to define health risk in childhood obesity: results from the CANPWR cross-sectional study. *Lancet Child Adolesc Health.* 2019;3(6):398–407

33. Kim Y, Cubbin C, Oh S. A systematic review of neighbourhood economic context on child obesity and obesity-related behaviours. *Obes Rev.* 2019; 20(3):420–431

34. Akinbami LJ, Rossen LM, Fakhouri THI, Simon AE, Kit BK. Contribution of weight status to asthma prevalence racial disparities, 2-19 year olds, 1988-2014. *Ann Epidemiol.* 2017;27(8):472–478.e3

35. Reinehr T, Kleber M, Toschke AM. Lifestyle intervention in obese children is associated with a decrease of the metabolic syndrome prevalence. *Atherosclerosis.* 2009;207(1):174–180

36. Dietz WH, Belay B, Bradley D, et al. *A Model Framework That Integrates Community and Clinical Systems for the Prevention and Management of Obesity and Other Chronic Diseases.* Washington, DC: National Academy of Medicine; 2017

37. Cardel MI, Newsome FA, Pearl RL, et al. Patient-centered care for obesity: how health care providers can treat obesity while actively addressing weight stigma and eating disorder risk. *J Acad Nutr Diet.* 2022;122(6):1089–1098

38. Eichen DM, Strong DR, Rhee KE, et al. Change in eating disorder symptoms following pediatric obesity treatment. *Int J Eat Disord.* 2019;52(3):299–303

39. Jebeile H, Gow ML, Baur LA, Garnett SP, Paxton SJ, Lister NB. Treatment of obesity, with a dietary component, and eating disorder risk in children and adolescents: a systematic review with meta-analysis. *Obes Rev.* 2019;20(9):1287–1298

40. American Psychological Association, Clinical Practice Guideline Panel. *Clinical Practice Guideline for Multicomponent Behavioral Treatment of Obesity and Overweight in Children and Adolescents: Current State of the Evidence and Research Needs.* Washington, DC: American Psychological Association; 2018

41. Rosenkranz RR, Bauer A, Dzewaltowski DA. Mother-daughter resemblance in BMI and obesity-related behaviors. *Int J Adolesc Med Health.* 2010;22(4):477–489

42. Spear BA, Barlow SE, Ervin C, et al. Recommendations for treatment of child and adolescent overweight and obesity. *Pediatrics.* 2007;120(suppl 4):S254–S288

43. van der Kruk JJ, Kortekaas F, Lucas C, Jager-Wittenaar H. Obesity: a systematic review on parental involvement in long-term European childhood weight control interventions with a nutritional focus. *Obes Rev.* 2013;14(9):745–760

44. Van Ryzin MJ, Nowicka P. Direct and indirect effects of a family-based intervention in early adolescence on parent-youth relationship quality, late adolescent health, and early adult obesity. *J Fam Psychol.* 2013;27(1): 106–116

45. Skinner AC, Staiano A, Armstrong S, et al. Appraisal of clinical care practices for child obesity prevention and treatment to inform quality improvement. Part I: interventions. *Pediatrics.* 2023;151(2):e2022060642

46. Armstrong SC, Bolling CF, Michalsky MP, Reichard KW; American Academy of Pediatrics, Section on Obesity, Section on Surgery. Pediatric metabolic and bariatric surgery: evidence, barriers, and best practices. *Pediatrics.* 2019;144(6): e20193223

APPENDIX 1 Algorithm for Screening, Diagnosis, Evaluation, and Treatment of Children and Adolescents with Obesity

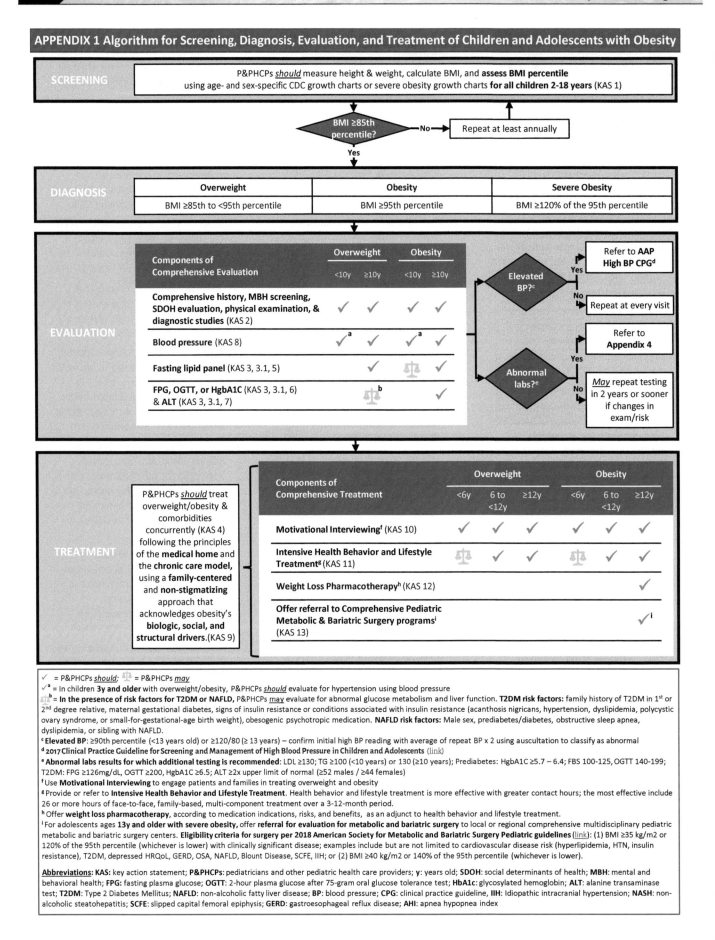

SCREENING

P&PHCPs *should* measure height & weight, calculate BMI, and **assess BMI percentile** using age- and sex-specific CDC growth charts or severe obesity growth charts **for all children 2-18 years** (KAS 1)

BMI ≥85th percentile? —No→ Repeat at least annually

Yes

DIAGNOSIS

Overweight	Obesity	Severe Obesity
BMI ≥85th to <95th percentile	BMI ≥95th percentile	BMI ≥120% of the 95th percentile

EVALUATION

Components of Comprehensive Evaluation	Overweight		Obesity	
	<10y	≥10y	<10y	≥10y
Comprehensive history, MBH screening, SDOH evaluation, physical examination, & diagnostic studies (KAS 2)	✓	✓	✓	✓
Blood pressure (KAS 8)	✓ᵃ	✓	✓ᵃ	✓
Fasting lipid panel (KAS 3, 3.1, 5)		⚖		✓
FPG, OGTT, or HgbA1C (KAS 3, 3.1, 6) & **ALT** (KAS 3, 3.1, 7)		⚖ᵇ		✓

Elevated BP?ᶜ —Yes→ Refer to **AAP High BP CPG**ᵈ

No→ Repeat at every visit

Abnormal labs?ᵉ —Yes→ Refer to **Appendix 4**

No→ *May* repeat testing in 2 years or sooner if changes in exam/risk

TREATMENT

P&PHCPs *should* treat overweight/obesity & comorbidities concurrently (KAS 4) following the principles of the **medical home** and the **chronic care model**, using a **family-centered** and **non-stigmatizing** approach that acknowledges obesity's **biologic, social, and structural drivers**.(KAS 9)

Components of Comprehensive Treatment	Overweight			Obesity		
	<6y	6 to <12y	≥12y	<6y	6 to <12y	≥12y
Motivational Interviewingᶠ (KAS 10)	✓	✓	✓	✓	✓	✓
Intensive Health Behavior and Lifestyle Treatmentᵍ (KAS 11)	⚖	✓	✓	⚖	✓	✓
Weight Loss Pharmacotherapyʰ (KAS 12)						✓
Offer referral to Comprehensive Pediatric Metabolic & Bariatric Surgery programsⁱ (KAS 13)						✓ⁱ

✓ = P&PHCPs *should*; ⚖ = P&PHCPs *may*

✓ᵃ = In children **3y and older** with overweight/obesity, P&PHCPs *should* evaluate for hypertension using blood pressure

⚖ᵇ = **In the presence of risk factors for T2DM or NAFLD**, P&PHCPs *may* evaluate for abnormal glucose metabolism and liver function. **T2DM risk factors:** family history of T2DM in 1ˢᵗ or 2ⁿᵈ degree relative, maternal gestational diabetes, signs of insulin resistance or conditions associated with insulin resistance (acanthosis nigricans, hypertension, dyslipidemia, polycystic ovary syndrome, or small-for-gestational-age birth weight), obesogenic psychotropic medication. **NAFLD risk factors:** Male sex, prediabetes/diabetes, obstructive sleep apnea, dyslipidemia, or sibling with NAFLD.

ᶜ **Elevated BP:** ≥90th percentile (<13 years old) or ≥120/80 (≥ 13 years) – confirm initial high BP reading with average of repeat BP x 2 using auscultation to classify as abnormal

ᵈ **2017 Clinical Practice Guideline for Screening and Management of High Blood Pressure in Children and Adolescents** (link)

ᵉ **Abnormal labs** results for which additional testing is recommended: LDL ≥130; TG ≥100 (<10 years) or 130 (≥10 years); Prediabetes: HgbA1C ≥5.7 – 6.4; FBS 100-125, OGTT 140-199; T2DM: FPG ≥126mg/dL, OGTT ≥200, HgbA1C ≥6.5; ALT ≥2x upper limit of normal (≥52 males / ≥44 females)

ᶠ Use **Motivational Interviewing** to engage patients and families in treating overweight and obesity

ᵍ Provide or refer to **Intensive Health Behavior and Lifestyle Treatment**. Health behavior and lifestyle treatment is more effective with greater contact hours; the most effective include 26 or more hours of face-to-face, family-based, multi-component treatment over a 3-12-month period.

ʰ Offer **weight loss pharmacotherapy**, according to medication indications, risks, and benefits, as an adjunct to health behavior and lifestyle treatment.

ⁱ For adolescents ages **13y and older with severe obesity**, offer **referral for evaluation for metabolic and bariatric surgery** to local or regional comprehensive multidisciplinary pediatric metabolic and bariatric surgery centers. Eligibility criteria for surgery per 2018 American Society for Metabolic and Bariatric Surgery Pediatric guidelines (link): (1) BMI ≥35 kg/m2 or 120% of the 95th percentile (whichever is lower) with clinically significant disease; examples include but are not limited to cardiovascular disease risk (hyperlipidemia, HTN, insulin resistance), T2DM, depressed HRQoL, GERD, OSA, NAFLD, Blount Disease, SCFE, IIH; or (2) BMI ≥40 kg/m2 or 140% of the 95th percentile (whichever is lower).

Abbreviations: KAS: key action statement; **P&PHCPs:** pediatricians and other pediatric health care providers; **y:** years old; **SDOH:** social determinants of health; **MBH:** mental and behavioral health; **FPG:** fasting plasma glucose; **OGTT:** 2-hour plasma glucose after 75-gram oral glucose tolerance test; **HbA1c:** glycosylated hemoglobin; **ALT:** alanine transaminase test; **T2DM:** Type 2 Diabetes Mellitus; **NAFLD:** non-alcoholic fatty liver disease; **BP:** blood pressure; **CPG:** clinical practice guideline; **IIH:** Idiopathic intracranial hypertension; **NASH:** non-alcoholic steatohepatitis; **SCFE:** slipped capital femoral epiphysis; **GERD:** gastroesophageal reflux disease; **AHI:** apnea hypopnea index

CLINICAL PRACTICE GUIDELINE Guidance for the Clinician in Rendering Pediatric Care

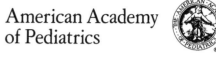

American Academy
of Pediatrics

DEDICATED TO THE HEALTH OF ALL CHILDREN™

Clinical Practice Guideline for the Evaluation and Treatment of Children and Adolescents With Obesity

Sarah E. Hampl, MD, FAAP,[a] Sandra G. Hassink, MD, FAAP,[b] Asheley C. Skinner, PhD,[c] Sarah C. Armstrong, MD, FAAP,[d] Sarah E. Barlow, MD, MPH, FAAP,[e] Christopher F. Bolling, MD, FAAP,[f] Kimberly C. Avila Edwards, MD, FAAP,[g] Ihuoma Eneli, MD, MS, FAAP,[h] Robin Hamre, MPH,[i] Madeline M. Joseph, MD, FAAP,[j] Doug Lunsford, MEd,[k] Eneida Mendonca, MD, PhD, FAAP,[l] Marc P. Michalsky, MD, MBA, FAAP,[m] Nazrat Mirza, MD, ScD, FAAP,[n] Eduardo R. Ochoa, Jr, MD, FAAP,[o] Mona Sharifi, MD, MPH, FAAP,[p] Amanda E. Staiano, PhD, MPP,[q] Ashley E. Weedn, MD, MPH, FAAP,[r] Susan K. Flinn, MA,[s] Jeanne Lindros, MPH,[t] Kymika Okechukwu, MPA[u]

[a]Children's Mercy Kansas City Center for Children's Healthy Lifestyles & Nutrition, University of Missouri-Kansas City School of Medicine, Kansas City, Missouri; [b]Medical Director, American Academy of Pediatrics, Institute for Healthy Childhood Weight, Wilmington, Delaware; [c]Department of Population Health Sciences, Duke University School of Medicine, Durham, North Carolina; [d]Departments of Pediatrics and Population Health Sciences, Duke Clinical Research Institute, Duke University, Durham, North Carolina; [e]Department of Pediatrics, University of Texas Southwestern Medical Center, Children's Medical Center of Dallas, Dallas, Texas; [f]Department of Pediatrics, University of Cincinnati College of Medicine, Cincinnati, Ohio; [g]Children's Health Policy & Advocacy, Ascension; Department of Pediatrics, Dell Medical School at The University of Texas at Austin, Austin, Texas; [h]Department of Pediatrics, The Ohio State University, Center for Healthy Weight and Nutrition, Nationwide Children's Hospital, Columbus, Ohio; [i]Centers for Disease Control and Prevention, Atlanta, Georgia; [j]Division of Pediatric Emergency Medicine, Department of Emergency Medicine, University of Florida College of Medicine–Jacksonville, University of Florida Health Sciences Center–Jacksonville, Jacksonville, Florida; [k]Family Representative; [l]Departments of Pediatrics and Biostatistics & Health Data Science, Indiana University School of Medicine, Indianapolis, Indiana; [m]Department of Pediatric Surgery, The Ohio State University, College of Medicine, Nationwide Children's Hospital, Columbus, Ohio; [n]Children's National Hospital, George Washington University, Washington, DC; [o]Department of Pediatrics, University of Arkansas for Medical Sciences, Arkansas Children's Hospital, Little Rock, Arkansas; [p]Department of Pediatrics, Yale School of Medicine, New Haven, Connecticut; [q]Louisiana State University Pennington Biomedical Research Center, Baton Rouge, Louisiana; [r]Department of Pediatrics, University of Oklahoma Health Sciences Center, Oklahoma City, Oklahoma; [s]Medical Writer/Consultant, Washington, DC; [t]American Academy of Pediatrics, Itasca, Illinois; and [u]American Academy of Pediatrics, Itasca, Illinois

Greetings

You have in your hands, or at your fingertips, the first edition of the American Academy of Pediatrics clinical practice guideline for evaluation and management of children and adolescents with overweight and obesity. Putting together this guideline was no small task, and the Academy is grateful to the efforts of all the professionals who contributed to the production of this document. This work is a true testament to their passion and dedication to combatting childhood and adolescent overweight and obesity.

The Subcommittee responsible for developing this guideline comprises a diverse group of professionals from a variety of disciplines representing both governmental entities and private institutions. Experts all, they are united by a common desire to provide the finest, most effective care and treatment to children and adolescents with overweight and obesity. Over the course of several months, the members of the Subcommittee reviewed the technical reports produced from the study review, then worked in concert to develop the Key Action Statements and Expert Consensus Recommendations contained within this guideline. These were crafted with meticulous care by the Subcommittee members, to align with current literature and to place appropriate emphasis on each statement.

While representing such a broad spectrum of perspectives, the members of this committee are all keenly aware of the multitude of barriers to treatment that patients and their families face. These barriers impact not only their access to treatment, but their ability to follow prescribed treatment plans. Whereas some patients are able to adopt the lifestyle changes and habitualize elements of their prescribed treatment plans, so many others struggle to do so for a wide variety of reasons. The members of the Subcommittee understand all of this. To assist with optimizing health equity and overcoming these barriers, guidance on a number of multilevel factors related to barriers to treatment have been included in this guideline. During the course of their work, members of the Subcommittee acknowledged that, although so much has been learned to advance the treatment of children and adolescents with overweight and obesity, there is still so much we have yet

To cite: Hampl SE, Hassink SG, Skinner AC, et al. Clinical Practice Guideline for the Evaluation and Treatment of Children and Adolescents With Obesity. *Pediatrics.* 2023;151(2): e2022060640

TECHNICAL REPORT

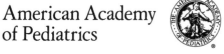

American Academy
of Pediatrics

DEDICATED TO THE HEALTH OF ALL CHILDREN™

Appraisal of Clinical Care Practices for Child Obesity Treatment. Part I: Interventions

Asheley C. Skinner, PhD,[a] Amanda E. Staiano, PhD, MPP,[b] Sarah C. Armstrong, MD, FAAP,[c] Shari L. Barkin, MD, MSHS,[d] Sandra G. Hassink, MD, FAAP,[e] Jennifer E. Moore, PhD, RN, FAAN,[f] Jennifer S. Savage, PhD,[g] Helene Vilme, DrPH,[h] Ashley E. Weedn, MD, MPH, FAAP,[i] Janice Liebhart, MS,[j] Jeanne Lindros, MPH,[k] Eileen M. Reilly, MSW[l]

The objective of this technical report is to provide clinicians with evidence-based, actionable information upon which to make assessment and treatment decisions for children and adolescents with obesity. In addition, this report will provide an evidence base to inform clinical practice guidelines for the management and treatment of overweight and obesity in children and adolescents.

To this end, the goal of this report was to identify all relevant studies to answer 2 overarching key questions: (KQ1) "What are clinically based, effective treatments for obesity?" and (KQ2) "What is the risk of comorbidities among children with obesity?" See Appendix 1 for the conceptual framework and a priori key questions.

abstract

[a]Department of Population Health Sciences, Duke University School of Medicine, Durham, North Carolina; [b]Louisiana State University Pennington Biomedical Research Center, Baton Rouge, Louisiana; [c]Departments of Pediatrics and Population Health Sciences, Duke Clinical Research Institute, Duke University, Durham, North Carolina; [d]Children's Hospital of Richmond at Virginia Commonwealth University, Richmond, Virginia; [e]Medical Director, American Academy of Pediatrics, Institute for Healthy Childhood Weight, Wilmington, Delaware; [f]Institute for Medicaid Innovation, University of Michigan Medical School, Ann Arbor, Michigan; [g]Center for Childhood Obesity Research, Pennsylvania State University, Department of Nutritional Sciences, Pennsylvania State University, University Park, Pennsylvania; [h]Department of Population Health Sciences, Duke University School of Medicine, Durham, North Carolina; [i]Department of Pediatrics, University of Oklahoma Health Sciences Center, Oklahoma City, Oklahoma; [j]American Academy of Pediatrics, Itasca, Illinois; [k]American Academy of Pediatrics, Itasca, Illinois; and [l]American Academy of Pediatrics, Itasca, Illinois

This document is copyrighted and is property of the American Academy of Pediatrics and its Board of Directors. All authors have filed conflict of interest statements with the American Academy of Pediatrics. Any conflicts have been resolved through a process approved by the Board of Directors. The American Academy of Pediatrics has neither solicited nor accepted any commercial involvement in the development of the content of this publication.

Technical reports from the American Academy of Pediatrics benefit from expertise and resources of liaisons and internal (AAP) and external reviewers. However, technical reports from the American Academy of Pediatrics may not reflect the views of the liaisons or the organizations or government agencies that they represent.

The guidance in this report does not indicate an exclusive course of treatment or serve as a standard of medical care. Variations,

Obesity is a common concern in pediatric practice. In caring for patients with obesity or patients who may be at risk for developing obesity, clinicians have many unanswered questions. Examples of these questions include: What is the best way to identify excess adiposity, and does the identification of obesity provide opportunities for treatment? If so, what evidence-based interventions for obesity treatment, delivered at least in part by clinicians in office-based settings, are most effective? Among children and adolescents identified as having obesity, does screening for comorbidities result in improved health outcomes?

Many previous studies, most notably the systematic review conducted for the US Preventive Services Task Force (USPSTF), have synthesized research regarding the efficacy of treatment of obesity, particularly in the context of prevention of future comorbidities.[1] However, some important gaps remain. First, the USPSTF recommended that obesity treatment should include at least ≥26 hours of face-to-face contact over 2 to 12 months. However, subsequent studies have failed to

To cite: Skinner AC, Staiano AE, Armstrong SC, et al. Appraisal of Clinical Care Practices for Child Obesity Treatment. Part I: Interventions. Pediatrics. 2023;151(2): e2022060642

TECHNICAL REPORT

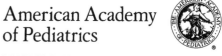

American Academy
of Pediatrics

DEDICATED TO THE HEALTH OF ALL CHILDREN™

Appraisal of Clinical Care Practices for Child Obesity Treatment. Part II: Comorbidities

Asheley C. Skinner, PhD,[a] Amanda E. Staiano, PhD, MPP,[b] Sarah C. Armstrong, MD, FAAP,[c] Shari L. Barkin, MD, MSHS,[d] Sandra G. Hassink, MD, FAAP,[e] Jennifer E. Moore, PhD, RN, FAAN,[f] Jennifer S. Savage, PhD,[g] Helene Vilme, DrPH,[h] Ashley E. Weedn, MD, MPH, FAAP,[i] Janice Liebhart, MS,[j] Jeanne Lindros, MPH,[k] Eileen M. Reilly, MSW[l]

The objective of this technical report is to provide clinicians with actionable evidence-based information upon which to make treatment decisions. In addition, this report will provide an evidence base on which to inform clinical practice guidelines for the management and treatment of overweight and obesity in children and adolescents.

To this end, the goal of this report was to identify all relevant studies to answer 2 overarching key questions: (KQ1) "What are effective clinically based treatments for obesity?" and (KQ2) "What is the risk of comorbidities among children with obesity?" See Appendix 1 for the conceptual framework and a priori Key Questions.

abstract

[a]Department of Population Health Sciences, Duke University School of Medicine, Durham, North Carolina; [b]Louisiana State University Pennington Biomedical Research Center, Baton Rouge, Louisiana; [c]Departments of Pediatrics and Population Health Sciences, Duke Clinical Research Institute, Duke University, Durham, North Carolina; [d]Children's Hospital of Richmond at Virginia Commonwealth University, Richmond, Virginia; [e]Medical Director, American Academy of Pediatrics, Institute for Healthy Childhood Weight, Wilmington, Delaware; [f]Institute for Medicaid Innovation, University of Michigan Medical School, Ann Arbor, Michigan; [g]Center for Childhood Obesity Research, Pennsylvania State University, Department of Nutritional Sciences, Pennsylvania State University, University Park, Pennsylvania; [h]Department of Population Health Sciences, Duke University School of Medicine, Durham, North Carolina; [i]Department of Pediatrics, University of Oklahoma Health Sciences Center, Oklahoma City, Oklahoma; [j]American Academy of Pediatrics, Itasca, Illinois; [k]American Academy of Pediatrics, Itasca, Illinois; and [l]American Academy of Pediatrics, Itasca, Illinois

Technical reports from the American Academy of Pediatrics benefit from expertise and resources of liaisons and internal (AAP) and external reviewers. However, technical reports from the American Academy of Pediatrics may not reflect the views of the liaisons or the organizations or government agencies that they represent.

The guidance in this report does not indicate an exclusive course of treatment or serve as a standard of medical care. Variations,

INTRODUCTION

Obesity is a common concern in pediatric practice. In caring for patients with obesity or patients who may be at risk for developing obesity, clinicians have many unanswered questions. Examples of these questions include: What is the best way to identify excess adiposity, and does the identification of obesity provide opportunities for treatment? If so, what evidence-based interventions for obesity treatment, delivered at least in part by clinicians in office-based settings, are most effective? Among children and adolescents identified as having obesity, does screening for comorbidities result in improved health outcomes?

Many previous studies, most notably conducted by the US Preventive Services Task Force, have synthesized research regarding the treatment of obesity.[1] Unfortunately, some important gaps remain unfilled. The US Preventive Services Task Force recommendation was that obesity treatment should include at least 26 hours of contact, including clinical care and other behavioral intervention (eg, guided physical activity).

To cite: Skinner AC, Staiano AE, Armstrong SC, et al. AAP Appraisal of Clinical Care Practices for Child Obesity Treatment. Part II: Comorbidities. *Pediatrics.* 2023;151(2): e2022060643

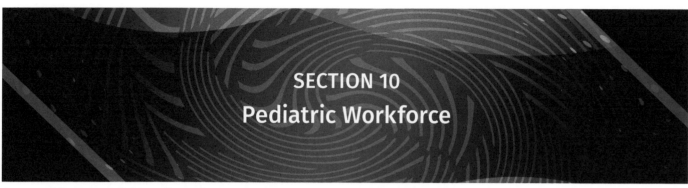

SECTION 10
Pediatric Workforce

Some articles are available online only; scan the QR code to access online content.

POLICY STATEMENT Organizational Principles to Guide and Define the Child Health
Care System and/or Improve the Health of all Children

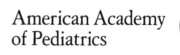

**American Academy
of Pediatrics**

DEDICATED TO THE HEALTH OF ALL CHILDREN™

Creating Work and Learning Environments Free of Gender-Based Harassment in Pediatric Health Care

Julie Story Byerley, MD, MPH, FAAP,[a] Nancy A. Dodson, MD, MPH, FAAP,[b] Tiffany St. Clair, MD, FAAP,[c] Valencia P. Walker, MD, MPH, FAAP,[d] and THE COMMITTEE ON PEDIATRIC WORKFORCE

Although gender harassment has long been a concern of the American Academy of Pediatrics, recent attention has helped to highlight the pervasive scope of the issue and identify previously under recognized harassment concerns for people of gender and sexual minorities. More subtle forms of harassment such as microaggressions have been recognized to contribute to significant negative outcomes for those who experience them. Patients and their families have also been recognized as potential perpetrators of harassment. Work and learning environments should support a clear no-tolerance policy regarding sexual harassment by employees or educators, and perpetrators should be held accountable for their actions. Sexual harassment that occurs with patients or family members as perpetrators, although more complicated given the nature of the caregiving relationship, should be stopped. Work and learning environments free of gender-based harassment support pediatric physicians, enhance vitality, advance equity, and improve patient care.

BACKGROUND INFORMATION

Sexual harassment is described by the United States Equal Employment Opportunity Commission (EEOC) in the following way: "It is unlawful to harass a person (an applicant or employee) because of that person's sex. Harassment can include "sexual harassment" or unwelcome sexual advances, requests for sexual favors, and other verbal or physical harassment of a sexual nature. Harassment does not have to be of a sexual nature, however, and can include offensive remarks about a person's sex or gender. For example, it is illegal to harass a woman by making offensive comments about women in general."[1] Although sexual harassment has been illegal for more than 50 years, there has been increased social awareness of the scope of the problem since the MeToo movement, including an increased awareness of the role of

[a]Professor of Pediatrics, President and Dean, Geisinger Commonwealth School of Medicine, Scranton, Pennsylvania; [b]Adolescent Medicine Pediatrician, Montefiore, Bronx, New York; [c]General Pediatrician, Cary Pediatric Center, Cary, North Carolina; and [d]Neonatologist, Nationwide Children's Hospital, Columbus, Ohio

Drs Byerley, Dodson, St. Clair, and Walker were each responsible for all aspects of writing and editing the document and reviewing and responding to questions and comments from reviewers and the Board of Directors.

To cite: Byerley JS, Dodson NA, St. Clair T, Walker VP; AAP Committee on Pediatric Workforce. Creating Work and Learning Environments Free of Gender-Based Harassment in Pediatric Health Care. *Pediatrics.* 2022;150(3):e2022058880

more subtle gender-based harassment.[2] Gender-based harassment includes not only behaviors that are meant to objectify or sexually exploit an individual but also behaviors or comments that are meant to reinforce harmful gender norms, perpetuate gender-based stereotypes, and degrade or disrespect a person on the basis of their sex (male, female, or intersex, assigned at birth), gender identity (how they perceive themselves), or sexual orientation (to whom they are attracted). A significant proportion of the burden of sexual harassment experienced by physicians originates from patients and families. Although sex-based harassment of women (and men, although with less frequency) is well-recognized, harassment of people of sexual and gender minorities remains an underrecognized and related problem. Much of the research on harassment has focused on cisgender women and men, and thus, the experiences of transgender and nonbinary people are not as well understood or described. Newer concepts have emerged that deepen our understanding of sexual harassment. Microaggressions are the everyday verbal, nonverbal, and environmental slights, snubs, or insults, whether intentional or unintentional, which communicate hostile, derogatory, or negative messages to target people based solely on their marginalized group membership.[3,4] These microaggressions may stem from conscious or unconscious bias. Examples of common microaggressions that relate to sexual harassment include the following[5]:

- Don't worry your pretty little head about it."
- That's women's work."
- Let a man take care of that for you."

- We understand you have pregnancy brain and can't keep up."
- Persistently (whether intentionally or unintentionally) using the wrong pronouns for a person who is nonbinary or transgender.
- Calling a woman doctor by her first name, but introducing a male colleague as "Dr."
- Referring to a woman colleague as "young and lovely."

Microaggressions are frequently accompanied by racial or ethnic overtones and typically are demeaning in their nature. "Intersectionality" refers to the unique patterns of compounding discrimination that reaches beyond a single minority status, noting the increased burden experienced by people who are members of 2 or more marginalized and/or minoritized groups. Harassment is more common where power differentials coexist, such as the traditional hierarchy observed in the medical profession. Thus, students and resident physicians are often much more likely than attending physicians to be victims. Nurses, medical assistants, and nonmedical administrative or support staff can face increased susceptibility to harassment as well.

Harassment regarding issues related to gender are not perpetrated only by men or limited to only women victims. It is well recognized that transgender individuals experience harassment at high rates with severe consequences.[6] As pediatric health care becomes a more women-dominated field, disparaging gender-based remarks directed at men warrant acknowledgment and recognition as potential harassment cases.

STATEMENT OF THE PROBLEM

Sexual harassment remains a prevalent problem for people of all genders, especially women, in many

fields of work, including medicine. Our understanding of what constitutes harassment and who is victimized has expanded significantly since the 2006 American Academy of Pediatrics policy statement "Prevention of Sexual Harassment in the Workplace and Educational Settings."[7]

EVIDENCE BASIS

The EEOC defines sexual harassment as unwelcomed sexual advances, requests for sexual favors, and other verbal or physical behavior of a sexual nature. However, the EEOC also highlights that sexual harassment is not always sexual. It can also include offensive remarks or behavior regarding a person's sex.[1] Sex and gender discrimination are recognized as forms of sexual harassment that violate Title VII of the Civil Rights Act of 1964.[8]

Harassment is known to produce negative consequences. A recent study on the extent of sexual harassment among pediatric, internal medicine, and general surgery resident physicians ($n = 1700$) found that sexual harassment was associated with lower levels of vitality (being energized by work) and higher rates of ethical and moral distress.[9] Resident physicians who experience mistreatment, including sexual harassment, are more likely than those who do not to report symptoms of burnout and also report higher stress levels and lower quality of life. In addition, resident physicians who experience harassment are less likely to believe that their program prioritizes collaboration, education, and mentoring.[10,11]

Despite decades of increased awareness, sexual harassment remains a common problem faced by health care professionals. Women resident physicians who identify as lesbian, gay, bisexual, transgender, queer, or questioning (LGBTQ) reported significantly higher rates of sexual harassment than those who did not identify as LGBTQ (19% vs 6.2%).[9] Using data from the spring 2019 Pediatric Resident Burnout and Resilience Consortium's online survey, a study of 1290 pediatric residents in 46 programs found that 5% of pediatric resident physicians reported sexual harassment.[12] In response to the Association of American Medical Colleges' 2017 Medical School Graduation Questionnaire, which surveyed graduating medical students at 140 medical schools, 14.8% of students reported that they had been subjected to offensive sexist remarks or names at least once, 4.3% reported unwanted sexual advances, and 0.3% reported they were asked to exchange sexual favors for grades or other awards.[13] According to the same questionnaire, only 21% of students who experienced harassment or other offensive behaviors reported these incidents to faculty members or medical school administrators. Among those who said that they experienced offensive behaviors, 28% said they did not report the incident because of a fear of reprisal.[14] A 2018 Medscape survey of 3700 physicians and medical residents reported that 27% of physicians have been sexually harassed by a patient, compared with 7% who reported being harassed by other medical personal or administrators in their workplace.[15] A systematic review and meta-analysis of 51 studies published in *Academic Medicine* revealed that 59% of medical trainees had experienced 1 form of harassment or discrimination during their training. The most reported source of harassment or discrimination was other physician consultants at 34%, followed by patients or patients' families at

22%.[16] Harassment has been long described as occurring with perpetrators such as teachers or supervising employers. More recently, the phenomenon of patients or their family members as perpetrators of mistreatment has been discussed in the literature.[17]

Microaggressions

Since the initial publication of the AAP's policy statement on sexual harassment in 2006, several concepts have emerged that have broadened and deepened our understanding of the nature of sexual harassment and its consequences. One such concept is that of microaggressions, which are subtle behaviors or hurtful or invalidating statements that may arise from unconscious biases or prejudice. Microaggressions were first described in relation to historically disadvantaged racial and ethnic groups[3] but have since been studied in women, people of gender and sexual minorities, and other marginalized groups.[18] Unlike more overt sexual or sexist aggressions, which may be intentional, openly hostile, and obvious, microaggressions are often unintentional and may appear innocuous or even invisible to a bystander. For members of marginalized groups, experiencing the cumulative effect of months or years of microaggressions can profoundly harm psychological well-being and contribute to adverse health outcomes.[19] This evidence supports antiracist activist and professor Ibram Kendi's supposition that the very term "microaggressions" understates the accumulation of these incidents as profoundly abusive and discriminatory.[20] Gender-based microaggressions in medical workplaces have been described as falling into 6 themes that women in medicine commonly experience: (1) encountering sexism;

(2) encountering pregnancy- and child care-related bias; (3) having one's abilities underestimated; (4) encountering sexually inappropriate comments; (5) being relegated to mundane tasks; and (6) feeling excluded or marginalized.[21]

Intersectionality

Since the initial publication of the AAP's policy on sexual harassment, we have become increasingly aware of the concept of intersectionality.[22] This framework was first introduced by professor and civil rights advocate Kimberle Crenshaw in 1989 to describe the dual burdens of sexism and racism experienced by Black women. It is now applied to individuals with more than 1 marginalized identity.[23] Specifically, the term "intersectionality" describes how a person possessing 2 or more marginalized identities can experience a distinct form of discrimination that reaches beyond the individual bounds of sexism, racism, or homophobia as they are commonly understood.[24] For example, Crenshaw described how African American women lived at the intersection of racism and sexism, rendering them nearly invisible in matters of equality, access to opportunities, and vulnerability to violence.[25] In science and medicine, minoritized women with marginalized racial and ethnic identities feel the effects of intersectional discrimination and report higher rates of feeling unsafe at work than White women, minoritized men with marginalized racial and ethnic identities, or White men.[26] Minoritized people with marginalized racial and ethnic identities who identify as LGBTQ and/or disabled may also experience uniquely complicated intersectional effects of racism, ableism, homophobia, or transphobia.

Harassment of Men

Men can be victims of gender-based harassment. Although attention to gender-based harassment typically focuses on men as perpetrators and women as victims, it is important to take a holistic approach to the issue, especially as a recognition for the workforce within the field of pediatrics. In 2017, nearly three quarters of pediatric resident physicians were women; nearly two thirds of practicing pediatricians were women, and just over half of pediatric academicians were women.[27] Many departments may comprise mostly women, and smaller divisions or private practices may have 1 or few men as trainees or faculty members. Even in environments with men in the majority, men may also experience gender-based harassment in the form of overt sexist comments, microaggressions, or sexualizing language. With the traditional gender power dynamics of leadership continuing to favor men, the skew of women as well as gender and sexual minorities as victims of harassment remains in place, even as the number of women physicians grows in pediatrics.

Patient Behavior

Although patient expectations are often stated about timeliness to the visit, payments for services rendered, and other activities involved in the clinical interaction, it is less common to see statements of patient expectations regarding respectful treatment of clinical staff. In many settings, this culture is changing in recognition that stating expectations for patient behavior helps to establish a healing-oriented culture. Furthermore, naming respectful treatment and nondiscrimination as expectations for patient and family behaviors supports clinicians' wellness and sustainability.

Culture

A key feature affecting patient safety is culture. The lag in leadership roles and positions of authority for people from marginalized and minoritized groups (race and ethnicity, gender, sexual orientation, etc.) demonstrates the pervasiveness of inequity in a patriarchal racialized culture.[28] Respect is an essential component of a culture that supports patient safety, and working in a culture that demonstrates respect is key to well-being.[29] A culture that protects clinician well-being has a positive effect on patient safety, clinician sustainability, and clinical productivity. A lack of psychological safety compromises learning and clinical care. Several tools exist to maintain respect, inclusion, and belonging, including bystander training and reporting mechanisms.

Bystander Training

Bystander training prepares people for how to respond when microaggressions and other forms of mistreatment and harassment occur to protect and promote a positive climate. Based on the idea that people of any gender can interrupt behavior that threatens safety, bystander training includes anticipating that these events will occur and preparing individuals for how to respond when they do. Optimal bystander training programs teach individuals that microaggressions or other mistreatment will occur and encourage people to intervene when they recognize such infractions. Individuals learn to address incidents in real time with comments and actions that support the victim and concurrently encourage a positive culture. When a bystander takes action to improve the situation, mitigate bias, and boost the culture toward equity,

they may be referred to as an "upstander." Strategies for upstander interventions may include redirecting attention from the negative behavior (distraction), interrupting through the appropriate use of wit, or directly confronting the behavior.[30]

Additionally, bystander training promotes shared accountability for the culture in a particular setting. Shared training experiences create a knowledge base and common language to address these repeated situations that occur. Such training can also re-establish social norms. In addition to bystander training regarding responding to microaggressions, there are culture-boosting programs that recruit allies and advocates for gender equity.[31,32]

The responsibility of clinicians to maintain a culture free from gender-based harassment encompasses considerations for the subtle, gender-based messages conveyed during our patient interactions. These behaviors can potentially foster an environment that normalizes gender-based maltreatment and allows it to flourish. Examples include rigid and excessive attention paid to binary gender classification of newborn infants, ascribing certain colors to delineate genders, and gender stereotypes reinforced through toy choices. These examples are in addition to the wider range of comments and behaviors that imply gender-based expectations. To create an equitable culture based on gender, we must consider the implications of our actions.[33,34]

Reporting

Victims of gender-based harassment are encouraged to report their experiences to the human resource or other authority bodies in their workplace.

Similarly, bystanders can report observed harassment to bolster accountability within the professional environment. Those in certain leadership positions are mandated to report incidents of gender-based harassment that are brought to their attention. Irrespective of the broadened definition for recognized gender harassment, egregious incidents of sexual harassment continue to occur. In addition to causing trauma, these incidents increase the risk of career sabotage that can result from the effects on performance, adverse impact on mental health, or as a consequence of retaliation against the reporter. Practical strategies for eliminating sexual and gender-based harassment provide supportive services for reporters, establish systematic management of complaints, and assure zero tolerance for retaliation against reporters.[35] Accountability, prevention from continued harm, and consequences for perpetrators of harassment are vital to successful elimination of harassment and mistreatment.[36]

CONCLUSIONS

Sexual and gender-based harassment is an ongoing problem in society, and medicine is not immune. Creating pediatric work and learning environments free of harassment supports wellness and sustainability for the workforce and the learners within it. Addressing sexual harassment and gender-based maltreatment is important to creating an environment where all can thrive.

RECOMMENDATIONS

Beyond a zero tolerance toward overt forms of sexual harassment, we must remain vigilant against subtle comments and actions that make people feel diminished,

sexualized, or excluded. We can teach victims and bystanders what to do in such moments and empower them to respond. Prioritizing these actions and the following recommendations help us create an environment that genuinely welcomes people of all genders.

1. Work and learning environments should not tolerate gender-based harassment by employees or educators. Employers and institutions should investigate reports of harassment by employees and act against the perpetrator when verified.
2. Perpetrators should be held accountable for their actions. Clear policies and practices in each place of employment and education should ensure no tolerance of harassment based on gender, gender identity, or sexual orientation as part of a broader antidiscrimination and harassment policy.
3. Gender-based harassment that occurs with patients or family members as perpetrators, although more complicated given the nature of the caregiving relationship, should also be acknowledged as a potential source of harassment and not tolerated.
4. Practices should establish a list of expected patient behaviors to protect from harassment of all care providers, including attending physicians, resident physicians, medical students, and all staff.
5. Practices should develop a protocol for managing harassment by patients.
6. Victims who report gender-based harassment deserve support and protection from retaliation.
7. Data regarding the incidence of harassment in a workplace should be transparently shared among staff to ensure

accountability. This information must be shared in a way that maintains confidentiality, especially to avoid retaliation.
8. Workplaces and educational institutions need to prioritize positive work environments where people feel respected as professionals and never sexually objectified.
9. To enhance the workplace culture, institutions should offer training to increase awareness of gender-based harassment and its consequences.
10. Bystander training should be provided to prepare those witnessing discrimination and/or harassment to respond and report appropriately.
11. Professionals should consider the gender-based messages conveyed through their personal interactions and the actions of their places of work.
12. Professional specialty groups within organized medicine, accreditation bodies, and leaders within health care organizations should accept their responsibilities to play active roles in creating safe, respectful environments and moving organizations toward equity.

LEAD AUTHORS

Julie Story Byerley, MD, MPH, FAAP
Nancy A. Dodson, MD, MPH, FAAP
Tiffany St. Clair, MD, FAAP
Valencia P. Walker, MD, MPH, FAAP

COMMITTEE ON PEDIATRIC WORKFORCE, 2020-2021

Harold K. Simon, MD, MBA, FAAP, Chairperson
Julie Story Byerley, MD, MPH, FAAP
Nancy A. Dodson, MD, FAAP
Eric N. Horowitz, MD, FAAP
Thomas W. Pendergrass, MD, MSPH, FAAP
Edward A. Pont, MD, FAAP
Kristin N. Ray, MD, FAAP

William B. Moskowitz, MD, FAAP, Immediate Past Chairperson

LIAISONS

Laurel K. Leslie, MD, MPH, FAAP – American Board of Pediatrics

STAFF

Lauren F. Barone, MPH

Address correspondence to Julie Story Byerley, MD, MPH, FAAP. E-mail: jbyerley1@som.geisinger.edu

PEDIATRICS (ISSN Numbers: Print, 0031-4005; Online, 1098-4275).

DOI: https://doi.org/10.1542/peds.2022-058880

Copyright © 2022 by the American Academy of Pediatrics

FINANCIAL/CONFLICT OF INTEREST DISCLOSURE: None.

REFERENCES

1. US Equal Employment Opportunity Commission. Sexual harassment. Available at: https://www.eeoc.gov/sexual-harassment. Accessed October 28, 2020

2. MeToo Movement. Me too movement. Available at: https://metoomvmt.org/. Accessed November 16, 2020

3. Sue DW, Capodilupo CM, Torino GC, et al. Racial microaggressions in everyday life: implications for clinical practice. *Am Psychol.* 2007;62(4):271–286

4. Sue DW. *Microaggressions and Marginality: Manifestation, Dynamics, and Impact.* Hoboken, NJ: John Wiley & Sons Inc; 2010

5. Barrett B; Forbes. The microaggressions towards black women you might be complicit in at work. Available at: https://www.forbes.com/sites/biancabarratt/2020/06/19/the-microaggressions-towards-black-women-you-might-be-complicit-in-at-work/?sh=37c50e8e2bda. Accessed August 26, 2021

6. Eliason MJ, Dibble SL, Robertson PA. Lesbian, gay, bisexual, and transgender (LGBT) physicians' experiences in the workplace. *J Homosex.* 2011;58(10):1355–1371

7. Pletcher BA; American Academy of Pediatrics Committee on Pediatric Workforce. Prevention of sexual harassment in the workplace and educational settings. *Pediatrics.* 2006;118(4):1752–1756

8. US Equal Employment Opportunity Commission. Title VII of the Civil Rights Act of 1964, 42 USC § 2000e et seq (1964). Available at: https://www.eeoc.gov/statutes/title-vii-civil-rights-act-1964. Accessed November 16, 2020

9. Pololi LH, Brennan RT, Civian JT, Shea S, Brennan-Wydra E, Evans AT; Sexual Harassment Within Academic Medicine in the United States. Us, too. sexual harassment within academic medicine in the United States. *Am J Med.* 2020;133(2):245–248

10. Kemper KJ, Schwartz A; Pediatric Resident Burnout-Resilience Study Consortium. Bullying, discrimination, sexual harassment and physical violence: common and associated with burnout in pediatric residents. *Acad Pediatr.* 2020;20(7):991–997

11. Young K, Punnett A, Suleman S. A little hurts a lot: exploring the impact of microaggressions in pediatric medical education. *Pediatrics.* 2020;146(1):e20201636

12. Pediatric Resident Burnout-Resilience Study Consortium. Spring 2019 pediatric resident burnout-resilience consortium study. Available at: https://pedsresresilience.com/. Accessed January 4, 2022

13. Binder R, Garcia P, Johnson B, Fuentes-Afflick E. Sexual harassment in medical schools: the challenge of covert retaliation as a barrier to reporting. *Acad Med.* 2018;93(12):1770–1773

14. Association of American Medical Colleges. 2017 Medical school graduation questionnaire. Available at: https://www.aamc.org/media/8746/download. Accessed May 28, 2021

15. Kane L. Patients sexually harassing physicians: report 2018. Available at: https://www.medscape.com/slideshow/patients-sexually-harassing-physicians-6010036. Accessed October 28, 2020

16. Fnais N, Soobiah C, Chen MH, et al. Harassment and discrimination in medical training: a systematic review and meta-analysis. *Acad Med.* 2014;89(5):817–827

17. Cyrus KD, Angoff NR, Illuzzi JL, Schwartz ML, Wilkins KM. When patients hurt us. *Med Teach.* 2018;40(12):1308–1309

18. Basford TE, Offermann LR, Behrend TS. Do you see what I see? perceptions of gender microaggressions in the workplace. *Psychol Women Q.* 2014;38(3):340–349

19. Pascoe EA, Smart Richman L. Perceived discrimination and health: a meta-analytic review. *Psychol Bull.* 2009;135(4):531–554

20. Kendi I. *How to Be an Antiracist.* London, England: The Bodley Head; 2019

21. Periyakoil VS, Chaudron L, Hill EV, Pellegrini V, Neri E, Kraemer HC. Common types of gender-based

microaggressions in medicine. *Acad Med.* 2020;95(3):450–457

22. Wilson Y, White A, Jefferson A, Danis M. Broadening the conversation about intersectionality in clinical medicine. *Am J Bioeth.* 2019;19(4):W1–W5

23. Crenshaw K. Demarginalizing the intersection of race and sex: a black feminist critique of antidiscrimination doctrine, feminist theory and antiracist politics. *Univ Chic Leg Forum.* 1989;(1):139–167

24. Walby S, Armstrong J, Strid S. Intersectionality: multiple inequalities in social theory. *Sociology.* 2012;46(2):224–240

25. Crenshaw K. Mapping the margins: intersectionality, identity politics, and violence against women of color. *Stanford Law Rev.* 1991;43(6):1241–1299

26. Golden SH. The perils of intersectionality: racial and sexual harassment in medicine. *J Clin Invest.* 2019;129(9):3465–3467

27. Spector ND, Asante PA, Marcelin JR, et al. Women in pediatrics: progress, barriers, and opportunities for equity, diversity, and inclusion. *Pediatrics.* 2019;144(5):e20192149

28. Morgan AU, Chaiyachati KH, Weissman GE, Liao JM. Eliminating gender-based bias in academic medicine: more than naming the "elephant in the room." *J Gen Intern Med.* 2018;33(6): 966–968

29. National Academies of Sciences, Engineering, and Medicine. *Taking Action Against Clinician Burnout: A Systems Approach to Professional Well-Being.* Washington, DC: National Academies Press; 2019

30. Goldenberg MN, Cyrus KD, Wilkins KM. ERASE: a new framework for faculty to manage patient mistreatment of trainees. *Acad Psychiatry.* 2019;43(4): 396–399

31. HeforShe. He for she. Available at: https://www.heforshe.org/en. Accessed August 26, 2021

32. The Ohio State University. The women's place. Available at: https://womensplace. osu.edu/initiatives-and-programs/ advocates-allies. Accessed August 26, 2021

33. Let Toys Be Toys. Available at: https:// www.lettoysbetoys.org.uk/. Accessed August 26, 2021

34. A Mighty Girl. Available at: https://www. amightygirl.com/. Accessed August 26, 2021

35. American Medical Association. Code of medical ethics opinion 9.1.3 sexual harassment in the practice of medicine. Available at: https://www. ama-assn.org/delivering-care/ethics/ sexual-harassment-practice-medicine. Accessed August 26, 2021

36. US Department of the Interior. Prevention and elimination of harassing conduct. Available at: https://www. doi.gov/employees/anti-harassment/ harassing-conduct. Accessed October 26, 2021

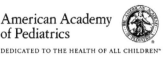

American Academy
of Pediatrics
DEDICATED TO THE HEALTH OF ALL CHILDREN™

Organizational Principles to Guide and Define the Child
Health Care System and/or Improve the Health of all Children

This Policy Statement was reaffirmed October 2015 and December 2022.

POLICY STATEMENT

Enhancing Pediatric Workforce Diversity and Providing Culturally Effective Pediatric Care: Implications for Practice, Education, and Policy Making

COMMITTEE ON PEDIATRIC WORKFORCE

KEY WORDS
pediatrician, workforce, diversity, health disparities, culturally
effective care, education

ABBREVIATIONS
AAP—American Academy of Pediatrics
CEHC—culturally effective health care
CME—continuing medical education
LGBT—lesbian, gay, bisexual, and transgender
URM—underrepresented in medicine

www.pediatrics.org/cgi/doi/10.1542/peds.2013-2268

doi:10.1542/peds.2013-2268

PEDIATRICS (ISSN Numbers: Print, 0031-4005; Online, 1098-4275).

Copyright © 2013 by the American Academy of Pediatrics

abstract

This policy statement serves to combine and update 2 previously independent but overlapping statements from the American Academy
of Pediatrics (AAP) on culturally effective health care (CEHC) and workforce diversity. The AAP has long recognized that with the ever-increasing
diversity of the pediatric population in the United States, the health of all
children depends on the ability of all pediatricians to practice culturally
effective care. CEHC can be defined as the delivery of care within the
context of appropriate physician knowledge, understanding, and appreciation of all cultural distinctions, leading to optimal health outcomes.
The AAP believes that CEHC is a critical social value and that the knowledge and skills necessary for providing CEHC can be taught and acquired
through focused curricula across the spectrum of lifelong learning.

This statement also addresses workforce diversity, health disparities,
and affirmative action. The discussion of diversity is broadened to include not only race, ethnicity, and language but also cultural attributes
such as gender, religious beliefs, sexual orientation, and disability,
which may affect the quality of health care. The AAP believes that
efforts must be supported through health policy and advocacy initiatives to promote the delivery of CEHC and to overcome educational,
organizational, and other barriers to improving workforce diversity.
Pediatrics 2013;132:e1105–e1116

INTRODUCTION

This policy statement serves to combine and update 2 previous
statements from the American Academy of Pediatrics (AAP) on culturally effective health care (CEHC)[1] and workforce diversity.[2] The
impetus to combine these independent policy statements comes from
the recognition that the provision of culturally effective care and
enhancing the diversity of the pediatrician workforce represent
parallel and often overlapping initiatives to improve care for pediatric
patients. This policy statement provides guidance for policy makers,
advocacy groups, medical educators, and physicians on the provision
of CEHC and enhancing the diversity of the pediatrician workforce.

CEHC can be defined as the delivery of care within the context of
appropriate physician knowledge, understanding, and appreciation of
all cultural distinctions, leading to optimal health outcomes, quality of life,

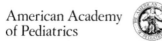

American Academy
of Pediatrics
DEDICATED TO THE HEALTH OF ALL CHILDREN™

POLICY STATEMENT

Nondiscrimination in Pediatric Health Care

Committee on Pediatric Workforce

Organizational Principles to Guide and
Define the Child Health Care System and/or
Improve the Health of All Children

This Policy Statement was reaffirmed June 2011 and May 2021.

ABSTRACT

This policy statement is a revision of a 2001 statement and articulates the positions of the American Academy of Pediatrics on nondiscrimination in pediatric health care. It addresses both pediatricians who provide health care and the infants, children, adolescents, and young adults whom they serve.

THE MISSION OF the American Academy of Pediatrics (AAP) is "to attain optimal physical, mental, and social health and well-being for all infants, children, adolescents and young adults."[1] In support of this mission, therefore, the AAP is opposed to discrimination in the care of any patient on the basis of race, ethnicity, ancestry, national origin, religion, gender, marital status, sexual orientation, gender identity or expression, age, veteran status, immigration status, or disability of the patient or patient's parent(s) or guardian(s). In addition, the AAP supports the right of pediatricians, pediatric medical subspecialists, pediatric surgical specialists, and other specialist physicians who care for pediatric patients in both educational and practice settings to participate in the delivery of health care without discrimination on the basis of race, ethnicity, ancestry, national origin, religion, gender, marital status, sexual orientation, gender identity or expression, age, veteran status, immigration status, or disability. Physicians with disabilities who maintain the ability to perform the essential functions of their jobs with or without "reasonable accommodation," as defined by the Americans With Disabilities Act (ADA),[2] should not be hindered from participating in such activities.

Regardless of the size of the practice, all pediatricians, whether employers or employees, are encouraged to have nondiscrimination policies and to review all their personnel policies and procedures to monitor how they are implemented to ensure that they do not have an adverse effect on any individual or group.[3] If one wishes to air a grievance concerning discrimination on the basis of any of the above-listed factors, they must be able to do so in an environment that is free of prejudice and discrimination so that the matter may be addressed and resolved expediently.

The AAP recognizes the value of diversity among patients and pediatricians and the importance of proactively establishing and adhering to nondiscrimination policies for both pediatricians (as employers and employees) and the patients in their care. The AAP recommends that both public and private insurers provide nondiscriminatory and continuous coverage of pediatric services. Finally, the AAP encourages its members to support these nondiscrimination principles consistently in their interactions with colleagues, patients, and the patient's parent(s) or guardian(s).

www.pediatrics.org/cgi/doi/10.1542/
peds.2007-2334

doi:10.1542/peds.2007-2334

All policy statements from the American Academy of Pediatrics automatically expire 5 years after publication unless reaffirmed, revised, or retired at or before that time.

Key Words
pediatric workforce

Abbreviation
AAP—American Academy of Pediatrics

PEDIATRICS (ISSN Numbers: Print, 0031-4005; Online, 1098-4275). Copyright © 2007 by the American Academy of Pediatrics

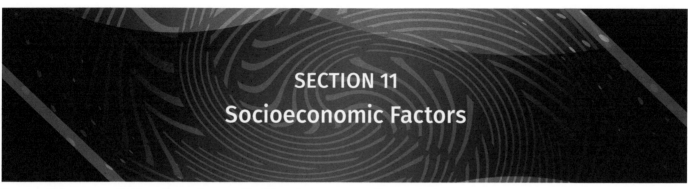

SECTION 11
Socioeconomic Factors

Some articles are available online only; scan the QR code to access online content.

POLICY STATEMENT Organizational Principles to Guide and Define the Child Health Care System and/or Improve the Health of all Children

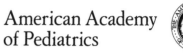

American Academy
of Pediatrics

DEDICATED TO THE HEALTH OF ALL CHILDREN™

Medicaid and the Children's Health Insurance Program: Optimization to Promote Equity in Child and Young Adult Health

Jennifer D. Kusma, MD, MS, FAAP,[a] Jean L. Raphael, MD, MPH, FAAP,[b] James M. Perrin, MD, FAAP,[c] Mark L. Hudak, MD, FAAP,[d]
COMMITTEE ON CHILD HEALTH FINANCING

The American Academy of Pediatrics envisions a child and adolescent health care system that provides individualized, family-centered, equitable, and comprehensive care that integrates with community resources to help each child and family achieve optimal growth, development, and well-being. All infants, children, adolescents, and young adults should have access to this system. Medicaid and the Children's Health Insurance Program (CHIP) provide critical support and foundation for this vision. Together, the programs currently serve about half of all children, many of whom are members of racial and ethnic minoritized populations or have complex medical conditions. Medicaid and CHIP have greatly improved the health and well-being of US infants, children, adolescents, and young adults. This statement reviews key program aspects and proposes both program reforms and enhancements to support a higher-quality, more comprehensive, family-oriented, and equitable system of care that increases access to services, reduces disparities, and improves health outcomes into adulthood. This statement recommends foundational changes in Medicaid and CHIP that can improve child health, achieve greater equity in health and health care, further dismantle structural racism within the programs, and reduce major state-by-state variations. The recommendations focus on (1) eligibility and duration of coverage; (2) standardization of covered services and quality of care; and (3) program financing and payment. In addition to proposed foundational changes in the Medicaid and CHIP program structure, the statement indicates stepwise, coordinated actions that regulation from the Centers for Medicare and Medicaid Services or federal legislation can accomplish in the shorter term. A separate technical report will address the origins and intents of the Medicaid and CHIP programs; the current state of the program including variations across states and payment structures; Medicaid for special populations; program innovations and waivers; and special Medicaid coverage and initiatives.

abstract

[a]Department of Pediatrics, Lurie Children's Hospital, Northwestern University School of Medicine, Chicago, Illinois; [b]Department of Pediatrics, Baylor College of Medicine, Houston, Texas; [c]Department of Pediatrics, Mass General Hospital for Children, Harvard Medical School, Boston, Massachusetts; and [d]Department of Pediatrics, University of Florida College of Medicine, Jacksonville, Florida

Dr Hudak wrote the initial draft of the revision of this policy statement; Drs Kusma, Raphael, and Perrin substantially revised that draft and incorporated valuable input from other members of the Committee on Child Health Financing, and revised the statement based on a broad review by other Sections, Committees, Councils, and Task Forces within the AAP.

To cite: Kusma JD, Raphael JL, Perrin JM, Hudak ML; American Academy of Pediatrics, Committee on Child Health Financing. Medicaid and the Children's Health Insurance Program: Optimization to Promote Equity in Child and Young Adult Health. *Pediatrics*. 2023;152(5):e2023064088

INTRODUCTION

The American Academy of Pediatrics (AAP) envisions a health care system in which all infants, children, adolescents, young adults, and families can access high-quality, comprehensive, family-centered, and equitable care. Such a system would link with other community resources to ensure optimal growth, development, and well-being of all infants, children, adolescents, and young adults (hereafter referred to as "children [0–26 years]"), regardless of where they live, emphasizing prevention and health promotion. This system must have adequate resources and incentives to achieve these goals. This vision builds on much AAP work and policy, including policy statements on the unique value proposition of pediatric health care,[1] principles for child health care financing,[2] guiding principles for managed care arrangements,[3] continuing on the path to equity,[4] the medical home,[5] and community pediatrics.[6] Approximately 50% of all US children receive care through Medicaid and/or the Children's Health Insurance Program (CHIP).[7] However, although children of African American/Black or Hispanic/Latino background represent 38.2% of US children, more than 60% of children from these backgrounds receive services through Medicaid and/or CHIP.[8,9] These 2 programs have historically provided fundamental support for the health care of millions of children who would otherwise have lacked any insurance.[10] Medicaid and CHIP provide an essential base from which to achieve the AAP vision. Much evidence documents the positive effects of Medicaid and CHIP on child health,[11,12] including timely access to care and reductions in neonatal and child mortality, emergency care utilization, and avoidable hospitalizations, as well as positive lifelong impacts such as less chronic disease in adulthood, lower rates of teenage pregnancy, higher rates of high school graduation, increased college enrollment, and higher future wages.[13] Medicaid specifically has several characteristics that make it a strong program for children, such as no waiting or special enrollment periods and no copays, entitlement to services for all eligible applicants, and coverage of all medically necessary services via the Early and Periodic Screening, Diagnostic, and Treatment (EPSDT) benefit.

The creation and evolution of Medicaid and CHIP reflect the key strengths and limitations of the programs. Since 1965, Medicaid has provided coverage to several populations: children from low-income families receiving government assistance; children and adults with disabilities; elderly low-income populations; and people with vision impairment lacking other health insurance. Over time, Medicaid expanded to include more populations, such as low-income pregnant people and children in foster care, and evolved into an essential safety net for children.[14] The Patient Protection and Affordable Care Act provided the most recent large-scale change to Medicaid by expanding eligibility to all children in households with income less than 138% of the federal poverty level (FPL).[15] The programs provide stability during economic downturns, pandemics, and catastrophic events.[16] Medicaid has joint federal-state financing (unlike Medicare, which has full federal funding). States receive a federal payment match, ranging from 50% to 77%, based on several state characteristics (federal medical assistance percentage).[17] This funding arrangement allows states broad discretion over eligibility, benefits, enrollment, and payments while meeting federal minimums and guidelines.

The Medicaid statute requires the broad EPSDT benefit for children insured by Medicaid to 21 years of age.[18] Most states use *Bright Futures: Guidelines for Health Supervision of Infants, Children, and Adolescents*[19,20] as their standard for pediatric preventive care visits. EPSDT requires states to cover any services identified during preventive screening needed for healthy growth and development, even if the state's Medicaid program does not normally cover that service (eg, behavioral health services).[21]

Medicaid state flexibility was intended to preserve state operational autonomy and programming. Indeed, many states have innovated in Medicaid eligibility, benefit, and payment design, particularly through 1115 waivers, which allow states to try innovations to improve care for beneficiaries. State flexibility, nonetheless, has also fostered wide variability and geographic inequities and further enabled ableism and structural racism.[22] From inception, state uptake and administration of Medicaid varied substantially, with less uptake particularly in states with large populations of African American people.[23] Substantial dependence on state revenues has led to low payment rates and cumbersome enrollment and renewal policies that effectively limit enrollment. These features both undervalue care and disincentivize providing care to the often minoritized populations the program serves. Variations in state implementation of EPSDT and limited federal enforcement of this and other requirements compromises quality of care for insured children, while further exacerbating inequities.[24,25]

Created as part of the Balanced Budget Act of 1997, CHIP was designed to insure children with household incomes above the state's Medicaid income eligibility threshold but too low to afford private insurance. States can use CHIP funds to create a separate CHIP program, expand their Medicaid program, or adopt a hybrid approach.[26] Medicaid and CHIP have similarities and differences in financing and operation. Both are federal-state matching programs, but the CHIP federal match rate is higher than the Medicaid match rate. Medicaid is an entitlement program, requiring states to enroll all eligible individuals who apply, with no limits on Medicaid's federal matching funds. CHIP, as a block grant, provides each state an annual capped allotment, such that eligible applicants can be denied coverage after the cap has been reached.[27] Relative to Medicaid, CHIP has more flexibility in benefit requirements and does not need to include the EPSDT benefit.[28] Although states usually cannot impose premiums and cost-sharing in Medicaid, both are permitted under CHIP. CHIP requires periodic congressional reauthorization, with current authorization through September 30, 2029.

Reform of Medicaid and CHIP will lead to a more equitable, higher quality, and more comprehensive family and community-centered health care system as laid out in the AAP vision. This system can better address health-related social needs and integrate mental health, including prevention and promotion, into pediatric care. (The term "mental" or "mental health" throughout this statement is intended to encompass "behavioral," "psychiatric," "psychological," "emotional," and "substance use" as well as family context and community-related concerns.) Reforms including decreasing major state-by-state variations in access and care, establishing and enforcing national standards of care, providing financing at least consistent with the higher of commercial or Medicare rates, and expanding eligibility will all strengthen public health insurance for children, reduce structural racism and ableism, and improve access to quality care.

This policy statement embraces the belief that greater investment and key reforms in Medicaid and CHIP represent strategic initiatives critical to the future of our nation. Improvement in the physical and mental health of children will achieve an immense long-term return on investment over the life span, including lower rates of disease, greater productivity from a healthier workforce, and reduced adult health care costs. Making investments in Medicaid and CHIP supports a necessary shift from a highly variable, state-by-state system that generates and exacerbates health disparities, to a more uniform program that fosters healthy young people and a productive adult population, allowing individuals to attain well-being, counteracts the effects of poverty, and reduces the likelihood of future incarceration,[29] with a multigenerational impact.[12,30]

GOALS AND FOUNDATIONAL POLICY CHANGES

The AAP calls for several foundational changes to Medicaid and CHIP that advance specific goals in eligibility and enrollment, coverage and care, and financing and payment. The AAP understands well that achievement of many goals will require legislation, regulation, and systems changes. The AAP calls for national standards for eligibility and enrollment, program implementation and benefit standards, and financing and payment. These goals could be achieved through increasing federal and state oversight, federal share of funding, and total investment in the programs. The Centers for Medicare and Medicaid Services (CMS) and state agencies should conduct regular equity impact assessments of the current implementation and proposed policy changes in line with the CMS framework for health equity.[31] Input from community and family members on program and policy changes that would improve their access and health should help drive change. The following changes will lead to

a more equitable program for all children (0–26 years) regardless of state lines, while also allowing state innovation, acknowledging differences in health needs across states.

Eligibility and Enrollment

Goal: *All children (0–26 years) in the United States should have access to health insurance coverage.*
   Proposed Foundational Changes:

1. Universal eligibility for all children up to age 26 years residing in the United States who lack other sources of health insurance, through a single program that combines Medicaid and CHIP.
2. Automatic enrollment in a combined Medicaid and CHIP program at birth of all infants born in the United States, with the option to opt out of coverage for those with other sources of insurance, to guarantee health insurance coverage without reverification of eligibility until age 6 years and no more than every 2 years thereafter.

Coverage and Care

Goal: *Children (0–26 years) insured by Medicaid/CHIP should have meaningful access to a consistent, high-quality set of services and supports that meets their health needs, including mental, dental, and preventive health services, regardless of their state of residence or their socioeconomic status.*
   Proposed Foundational Changes:

1. Uniform Medicaid or CHIP program and benefit design and implementation that effectively supports the needs of children, youth, and families with uniform access across all states.
2. Implementation of a federal Medicaid/CHIP core drug benefit setting minimum requirements for state formularies.

Financing

Goal: *Medicaid program financing should facilitate a robust, high-quality network of providers, services, and supports.*
   Proposed Foundational Changes:

1. Major increases in the federal share of funding of the Medicaid/CHIP programs, especially for all direct patient care, to eliminate state variations that contribute to unequal access to care.
2. A federal minimum rate schedule with an end to undervalued Medicaid payment, with rates at least comparable to prevailing Medicare rates and that support the full range of services needed to provide comprehensive care to children.

The next section elaborates on these proposed foundational changes and articulates incremental strategies that could lead to these foundational goals.

ELIGIBILITY AND ENROLLMENT

Goal: All children (0–26 years) in the United States should have access to health insurance coverage.

Background

The AAP recommends universal eligibility and automatic enrollment for Medicaid/CHIP for all children (0–26 years) lacking other sources of health insurance. Uniform eligibility levels and enrollment and retention policies will help ensure equitable and continuous access to coverage. Currently, states determine Medicaid/CHIP eligibility for children based on age, household income, and other special circumstances (eg, foster care or special health care needs). States now must meet the minimum federal Medicaid income eligibility level for children (currently 138% of FPL), but many states use higher income thresholds, leading to significant state variation in income eligibility.[32] Although current statute allows states to increase the age threshold to 20 years, most states limit eligibility to ages 0 to 18 years. States also can vary the income threshold by age.[32]

Furthermore, after establishing eligibility, each state can impose administrative burdens related to enrollment (eg, required documentation, complex applications, periodic data checks[33,34]) or alternatively, provide support to facilitate enrollment, such as supporting different language preferences or health literacy levels. Frequent redeterminations often lead eligible recipients to lose coverage because of documentation or other problems. These variations exacerbate inequities, perpetuate systemic racism, and lead to disproportionate underutilization of vital services and programs by the populations Medicaid and CHIP are intended to benefit.[35]

Proposed Foundational Changes

1. **Universal eligibility for all children residing in the United States up to age 26 years through a single program that combines Medicaid and CHIP.**

   Universal eligibility would eliminate coverage gaps and the types of state variation described above. The proposed age range also aligns with the availability of dependent coverage for individuals up to age 26 years in the commercial market. Ensuring eligibility through a single program that combines Medicaid and CHIP also addresses avoidable variations in care and access among children, particularly as household income fluctuates. Parents or guardians could opt out of Medicaid/CHIP if they have other coverage.

2. **Automatic enrollment of all newborn infants at birth to guarantee health insurance coverage.**

   All newborn infants should have health insurance in place at birth that will ensure access to health care benefits during critical newborn hospitalization and postdischarge periods. Enrollment in Medicaid/CHIP should be automatic, with the option to opt out of coverage if the infant has another source of health insurance.

Additional Strategies

Until the above foundational changes are achieved, the AAP recommends interim strategies to augment Medicaid and CHIP eligibility and promote continuity of coverage:

1. **Continuous eligibility:** Continuous eligibility helps to ensure health care access and limits disenrollment of eligible recipients. The AAP recommends required continuous eligibility of all individuals from the newborn period to age 6 years, and a minimum period of 2-year continuous eligibility without renewal requirement for individuals ages 6 years to up to age 26 years. Medicaid coverage for pregnant individuals should be extended from 60 days to 1 year postpartum[36,37] nationwide, consistent with policy many states have already implemented. Such changes will reduce the number of eligibility redeterminations and temporary losses of Medicaid coverage, while improving infant and maternal health and outcomes.

2. **Medicaid and CHIP alignment:** Even without combining the programs, Medicaid and CHIP can operate in a more aligned fashion by allowing seamless, continuous coverage for children (0–26 years) as they transition between the 2 programs because of family income fluctuations.

3. **Broader eligibility standards:** The federal minimum income eligibility for all children (0–26 years) in Medicaid/CHIP should increase to 400% of FPL. This income eligibility level will ensure affordable health insurance coverage for children (0–26 years), regardless of whether they qualify for coverage under an Affordable Care Act marketplace plan or have access to an employer-sponsored plan.

4. **Expanded eligibility for children in immigrant families:** Children (0–26 years) in immigrant families are at particular risk for uninsurance and access gaps. Given this risk, Medicaid/CHIP eligibility should be extended to all immigrant children irrespective of immigration status to age 26 years. Short of this change, policy should include extending Medicaid/CHIP eligibility to all individuals in the Deferred Action for Childhood Arrivals program and those seeking humanitarian protection and removing the 5-year bar for lawfully present children and/or pregnant individuals at the federal level.

5. **Enrollment and retention supports:** States and CMS should provide adequate funding to simplify enrollment and retention for children (0–26 years) and families, including outreach and enrollment assistance, especially to populations at high risk of uninsurance. States should have (1) multiple sites for enrollment, including online and paper enrollment and joint applications with other public assistance programs; (2) community-based enrollment navigators; (3) income tax filing prompts for eligibility and enrollment options; and (4) continuous enrollment availability without lockout periods.[38]

6. **Presumptive enrollment:** Implement presumptive eligibility for re-enrollment for families who had previously submitted evidence of fiscal income eligibility but face challenges in providing timely current income data. This policy helps to minimize coverage disruptions and access gaps.

7. **Cross-state coverage support:** Limit disruptions in Medicaid/CHIP coverage when children (0–26 years) move across state lines. The previous state should provide seamless coverage until it notifies the new state about termination, and the new state should then grant presumptive eligibility. Additionally, services feasibly accessed only by crossing state lines, such as subspecialist care, should be covered without any interruptions. This should also apply across counties for children enrolled in managed care plans.

COVERAGE AND CARE

Goal: Children (0–26 years) should have access to a consistent, high-quality set of services and supports that address their clinical needs regardless of their state of residence or their socioeconomic status.

Background

Federal guidelines mandate a core set of benefits and covered services in Medicaid/CHIP, although states have wide discretion and minimal oversight regarding which optional services to cover as well as the design of their benefits. For example, states must provide inpatient care but can limit the number of allowable days per year or provide similar limits on specialized therapies. States can also limit providers eligible to offer various services, such as restricting payment for provision of mental health and developmental preventive and treatment services to professionals licensed in those fields or can deny payment for both medical and mental health services provided to the same patient on the same day. Especially given the high rates of mental health conditions among children, these limits hinder opportunities for primary care pediatricians to assess and manage common behavioral conditions, such as emotional dysregulation, anxiety, depression, and attention-deficit/hyperactive disorder. The Medicaid statute provides a clear standard of care for children through the "equal access" provision and through EPSDT; however, federal monitoring and enforcement of enrollees' access to care and of state EPSDT implementation has been limited, leading to inequities across states in the services enrollees can access in a timely way, as well as what medically necessary services are covered.

Proposed Foundational Changes

1. **Uniform Medicaid/CHIP program design and implementation that effectively supports the complex needs of children, youth, and their families.**

   The AAP calls for the consistent application of national Medicaid standards that ensure a common and equitable approach to benefits (scope and duration) and quality across states. Although several current federal requirements for Medicaid programs address benefits and administration, current requirements and federal enforcement still enable substantial state-by-state variation. The AAP calls for stronger national standards, based on EPSDT, to ensure that every child, regardless of where they live, can access the same types of services and quality of care. Stronger benefit standards would require consistent scope and duration and permit the same set of provider types across state lines. Consistent and enforceable national standards will better support the modern-day complex clinical, social, developmental, dental, and mental health needs of children, youth, and their families as well as the health providers who care for them. States would continue to have sufficient flexibility to experiment with and test different models of care for their local populations.

2. **Implementation of federal core Medicaid/CHIP drug set.**

   Pharmacy, durable medical equipment, and specialty formula benefits must ensure access to all needed medicines and equipment for all children (0–26 years), including those with special health care needs and/or rare diseases. Pharmacy benefits must allow for the fact that children often require off-label use of medications, despite not being able to be in a formulary. The federal government should mandate the Medicaid/CHIP program adopt a uniform base of pediatric drugs across states and managed care entities within states, as states and plans develop their formularies. This core should allow for generic and biosimilar substitutions and cover over-the-counter medications, reducing variation across programs and states and decreasing the prior authorization burden.

Additional Strategies

Until the above foundational changes are achieved, the AAP recommends interim strategies to ensure high-quality coverage for all children:

1. **Full implementation and monitoring of the EPSDT benefit in Medicaid and CHIP:** At minimum, states should cover all benefits and services outlined in the AAP statement on scope of health care benefits.[18] The EPSDT benefit should also be mandated as standard within CHIP.

2. **Standard medical necessity definition:** Ensuring a national standard of care through EPSDT makes clear the need to formalize the definition and coverage of medically necessary services, including preventive care or periodicity[19,20] and immunization schedules consistent with national guidelines.[39] See the AAP statement on medical necessity.[40]

3. **Standard measure set:** States and the federal government must ensure quality and accountability in the Medicaid/CHIP programs, using measures appropriate

for children (0–26 years) and young families with goals of enhancing care and outcomes. Quality measurement should identify racial disparities and other areas of potential health inequities. Measures included in the Medicaid Child Core Set should be frequently reviewed and updated to align with AAP recommendations and advances in measurement science.[41] States should provide incentives to encourage practices[42] to achieve predefined quality and performance metrics that reflect pediatric clinical priorities.

4. **Incorporate racial and health equity analysis into the development and evaluation of Medicaid and CHIP Policies:** Optimizing Medicaid/CHIP for equity will benefit from systems of accountability that help avoid introducing new harms and barriers, as well as perpetuating existing damage. Existing analysis tools, including community input, should be incorporated early in Medicaid and CHIP policy and budget development, as well as implementation and evaluation.

5. **Medicaid Claims Database:** CMS should enhance national Medicaid claims data resources and require state Medicaid plans and Medicaid managed care organizations (MCOs) to participate fully in reporting encounter data, with a standardized approach to collecting and reporting race and ethnicity and language data.[43-45] This database will allow health policy analysts and researchers in government, academia, and the private sector to examine regional patterns of utilization, denials, access to care, and quality of care to provide accountability and inform efforts to construct "best practice" models of care.[46,47]

FINANCING AND PAYMENT

Goal: Medicaid program financing should facilitate a robust, high-quality network of providers, services, and supports.

Background

Medicaid and CHIP are based on a complex federal-state financing partnership that promotes wide state variation in all program aspects, including financing and payments. State variations in payment help to perpetuate racial and geographic inequities. Most states contract with MCOs to implement their Medicaid/CHIP programs, and MCOs now cover the large majority of children[48]; differences across MCOs create further heterogeneity within states. In addition, persistently undervalued payment rates by Medicaid and CHIP have disincentivized physician and other provider participation in these programs, limiting the number of accessible health care options.

Proposed Foundational Changes

1. **Federal assumption of most funding for Medicaid/ CHIP beneficiaries up to age 26 years, especially all direct patient care, to eliminate state variations that contribute to unequal access to care.**

The federal government should assume substantially more patient care financing costs of Medicaid/CHIP, leading to program uniformity as described in the previous section and ensure children receive the same services and supports in all states while allowing for some state flexibility in funding and innovation.

2. **A federal minimum rate schedule with an end to undervalued Medicaid payment, with rates at least comparable to prevailing Medicare rates and that support the full range of services needed to provide comprehensive care to children.[49,50]**

The AAP recommends a federal minimum rate schedule that ends undervaluing in Medicaid rates and provides rates at least comparable to prevailing Medicare schedules expanded to include pediatric-specific services that Medicare payers may not cover. Where no Medicare equivalents exist, payment rates should be made consistent with commercial rates. Where no payment standard exists, pediatric physicians should be consulted in determining adequate payment. Payments must support both the goods and services involved in caring for children and related work and practice expenses and also provide a return sufficient to ensure economic feasibility and continued operation of a practice or facility. Payments should also be sufficient and timely to recruit and maintain an adequate supply of team providers, including physicians, nurses, mental health and developmental clinicians, community health work, as well as specialized pediatric service providers and facilities to ensure Medicaid and CHIP recipients have access to primary and specialty care and services equal to access experienced by commercially insured patients in that geographic region. Participation and quality care depend on adequate payment for staff, space, and material to provide high-quality patient care.

Additional Strategies

Until the above foundational changes are achieved, the AAP recommends interim strategies to improve adequate Medicaid/CHIP program financing:

1. **Expand federal oversight:** Change the statutory relationships between CMS and the states so that CMS has expanded authority to ensure national standards for eligibility, enrollment, benefits, quality, and payment.

2. **Restructure CHIP as an entitlement program:** Transform CHIP to an entitlement program similar to Medicaid to eliminate the impact of potential lapses in funding resulting from congressional inaction. Prohibit states from freezing or capping enrollments.

3. **Augment resources and adjust payments for health-related social needs:** Payment rates should recognize

the costs of supporting families and their complex social, developmental, and economic needs, including the extra resources needed to promote healthy mental and emotional development and screening for and addressing social influencers of health. Payment models should account for elevated costs associated with caring for children with varied special needs, such as chronic and complex medical conditions, mental health concerns, and health-related social needs. Risk adjustment models that rely on previous utilization may not fully account for needs, in part because children, especially in less-resourced households or neighborhoods or who face systemic racism, may underutilize care.[51] Further, payments should be adjusted for the health and/or mental health of family caregivers, whose health and well-being greatly influence needs and health care use by children.[52]

4. **Enable access to integrated mental health supports regardless of diagnosis:** Payment must be adequate to allow for access to needed mental health preventive and treatment services, including therapy in addition to medication management, even without a specific diagnosis. All Medicaid and CHIP programs should enable children (0–26 years) to access mental health supports without a formal diagnosis.[53] The growing mental health needs among children (0–26 years) create an urgent need to support mental health integration in pediatric care, including incentives for primary care pediatricians to provide needed services.

CONCLUSIONS

Medicaid and CHIP currently provide essential health coverage for over half of all US children, who reflect the racial and ethnic diversity of the United States. These critical programs provide substantial pediatric-specific benefits and care that have had major positive impacts for children, youth, and families. Transformational reform and enhancements of Medicaid and CHIP have the potential to build a national system of care that fully addresses the clinical, developmental, social, and mental health needs of diverse, low-income children, youth, and their families. This AAP statement outlines goals and strategies to ensure health equity, quality of care, and access to vital health care services while dismantling the longstanding impacts of systemic racism within public insurance programs for children. The statement clarifies ways to expand on current program strengths, but the AAP recognizes the need for more foundational and lasting reform to meet the needs of children, advance health equity, and ensure healthy and productive adults in the future. Regular health equity assessments will check that changes made improve equitable access, with modifications made if health equity goals are not met. Changes outlined in this statement will improve health care and access for all children. The technical report will describe how Medicaid supports the needs of several special populations in more detail. Proposed reforms in Medicaid/CHIP include a federal standard that expands eligibility and improves enrollment and retention and promotes innovative payment structures; makes EPSDT the standard for both Medicaid/CHIP with enforcement by CMS[54]; regulates standards and decreases state-by-state variation; and ensures adequate payment while still allowing, encouraging, and supporting continued state innovation.

LEAD AUTHORS

Jennifer D. Kusma, MD, MS, FAAP
Jean L. Raphael, MD, MPH, FAAP
James M. Perrin, MD, FAAP
Mark L. Hudak, MD, FAAP

COMMITTEE ON CHILD HEALTH FINANCING, 2022–2023

James M. Perrin, MD, FAAP, Chairperson
Lisa Chamberlain, MD, MPH, FAAP
Jennifer D. Kusma, MD, MS, FAAP
William Bernard Moskowitz, MD, FAAP
Alison Amidei Galbraith, MD, FAAP
Jean L. Raphael, MD, MPH, FAAP
Renee M. Turchi, MD, MPH, FAAP

LIAISONS

Angelo P. Giardino, MD, FAAP – Medicaid and CHIP Payment and Access Commission
Mike Chen, MD, FAAP – Section on Surgery
Todd Wolynn, MD, MMM, FAAP – Section on Administration and Practice Management

CONSULTANTS

Hope Glassberg
Elizabeth Patchias

STAFF

Sunnah Kim
Stephanie Glier
Dan Walter
Todd Fraley
Nicholas Wallace

ABBREVIATIONS

AAP: American Academy of Pediatrics
CHIP: Children's Health Insurance Program
CMS: Centers for Medicare and Medicaid Services
EPSDT: Early and Periodic Screening, Diagnostic, and Treatment
FPL: federal poverty level
MCO: managed care organization

DOI: https://doi.org/10.1542/peds.2023-064088

Address correspondence to Jennifer D. Kusma, MD, MS, FAAP. E-mail: jkusma@luriechildrens.org

PEDIATRICS (ISSN Numbers: Print, 0031-4005; Online, 1098-4275).

FUNDING: No external funding.

CONFLICT OF INTEREST DISCLOSURES: The authors have indicated they have no potential conflicts of interest to disclose.

REFERENCES

1. Perrin JM, Flanagan P, Katkin J, Barabell G, Price J; Committee on Child Health Financing. The unique value proposition of pediatric health care. *Pediatrics*. 2023;151(2):e2022060681

2. Hudak ML, Helm ME, White PH; American Academy of Pediatrics, Committee on Child Health Financing. Principles of child health care financing. *Pediatrics*. 2017;140(3):e20172098

3. Carlson KM, Berman SK, Price J; American Academy of Pediatrics, Committee on Child Health Financing. Guiding principles for managed care arrangements for the health of newborns, infants, children, adolescents and young adults. *Pediatrics*. 2022; 150(2):e2022058396

4. American Academy of Pediatrics Board of Directors. Truth, reconciliation, and transformation: continuing on the path to equity. *Pediatrics*. 2020;146(3):e2020019794

5. American Academy of Pediatrics, Medical Home Initiatives for Children With Special Needs Project Advisory Committee. The medical home. *Pediatrics*. 2002;110(1 Pt 1):184–186

6. American Academy of Pediatrics, Council on Community Pediatrics. Navigating the intersection of medicine, public health, and social determinants of children's health. *Pediatrics*. 2013;131(3): 623–628

7. Alker J, Brooks T. Millions of children may lose Medicaid: what can be done to help prevent them from becoming uninsured?. Available at: https://ccf.georgetown.edu/2022/02/17/millions-of-children-may-lose-medicaid-what-can-be-done-to-help-prevent-them-from-becoming-uninsured/. Accessed July 18, 2023

8. Cohen RA, Cha AE. Health insurance coverage: early release of estimates from the National Health Interview Survey, January–June 2022. Available at: https://www.cdc.gov/nchs/data/nhis/earlyrelease/insur202212.pdf. Accessed July 18, 2023

9. KFF. Population distribution of children by race/ethnicity. Available at: https://www.kff.org/other/state-indicator/children-by-raceethnicity/?currentTimeframe=0&sortModel=%7B%22colId%22:%22Location%22,%22sort%22:%22asc%22%7D. Accessed July 18, 2023

10. Paradise J. The impact of the Children's Health Insurance Program (CHIP): what does the research tell us?. Available at: https://www.kff.org/report-section/the-impact-of-the-childrens-health-insurance-program-chip-issue-brief/. Accessed July 18, 2023

11. Hakim RB, Boben PJ, Bonney JB. Medicaid and the health of children. *Health Care Financ Rev*. 2000;22(1):133–140

12. Currie J, Chorniy A. Medicaid and Child Health Insurance Program improve child health and reduce poverty but face threats. *Acad Pediatr*. 2021;21(8S Suppl):S146–S153

13. Medicaid KFF. A primer – key information on the nation's health coverage program for low-income people. Available at: https://www.kff.org/medicaid/issue-brief/medicaid-a-primer/. Accessed July 18, 2023

14. The Future of Children. Historical overview of children's health care coverage. Available at: https://ccf.georgetown.edu/wp-content/uploads/2012/03/Uninsured_historical-overview.pdf. Accessed July 18, 2023

15. Mann C, Rowland D, Garfield R. Children's health coverage: Medicaid, CHIP, and the ACA. Available at: https://www.kff.org/health-reform/issue-brief/childrens-health-coverage-medicaid-chip-and-the-aca/. Accessed July 18, 2023

16. Jacobs PD, Moriya AS. Changes in health coverage during the COVID-19 pandemic. *Health Aff (Millwood)*. 2023;42(5):721–726

17. KFF. Federal medical assistance percentage (FMAP) for Medicaid and multiplier. Available at: https://www.kff.org/medicaid/state-indicator/federal-matching-rate-and-multiplier/?currentTimeframe=0&sortModel=%7B%22colId%22:%22FMAP%20Percentage%22,%22sort%22:%22desc%22%7D. Accessed July 18, 2023

18. Hudak ML; American Academy of Pediatrics, Committee on Child Health Financing. Scope of health care benefits for neonates, infants, children, adolescents, and young adults through age 26. *Pediatrics*. 2022;150(3):e2022058881

19. Hagan JF Jr, Shaw JS, Duncan PM, eds. *Bright Futures: Guidelines for Health Supervision of Infants, Children, and Adolescents*. 4th ed. American Academy of Pediatrics; 2017

20. American Academy of Pediatrics, Committee on Practice and Ambulatory Medicine; Bright Futures Periodicity Schedule Workgroup. 2023 Recommendations for preventive pediatric health care. *Pediatrics*. 2023;151(4):e2023061451

21. Centers for Medicare and Medicaid Services. EPSDT - a guide for states: coverage in the Medicaid benefit for children and adolescents. Available at: https://www.medicaid.gov/sites/default/files/2019-12/epsdt_coverage_guide.pdf. Accessed September 11, 2023

22. Michener JD. Politics, pandemic, and racial justice through the lens of Medicaid. *Am J Public Health*. 2021;111(4):643–646

23. Somers S, Perkins J. The ongoing racial paradox of the Medicaid program. *J Health Life Sci Law*. 2022;16(1):98–111

24. US Government Accountability Office. Medicaid. Additional CMS data and oversight needed to help ensure children receive recommended screenings. Available at: https://www.gao.gov/assets/gao-19-481.pdf. Accessed July 18, 2023

25. US Government Accountability Office. Medicaid. Stronger efforts needed to ensure children's access to health screening services. Available at: https://www.gao.gov/assets/gao-01-749.pdf. Accessed July 18, 2023

26. Medicaid and CHIP Payment and Access Commission. Key CHIP design features. Available at: https://www.macpac.gov/subtopic/key-design-features/. Accessed July 18, 2023

27. Artiga S, Ubri P. Key issues in children's health coverage. Available at: https://www.kff.org/medicaid/issue-brief/key-issues-in-childrens-health-coverage/. Accessed July 18, 2023

28. Health Resources and Services Administration, Maternal and Child Health. Early periodic screening, diagnosis, and treatment. Available at: https://mchb.hrsa.gov/programs-impact/early-periodic-screening-diagnosis-treatment. Accessed July 18, 2023

29. Arenberg S, Neller S, Stripling S. The impact of youth Medicaid eligibility on adult incarceration. Available at: https://www.aeaweb.org/articles?id=10.1257/app.20200785&from=f. Accessed August 17, 2023

30. US Department of Health and Human Services, Administration for Children and Families, Office of Family Assistance, Peer TA. Report: Medicaid and intergenerational economic mobility. Available at: https://peerta.acf.hhs.gov/content/medicaid-and-intergenerational-economic-mobility. Accessed August 17, 2023

31. Centers for Medicare and Medicaid Services. CMS framework for health equity 2022-2032. Available at: https://www.cms.gov/files/document/cms-framework-health-equity-2022.pdf. Accessed August 17, 2023

32. KFF. Medicaid and CHIP income eligibility limits for children as a percent of the federal poverty level. Available at: https://www.kff.org/health-reform/state-indicator/medicaid-and-chip-income-eligibility-limits-for-children-as-a-percent-of-the-federal-poverty-level/?currentTimeframe=0&sortModel=%7B%22colId%22:%22Medicaid%20Coverage%20for%20Children%20Ages%201-5__Medicaid%20Funded%22,%22sort%22:%22desc%22%7D. Accessed July 18, 2023

33. Swartz K, Short PF, Graefe DR, Uberoi N. Reducing Medicaid churning: extending eligibility for twelve months or to end of calendar year is most effective. *Health Aff (Millwood)*. 2015;34(7):1180–1187

34. Georgetown University Health Policy Institute, Center for Children and Families. Medicaid and CHIP continuous coverage for children. Available at: https://ccf.georgetown.edu/2022/10/07/medicaid-and-chip-continuous-coverage-for-children/. Accessed July 18, 2023

35. Wikle S, Wagner J, Erzouki F, Sullivan J. States can reduce Medicaid's administrative burdens to advance health and racial equity. Available at: https://www.cbpp.org/research/health/states-can-reduce-medicaids-administrative-burdens-to-advance-health-and-racial. Accessed July 18, 2023

36. Johnson K, Rosenbaum S, Handley M. The next steps to advance maternal and child health in Medicaid: filling gaps in postpartum coverage and newborn enrollment. Available at: https://www.healthaffairs.org/do/10.1377/hblog20191230.967912/full/. Accessed July 18, 2023

37. KFF. Medicaid postpartum coverage extension tracker July 2023. Available at: https://www.kff.org/medicaid/issue-brief/medicaid-postpartum-coverage-extension-tracker/. Accessed July 18, 2023

38. Garcia Mosqueira A, Sommers BD. Better outreach critical to ACA enrollment, particularly for Latinos. Available at: https://www.commonwealthfund.org/blog/2016/better-outreach-critical-aca-enrollment-particularly-latinos. Accessed May 5, 2020

39. Ezeanolue E, Harriman K, Hunter P, Kroger A, Pellegrini C; Centers for Disease Control and Prevention. General best practice guidelines for immunization: best practices guidance of the Advisory Committee on Immunization Practices (ACIP). Available at: https://www.cdc.gov/vaccines/hcp/acip-recs/general-recs/index.html. Accessed May 5, 2020

40. Giardino AP, Hudak ML, Sood BG, Pearlman SA; American Academy of Pediatrics, Committee on Child Health Financing. Considerations in the determination of medical necessity in children: application to contractual language. *Pediatrics*. 2022;150(3):e2022058882

41. Medicaid.gov. Children's health care quality measures. Core set of children's health care quality measures. Available at: https://www.medicaid.gov/medicaid/quality-of-care/performance-measurement/adult-and-child-health-care-quality-measures/childrens-health-care-quality-measures/index.html#:~:text=Children%27s%20Health%20Care%20Quality%20Measures%201%20Core%20Set,Medicaid%20and%20CHIP%20 ... %204%20Related%20Initiatives%20. Accessed July 18, 2023

42. Adirim T, Meade K, Mistry K; American Academy of Pediatrics, Council on Quality Improvement and Patient Safety; Committee on Practice and Ambulatory Management. A new era in quality measurement: the development and application of quality measures. *Pediatrics*. 2017;139(1):e20163442

43. Medicaid and CHIP Payment and Access Commission. Re: CMS-2440-P: Medicaid Program and CHIP; mandatory Medicaid and Children's Health Insurance Program (CHIP) core set reporting. Letter to the Honorable Chiquita Brooks-LaSure, Administrator, Centers for Medicare & Medicaid Services, US Department of Health and Human Services. Available at: https://www.macpac.gov/wp-content/uploads/2022/10/Medicaid-and-CHIP-Core-Set-Reporting-Comment-Letter-Final.pdf. Accessed July 18, 2023

44. Hu J-C, Cummings JR, Ji X, Wilk AS. Evaluating Medicaid managed care network adequacy standards and associations with specialty care access for children. *Health Aff (Millwood)*. 2023;42(6):759–769

45. National Health Law Program. Exceptions to network adequacy rules may exacerbate health disparities in Medi-Cal managed care. Available at: https://healthlaw.org/exceptions-to-network-adequacy-rules-may-exacerbate-health-disparities-in-medi-cal-managed-care/. Accessed July 18, 2023

46. Medicaid.gov. Transformed Medicaid Statistical Information System (T-MSIS). Available at: https://www.medicaid.gov/medicaid/data-systems/macbis/transformed-medicaid-statistical-information-system-t-msis/index.html. Accessed July 18, 2023

47. Medicaid and CHIP Payment and Access Commission. Update on Transformed Medicaid Statistical Information System (T-MSIS). Available at: https://www.macpac.gov/wp-content/uploads/2021/

04/Update-on-Transformed-Medicaid-Statistical-Information-System-T-MSIS.pdf. Accessed July 18, 2023

48. Centers for Medicare and Medicaid Services. 2017 Managed care enrollment summary. Available at: https://data.medicaid.gov/Enrollment/2017-Managed-Care-Enrollment-Summary/uw3d-3r25. Accessed May 5, 2020

49. Mann C, Striar A. How differences in Medicaid, Medicare, and commercial health insurance payment rates impact access, health equity, and cost. Available at: https://www.commonwealthfund.org/blog/2022/how-differences-medicaid-medicare-and-commercial-health-insurance-payment-rates-impact. Accessed July 18, 2023

50. Berman S, Dolins J, Tang SF, Yudkowsky B. Factors that influence the willingness of private primary care pediatricians to accept more Medicaid patients. *Pediatrics*. 2002;110(2 Pt 1):239–248

51. Mass.gov. Reports on health care cost trends and cost drivers. Available at: https://www.mass.gov/lists/reports-on-health-care-cost-trends-and-cost-drivers. Accessed July 18, 2023

52. McWilliams JM, Weinreb G, Ding L, Ndumele CD, Wallace J. Risk adjustment and promoting health equity in population-based payment: concepts and evidence. *Health Aff (Millwood)*. 2023;42(1):105–114

53. West-Bey N. California's Medicaid family therapy benefit reimagines medical necessity. Available at: https://www.clasp.org/blog/californias-medicaid-family-therapy-benefit-reimagines-medical-necessity/. Accessed July 18, 2023

54. Rosenbaum S, Johnson K. A twenty-first century Medicaid child health policy: modernizing EPSDT [opinion]. Available at: https://www.milbank.org/quarterly/opinions/a-twenty-first-century-medicaid-child-health-policy-modernizing-epsdt/. Accessed July 18, 2023

POLICY STATEMENT Organizational Principles to Guide and Define the Child Health
Care System and/or Improve the Health of all Children

American Academy
of Pediatrics

DEDICATED TO THE HEALTH OF ALL CHILDREN™

This Policy Statement was reaffirmed April 2021.

Poverty and Child Health in the United States

COUNCIL ON COMMUNITY PEDIATRICS

abstract

Almost half of young children in the United States live in poverty or near poverty. The American Academy of Pediatrics is committed to reducing and ultimately eliminating child poverty in the United States. Poverty and related social determinants of health can lead to adverse health outcomes in childhood and across the life course, negatively affecting physical health, socioemotional development, and educational achievement. The American Academy of Pediatrics advocates for programs and policies that have been shown to improve the quality of life and health outcomes for children and families living in poverty. With an awareness and understanding of the effects of poverty on children, pediatricians and other pediatric health practitioners in a family-centered medical home can assess the financial stability of families, link families to resources, and coordinate care with community partners. Further research, advocacy, and continuing education will improve the ability of pediatricians to address the social determinants of health when caring for children who live in poverty. Accompanying this policy statement is a technical report that describes current knowledge on child poverty and the mechanisms by which poverty influences the health and well-being of children.

DOI: 10.1542/peds.2016-0339

PEDIATRICS (ISSN Numbers: Print, 0031-4005; Online, 1098-4275).

To cite: AAP COUNCIL ON COMMUNITY PEDIATRICS. Poverty and Child Health in the United States. *Pediatrics*. 2016; 137(4):e20160339

STATEMENT OF THE PROBLEM

Poverty is an important social determinant of health and contributes to child health disparities. Children who experience poverty, particularly during early life or for an extended period, are at risk of a host of adverse health and developmental outcomes through their life course.[1] Poverty has a profound effect on specific circumstances, such as birth weight, infant mortality, language development, chronic illness, environmental exposure, nutrition, and injury. Child poverty also influences genomic function and brain development by exposure to toxic stress,[2] a condition characterized by "excessive or prolonged activation of the physiologic stress response systems in the absence of the buffering protection afforded by stable, responsive relationships."[3] Children living in poverty

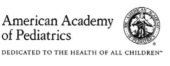

American Academy
of Pediatrics
DEDICATED TO THE HEALTH OF ALL CHILDREN™

Organizational Principles to Guide and Define the Child
Health Care System and/or Improve the Health of all Children

This Policy Statement was reaffirmed October 2016 and February 2022.

POLICY STATEMENT

Providing Care for Children and Adolescents Facing Homelessness and Housing Insecurity

abstract

Child health and housing security are closely intertwined, and children without homes are more likely to suffer from chronic disease, hunger, and malnutrition than are children with homes. Homeless children and youth often have significant psychosocial development issues, and their education is frequently interrupted. Given the overall effects that homelessness can have on a child's health and potential, it is important for pediatricians to recognize the factors that lead to homelessness, understand the ways that homelessness and its causes can lead to poor health outcomes, and when possible, help children and families mitigate some of the effects of homelessness. Through practice change, partnership with community resources, awareness, and advocacy, pediatricians can help optimize the health and well-being of children affected by homelessness. *Pediatrics* 2013;131:1206–1210

INTRODUCTION

An estimated 1.6 million children, or nearly 1 in 45 American children, experienced homelessness in 2010.[1] Although a national economic downturn and an increase in housing foreclosures contribute to family homelessness, additional adversity and risk factors often contribute to this complex problem. Children affected by homelessness may experience a variety of challenges to their health because of difficulty accessing health care, inadequate nutrition, education interruptions, trauma, and family dynamics. By recognizing these challenges, pediatricians can help improve the care of these children in practices and communities.

DEFINING AND MEASURING HOMELESSNESS

The US Department of Education defines a homeless individual as "(A) an individual who lacks a fixed, regular, and adequate nighttime residence . . . and (B) includes (i) children and youths who are sharing the housing of other persons due to loss of housing, economic hardship, or a similar reason; are living in motels, hotels, trailer parks, or camping grounds due to the lack of alternative accommodations; are living in emergency or transitional shelters; are abandoned in hospitals; or are awaiting foster care placement; (ii) children and youths who have a primary nighttime residence that is a public or private place not designed for or ordinarily used as

COUNCIL ON COMMUNITY PEDIATRICS

KEY WORDS
homelessness, housing insecurity, children, adolescents, pediatrician, health, poverty, toxic stress

This article was written by members of the American Academy of Pediatrics. It does not represent the views of the US government or any US government agency.

www.pediatrics.org/cgi/doi/10.1542/peds.2013-0645

doi:10.1542/peds.2013-0645

PEDIATRICS (ISSN Numbers: Print, 0031-4005; Online, 1098-4275).

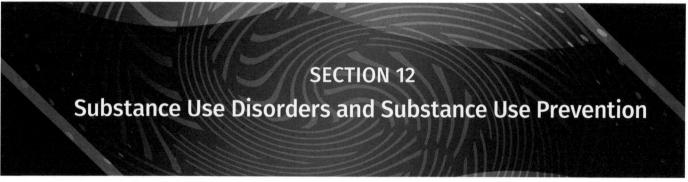

SECTION 12
Substance Use Disorders and Substance Use Prevention

Some articles are available online only; scan the QR code to access online content.

POLICY STATEMENT Organizational Principles to Guide and Define the Child Health Care System and/or Improve the Health of all Children

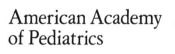

American Academy of Pediatrics

DEDICATED TO THE HEALTH OF ALL CHILDREN™

Protecting Children and Adolescents From Tobacco and Nicotine

Brian P. Jenssen, MD, FAAP,[a] Susan C. Walley, MD, FAAP,[b] Rachel Boykan, MD, FAAP,[c] Alice Little Caldwell, MD, MPH, IBCLC, FAAP,[d] Deepa Camenga, MD, FAAP[e]

SECTION ON NICOTINE AND TOBACCO PREVENTION AND TREATMENT, COMMITTEE ON SUBSTANCE USE AND PREVENTION

abstract

Tobacco use remains the leading preventable cause of disease and death for adults in the United States. Significant strides have been made in reducing rates of cigarette smoking among adolescents in the United States. However, rates of e-cigarette and similar device use among youth are high, and rates of other tobacco product use, such as cigars and hookahs, have not declined. Public policy actions to protect children and adolescents from tobacco and nicotine use, as well as tobacco smoke and aerosol exposure, have proven effective in reducing harm. Effective public health approaches need to be both extended to include e-cigarettes, similar devices, and other and emerging tobacco products and expanded to reduce the toll that the tobacco epidemic takes on children and adolescents.

[a]Children's Hospital of Philadelphia (CHOP), University of Pennsylvania Perelman School of Medicine, Philadelphia, Pennsylvania; [b]Children's National Hospital, George Washington University School of Medicine and Health Sciences, Washington, District of Columbia; [c]Renaissance School of Medicine at Stony Brook University, Stony Brook Children's Hospital, Stony Brook, New York; [d]Medical College of Georgia, Augusta University Medical Center, Augusta, Georgia; and [e]Pediatrics and Public Health, Yale Program in Addiction Medicine, Yale Schools of Medicine and Public Health, New Haven, Connecticut

Policy statements from the American Academy of Pediatrics benefit from expertise and resources of liaisons and internal (AAP) and external reviewers. However, policy statements from the American Academy of Pediatrics may not reflect the views of the liaisons or the organizations or government agencies that they represent.

The guidance in this statement does not indicate an exclusive course of treatment or serve as a standard of medical care. Variations, taking into account individual circumstances, may be appropriate.

All policy statements from the American Academy of Pediatrics automatically expire 5 years after publication unless reaffirmed, revised, or retired at or before that time.

COMPANION PAPERS: Companions to this article can be found online at www.pediatrics.org/cgi/doi/10.1542/peds.2023-061805 and www.pediatrics.org/cgi/doi/10.1542/peds.2023-061806.

DOI: https://doi.org/10.1542/peds.2023-061804

To cite: Jenssen BP, Walley SC, Boykan R, et al; AAP Section on Nicotine and Tobacco Prevention and Treatment, Committee on Substance Use and Prevention. Protecting Children and Adolescents From Tobacco and Nicotine. Pediatrics. 2023; 151(5):e2023061804

DEFINITIONS

Tobacco product: Any product or device that can deliver nicotine to the human brain, whether derived from tobacco or another source, except for safe and effective nicotine replacement therapies approved by the US Food and Drug Administration (FDA) for tobacco cessation. Tobacco products include, but are not limited to, e-cigarettes, cigarettes, cigars, smokeless tobacco, hookahs, pipe tobacco, heated tobacco products, and nicotine "tobacco-free" pouches.

Secondhand smoke: Smoke emitted from a tobacco product or exhaled from a person who smokes that is inhaled by a person who does not smoke.

Thirdhand smoke: Tobacco smoke that is absorbed onto surfaces and exposes a person who does not use tobacco to its components by direct contact and dermal absorption, ingestion, and/or off-gassing and inhalation. Thirdhand smoke may react with oxidants and other compounds in the environment to yield secondary pollutants.

Tobacco smoke exposure: Tobacco smoke exposure among people who do not use tobacco, which includes both secondhand and thirdhand exposure.

E-cigarettes: Handheld devices that come in a variety of shapes and sizes. Most have a battery, a heating element, and a container to hold a solution that can contain nicotine, flavorings, and other chemicals. E-cigarettes are known by many different names. They are sometimes called e-cigs, e-hookahs, mods, pods, vapes, vape pens, tank systems, and electronic nicotine delivery systems or referred to by brand name, including Juul or Puff Bar.

Aerosol exposure: The emissions from e-cigarettes to which people who do not use e-cigarettes are exposed, including secondhand and thirdhand exposure.

Tobacco use disorder: A clinical diagnosis for which treatment is within the scope of practice of pediatric providers. Moderate or severe tobacco use disorder is defined as having 4 or more symptoms that arise from tobacco use (eg, craving; withdrawal; tolerance; increasing use over time; social, occupational, or health consequences from nicotine use).

INTRODUCTION

This policy statement accompanies the clinical report and technical report on protecting children and adolescents from tobacco and nicotine.[1,2] It builds on, strengthens, and expands American Academy of Pediatrics (AAP) recommendations from the 2015 policy statement.[3] Although many evidence-based recommendations from the 2015 policy statement remain relevant, this revision expands on and adds policy recommendations on the basis of new evidence since the last summative

review. The approach to the evidence review and grading evidence quality are described in the accompanying technical report.[2] Policy recommendations were developed using the evidence-based approach as detailed by the AAP.[4,5] In addition to a "quality of evidence" summary,[2] a brief "strength of recommendation" summary is provided, using the "strong recommendation," "recommendation," "option," or "no recommendation" classification system.[4,5] For a summary of AAP clinical reports, policy statements, and other resources for tobacco and e-cigarettes, see Table 1.

PUBLIC POLICY RECOMMENDATIONS

1. The FDA Should Regulate all Tobacco and Nicotine Products to Protect Public Health

Strength of Recommendation: Strong

The FDA is charged with protecting consumers and enhancing public health by maximizing compliance of FDA-regulated products and minimizing risks associated with those products. The FDA Center for Tobacco Products is responsible for enforcing the Family Smoking Prevention and Tobacco Control Act, passed in 2009 in an effort to protect the public and create a healthier future for all Americans.[6] Tobacco products include, but are not limited to, e-cigarettes, cigarettes, cigars, smokeless tobacco, hookahs, pipe tobacco, and heated tobacco products. The Family Smoking Prevention and Tobacco Control Act put in place restrictions on marketing tobacco products to children and adolescents, and gave the FDA the authority to further regulate tobacco products to protect public health. Some of the agency's responsibilities under the law include establishing product standards, reviewing premarketing applications for new and modified-risk tobacco products, and requiring new warning labels for tobacco

products.[7] The FDA is required by law to conduct reviews of e-cigarettes and other new tobacco products to ensure that products are not marketed unless they are "appropriate for the protection of the public health."[6] The AAP and other public health organizations initiated a successful legal challenge to the long FDA delays in conducting these public health reviews for e-cigarettes. A resulting federal court order required the FDA to act in 2021. As of 2022, the FDA has authorized several tobacco-flavored e-cigarette products for marketing and has denied marketing authorization to thousands of flavored e-cigarette products. At the time of publication, the legal status of a market-leading product, JUUL, remains in limbo. However, the FDA has yet to render decisions on many market-leading products and has deferred action on a number of applications for menthol-flavored products. Products with pending applications remain on the market because the FDA has declined to take enforcement action against them during application review. The FDA must monitor postmarketing data from any authorized tobacco products to ensure that these products are not used by youth.

2. Tobacco Use Prevention, Screening, and Treatment Should be Adequately Funded and Specifically Designated for Pediatric Populations

Quality of Evidence: High

Strength of Recommendation: Strong

Tobacco use treatment should be available to all individuals who use tobacco products, including adolescents and, specifically, youth from communities that have historically experienced high levels of discrimination and stigma. The Centers for Disease Control and Prevention (CDC) Community Preventive Services Task Force evidence review found strong

TABLE 1 AAP Policy Statements and Other Resources for Tobacco and E-Cigarettes

Resources for Decreasing Tobacco Exposure at the Individual Practice Level	Evidence Base for Tobacco Control	E-Cigarette and Vaping Resources	Advocacy and Policy Resources
"Protecting Children and Adolescents From Tobacco and Nicotine" (AAP clinical report)	"Protecting Children and Adolescents From Tobacco and Nicotine" (AAP technical report)	"E-Cigarettes and Similar Devices" (AAP policy statement)	"Health Disparities in Tobacco Use and Exposure: A Structural Competency Approach" (AAP clinical report)
CEASE Resources (Massachusetts General Hospital Web site; www.massgeneral.org/children/cease-tobacco)		Vaping, JUUL, and E-Cigarettes Presentation Toolkit (Julius B. Richmond Center of Excellence; www.aap.org/en/patient-care/tobacco-control-and-prevention/e-cigarettes-and-vaping/vaping-juul-and-e-cigarettes-presentation-toolkit)	Tobacco Prevention Policy Tool (Julius B. Richmond Center of Excellence; www.aap.org/en/patient-care/tobacco-control-and-prevention/policy-and-advocacy/tobacco-prevention-policy-tool)
Pediatric Environmental Health (AAP policy manual)			
"Substance Use Screening, Brief Intervention, and Referral to Treatment" (AAP clinical report)			Tobacco Education Resources for Kids & Teens (HealthyChildren.org)
Tobacco Use: Considerations for Clinicians resource (www.aap.org/cessation)			

support for the effectiveness of comprehensive tobacco control prevention and treatment programs in reducing tobacco use and secondhand smoke (SHS) exposure, independent of increases in tobacco product prices or adoption of smoke-free policies.[8] These programs reduce the prevalence of tobacco use among adults and young people, reduce tobacco product consumption, increase quitting, and contribute to reductions in tobacco-related diseases and deaths. The CDC outlines optimal funding levels for these programs, as well as evidence that program effectiveness increases with adequate funding.[9] States do not fund these programs at anywhere near the level suggested by the CDC.[10] Further, despite receiving billions of dollars each year (estimated at approximately $27 billion in 2021) through tobacco settlement money and tobacco taxes, most states only use a small percentage of these funds to support tobacco prevention and treatment programs.[11] Rather than support efforts to reduce the enormous public health toll caused by tobacco use as promised in the 1998 Master

Settlement Agreement between 46 states and several US territories and major tobacco companies, these funds are often used for unrelated efforts, including balancing state budgets.

Given the important benefits to society of reducing tobacco use, cost should not be a barrier to receiving tobacco cessation services. The Affordable Care Act requires most private health plans to cover, without cost-sharing, tobacco cessation services.[12] The Departments of Health and Human Services, Labor, and the Treasury define adequate insurance coverage for cessation services as those which include, without cost-sharing or previous authorization, both counseling and medication for up to 2 quit attempts a year.[13] Although many Medicaid and Children's Health Insurance Program plans cover tobacco use treatment, they are not required to do so by law, so comprehensive coverage is not universal.[14] Further, many insurers do not cover tobacco treatment of people younger than 18. The AAP policy statement, "Improving Substance Use Prevention, Assessment, and

Treatment Financing to Enhance Equity and Improve Outcomes Among Children, Adolescents, and Young Adults," recommends appropriate insurance coverage and payment for provider time spent counseling and prescribing tobacco cessation services to facilitate greater availability of tobacco cessation treatment of all, including adolescents and young adults.[15]

3. Tobacco Control Research Should be Considered a High Priority and Funded Accordingly From Both Government and Private Sources

Quality of Evidence: High

Strength of Recommendation: Strong

Tobacco use remains one of the leading preventable causes of disease and death in the United States.[16] Use of any tobacco product by youth is unsafe, regardless of the form of use.[17] Tobacco use is a pediatric epidemic, because tobacco use disorder almost always starts in childhood or adolescence.[18] Tobacco control research funding should be specifically designated for clinical and policy interventions for pediatric populations, including those who are from communities that have historically experienced high levels of discrimination and stigma or have been traditionally underrepresented in research but highly impacted by tobacco use. Research is needed, in particular, to identify effective behavioral and/or pharmacotherapy interventions for tobacco cessation for youth[19] and pregnant persons.[20] Tobacco industry funding should not be used for this purpose. The tobacco industry has a long and well-documented history of using industry-funded programs to divert attention away from effective tobacco control programs and research, as well as misusing health care providers and academia to thwart attempts at tobacco control.[17]

4. Tobacco and Nicotine Product Prices Should be Increased to Reduce Child and Adolescent Tobacco use Initiation

Quality of Evidence: High

Strength of Recommendation: Strong

According to the 2014 Surgeon General's report, "the evidence is sufficient to conclude that increases in the prices of tobacco products, including those resulting from excise tax increases, prevent initiation of tobacco use, promote cessation, and reduce the prevalence and intensity of tobacco use among youth and adults."[17] As such, increasing the price of all tobacco products is one of the most effective methods to prevent or reduce tobacco use.[17] Youth are particularly sensitive to tobacco product price increases, with research suggesting that youth and young adults are 2 to 3 times as responsive to changes in price compared with adults.[17] Increasing excise taxes on tobacco products is especially effective in discouraging initiation among young people who have not developed tobacco use disorder, thus protecting their

health and increasing their likelihood of remaining tobacco-free.[21] Increasing the tobacco tax has the benefit of both raising the price and providing a source of funds that can be used for tobacco control programs, helping states capture health care–related cost savings from reductions in associated financial costs from death and disease because of tobacco use.[9] As of January 2023, e-cigarettes are not currently taxed at the federal level and other types of tobacco products are taxed at different levels. Taxes should be instituted for e-cigarettes and all tobacco products should be taxed at comparable levels to prevent substitution.

5. Enforce the Tobacco Product Sales Age of 21 Years

Quality of Evidence: High

Strength of Recommendation: Strong

In December 2019, Congress passed a federal law to raise the sales age for all tobacco products to 21 years.[22] The new federal minimum age of sale applies to all retail establishments and persons, with no exceptions. The law penalizes retailers for selling tobacco products to youth. The law does not penalize youth who purchase, possess, or use tobacco products. The law was the culmination of research identifying these laws as effective with high levels of public support. A 2015 Institute of Medicine report summarized the evidence of effectiveness and provided evidence from two different simulation models that increasing the minimum age to 21 years would lead to a 12% reduction in smoking prevalence.[23] Survey data identified that the vast majority of Americans supported the adoption of a federal "Tobacco 21" law, with support extending across sociodemographic groups, including age, gender, race,

ethnicity, and socioeconomic status, as well as political affiliation and smoking status.[24]

Enforcement activities are important for age-of-purchase laws to be effective. A Cochrane review on interventions for preventing tobacco sales to minors found that active enforcement, including media coverage of that enforcement, was much more effective than educational programs alone.[25] A 2011 review found that enforcement programs that disrupted the sale of tobacco to minors reduced smoking among youth, whereas merely enacting a law without sufficient enforcement had minimal, if any, impact on youth tobacco use.[26]

6. All Flavor Ingredients, Including Menthol, Should be Prohibited in all Tobacco and Nicotine Products

Quality of Evidence: High

Strength of Recommendation: Strong

Across a range of tobacco products, flavorings are one of the main reasons that youth initiate tobacco use. More than 80% of adolescents and young adults who have tried tobacco report that their first product was flavored.[27] When asked why they use tobacco, young people consistently say it is because they like the flavors.[28] E-cigarette solutions are often flavored, with thousands of unique flavors advertised.[29] The 2016 Surgeon General's report on e-cigarettes concluded that flavors are among the most commonly cited reasons for using e-cigarettes among youth and young adults.[30] In 2021, flavored e-liquids were used by 84.7% of youth who reported current e-cigarette use.[31] Cigars and little cigars are also flavored, and it has been hypothesized that the flavors in these products mask the harshness of the cigar smoke, making the smoking experience more tolerable and enjoyable for young people.

Flavorings (other than menthol) have been banned in conventional cigarettes since the Family Smoking Prevention and Tobacco Control Act of 2009 because flavorings encourage cigarette experimentation and regular use, which can lead to tobacco use disorder.[18,32,33] The cigarette flavor ban appears to be working, as it has been associated with a 58% decrease in the number of cigarettes smoked among youth and a 17% decrease in the likelihood of smoking cigarettes overall in this age group.[33] However, these effects are likely diminished by the continued availability of menthol cigarettes and other flavored tobacco and nicotine products. Small cigars, e-cigarettes, and similar devices often contain flavors but are not subject to the same regulations as cigarettes. To fully protect youth from the harms of tobacco, it is necessary to prohibit all flavor ingredients, including menthol, in all tobacco and nicotine products. Emerging evidence suggests that focusing on "characterizing" flavors rather than any flavor ingredient creates potential policy loopholes that are exploited by tobacco companies to circumvent tobacco flavor bans.[34] Tobacco companies have historically used flavored products to target youth and, in particular, youth from communities that have experienced high levels of discrimination and stigma; for example, the targeting of Black communities with menthol cigarette advertising and promotions.[18,35] Thus, prohibiting all flavors in all tobacco and nicotine products is a policy approach that promotes social justice and racial equity, in support of the AAP Equity Agenda.

7. Comprehensive Tobacco-Free Laws that Prohibit use of all Tobacco and Nicotine Products (Including Cigarettes, E-Cigarettes, and Similar Devices) Should be Enacted in all Places Where Children and Adolescents Live, Learn, Play, Work, and Visit

Quality of Evidence: High

Strength of Recommendation: Strong

Enhanced and equitable implementation of comprehensive smoke-free laws and policies for indoor public places, workplaces, cars, and multiunit housing can dramatically reduce SHS exposure. The 2006 Surgeon General's report concluded that smoking bans in workplaces, hospitals, restaurants, bars, and offices substantially reduce SHS exposure. Further, the report highlighted that "evidence from multiple peer-reviewed studies shows that smoke-free policies and regulations do not have an adverse economic impact on the hospitality industry."[36] The 2020 Surgeon General's report on smoking cessation also found that there is sufficient evidence "to infer that smoke-free policies reduce smoking prevalence, reduce cigarette consumption, and increase smoking cessation."[37]

Smoke-free laws are associated with improved child health outcomes. For example, implementation of smoke-free laws in England, Canada, and Scotland was associated with decreases in childhood asthma hospitalizations.[38,39] Similar laws in Kentucky were associated with decreased emergency department visits for asthma.[40] Implementation of smoke-free laws in Belgium, Scotland, and England have been associated with decreased rates of preterm births.[41,42] A study in England also found a significantly decreased risk of infants being of low birth weight and small for gestational age after

implementation of smoke-free legislation.[43]

Smoke-free policies for cars can also reduce SHS exposure and should be promoted in an equitable manner. Studies of tobacco smoking in automobiles found that a significant amount of tobacco smoke remains in the vehicle, even with the windows open.[44] Studies have found that nonsmoking passengers have substantially elevated levels of cotinine (a nicotine metabolite and measure of nicotine exposure), other tobacco-related toxicants, and carcinogens after sitting in a parked car with an open window while a person smoked 3 cigarettes over 1 hour.[45,46] A 2021 systematic review and meta-analysis found smoke-free car policies were associated with reductions in reported child tobacco smoke exposure in cars (risk ratio, 0.69; 95% confidence interval [CI], 0.55–0.87; $n = 161\,466$ participants in 4 studies).[47]

Multi-unit housing represents another potential source of SHS exposure for a large portion of US children and adults. Smoking in one unit involuntarily exposes those in nearby units.[48–50] Among multiunit housing residents, surveys suggest a majority of respondents support smoking bans in common areas and within individual units, with increased support among individuals who reside with children.[51,52] In 2016, the US Department of Housing and Urban Development announced regulations to require public housing agencies across the country to implement smoke-free policies.[53] Evaluation of the effectiveness of this regulation is ongoing.[54,55] Smoke-free policies for homes should be promoted in an equitable manner.

Evidence also supports the inclusion of e-cigarettes and similar devices in comprehensive smoke-free laws and policies.

E-cigarette aerosol contains known harmful toxicants and carcinogens that can be discharged directly into the surrounding environment and deposited on surface areas.[30,56] Bystanders are exposed to this secondhand and thirdhand aerosol in a manner similar to that of secondhand and thirdhand cigarette smoke. Lessons learned from existing smoke-free policies, which include combustible cigarettes, along with available e-cigarette research, supports the inclusion of e-cigarettes into tobacco-free laws and ordinances where children and adolescents live, learn, play, work, and visit.[29]

8. All Tobacco and Nicotine Product Advertising and Promotion in Forms That Are Accessible to Children and Adolescents Should be Prohibited

Quality of Evidence: Moderate

Strength of Recommendation: Strong

The 2012 Surgeon General's report concluded, "Advertising and promotional activities by tobacco companies have been shown to cause the onset and continuation of smoking among adolescents and young adults."[18,30] Further, the report concluded that "evidence is suggestive but not sufficient, to conclude that tobacco companies have changed the packaging and design of their products in ways that have increased these products' appeal to adolescents and young adults."[18] Studies also suggest exposure to e-cigarette advertising on social media sites is associated with e-cigarette use among adolescents[57,58] and young adults.[59] Recently, e-cigarette and other tobacco product advertisements have increased dramatically on social media platforms.[60,61] Exposure to TV advertisements is associated with increased intentions to use e-cigarettes,[62] and exposure to a range of advertisement modalities (including Internet, print, retail, and TV/movies) is associated with current e-cigarette use,[63] with increasing

exposure being associated with increased odds of use.[64,65] Therefore, reducing exposure to pro-tobacco advertising is an important component of comprehensive tobacco control strategies to prevent tobacco and nicotine initiation among youth.[18] For example, social media companies should create policies to limit children's exposure to tobacco content online, including prohibiting tobacco/e-cigarette companies from advertising on their platforms to children younger than 21 years.

9. Point-of-Sale Tobacco and Nicotine Product Advertising and Product Placement That Can be Viewed by Children and Adolescents Should be Prohibited

Quality of Evidence: Moderate

Strength of Recommendation: Strong

Point-of-sale (POS) advertising increases tobacco initiation and tobacco product use among youth. POS advertising refers to a variety of marketing and promotion activities, including signs on the interior and exterior of retail stores, functional items like counter mats and change cups, shelving displays, and coupons and other price discounts that reduce the price for the consumer. It also includes promotional payments to retailers by tobacco companies to have their products placed in specific store locations, making it more likely that consumers will see them.[66] Tobacco companies spend the vast majority of their total marketing expenditures on price-related strategies at the POS.[67] Evidence suggests POS display bans reduce youth smoking susceptibility and denormalize smoking.[68-70] According to a 2016 meta-analysis, the odds of having tried smoking are around 1.6 times higher for children and youth who are frequently exposed to POS tobacco promotion, compared with those who are less frequently exposed.[71] A virtual store experiment found that youth 13 to

17 years of age were substantially less likely to try purchasing tobacco products when tobacco products were not displayed (odds ratio, 0.30; 95% CI, 0.13–0.67).[35,72]

E-cigarette companies, the vast majority of which are owned by tobacco companies, use a wide variety of product placement strategies. The AAP policy statement "E-Cigarettes and Similar Devices" outlined e-cigarette POS advertising at various retail outlets, as well as the ability for youth to purchase these products through online vendors.[29]

E-cigarette advertisements are also placed within music, entertainment, and sport venues, and on social media and streaming media.[73] Additionally, e-cigarettes have been marketed through celebrity endorsements and sponsorships and free samples at youth-oriented events.[74] These product placement strategies are illegal for conventional cigarettes, because they promote youth initiation and progression to traditional tobacco product use.[18,30]

Venues for unsupervised purchase of tobacco and nicotine products, such as vending machines and online merchants, should be eliminated. All tobacco and nicotine products should be placed behind sales counters to reduce shoplifting. Sales of tobacco and nicotine products should be eliminated from schools, health care facilities, military bases, pharmacies, and other sites that serve youth. The promotional distribution of tobacco and nicotine products should be prohibited.

10. Depictions of Tobacco and Nicotine Products in Movies and Other Media, such as Content Through Streaming Platforms, That Can be viewed by Children and Adolescents Should be Restricted

Quality of Evidence: High

Strength of Recommendation: Strong

Depictions of smoking in movies have been repeatedly shown to increase rates of smoking initiation among adolescents both in the United States and globally. The 2012 Surgeon General's report concluded, "The evidence is sufficient to conclude that there is a causal relationship between depictions of smoking in the movies and the initiation of smoking among young people."[18] Numerous prospective studies of adolescents across the world have shown that exposure to depictions of smoking in movies is associated with smoking initiation.[75-77] One estimate suggests that reducing adolescent exposure to smoking depictions in movies from a current median of about 275 annual exposures per adolescent from PG-13 movies down to approximately 10 or less would reduce the prevalence of adolescent smoking by 18% (95% CI, 14%–21%).[78] According to the 2014 Surgeon General's report, "actions that would eliminate depiction of tobacco use in movies that are produced and rated as appropriate for children and adolescents could have a significant effect toward preventing youth from becoming tobacco users."[17] With the rise of depictions of e-cigarettes in movies and episodic programs (defined as programs aired as a series on streaming platforms or broadcast or cable TV) and preliminary evidence suggesting a dose-response relationship between depictions and e-cigarette initiation among youth,[79] it is reasonable to have these recommendations apply to all depictions of tobacco and nicotine products.

11. Tobacco Industry-Sponsored Mass Media and School-Based Tobacco Control Programs Should be Prohibited

Quality of Evidence: High

Strength of Recommendation: Strong

Mass media and school-based tobacco control programs are often funded by federal, state, and nonprofit entities. These programs have been shown to reduce the initiation of tobacco use and increase cessation by denormalizing

tobacco and nicotine product use.[9,18,80] Tobacco industry-sponsored programs do not use the same strategies, are not effective in preventing tobacco use among youth, and are counterproductive, potentially undermining effective tobacco control efforts.[18] This recommendation remains relevant with the recent efforts by JUUL Laboratories to target school-aged children with youth prevention programs. A 2018 study found that the JUUL curriculum was not evidence-based and failed to adequately address the harms of e-cigarettes, youth susceptibility to the addictive nature of nicotine, or the role that targeted tobacco industry marketing plays in youth use of e-cigarettes.[81]

12. Child and Adolescent Tobacco Control Programs Should Incorporate Antitobacco Themes of Health Effects and Industry Manipulation

Quality of Evidence: Moderate

Strength of Recommendation: Strong

Mass-reach health communication interventions can be powerful tools for preventing the initiation of tobacco use, promoting and facilitating cessation, and shaping social norms related to tobacco use.[9] The Community Preventive Services Task Force recommends mass-reach health communication interventions based on strong evidence of effectiveness in decreasing the prevalence and initiation of tobacco use among young people and increasing cessation and use of available services such as quitlines.[8] According to a 2017 Cochrane review of mass media campaigns directed at youth, there is some evidence that certain types of media campaigns can be effective in preventing the uptake of smoking in young people.[82] Adolescents and young adults are very sensitive to perceived social norms and media presentations of smoking behavior. Campaigns, such as those organized by the Truth Initiative, which focus on raising awareness of tobacco

companies' targeting and manipulating of youth, has been estimated to help significant portions of youth reject tobacco, including more than 450 000 adolescents in one 4-year span.[83,84] The Florida Tobacco Pilot Program, the major component of which was a youth-oriented, counter-marketing media campaign developed to reduce the allure of smoking, was associated with a significant decline (approximately 2% to 3%) in smoking among middle and high school students.[85]

Pictorial health warnings improve adolescents' awareness of the harms of smoking and decrease their perceptions of the social appeal of smoking.[86,87] According to the 2020 Surgeon General's report on smoking cessation, "The evidence is sufficient to infer that large, pictorial (also known as graphic) health warnings increase smokers' knowledge about the health harms of smoking, interest in quitting, and quit attempts, and decrease smoking prevalence."[37]

13. Children and Adolescents Should be Legally Prohibited From Working on Tobacco Farms and in Tobacco Production

Quality of Evidence: Moderate

Strength of Recommendation: Strong

Children and adolescents can be harmed from absorption of tobacco toxins when they participate in tobacco production.[88,89] Green tobacco sickness, or nicotine poisoning that occurs while handling tobacco plants, is well described. Dermal absorption of nicotine from moist tobacco plants can lead to symptoms of severe nicotine poisoning, including weakness, headache, nausea, vomiting, dizziness, abdominal cramps, breathing difficulty, pallor, diarrhea, chills, fluctuations in blood pressure or heart rate, seizures, and increased perspiration and excessive salivation.[89-91]

14. Any Tobacco or Nicotine Products Legally sold to Adults Aged 21 Years and Above, Including E-Cigarettes, Cigarettes, and Other Tobacco Products, Should Meet a Product Standard That Makes the Product Both Minimally Addictive for Adults and Highly Unlikely to Promote Initiation and Continued use Among Children and Adolescents

Quality of Evidence: Low

Strength of Recommendation: Recommendation

Reducing nicotine content in cigarettes has been suggested as a potential strategy to make them less addictive[92] or less reinforcing (eg, at a dose least likely to increase or maintain nicotine self-administration behaviors).[93] This strategy has been linked to cigarette smoking reduction and cessation in adults, both of which can substantially reduce tobacco-related morbidity and mortality.[94] For example, studies have shown that, when adults switch from cigarettes with regular nicotine content to cigarettes with very low nicotine content (≤ 0.4 mg/g), they experience reductions in biomarkers of nicotine exposure, cigarettes smoked/day, and symptoms of tobacco use disorder.[95,96] No clinical studies have assessed how nicotine reduction affects adolescents' experiences with cigarette smoking or intentions to smoke; however, preclinical studies have shown that adolescent rats are more sensitive to lower doses of nicotine than adults.[95] In 2018, the FDA announced its intent to develop a tobacco product standard to set the maximum nicotine level for cigarettes.[97] At the time of this publication, however, the FDA has not put forth specific regulations.

The United Kingdom and Europe have adopted nicotine limits for nicotine-containing e-liquids at 20 mg/mL.[98] With the emergence of e-cigarettes, some have argued that enough nicotine needs to be available in these noncombusted products to facilitate adults' transition from combusted to noncombusted forms of nicotine and mitigate the emergence of an illicit market of tobacco products with high nicotine content. In the United States, e-cigarettes have evolved over the past decade to have high levels of nicotine content, as well as salt-based nicotine solutions, which are more palatable than the free-based nicotine used in earlier generations of e-cigarettes.[99] These features are marketed to assist with the transition from cigarette smoking to noncombusted tobacco products; however, data show that these features may sustain long-term e-cigarette use among adults (rather than cessation) and also appeal to adolescents who do not smoke cigarettes.[95] To best minimize health harms to children when formulating a comprehensive regulatory framework for the nicotine content of cigarettes in the United States, policymakers must also create a standard that minimizes long-term use of e-cigarettes and other tobacco products by adults (which adversely impacts children through the mechanisms listed above), as well as initiation of nicotine and maintenance of tobacco use among youth.

15. Tobacco Control Research and Advocacy Priorities Should be Grounded in "Tobacco Endgame" Strategies, a Framework to Prevent new Addiction and End the Tobacco Epidemic

Quality of Evidence: Low

Strength of Recommendation: Recommendation

The "tobacco endgame" reorients tobacco policy and guidelines toward plans for ending the tobacco epidemic and envisions a tobacco-free future. A variety of policy approaches have been outlined, including product-focused, user-focused, market-supply focused, and institutional structure-focused proposals.[100] The tobacco endgame has been discussed by the CDC and the Surgeon General.[37] In 2021, California formally adopted an endgame policy initiative, with a commitment toward ending the commercial tobacco epidemic in the state by 2035.[101] The National Institutes of Health and the FDA, as well as the whole of government, should endorse and support tobacco endgame goals, and tobacco control researchers should consistently recognize and frame our research findings in alignment with endgame policies to prevent new addiction and to end the tobacco epidemic. Finally, considering how tobacco use disproportionately affects youth from communities that have historically experienced high levels of discrimination and stigma, endgame strategies should incorporate policies targeted at reducing these disparities; for example, through special outreach to these populations.

CONCLUSIONS

Tobacco use almost always starts in childhood or adolescence. The tobacco epidemic takes a substantial toll on the health of all pediatric populations. Public policy actions to protect infants, children, adolescents, and young adults from tobacco have proven effective in reducing harm. Effective public health approaches need to be both extended to include e-cigarettes, similar devices, and other and emerging tobacco and nicotine products, and expanded to reduce the toll that the tobacco epidemic takes on our children.

For further reading and a summary of AAP clinical reports, policy statements, and other resources for tobacco and e-cigarettes, see Table 1.

LEAD AUTHORS

Brian P. Jenssen, MD, FAAP
Susan C. Walley, MD, FAAP
Rachel Boykan, MD, FAAP
Alice Little Caldwell, MD, FAAP
Deepa Camenga, MD, FAAP

ABBREVIATIONS

AAP: American Academy of Pediatrics
CDC: Centers for Disease Control and Prevention
CI: confidence interval
FDA: US Food and Drug Administration
POS: point of sale
SHS: secondhand smoke

Address correspondence to Brian P. Jenssen, MD, FAAP. E-mail: JenssenB@chop.edu

PEDIATRICS (ISSN Numbers: Print, 0031-4005; Online, 1098-4275).

REFERENCES

1. Jenssen BP, Walley SC, Boykan R, Little Caldwell A, Camenga D. American Academy of Pediatrics, Section on Nicotine and Tobacco Prevention and Treatment, Committee on Substance Use Prevention. Clinical report. Protecting children and adolescents from tobacco and nicotine. *Pediatrics*. 2023;151(5): e2023061805

2. Jenssen BP, Walley SC, Boykan R, Little Caldwell A, Camenga D. American Academy of Pediatrics, Section on Nicotine and Tobacco Prevention and Treatment, Committee on Substance Use Prevention. Technical report. Protecting children and adolescents from tobacco and nicotine. *Pediatrics*. 2023;151(5): e2023061806

3. Farber HJ, Nelson KE, Groner JA, Walley SC. Section on Tobacco Control. Public policy to protect children from tobacco, nicotine, and tobacco smoke. *Pediatrics*. 2015;136(5):998–1007

4. American Academy of Pediatrics Steering Committee on Quality Improvement and Management.

Classifying recommendations for clinical practice guidelines. *Pediatrics*. 2004;114(3):874–877

5. Shiffman RN, Marcuse EK, Moyer VA, et al. American Academy of Pediatrics Steering Committee on Quality Improvement and Management. Toward transparent clinical policies. *Pediatrics*. 2008;121(3):643–646

6. U.S. Government Publishing Office. Family smoking prevention and tobacco control and federal retirement reform. Available at: https://www.govinfo.gov/content/pkg/PLAW-111publ31/pdf/PLAW-111publ31.pdf. Accessed February 2, 2023

7. US Food and Drug Administration. Center for Tobacco Products. Available at: https://www.fda.gov/about-fda/fda-organization/center-tobacco-products. Accessed February 2, 2023

8. Community Preventive Services Task Force. The guide to community preventive services. Reducing tobacco use and secondhand smoke exposure: comprehensive tobacco control programs. Task force finding and rationale statement. Available at: https://www.

thecommunityguide.org/findings/tobacco-use-comprehensive-tobacco-control-programs.html. Accessed February 2, 2023

9. Centers for Disease Control and Prevention. Smoking and tobacco use. Best practices for comprehensive tobacco control programs–2014. Available at: https://www.cdc.gov/tobacco/stateandcommunity/guides/pdfs/2014/comprehensive.pdf. Accessed February 2, 2023

10. American Lung Association. State of tobacco control 2023. Available at: https://www.lung.org/research/sotc. Accessed February 2, 2023

11. Campaign for Tobacco-Free Kids. Broken promises to our children. A state-by-state look at the 1998 tobacco settlement 23 years later. Available at: https://www.tobaccofreekids.org/what-we-do/us/statereport/. Accessed February 2, 2023

12. Krist AH, Davidson KW, Mangione CM, et al. US Preventive Services Task Force. Interventions for tobacco smoking cessation in adults, including

pregnant persons: US Preventive Services Task Force recommendation statement. *JAMA.* 2021;325(3):265–279

13. McAfee T, Babb S, McNabb S, Fiore MC. Helping smokers quit–opportunities created by the Affordable Care Act. *N Engl J Med.* 2015;372(1):5–7

14. DiGiulio A, Jump Z, Babb S, et al. State Medicaid coverage for tobacco cessation treatments and barriers to accessing treatments–United States, 2008–2018. *MMWR Morb Mortal Wkly Rep.* 2020;69(6):155–160

15. Camenga DR, Hammer LD. Committee on Substance Use and Prevention, and Committee on Child Health Financing. Improving substance use prevention, assessment, and treatment financing to enhance equity and improve outcomes among children, adolescents, and young adults. *Pediatrics.* 2022;150(1):e2022057992

16. Mokdad AH, Ballestros K, Echko M, et al. US Burden of Disease Collaborators. The state of US health, 1990–2016: burden of diseases, injuries, and risk factors among US states. *JAMA.* 2018;319(14):1444–1472

17. US Department of Health and Human Services; Centers for Disease Control and Prevention; National Center for Chronic Disease Prevention and Health Promotion; Office on Smoking and Health. The health consequences of smoking–50 years of progress: a report of the surgeon general, 2014. Available at: https://www.ncbi.nlm.nih.gov/books/NBK179276/. Accessed February 2, 2023

18. US Department of Health and Human Services; Centers for Disease Control and Prevention, Office on Smoking and Health. Preventing tobacco use among youth and young adults: a report of the surgeon general. Atlanta, GA: Centers for Disease Control and Prevention; 2012

19. Selph S, Patnode C, Bailey SR, Pappas M, Stoner R, Chou R. Primary care-relevant interventions for tobacco and nicotine use prevention and cessation in children and adolescents: updated evidence report and systematic review for the US Preventive Services Task Force. *JAMA.* 2020;323(16):1599–1608

20. Patnode CD, Henderson JT, Coppola EL, Melnikow J, Durbin S, Thomas RG. Interventions for tobacco cessation in adults, including pregnant persons: updated evidence report and systematic review for the US Preventive Services Task Force. *JAMA.* 2021;325(3):280–298

21. Centers for Disease Control and Prevention. STATE system excise tax fact sheet. Available at: https://www.cdc.gov/statesystem/factsheets/excisetax/ExciseTax.html. Accessed February 2, 2023

22. US Food and Drug Administration. Tobacco 21. Available at: https://www.fda.gov/tobacco-products/retail-sales-tobacco-products/tobacco-21. Accessed February 2, 2023

23. Institute of Medicine. *Public Health Implications of Raising the Minimum Age of Legal Access to Tobacco Products.* Washington, DC: National Academies Press; 2015

24. Morain SR, Winickoff JP, Mello MM. Have tobacco 21 laws come of age? *N Engl J Med.* 2016;374(17):1601–1604

25. Stead LF, Lancaster T. Interventions for preventing tobacco sales to minors. *Cochrane Database Syst Rev.* 2005;(1): CD001497

26. DiFranza JR. Which interventions against the sale of tobacco to minors can be expected to reduce smoking? *Tob Control.* 2012;21(4):436–442

27. Villanti AC, Johnson AL, Ambrose BK, et al. Flavored tobacco product use in youth and adults: findings from the first wave of the PATH Study (2013–2014). *Am J Prev Med.* 2017; 53(2):139–151

28. Ambrose BK, Day HR, Rostron B, et al. Flavored tobacco product use among US Youth aged 12–17 years, 2013–2014. *JAMA.* 2015;314(17):1871–1873

29. Jenssen BP, Walley SC. Section on Tobacco Control. E-cigarettes and similar devices. *Pediatrics.* 2019;143(2): e20183652

30. US Department of Health and Human Services. *E-Cigarette Use Among Youth and Young Adults. A Report of the Surgeon General.* Atlanta, GA: US Department of Health and Human Services, Centers for Disease Control and Prevention, National Center for Chronic Disease Prevention and Health Promotion, Office on Smoking and Health; 2016

31. Park-Lee E, Ren C, Sawdey MD, et al. Notes from the field: e-cigarette use among middle and high school students–National Youth Tobacco Survey, United States, 2021. *MMWR Morb Mortal Wkly Rep.* 2021;70(39):1387–1389

32. Deyton L, Sharfstein J, Hamburg M. Tobacco product regulation–a public health approach. *N Engl J Med.* 2010;362(19):1753–1756

33. Courtemanche CJ, Palmer MK, Pesko MF. Influence of the flavored cigarette ban on adolescent tobacco use. *Am J Prev Med.* 2017;52(5):e139–e146

34. Brink AL, Glahn AS, Kjaer NT. Tobacco companies' exploitation of loopholes in the EU ban on menthol cigarettes: a case study from Denmark [Published online ahead of print March 21, 2022]. *Tob Control.* 2022. 10.1136/tobaccocontrol-2021-057213

35. Dauphinee AL, Doxey JR, Schleicher NC, Fortmann SP, Henriksen L. Racial differences in cigarette brand recognition and impact on youth smoking. *BMC Public Health.* 2013;13:170

36. Centers for Disease Control and Prevention, Office on Smoking and Health. The health consequences of involuntary exposure to tobacco smoke: a report of the surgeon general. Available at: www.ncbi.nlm.nih.gov/books/NBK44324/. Accessed February 2, 2023

37. US Department of Health and Human Services. *Smoking Cessation: A Report of the Surgeon General.* Atlanta, GA: US Department of Health and Human Services, Centers for Disease Control and Prevention, National Center for Chronic Disease Prevention and Health Promotion, Office on Smoking and Health; 2020

38. Mackay D, Haw S, Ayres JG, Fischbacher C, Pell JP. Smoke-free legislation and hospitalizations for childhood asthma. *N Engl J Med.* 2010;363(12): 1139–1145

39. Naiman A, Glazier RH, Moineddin R. Association of anti-smoking legislation with rates of hospital admission for cardiovascular and respiratory conditions. *CMAJ.* 2010;182(8):761–767

40. Rayens MK, Burkhart PV, Zhang M, et al. Reduction in asthma-related emergency department visits after implementation of a smoke-free law.

J Allergy Clin Immunol. 2008;122(3): 537–41.e3

41. Cox B, Martens E, Nemery B, Vangronsveld J, Nawrot TS. Impact of a stepwise introduction of smoke-free legislation on the rate of preterm births: analysis of routinely collected birth data. *BMJ.* 2013; 346:f441

42. Mackay DF, Nelson SM, Haw SJ, Pell JP. Impact of Scotland's smoke-free legislation on pregnancy complications: retrospective cohort study. *PLoS Med.* 2012;9(3):e1001175

43. Bakolis I, Kelly R, Fecht D, et al. Protective effects of smoke-free legislation on birth outcomes in England: a regression discontinuity design. *Epidemiology.* 2016;27(6):810–818

44. Ott W, Klepeis N, Switzer P. Air change rates of motor vehicles and in-vehicle pollutant concentrations from secondhand smoke. *J Expo Sci Environ Epidemiol.* 2008;18(3):312–325

45. St Helen G, Jacob P III, Peng M, Dempsey DA, Hammond SK, Benowitz NL. Intake of toxic and carcinogenic volatile organic compounds from secondhand smoke in motor vehicles. *Cancer Epidemiol Biomarkers Prev.* 2014;23(12): 2774–2782

46. Jones IA, St Helen G, Meyers MJ, et al. Biomarkers of secondhand smoke exposure in automobiles. *Tob Control.* 2014;23(1):51–57

47. Radó MK, Mölenberg FJM, Westenberg LEH, et al. Effect of smoke-free policies in outdoor areas and private places on children's tobacco smoke exposure and respiratory health: a systematic review and meta-analysis. *Lancet Public Health.* 2021;6(8):e566–e578

48. Hewett MJ, Ortland WH, Brock BE, Heim CJ. Secondhand smoke and smokefree policies in owner-occupied multi-unit housing. *Am J Prev Med.* 2012;43(5 Suppl 3):S187–S196

49. Kraev TA, Adamkiewicz G, Hammond SK, Spengler JD. Indoor concentrations of nicotine in low-income, multi-unit housing: associations with smoking behaviors and housing characteristics. *Tob Control.* 2009;18(6):438–444

50. Wilson KM, Klein JD, Blumkin AK, Gottlieb M, Winickoff JP. Tobacco-smoke exposure in children who live in

multiunit housing. *Pediatrics.* 2011;127(1):85–92

51. King BA, Cummings KM, Mahoney MC, Juster HR, Hyland AJ. Multiunit housing residents' experiences and attitudes toward smoke-free policies. *Nicotine Tob Res.* 2010;12(6):598–605

52. Hood NE, Ferketich AK, Klein EG, Wewers ME, Pirie P. Individual, social, and environmental factors associated with support for smoke-free housing policies among subsidized multiunit housing tenants. *Nicotine Tob Res.* 2013;15(6):1075–1083

53. US Department of Housing and Urban Development. HUD Secretary Castro announces new rule making public housing smoke-free. Available at: https://archives.hud.gov/news/2016/pr16-184.cfm. Accessed February 2, 2023

54. Anastasiou E, Feinberg A, Tovar A, et al. Secondhand smoke exposure in public and private high-rise multiunit housing serving low-income residents in New York City prior to federal smoking ban in public housing, 2018. *Sci Total Environ.* 2020;704:135322

55. Thorpe LE, Anastasiou E, Wyka K, et al. Evaluation of secondhand smoke exposure in New York City public housing after implementation of the 2018 Federal Smoke-Free Housing Policy. *JAMA Netw Open.* 2020;3(11):e2024385

56. *National Academies of Sciences, Engineering, and Medicine. Public Health Consequences of E-Cigarettes.* Washington, DC: National Academies Press; 2018

57. Camenga D, Gutierrez KM, Kong G, Cavallo D, Simon P, Krishnan-Sarin S. E-cigarette advertising exposure in e-cigarette naïve adolescents and subsequent e-cigarette use: a longitudinal cohort study. *Addict Behav.* 2018;81: 78–83

58. Vogel EA, Ramo DE, Rubinstein ML, et al. Effects of social media on adolescents' willingness and intention to use e-cigarettes: an experimental investigation. *Nicotine Tob Res.* 2021;23(4): 694–701

59. Pokhrel P, Fagan P, Herzog TA, et al. Social media e-cigarette exposure and e-cigarette expectancies and use

among young adults. *Addict Behav.* 2018;78:51–58

60. Czaplicki L, Kostygina G, Kim Y, et al. Characterizing JUUL-related posts on Instagram. *Tob Control.* 2020;29(6): 612–617

61. O'Brien EK, Hoffman L, Navarro MA, Ganz O. Social media use by leading US e-cigarette, cigarette, smokeless tobacco, cigar, and hookah brands. *Tob Control.* 2020;29(e1):e87–e97

62. Farrelly MC, Duke JC, Crankshaw EC, et al. A randomized trial of the effect of e-cigarette TV advertisements on intentions to use e-cigarettes. *Am J Prev Med.* 2015;49(5):686–693

63. Hammig B, Daniel-Dobbs P, Blunt-Vinti H. Electronic cigarette initiation among minority youth in the United States. *Am J Drug Alcohol Abuse.* 2017;43(3): 306–310

64. Singh T, Agaku IT, Arrazola RA, et al. Exposure to advertisements and electronic cigarette use among us middle and high school students. *Pediatrics.* 2016;137(5):e20154155

65. Mantey DS, Cooper MR, Clendennen SL, Pasch KE, Perry CL. E-cigarette marketing exposure is associated with e-cigarette use among us youth. *J Adolesc Health.* 2016;58(6):686–690

66. Campaign for Tobacco-Free Kids. Fact sheets. Available at: https://www.tobaccofreekids.org/fact-sheets/tobaccos-toll-health-harms-and-cost/tobacco-and-kids-marketing. Accessed February 2, 2023

67. US Federal Trade Commission. Federal Trade Commission cigarette report for 2019. Available at: https://www.ftc.gov/system/files/documents/reports/federal-trade-commission-cigarette-report-2019-smokeless-tobacco-report-2019/cigarette_report_for_2019.pdf. Accessed February 2, 2023

68. Dunlop S, Kite J, Grunseit AC, et al. Out of sight and out of mind? Evaluating the impact of point-of-sale tobacco display bans on smoking-related beliefs and behaviors in a sample of Australian adolescents and young adults. *Nicotine Tob Res.* 2015;17(7): 761–768

69. McNeill A, Lewis S, Quinn C, et al. Evaluation of the removal of point-of-sale

tobacco displays in Ireland. *Tob Control.* 2011;20(2):137–143

70. Ford A, MacKintosh AM, Moodie C, Kuipers MAG, Hastings GB, Bauld L. Impact of a ban on the open display of tobacco products in retail outlets on never smoking youth in the UK: findings from a repeat cross-sectional survey before, during, and after implementation. *Tob Control.* 2020; 29(3):282–288

71. Robertson L, Cameron C, McGee R, Marsh L, Hoek J. Point-of-sale tobacco promotion and youth smoking: a meta-analysis. *Tob Control.* 2016;25(e2): e83–e89

72. Kim AE, Nonnemaker JM, Loomis BR, et al. Influence of tobacco displays and ads on youth: a virtual store experiment. *Pediatrics.* 2013;131(1):e88–e95

73. McCausland K, Maycock B, Leaver T, Jancey J. The messages presented in electronic cigarette–related social media promotions and discussion: scoping review. *J Med Internet Res.* 2019;21(2):e11953

74. Truth Initiative. E-cigarettes industry marketing and youth targeting. Available at: https://truthinitiative.org/sites/default/files/media/files/2021/06/Truth_E-Cigarette%20Factsheet_MARKETING_FINAL.pdf. Accessed February 2, 2023

75. Tanski SE, Stoolmiller M, Dal Cin S, Worth K, Gibson J, Sargent JD. Movie character smoking and adolescent smoking: who matters more, good guys or bad guys? *Pediatrics.* 2009;124(1):135–143

76. Morgenstern M, Sargent JD, Engels RCME, et al. Smoking in movies and adolescent smoking initiation: longitudinal study in six European countries. *Am J Prev Med.* 2013;44(4):339–344

77. Arora M, Mathur N, Gupta VK, Nazar GP, Reddy KS, Sargent JD. Tobacco use in Bollywood movies, tobacco promotional activities and their association with tobacco use among Indian adolescents. *Tob Control.* 2012;21(5):482–487

78. Sargent JD, Tanski S, Stoolmiller M. Influence of motion picture rating on adolescent response to movie smoking. *Pediatrics.* 2012;130(2):228–236

79. Bennett M, Hair EC, Liu M, Pitzer L, Rath JM, Vallone DM. Exposure to tobacco content in episodic programs and tobacco and E-cigarette initiation. *Prev Med.* 2020;139:106169

80. Stevens EM, Hébert ET, Keller-Hamilton B, et al. Associations between exposure to the real cost campaign, pro-tobacco advertisements, and tobacco use among youth in the United States. *Am J Prev Med.* 2021;60(5):706–710

81. Liu J, Halpern-Felsher B. The Juul curriculum is not the jewel of tobacco prevention education. *J Adolesc Health.* 2018;63(5):527–528

82. Carson KV, Ameer F, Sayehmiri K, et al. Mass media interventions for preventing smoking in young people. *Cochrane Database Syst Rev.* 2017;6(6):CD001006

83. Farrelly MC, Nonnemaker J, Davis KC, Hussin A. The Influence of the National truth campaign on smoking initiation. *Am J Prev Med.* 2009;36(5):379–384

84. Vallone D, Cantrell J, Bennett M, et al. Evidence of the impact of the truth FinishIt campaign. *Nicotine Tob Res.* 2018;20(5):543–551

85. Centers for Disease Control and Prevention (CDC). Tobacco use among middle and high school students—Florida, 1998 and 1999. *MMWR Morb Mortal Wkly Rep.* 1999;48(12):248–253

86. Hammond D. Health warning messages on tobacco products: a review. *Tob Control.* 2011;20(5):327–337

87. Drovandi A, Teague PA, Glass B, Malau-Aduli B. A systematic review of the perceptions of adolescents on graphic health warnings and plain packaging of cigarettes. *Syst Rev.* 2019;8(1):25

88. Lando HA, Hipple BJ, Muramoto M, et al. Tobacco control and children: an international perspective. *Pediatr Allergy Immunol Pulmonol.* 2010;23(2):99–103

89. McKnight RH, Spiller HA. Green tobacco sickness in children and adolescents. *Public Health Rep.* 2005;120(6): 602–605

90. McBride JS, Altman DG, Klein M, White W. Green tobacco sickness. *Tob Control.* 1998;7(3):294–298

91. McKnight RH, Levine EJ, Rodgers GC Jr. Detection of green tobacco sickness by a regional poison center. *Vet Hum Toxicol.* 1994;36(6):505–510

92. Benowitz NL, Henningfield JE. Establishing a nicotine threshold for addiction. The implications for tobacco regulation. *N Engl J Med.* 1994;331(2):123–125

93. Sofuoglu M, LeSage MG. The reinforcement threshold for nicotine as a target for tobacco control. *Drug Alcohol Depend.* 2012;125(1-2):1–7

94. Apelberg BJ, Feirman SP, Salazar E, et al. Potential public health effects of reducing nicotine levels in cigarettes in the United States. *N Engl J Med.* 2018;378(18):1725–1733

95. Donny EC, White CM. A review of the evidence on cigarettes with reduced addictiveness potential. *Int J Drug Policy.* 2022;99:103436

96. Berman ML, Glasser AM. Nicotine reduction in cigarettes: literature review and gap analysis. *Nicotine Tob Res.* 2019;21(Suppl 1):S133–S144

97. Regulations.gov. Tobacco product standard for nicotine level of combusted cigarettes. Available at: https://www.regulations.gov/document/FDA-2017-N-6189-0001. Accessed February 2, 2023

98. EUR-Lex. Directive 2014/40/EU of the European Parliament and of the Council of April 3, 2014, on the approximation of the laws, regulations and administrative provisions of the Member States concerning the manufacture, presentation, and sale of tobacco and related products and repealing Directive 2001/37/EC-Text with EEA relevance. Available at: https://eur-lex.europa.eu/legal-content/EN/TXT/?uri=celex:32014L0040. Accessed February 2, 2023

99. Jackler RK, Ramamurthi D. Nicotine arms race: JUUL and the high-nicotine product market. *Tob Control.* 2019;28(6):623–628

100. McDaniel PA, Smith EA, Malone RE. The tobacco endgame: a qualitative review and synthesis. *Tob Control.* 2016;25(5):594–604

101. Tobacco-Related Disease Research Program. California endgame resources. Available at: https://www.trdrp.org/about/ca-endgame-resources.html. Accessed February 2, 2023

CLINICAL REPORT Guidance for the Clinician in Rendering Pediatric Care

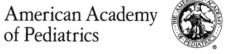

Protecting Children and Adolescents From Tobacco and Nicotine

Brian P. Jenssen, MD, FAAP,[a] Susan C. Walley, MD, FAAP,[b] Rachel Boykan, MD, FAAP,[c]
Alice Little Caldwell, MD, MPH, IBCLC, FAAP,[d] Deepa Camenga, MD, FAAP[e]
SECTION ON NICOTINE AND TOBACCO PREVENTION AND TREATMENT, COMMITTEE ON SUBSTANCE USE AND PREVENTION

abstract

Significant strides have been made in reducing rates of cigarette smoking among adolescents in the United States. However, rates of e-cigarette and similar device use among youth are high, and rates of other tobacco product use, such as cigars and hookahs, have not declined. In addition, almost 40% of children 3 to 11 years of age are regularly exposed to secondhand tobacco smoke, and rates of secondhand exposure to e-cigarette aerosol have increased over the last decade. Pediatricians are uniquely positioned to help children, adolescents, and their families live tobacco-free lives. Actions by pediatricians can help reduce children's risk of developing tobacco and nicotine use disorder and reduce children's tobacco smoke and/or aerosol exposure.

[a]Children's Hospital of Philadelphia (CHOP), University of Pennsylvania Perelman School of Medicine, Philadelphia, Pennsylvania; [b]Children's National Hospital, George Washington University School of Medicine and Health Sciences, Washington, District of Columbia; [c]Renaissance School of Medicine at Stony Brook University, Stony Brook Children's Hospital, Stony Brook, New York; [d]Medical College of Georgia, Augusta University Medical Center, Augusta, Georgia; and [e]Pediatrics and Public Health, Yale Program in Addiction Medicine, Yale Schools of Medicine and Public Health, New Haven, Connecticut

This document is copyrighted and is property of the American Academy of Pediatrics and its Board of Directors. All authors have filed conflict of interest statements with the American Academy of Pediatrics. Any conflicts have been resolved through a process approved by the Board of Directors. The American Academy of Pediatrics has neither solicited nor accepted any commercial involvement in the development of the content of this publication.

Clinical reports from the American Academy of Pediatrics benefit from expertise and resources of liaisons and internal (AAP) and external reviewers. However, clinical reports from the American Academy of Pediatrics may not reflect the views of the liaisons or the organizations or government agencies that they represent.

The guidance in this report does not indicate an exclusive course of treatment or serve as a standard of medical care. Variations, taking into account individual circumstances, may be appropriate.

All clinical reports from the American Academy of Pediatrics automatically expire 5 years after publication unless reaffirmed, revised, or retired at or before that time.

DOI: https://doi.org/10.1542/peds.2023-061805

Address correspondence to Brian P. Jenssen, MD, FAAP. E-mail: JenssenB@chop.edu

PEDIATRICS (ISSN Numbers: Print, 0031-4005; Online, 1098-4275).

DEFINITIONS

Tobacco product: Any product or device that can deliver nicotine to the human brain, whether derived from tobacco or another source, except for safe and effective nicotine replacement therapies approved by the US Food and Drug Administration (FDA) for tobacco cessation. Tobacco products include, but are not limited to, e-cigarettes, cigarettes, cigars, smokeless tobacco, hookahs, pipe tobacco, heated tobacco products, and nicotine "tobacco-free" pouches.

Secondhand smoke: Smoke emitted from a tobacco product or exhaled from a person who smokes that is inhaled by a person who does not smoke.

Thirdhand smoke: Tobacco smoke that is absorbed onto surfaces and exposes a person who does not use tobacco to its components by direct contact and dermal absorption, ingestion, and/or off-gassing and inhalation. Thirdhand smoke may react with oxidants and other compounds in the environment to yield secondary pollutants.

To cite: Jenssen BP, Walley SC, Boykan R, et al; AAP Section on Nicotine and Tobacco Prevention and Treatment, Committee on Substance Use and Prevention. Protecting Children and Adolescents From Tobacco and Nicotine. *Pediatrics.* 2023; 151(5):e2023061805

Tobacco smoke exposure: Tobacco smoke exposure among people who do not use tobacco, which includes both secondhand and thirdhand exposure.

E-cigarettes: Handheld devices that come in a variety of shapes and sizes. Most have a battery, a heating element, and a container to hold a solution that can contain nicotine, flavorings, and other chemicals. E-cigarettes are known by many different names. They are sometimes called e-cigs, e-hookahs, mods, pods, vapes, vape pens, tank systems, and electronic nicotine delivery systems (ENDS) or referred to by brand name, including Juul or Puff Bar.

Aerosol exposure: The emissions from e-cigarettes to which people who do not use e-cigarettes are exposed, including secondhand and thirdhand exposure.

Tobacco use disorder: A clinical diagnosis for which treatment is within the scope of practice of pediatric providers. Moderate or severe tobacco use disorder is defined as having 4 or more symptoms that arise from tobacco use (eg, craving; withdrawal; tolerance; increasing use over time; social, occupational, or health consequences from nicotine use).

INTRODUCTION

This clinical report accompanies a policy statement and technical report[1,2] and builds on, strengthens, and expands recommendations from the 2015 clinical report from the American Academy of Pediatrics (AAP).[3] Although many evidence-based recommendations from the 2015 report remain relevant, this revision expands on and adds clinical recommendations based on new evidence since the last summative review. The approach to the evidence review and grading evidence quality are described in the accompanying

technical report.[2] Clinical recommendations were developed using the evidence-based approach as detailed by the AAP.[4,5] In addition to a "quality of evidence" summary,[2] a brief "strength of recommendation" summary is provided, using the "strong recommendation," "recommendation," "option," or "no recommendation" classification system.[4,5] For a summary of AAP clinical reports, policy statements, and other resources for tobacco and e-cigarettes, see Table 1.

RECOMMENDED ACTIONS FOR PEDIATRICIANS: PREVENT AND TREAT TOBACCO AND NICOTINE USE AMONG PATIENTS (CHILDREN AND ADOLESCENTS)

1. Screen all Adolescents for Tobacco and Nicotine Use as Part of Health Supervision Visits

Quality of Evidence: Moderate
Strength of Recommendation: Strong

It is important to screen for tobacco use so that appropriate interventions can be offered to either prevent tobacco use or promote tobacco cessation. Tobacco use screening is recommended as part of the HEADSS (home, education [ie, school], activities/employment, drugs, suicidality, and sex)[6] or SSHADESS (strengths, school, home, activities, drugs/substance use, emotions/eating/depression, sexuality, safety),[7] both of which are psychosocial interview frameworks that assess strengths and risks in adolescents. The AAP clinical report on substance use screening, brief intervention, and referral to treatment discusses the approach to screening and the application of brief interventions based on screening results.[8] The Car-Relax-Alone-Forget-Friends-Trouble 2.1 + N is a widely used substance use screening tool that can identify tobacco and nicotine use, including e-cigarette use.[9] Overall, there are few well-designed studies examining the utility of screening in detecting tobacco use; however, although not

diagnostic tools, both the Brief Screener for Tobacco, Alcohol, and other Drugs[10] and the Screening to Brief Intervention[11] are scientifically valid screening tools for adolescent tobacco use. A study of 525 adolescents in primary care found that the Brief Screener for Tobacco, Alcohol, and other Drugs had 95% specificity and 97% sensitivity in detecting tobacco use disorder, as defined by the *Diagnostic and Statistical Manual of Mental Disorders, Fifth Edition*.[10] Similarly, the Screening to Brief Intervention detects nicotine use disorder with 75% specificity and 98% sensitivity.[11] The US Public Health Service clinical practice guideline "Treating Tobacco Use and Dependence: 2008 Update" recommends that clinicians ask pediatric and adolescent patients about tobacco use and provide a strong message regarding the importance of abstaining from tobacco use.[12]

2. Include Tobacco and Nicotine Use Prevention as Part of Anticipatory Guidance for Children and Adolescents

Quality of Evidence: Moderate
Strength of Recommendation: Strong

It is much easier to prevent tobacco use initiation among youth than it is to effectively treat tobacco use disorder (as detailed below). The US Preventive Services Task Force (USPSTF) recommends in its 2020 recommendation statement that pediatricians provide education or brief counseling to prevent initiation of tobacco use among school-aged children and adolescents.[13] Prevention interventions, including face-to-face counseling, telephone counseling, and computer-based and print-based interventions, consistently find small but clinically meaningful reductions in smoking initiation. In the USPSTF statement's accompanying meta-analysis, behavioral interventions were associated with statistically significant reductions in smoking initiation rates compared with controls at 7 to 36 months' follow-up (13 trials;

TABLE 1 AAP Policy Statements and Other Resources for Tobacco and E-cigarettes

Resources for Decreasing Tobacco Exposure at the Individual Practice Level	Evidence Base for Tobacco Control	E-Cigarette and Vaping Resources	Advocacy and Policy Resources
CEASE Resources (Massachusetts General Hospital Web site; www.massgeneral.org/ children/cease-tobacco) *Pediatric Environmental Health* (AAP policy manual) "Substance Use Screening, Brief Intervention, and Referral to Treatment" (AAP clinical report) Tobacco Use: Considerations for Clinicians resource (www.aap. org/cessation)	"Protecting Children From Tobacco, Nicotine, and Tobacco Smoke" (AAP technical report)	"E-Cigarettes and Similar Devices" (AAP policy statement) Vaping, JUUL, and E-Cigarettes Presentation Toolkit (Julius B. Richmond Center of Excellence; www.aap.org/en/ patient-care/tobacco-control-and-prevention/ e-cigarettes-and-vaping/vaping-juul-and-e-cigarettes-presentation-toolkit)	"Protecting Children From Tobacco, Nicotine, and Tobacco Smoke" (AAP policy statement) "Health Disparities in Tobacco Use and Exposure: A Structural Competency Approach" (AAP clinical report) Tobacco Prevention Policy Tool (Julius B. Richmond Center of Excellence; www.aap. org/en/patient-care/ tobacco-control-and-prevention/policy-and-advocacy/tobacco-prevention-policy-tool/) Tobacco Education Resources for Kids & Teens (HealthyChildren.org)

$n = 21\,700$; 7.4% vs 9.2%; relative risk [RR], 0.82; 95% confidence interval [CI], 0.73–0.92; $I^2 = 15$%). Further, no specific component of behavioral counseling interventions meaningfully altered intervention effectiveness, including intervention modality, target audience, duration, or setting.[14] On the basis of that information, the USPSTF recommends clinicians provide prevention counseling to all youth, regardless of the presence or absence of risk factors.[13] According to the US Surgeon General, tobacco prevention efforts should focus on both adolescents and young adults,[15] and health care professionals should warn youth of the health risks of e-cigarettes and other nicotine-containing products.[16]

The USPSTF also concluded that the evidence on interventions to prevent cigarette smoking could be applied to prevention of e-cigarette use as well, given the similar contextual and cultural issues currently surrounding the use of e-cigarettes in youth and the inclusion of e-cigarettes as a tobacco product by the FDA.

Similarly, the USPSTF concluded that the evidence could be applied to prevention of cigar use, which includes cigarillos and little cigars.[13]

Tobacco prevention messages should be clear, personally relevant, and developmentally appropriate. Messages can start as soon as children can understand them. Tobacco prevention messaging should start no later than 11 or 12 years of age, as approximately 3% to 7% of middle school students report current tobacco or nicotine product use.[17,18] One of the most important things a child can do to prepare for a healthy life is not starting use of tobacco. Messages that may resonate more with children and adolescents include the effects of tobacco use on appearance, breath, and sports performance; lack of benefit for weight loss[15]; how much money is spent on tobacco use disorder; and how the tobacco industry deceives and tries to manipulate them. The pediatric clinician should ask children and adolescents to make a

commitment to be tobacco free and help them to identify their own reasons for being tobacco free. The AAP policy statement "Improving Substance Use Prevention, Assessment, and Treatment Financing to Enhance Equity and Improve Outcomes Among Children, Adolescents, and Young Adults"[19] recommends that payers provide appropriate coverage and reimbursement for tobacco and nicotine prevention counseling.

3. Offer Treatment to Patients Who Use Tobacco Products

a. Pediatricians Should Refer Adolescents Who Want to Quit Using Tobacco to Behavioral Interventions.

Quality of Evidence: Moderate

Strength of Recommendation: Strong

Tobacco use disorder arises from a complex interaction of neurobiologic, behavioral, and social-environmental factors. Behavioral interventions are a cornerstone for tobacco use disorder treatment and can strengthen skills around coping with emotional, social, and environmental triggers; managing cravings; and coping with withdrawal symptoms. Substantial evidence supports the benefits of behavioral interventions for smoking cessation among adults in primary care.[20,21] Few studies examine the effectiveness of behavioral interventions in children and adolescents. As a result, the USPSTF concluded in 2020 that the evidence is currently insufficient to assess the risks and benefits of primary care-based tobacco cessation interventions for school-aged children and adolescents younger than 18 years.[13] In the USPSTF evidence review, 9 studies examined the effectiveness of behavioral interventions for cigarette smoking cessation. These primary care-based interventions used a variety of modalities, including face-to-face counseling, telephone counseling, text messaging, print materials, and computer-delivered counseling.[14] A meta-analysis of these studies found no statistically significant difference between behavioral interventions versus control conditions in likelihood of continued smoking at 6 to 12 months (9 trials; $n = 2516$; 80.6% vs 84.1%; RR, 0.97; 95% CI, 0.93–1.01; $I^2 = 29\%$).[14] However, limited evidence suggests that physician communication around smoking is associated with more negative attitudes about smoking, increased intention to quit, and more quit attempts.[22–26]

A 2017 Cochrane review presented evidence that group counseling is effective in increasing smoking cessation among adolescents.[27] This systematic review of primary care-and school-based tobacco cessation interventions for young people had broader inclusion criteria than the 2020 USPSTF review. It included trials of a range

of interventions for smoking cessation (eg, behavioral interventions, pharmacotherapy, and complex programs targeting families, schools, or communities) with participants younger than 20 years of age who smoked cigarettes regularly. In the meta-analysis, there was evidence of an intervention effect for group counseling (9 studies; RR, 1.35; 95% CI, 1.03–1.77), but not for individual counseling (7 studies; RR 1.07; 95% CI, 0.83–1.39), mixed delivery methods (8 studies; RR, 1.26; 95% CI, 0.95–1.66), or computer or messaging interventions (pooled RRs between 0.79 and 1.18; 9 studies in total).[27] As a group counseling example, Project EX (an 8-session, school-based clinic tobacco use cessation program for adolescents that includes enjoyable, motivating activities) was highlighted in the review. Although trials evaluating the Project EX program were noted to have a high risk of bias because of notable limitations (eg, institutional and participant-level dropout, high variability in control arm quit rates), several studies, both of Project EX within the United States and internationally, have found a beneficial effect on smoking cessation.[27]

Overall, the 2020 Surgeon General's report on smoking cessation emphasized that smoking cessation is beneficial at any age, reducing the risk of premature death, adding as much as a decade to life expectancy, while also reducing the risk of many adverse health effects.[21] More than half of adolescents who use tobacco products report that they want to quit, and more than half report making at least 1 quit attempt in the past year.[28] It is, therefore, reasonable to offer referral and/or treatment to adolescents who want to stop cigarette smoking, e-

cigarette use, or other tobacco product use.[21] Adolescents who want to stop smoking cigarettes should not be recommended to use e-cigarettes for tobacco cessation (see below for additional information). Best practices in brief intervention, motivational interviewing, and referral to treatment are covered in a separate AAP clinical report.[8]

Further, neither the 2017 Cochrane nor the 2020 USPSTF review identified any studies that examined behavioral interventions for e-cigarette cessation. Recent research, however, has examined text messaging for e-cigarette cessation. A randomized controlled trial (RCT) compared the effectiveness of tailored and intensive text messages ("This is Quitting") to an attention-only control condition on e-cigarette cessation outcomes among 2588 young adults who used e-cigarettes (mean age, 20.4 years). At the 7-month postrandomization follow-up, 24.1% (95% CI, 21.8%–26.5%) of intervention group participants self-reported abstinence compared with 18.6% (95% CI, 16.7%–20.8%) of control group participants (odds ratio [OR], 1.39; 95% CI, 1.15–1.68; $P < .001$).[25] Thus, for adolescents who want to stop e-cigarette use, it may be reasonable to refer them to text-messaging cessation supports.

b. Tobacco Use Pharmacotherapy Can be Considered for the Treatment of Moderate to Severe Tobacco Use Disorder in Adolescents Who Want to Quit Tobacco Products.

Quality of Evidence: Low

Strength of Recommendation: Option

The "low" quality of evidence rating for this recommendation is largely driven by the availability of only a few well-designed studies that examine the efficacy of pharmacotherapy for tobacco cessation in adolescents. The limited number of studies to date reflects challenges with enrollment, adherence, and retention of adolescents in well-designed clinical trials.[29,30] It should be noted that the evidence supports the safety of nicotine replacement therapy (NRT) in adolescents.

Only 3 studies in the USPSTF review evaluated the effectiveness of pharmacotherapy for cigarette smoking cessation among adolescents younger than 18 years. These studies included trials of bupropion sustained release versus control in 2 studies and NRT versus control in the third. In all 3 trials, there were no significant differences between intervention and control groups for cigarette smoking quit rates.[14] Additionally, a double-blind RCT comparing varenicline and placebo for cigarette smoking cessation among 157 adolescents found that the varenicline and placebo groups did not differ in the primary outcome of cotinine-confirmed self-reported 7-day abstinence at the end of treatment.[31] The USPSTF review was unable to identify any studies that evaluated primary care-based e-cigarette prevention or cessation interventions for children and adolescents.[14]

Again, the 2020 Surgeon General's report on smoking cessation emphasized that smoking cessation is beneficial at any age. Both the 2020 Surgeon General's report and the USPTF recommend NRT for smoking cessation in adults 18 years and older and that it is most effective when used in combination with behavioral interventions.[21,32,33] The labeling on many over-the-counter NRT products states that an individual younger than 18 years should consult with their doctor before using the product for tobacco cessation. Given the safety profile of NRT and the well-known consequences of untreated tobacco use, it is reasonable for pediatric providers to recommend and prescribe NRT to adolescents with moderate or severe tobacco use disorder. Moderate or severe tobacco use disorder is defined by the *Diagnostic and Statistical Manual of Mental Disorders, fifth Edition* as having 4 or more symptoms that arise from tobacco use (eg, craving; withdrawal; tolerance; increasing use over time; social, occupational, or health consequences from nicotine use).[34] Tobacco use disorder is a clinical diagnosis for which treatment is within the scope of practice of pediatric providers. Although only a few studies have examined NRT for tobacco cessation in individuals younger than 18 years,[13] NRT is safe with low potential for nonmedical use.[33]

AAP clinical resources for youth tobacco cessation can be found at Tobacco Use: Considerations for Clinicians (www.aap.org/cessation). This guide is based on expert consensus and reflects as robust a review of the current evidence as possible. All of the AAP clinical and policy resources on tobacco are available at www.aap.org/tobacco. Further, the AAP policy statement "Improving Substance Use Prevention, Assessment, and Treatment Financing for Children, Adolescents, and Young Adults"[19] outlines recommendations for adequate coverage and payment of tobacco use disorder treatment of pediatric providers caring for children, adolescents, and young adults. Finally, more information on coding for adolescent tobacco use counseling and treatment can be found at https://downloads. aap.org/AAP/PDF/ coding_factsheet_tobacco.pdf.

RECOMMENDED ACTIONS FOR PEDIATRICIANS: ADDRESS PARENT OR CAREGIVER TOBACCO USE AS PART OF PEDIATRIC HEALTH CARE

1. Inquire About Tobacco Use and Tobacco Smoke Exposure as Part of Health Supervision Visits and Visits for Diseases That May Be Caused or Exacerbated by Tobacco Smoke Exposure and Recommend Tobacco Use Treatment of Caregivers Who Smoke or Use Other Tobacco Products

Quality of Evidence: High

Strength of Recommendation: Strong

When parents quit smoking, they significantly increase their own life expectancy,[35,36] eliminate the majority of their children's secondhand smoke exposure,[37–39] and decrease the risk of smoking initiation among their children.[40] The 2021 USPSTF statement on smoking cessation recommends that clinicians ask all adults (18 years or older) about tobacco use, advise them to stop using tobacco, and provide behavioral interventions and FDA-approved pharmacotherapy for cessation to nonpregnant adults who use tobacco.[32] This recommendation is further emphasized by Healthy People 2030,[41] the US Department of Health and Human Services,[12] and the US Surgeon General.[21]

Pediatricians are uniquely positioned to protect children and their parents from tobacco. Parents expect their children's pediatrician to ask about their smoking status and are receptive to pediatrician interventions, including prescribing cessation medications and connecting to treatment resources.[42–44] Questions for parents that can be used to identify tobacco use and exposure include:

- Does your child live with anyone who uses tobacco?
- Does anyone who provides care for your child smoke or use other tobacco products?
- Does your child visit places where people smoke or use tobacco products?
- Does anyone ever smoke or use tobacco products in your home?

Tobacco use treatment messages that emphasize to parents the impact of their smoking on their child may increase acceptance of cessation treatment.[45,46] A 2018 Cochrane systematic review found that parent-facing clinical interventions delivered by pediatric clinicians can reduce children's tobacco smoke exposure and improve children's health. However, there was insufficient evidence to support one strategy over another to reduce the prevalence or level of children's tobacco smoke exposure.[47]

2. Implement Systems to Identify, Counsel, Treat, and Refer Caregivers Who Smoke or Use Other Tobacco Products

Quality of Evidence: Moderate

Strength of Recommendation: Strong

In adult health care settings, clinic or systemwide approaches can increase the delivery of evidence-based cessation treatment, routinizing identification, treatment, and referral for adults who smoke or use other tobacco products.[21] Strategies that are effective in the adult health care setting, however, have not easily translated to the pediatric setting.[47] To address this issue, practical systems have been developed and validated to address parental tobacco use as part of the child's health care. The Clinical Effort Against Secondhand Smoke Exposure (CEASE) program systematically identifies parents who smoke, actively enrolls them in quitlines, and provides them with printed prescriptions for

nicotine replacement therapy. In a cluster RCT comparing CEASE to standard of care, the CEASE intervention was associated with a practice-level reduction of parental smoking prevalence of 2.7%, a finding that was confirmed by cotinine measurements in individuals who reported quitting.[48] Electronic health record-embedded interventions can also be used to address parental tobacco use.[49-52] Clinician decision support (CDS) systems (electronic health record systems that enhance decision-making in the clinical workflow) have been associated with a 13-fold increase in the proportion of adults who successfully enrolled in smoking cessation treatment through state quitlines.[53] In pediatric settings, CDS systems can help pediatricians screen for secondhand smoke exposure and, similarly, effectively connect parents to treatment, including state quitlines.[54,55] Emerging evidence suggests that pediatric-based CDS systems that incorporate previsit questionnaires can support parent tobacco use screening, counseling, and treatment through more streamlined incorporation into office clinical workflows.[56]

Pediatricians can recommend and prescribe FDA approved medications as part of a treatment plan for parental tobacco cessation.[20,21] A prescription for tobacco cessation medications may be needed for insurance coverage. Breastfeeding people who smoke should be advised to quit tobacco use and connected with behavioral therapy and, if interested, pharmacotherapy.[57] When prescribing, pediatric clinicians should conduct an appropriate assessment of tobacco use, consider possible contraindications to the medications, counsel about risks and benefits, offer

recommendations for follow-up, and provide appropriate treatment. Follow-up is important to monitor for adherence to treatment recommendations, any adverse effects, correct technique for use of the recommended treatments, and adequacy of treatment in controlling nicotine withdrawal symptoms. Pediatricians should follow state regulations and institutional policies for charting on care provided to parents and caregivers to benefit the health of the child. More information on coding for caregiver tobacco use counseling and treatment can be found at https://downloads.aap. org/AAP/PDF/coding_ factsheet_tobacco.pdf.

3. Do Not Recommend E-Cigarettes for Tobacco Cessation

Quality of Evidence: Moderate

Strength of Recommendation: Strong

E-cigarettes are not FDA approved for tobacco cessation treatment. According to the 2021 USPSTF recommendation statement, current evidence is insufficient to assess the balance of benefits and harms of e-cigarettes or other vaping devices for tobacco cessation in adults, including pregnant people. Further, the USPSTF recommends that clinicians direct patients who use tobacco to other tobacco cessation interventions with proven effectiveness and established safety.[32] In contrast to the robust evidence on pharmacotherapy and behavioral interventions for smoking cessation, evidence on the use of e-cigarettes as an intervention to quit conventional smoking is lacking. According to the 2020 Surgeon General's report on smoking cessation, there is inadequate evidence to conclude that e-cigarettes, in general, increase smoking cessation and, because e-cigarettes and vaping devices are a heterogenous group of products, it is difficult to make generalizations about efficacy for cessation based on clinical trials involving a particular e-cigarette.[21] According to the systematic review conducted for the 2021 USPSTF recommendation statement, no studies on the use of e-cigarettes as tobacco cessation interventions reported health outcomes, and few trials reported on the potential adverse events of e-cigarette use when used in attempts to quit smoking.[20] This lack of evidence is of particular concern because of both the longer-term use of e-cigarettes for cessation compared with FDA-approved pharmacotherapy in the most rigorous trial to date[58] and the nationwide outbreak of e-cigarette or vaping product use-associated lung injury.[59] Further, there is a lack of long-term epidemiologic studies and large clinical trials examining the associations between e-cigarette use and morbidity and mortality.[60] Given the current state of the evidence, pediatricians should not recommend e-cigarettes and instead guide caregivers toward evidence-based, safe, and effective treatments, including behavioral counseling and FDA-approved medications for pharmacotherapy.[61]

4. If The Sources of a Child's Tobacco Smoke or Aerosol Exposure Cannot be Eliminated Through Parent or Caregiver Tobacco Use Treatment, Provide Counseling About Strategies to Reduce the Child's Exposure

Quality of Evidence: Low

Strength of Recommendation: Option

Individual family smoking bans in the home and cars and avoiding places where individuals use cigarettes or e-cigarettes should be recommended if parents and caregivers are not ready to stop smoking or start tobacco use treatment. Counseling about smoke-free homes and cars may reduce but is unlikely to eliminate a child's tobacco smoke exposure as long as household members and caregivers continue to smoke.[46,62]

RECOMMENDED ACTIONS FOR PEDIATRIC MEDICAL EDUCATION

1. Tobacco Prevention and Treatment Should be Included as Part of the Core Pediatric Residency and Medical School Curricula and Assessed on Pediatrics Board Certification and Maintenance of Certification Examinations

Quality of Evidence: Moderate

Strength of Recommendation: Strong

Because tobacco use disorder is one of the most common chronic diseases, it is imperative that there be adequate funding to train pediatric clinicians in treating tobacco use disorder. Training in tobacco use treatment enhances both pediatricians' self-efficacy for and likelihood of addressing tobacco prevention and control.[63–65] Many medical schools and pediatric residency programs have made strides in addressing knowledge about harms of tobacco smoke exposure and tobacco use disorder, but they do not promote active learning to teach tobacco intervention skills or encourage use of NRT for adolescents or parents.[66,67] As such, surveys of pediatricians reveal most do not provide quitting materials, discuss quitting techniques, recommend medications, or refer patients or parents who use tobacco to quitlines.[68] Tobacco prevention and treatment should be included as part of the core pediatric residency curriculum and medical school curriculum and assessed on pediatrics board certification and maintenance of certification examinations. This training is especially important for primary care clinicians and for medical subspecialists who treat tobacco-related diseases. Training of physicians and allied health professionals in

tobacco use treatment should be adequately funded.

CONCLUSIONS

Tobacco use almost always starts in childhood or adolescence. The tobacco epidemic takes a substantial toll on the health of all pediatric populations, including infants, children, adolescents, and young adults. Actions by pediatricians can help to reduce the risk of developing tobacco use disorder and reduce tobacco smoke exposure.

For further reading and a summary of AAP clinical reports, policy statements, and other resources for tobacco and e-cigarettes, see Table 1.

LEAD AUTHORS

Brian P. Jenssen, MD, FAAP
Susan C. Walley, MD, FAAP
Rachel Boykan, MD, FAAP
Alice Little Caldwell, MD, FAAP
Deepa Camenga, MD, FAAP

SECTION ON NICOTINE AND TOBACCO PREVENTION AND TREATMENT, 2021–2022

Susan C. Walley, MD, FAAP, Chairperson
Rachel Boykan, MD, FAAP
Judith A. Groner, MD, FAAP
Brian P. Jenssen, MD, FAAP
Jyothi N. Marbin, MD, FAAP
Bryan Mih, MD, MPH, FAAP

EX-OFFICIO MEMBER

Alice Little Caldwell, MD, FAAP

LIAISONS

Lily Rabinow, MD – Section on Pediatric Trainees
Gregory H. Blake, MD – American Academy of Family Physicians

STAFF

Karen S. Smith, Manager
James D. Baumberger, MPP, Sr Director, Federal Advocacy

COMMITTEE ON SUBSTANCE USE AND PREVENTION, 2021–2022

Lucien Gonzalez, MD, MS, FAAP, Chairperson

Rita Agarwal, MD, FAAP

Deepa R. Camenga, MD, MHS, FAAP

Joanna Quigley, MD, FAAP

Kenneth Zoucha, MD, FAAP

LIAISONS

Christine Kurien, DO – Section on Pediatric Trainees
Rebecca Ba'Gah, MD, FAAP – American Academy of Child and Adolescent Psychiatry

STAFF

Renee Jarrett, MPH

ABBREVIATIONS

AAP: American Academy of Pediatrics
CDS: clinical decision support
FDA: US Food and Drug Administration
NRT: nicotine replacement therapy
RCT: randomized controlled trial
USPSTF: US Preventive Services Task Force

COMPANION PAPERS: Companions to this article can be found online at www.pediatrics.org/cgi/doi/10.1542/peds.2023-061804 and www.pediatrics.org/cgi/doi/10.1542/peds.2023-061806.

REFERENCES

1. Jenssen BP, Walley SC, Boykan R, et al; American Academy of Pediatrics, Section on Nicotine and Tobacco Prevention and Treatment, Committee on Substance Use Prevention. Policy statement. Protecting children and adolescents from tobacco and nicotine. *Pediatrics*. 2023;151(5):e2023061804

2. Jenssen BP, Walley SC, Boykan R, et al; American Academy of Pediatrics, Section on Nicotine and Tobacco Prevention and Treatment, Committee on Substance Use Prevention. Technical report. Protecting children and adolescents from tobacco and nicotine. *Pediatrics*. 2023;151(5):e2023061806

3. Farber HJ, Walley SC, Groner JA, Nelson KE; Section on Tobacco Control. Clinical practice policy to protect children from tobacco, nicotine, and tobacco smoke. *Pediatrics*. 2015;136(5):1008–1017

4. American Academy of Pediatrics Steering Committee on Quality Improvement and Management. Classifying recommendations for clinical practice guidelines. *Pediatrics*. 2004;114(3):874–877

5. Shiffman RN, Marcuse EK, Moyer VA, et al; American Academy of Pediatrics Steering Committee on Quality Improvement and Management. Toward transparent clinical policies. *Pediatrics*. 2008;121(3):643–646

6. Cohen E, Mackenzie RG, Yates GL. HEADSS, a psychosocial risk assessment instrument: implications for designing effective intervention programs for runaway youth. *J Adolesc Health*. 1991;12(7):539–544

7. Ginsburg KR. *From Reaching Teens: Strength-Based Communication Strategies to Build Resilience and Support Healthy Adolescent Development*. Elk Grove Village, IL: American Academy of Pediatrics; 2013:139–144

8. Levy SJL, Williams JF; Committee on Substance and Prevention. Clinical report. Substance use screening, brief intervention, and referral to treatment. *Pediatrics*. 2016;138(1):e20161211

9. Harris SK, Knight JR Jr, Van Hook S, et al. Adolescent substance use screening in primary care: validity of computer self-administered versus clinician-administered screening. *Subst Abus*. 2016;37(1):197–203

10. Kelly SM, Gryczynski J, Mitchell SG, et al. Validity of brief screening instrument for adolescent tobacco, alcohol, and drug use. *Pediatrics*. 2014;133(5):819–826

11. Levy S, Weiss R, Sherritt L, et al. An electronic screen for triaging adolescent substance use by risk levels. *JAMA Pediatr*. 2014;168(9):822–828

12. Fiore MC, Jaén CR, Baker TB, et al. *Treating Tobacco Use and Dependence: 2008 Update. Clinical Practice Guideline*. Washington, DC: US Department of Health and Human Services. Public Health Service; 2008

13. Owens DK, Davidson KW, Krist AH, et al; US Preventive Services Task Force. Primary care interventions for prevention and cessation of tobacco use in children and adolescents: US Preventive Services Task Force recommendation statement. *JAMA*. 2020;323(16):1590–1598

14. Selph S, Patnode C, Bailey SR, et al. Primary care-relevant interventions for tobacco and nicotine use prevention and cessation in children and adolescents: updated evidence report and systematic review for the US Preventive Services Task Force. *JAMA*. 2020;323(16):1599–1608

15. US Department of Health and Human Services. *Preventing Tobacco Use Among Youth and Young Adults: A Report of the Surgeon General*. Atlanta, GA: US Department of Health and Human Services, Centers for Disease Control and Prevention, Office on Smoking and Health; 2012

16. US Department of Health and Human Services. *E-Cigarette Use Among Youth and Young Adults. A Report of the Surgeon General*. Atlanta, GA: US Department of Health and Human Services, Centers for Disease Control and Prevention, National Center for Chronic Disease Prevention and Health Promotion, Office on Smoking and Health; 2016

17. Creamer MR, Everett Jones S, Gentzke AS, et al. Tobacco product use among high school students—Youth Risk

Behavior Survey, United States, 2019. *MMWR Suppl.* 2020;69(1):56–63

18. Park-Lee E, Ren C, Sawdey MD, et al. Notes from the field: e-cigarette use among middle and high school students—National Youth Tobacco Survey, United States, 2021. *MMWR Morb Mortal Wkly Rep.* 2021;70(39):1387–1389

19. Camenga DR, Hammer LD; Committee on Substance Use and Prevention, and Committee on Child Health Financing. Improving substance use prevention, assessment, and treatment financing to enhance equity and improve outcomes among children, adolescents, and young adults. *Pediatrics.* 2022;150(1):e2022057992

20. Patnode CD, Henderson JT, Melnikow J, et al. *Interventions for Tobacco Cessation in Adults, Including Pregnant Women: An Evidence Update for the U.S. Preventive Services Task Force.* Rockville, MD: Agency for Healthcare Research and Quality; 2021

21. US Department of Health and Human Services. *Smoking Cessation: A Report of the Surgeon General.* Atlanta, GA: US Department of Health and Human Services, Centers for Disease Control and Prevention, National Center for Chronic Disease Prevention and Health Promotion, Office on Smoking and Health; 2020

22. Hum AM, Robinson LA, Jackson AA, Ali KS. Physician communication regarding smoking and adolescent tobacco use. *Pediatrics.* 2011;127(6):e1368–e1374

23. Shelley D, Cantrell J, Faulkner D, et al. Physician and dentist tobacco use counseling and adolescent smoking behavior: results from the 2000 National Youth Tobacco Survey. *Pediatrics.* 2005;115(3):719–725

24. Schauer GL, Agaku IT, King BA, Malarcher AM. Health care provider advice for adolescent tobacco use: results from the 2011 National Youth Tobacco Survey. *Pediatrics.* 2014;134(3):446–455

25. Graham AL, Amato MS, Cha S, et al. Effectiveness of a vaping cessation text message program among young adult e-cigarette users: a randomized clinical trial. *JAMA Intern Med.* 2021;181(7):923–930

26. American Academy of Pediatrics. Behavioral cessation supports for youth and young adults. Available at: www.aap.

org/en/patient-care/tobacco-control-and-prevention/youth-tobacco-cessation/behavioral-cessation-supports-for-youth/. Accessed February 2, 2023

27. Fanshawe TR, Halliwell W, Lindson N, et al. Tobacco cessation interventions for young people. *Cochrane Database Syst Rev.* 2017;11(11):CD003289

28. Wang TW, Gentzke AS, Creamer MR, et al. Tobacco product use and associated factors among middle and high school students—United States, 2019. *MMWR Surveill Summ.* 2019;68(12):1–22

29. Thrul J, Stemmler M, Goecke M, Bühler A. Are you in or out? Recruitment of adolescent smokers into a behavioral smoking cessation intervention. *Addict Behav.* 2015;45:150–155

30. Piper ME, Mermelstein R, Baker TB. Progress in treating youth smoking: imperative, difficult, slow. *JAMA Pediatr.* 2019;173(12):1131–1132

31. Gray KM, Baker NL, McClure EA, et al. Efficacy and safety of varenicline for adolescent smoking cessation: a randomized clinical trial. *JAMA Pediatr.* 2019;173(12):1146–1153

32. Krist AH, Davidson KW, Mangione CM, et al; US Preventive Services Task Force. Interventions for tobacco smoking cessation in adults, including pregnant persons: US Preventive Services Task Force recommendation statement. *JAMA.* 2021;325(3):265–279

33. Patnode CD, Henderson JT, Coppola EL, et al. Interventions for tobacco cessation in adults, including pregnant persons: updated evidence report and systematic review for the US Preventive Services Task Force. *JAMA.* 2021;325(3):280–298

34. American Psychiatric Association. *Diagnostic and Statistical Manual of Mental Disorders,* 5th Edition, Text Revision. Washington, DC: American Psychiatric Publishing; 2022

35. US Department of Health and Human Services. *The Health Consequences of Smoking—50 Years of Progress: A Report of the Surgeon General, 2014.* Atlanta, GA: US Department of Health and Human Services, Centers for Disease Control and Prevention, National Center for Chronic Disease Prevention and Health Promotion, Office on Smoking

and Health; 2014. Available at: https://www.ncbi.nlm.nih.gov/books/NBK179276/. Accessed February 2, 2023

36. Jha P, Ramasundarahettige C, Landsman V, et al. 21st-century hazards of smoking and benefits of cessation in the United States. *N Engl J Med.* 2013;368(4):341–350

37. US Department of Health and Human Services. *Health Consequences of Involuntary Exposure to Tobacco Smoke: A Report of the Surgeon General.* Washington, DC: US Government Printing Office; 2006

38. Wilson KM, Klein JD, Blumkin AK, et al. Tobacco-smoke exposure in children who live in multiunit housing. *Pediatrics.* 2011;127(1):85–92

39. Johansson A, Hermansson G, Ludvigsson J. How should parents protect their children from environmental tobacco-smoke exposure in the home? *Pediatrics.* 2004;113(4):e291–e295

40. den Exter Blokland EAW, Engels RCME, Hale WW III, et al. Lifetime parental smoking history and cessation and early adolescent smoking behavior. *Prev Med.* 2004;38(3):359–368

41. Healthy People 2030. Tobacco use. Available at: https://health.gov/healthypeople/objectives-and-data/browse-objectives/tobacco-use. Accessed February 2, 2023

42. Moss D, Cluss PA, Mesiano M, Kip KE. Accessing adult smokers in the pediatric setting: what do parents think? *Nicotine Tob Res.* 2006;8(1):67–75

43. Winickoff JP, Tanski SE, McMillen RC, et al. Child health care clinicians' use of medications to help parents quit smoking: a national parent survey. *Pediatrics.* 2005;115(4):1013–1017

44. Winickoff JP, Tanski SE, McMillen RC, et al. A national survey of the acceptability of quitlines to help parents quit smoking. *Pediatrics.* 2006;117(4):e695–e700

45. Jenssen BP, Kelly MK, Faerber J, et al. Parent preferences for pediatric clinician messaging to promote smoking cessation treatment. *Pediatrics.* 2020;146(1):e20193901

46. Jenssen BP, Kelly MK, Faerber J, et al. Pediatrician delivered smoking cessation messages for parents: a latent

class approach to behavioral phenotyping. *Acad Pediatr.* 2021;21(1):129–138

47. Behbod B, Sharma M, Baxi R, et al. Family and carer smoking control programmes for reducing children's exposure to environmental tobacco smoke. *Cochrane Database Syst Rev.* 2018;1(1):CD001746

48. Nabi-Burza E, Drehmer JE, Hipple Walters B, et al. Treating parents for tobacco use in the pediatric setting: the clinical effort against secondhand smoke exposure cluster randomized clinical trial. *JAMA Pediatr.* 2019; 173(10):931–939

49. Stead LF, Hartmann-Boyce J, Perera R, Lancaster T. Telephone counselling for smoking cessation. *Cochrane Database Syst Rev.* 2013;(8):CD002850

50. Boyle R, Solberg L, Fiore M. Use of electronic health records to support smoking cessation. *Cochrane Database Syst Rev.* 2014;2014(12):CD008743

51. Kruger J, O'Halloran A, Rosenthal AC, Babb SD, Fiore MC. Receipt of evidence-based brief cessation interventions by health professionals and use of cessation assisted treatments among current adult cigarette-only smokers: National Adult Tobacco Survey, 2009-2010. *BMC Public Health.* 2016;16(1):141

52. Schauer GL, Malarcher AM, Zhang L, Engstrom MC, Zhu SH. Prevalence and correlates of quitline awareness and utilization in the United States: an update from the 2009-2010 National Adult Tobacco Survey. *Nicotine Tob Res.* 2014;16(5):544–553

53. Vidrine JI, Shete S, Cao Y, et al. Ask-Advise-Connect: a new approach to smoking treatment delivery in health care

settings. *JAMA Intern Med.* 2013;173(6): 458–464

54. Sharifi M, Adams WG, Winickoff JP, et al. Enhancing the electronic health record to increase counseling and quit-line referral for parents who smoke. *Acad Pediatr.* 2014;14(5):478–484

55. Jenssen BP, Muthu N, Kelly MK, et al. Parent ereferral to tobacco quitline: a pragmatic randomized trial in pediatric primary care. *Am J Prev Med.* 2019;57(1):32–40

56. Jenssen BP, Karavite DJ, Kelleher S, et al. Electronic health record-embedded, behavioral science-informed system for smoking cessation for the parents of pediatric patients. *Appl Clin Inform.* 2022;13(2):504–515

57. Sachs HC; Committee On Drugs. The transfer of drugs and therapeutics into human breast milk: an update on selected topics. *Pediatrics.* 2013;132(3): e796–e809

58. Hajek P, Phillips-Waller A, Przulj D, et al. A randomized trial of e-cigarettes versus nicotine-replacement therapy. *N Engl J Med.* 2019;380(7):629–637

59. Krishnasamy VP, Hallowell BD, Ko JY, et al; Lung Injury Response Epidemiology/Surveillance Task Force. Update: characteristics of a nationwide outbreak of e-cigarette, or vaping, product use-associated lung injury—United States, August 2019–January 2020. *MMWR Morb Mortal Wkly Rep.* 2020;69(3):90–94

60. National Academies of Sciences, Engineering, and Medicine. *Public Health Consequences of E-Cigarettes.* Washington, DC: National Academies Press; 2018

61. Jenssen BP, Walley SC; Section on Tobacco Control. Policy statement. E-cigarettes and similar devices. *Pediatrics.* 2019;143(2):e20183652

62. Daly JB, Mackenzie LJ, Freund M, et al. Interventions by health care professionals who provide routine child health care to reduce tobacco smoke exposure in children: a review and meta-analysis. *JAMA Pediatr.* 2016;170(2):138–147

63. Cabana MD, Rand C, Slish K, et al. Pediatrician self-efficacy for counseling parents of asthmatic children to quit smoking. *Pediatrics.* 2004;113(1 Pt 1):78–81

64. Hartmann KE, Espy A, McPheeters M, Kinsinger LS. Physicians taught as residents to conduct smoking cessation intervention: a follow-up study. *Prev Med.* 2004;39(2):344–350

65. Victor JC, Brewster JM, Ferrence R, et al. Tobacco-related medical education and physician interventions with parents who smoke: survey of Canadian family physicians and pediatricians. *Can Fam Physician.* 2010;56(2): 157–163

66. Hymowitz N, Schwab JV. Pediatric residency training director tobacco survey II. *Pediatrics.* 2012;130(4):712–716

67. Boykan R, Gorzkowski J, Wellman RJ, et al. Pediatric resident training in tobacco control and the electronic health record. *Am J Prev Med.* 2021;60(3): 446–452

68. McMillen R, O'Connor KG, Groner J, et al. Changes and factors associated with tobacco counseling: results from the AAP Periodic Survey. *Acad Pediatr.* 2017;17(5):504–514

POLICY STATEMENT Organizational Principles to Guide and Define the Child Health Care System and/or Improve the Health of all Children

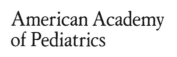

American Academy
of Pediatrics

DEDICATED TO THE HEALTH OF ALL CHILDREN™

Improving Substance Use Prevention, Assessment, and Treatment Financing to Enhance Equity and Improve Outcomes Among Children, Adolescents, and Young Adults

Deepa R. Camenga, MD, MHS, FAAP,[a,b] Lawrence D. Hammer, MD, FAAP,[c] and the Committee on Substance Use and Prevention, and Committee on Child Health Financing

Access to timely prevention and treatment services remains challenging for many children, adolescents, young adults, and families affected by substance use. The American Academy of Pediatrics recognizes the scope and urgency of this problem and has developed this policy statement for consideration by Congress, federal and state policy makers, and public and private payers. This policy statement updates the 2001 policy statement "Improving Substance Abuse Prevention, Assessment, and Treatment Financing for Children and Adolescents" and provides recommendations for financing substance use prevention, assessment, and treatment of children, adolescents, and young adults.

abstract

[a]Department of Emergency Medicine, Yale School of Medicine, Yale University, New Haven, Connecticut; [b]Department of Pediatrics, Yale School of Medicine, Yale University, New Haven, Connecticut; and [c]Department of Pediatrics, Stanford University School of Medicine, Stanford University, Stanford, California

Drs Camenga and Hammer drafted the article, and all authors participated in conception and design of the report, data interpretation, and critical revision of the article, and approved the final manuscript as submitted.

The guidance in this statement does not indicate an exclusive course of treatment or serve as a standard of medical care. Variations, taking into account individual circumstances, may be appropriate.

Policy statements from the American Academy of Pediatrics benefit from expertise and resources of liaisons and internal (AAP) and external reviewers. However, policy statements from the American Academy of Pediatrics may not reflect the views of the liaisons or the organizations or government agencies that they represent.

To cite: Camenga DR, Hammer LD; AAP Committee on Substance Use and Prevention, AAP Committee on Child Health Financing. Improving Substance Use Prevention, Assessment, and Treatment Financing to Enhance Equity and Improve Outcomes Among Children, Adolescents, and Young Adults. *Pediatrics.* 2022;150(1):e2022057992

Prevention, early identification, and treatment of substance use during childhood, adolescence, and young adulthood is key in promoting the sustained health and well-being of these populations.[1] Failure to intervene early or provide age-appropriate substance use services can result in substantial and long-term individual, familial, and intergenerational adverse consequences.[2] Unfortunately, the availability and financing of substance use prevention, assessment, and treatment services does not meet the needs of young people. According to 2019 data from the National Survey on Drug Use and Health, only 8% of adolescents and young adults who needed treatment of substance use actually received substance use treatment.[3] Racial/ethnic disparities in treatment access are linked to social, economic, and criminal justice inequities as well as stigma toward substance use within the health care system.[4–6] Black and Hispanic adolescents and young adults with substance use disorders (SUDs) are disproportionately affected by these inequities and, as of 2021, were less likely than non-Hispanic White youth to receive specialty substance use treatment.[7,8] The majority of adolescents and young adults with opioid use disorder (OUD) do not receive OUD medications, and non-Hispanic Black and Hispanic youth are less likely to receive medications than non-Hispanic White youth.[9-13] Additional training and workforce development around substance use and health equity is necessary if pediatric clinicians are to meet the need for these services in their practice settings. Parallel to this, it is also essential to improve coverage and payment for substance use prevention, assessment, and treatment services for the pediatric population.

PREVALENCE OF SUBSTANCE USE AMONG CHILDREN, ADOLESCENTS, AND YOUNG ADULTS

Substance use affects all age groups across the lifespan. In 2017, approximately 1 in 8 children in the United States lived with at least 1 parent with an SUD.[14] The 2021 Monitoring the Future Study, a long-term study that tracks substance use trends in the United States, shows that rates of substance use among adolescents have been trending downward over the past 4 decades.[15] However, substance use remains common, with alcohol, cannabis, and tobacco being the most frequently used substances by adolescents.[15] In 2021, 11.8% of 12th graders and 4.5% of eighth graders reported binge drinking at least once in the past 2 weeks. Rates of using e-cigarettes (vaping) have increased exponentially over the past decade; in 2021, up to 26.6% of 12th graders reported vaping nicotine and 18.3% reported vaping cannabis in the past year. As many as 19.5% of high school seniors and 4.1% of eighth graders reported using cannabis in the past 30 days. In addition, 12.8% of 12th graders had tried an illicit

drug other than cannabis (such as methamphetamines, cocaine, or heroin) at least once in the past year. In 2019, more than 5.9 million adolescents and young adults had an SUD, of which more than 300 000 had an OUD.[3]

Differences in exposure to social-environmental risk and protective factors contribute to disparities in rates of substance use between groups. Examples of substance use risk and protective factors include those related to the social determinants of health (eg, access to quality education, employment, health care, prosocial and faith-based activities), exposure to alcohol and tobacco use and marketing, and social connectedness with family and community.[16] Unique combinations of these social-environmental influences, as well as differences in exposures to generational trauma, childhood trauma, discrimination, racism, and marginalization, contribute to disparities in substance use.[17,18] For example, rates of substance use are higher among sexual and gender minority youth than among heterosexual and cisgender youth.[19] American Indian/Alaska Native adolescents living on or near reservations have rates of alcohol, cannabis, and other drug use that are higher than the national average.[20,21] Rates of alcohol and tobacco use are higher among non-Hispanic White youth than Black or Hispanic youth; however, by adulthood, rates between groups are more similar.[19,22,23] Further, youth with intersectional identities, or those with multiple identities with varying susceptibilities to disadvantage and privilege (eg, sex, age, class, gender identity),[24] have higher risk of developing substance use-related problems than those without. These disparities highlight the importance of fortifying protective factors, such as equitable access to substance use prevention and

treatment services, through national, state, and local policy initiatives.

Adolescence and young adulthood are vulnerable developmental periods for the onset of both SUDs and other mental health disorders. Among adolescents and young adults presenting for substance use treatment, up to ~75% also have another co-occurring mental health diagnosis.[25,26] Mental health disorders that commonly co-occur with SUDs in adolescents and young adults include attention deficit/hyperactivity disorder, conduct disorder, and/or depression.[27] Earlier age of onset of substance use is associated with a higher likelihood of developing SUDs and co-occurring mental health diagnoses, highlighting the need for prevention and early intervention services that begin in childhood.[28]

PREVENTION, EARLY INTERVENTION, AND TREATMENT OF SUBSTANCE USE AMONG CHILDREN, ADOLESCENTS, AND YOUNG ADULTS

There is growing evidence that primary prevention, early intervention, and treatment carries significant benefit for the individual and society.[1,29] Substance use primary prevention strategies include those that begin in early childhood; for example, family-based prevention programs such as Triple P, Family Check-up, and the Incredible Years have been shown to enhance protective factors that decrease substance use initiation risk.[30] Both Triple P and the Incredible Years are feasible to implement in primary care settings.[31,32] Family-based primary prevention programs for school-aged children and early adolescents, such as the Strong African-American Families Program, Strengthening Families, and Familias Unidas Preventive Interventions, have been shown to reduce substance use during adolescence.[30]

Indicated prevention interventions (those that are targeted toward adolescents showing early signs of behavioral problems), such as Functional Family Therapy or Multisystemic Therapy, have also been shown to reduce substance use. The American Academy of Pediatrics (AAP) published a clinical report and policy statement that addresses universal screening, brief intervention, and referral to treatment (SBIRT). SBIRT allows clinicians to intervene early with adolescents and young adults who use substances and link them to appropriate treatment interventions.[33] Lack of access to appropriate treatment sources is a major barrier to SBIRT implementation. Integrated behavioral health care, wherein both behavioral and medical providers function together as members of the care team, is an evidence-based strategy for delivering substance use services within primary care.[34] Research has shown that brief interventions delivered by behavioral health clinicians embedded in primary care are effective in reducing substance use and improving treatment initiation among adolescents.[35,36]

Cognitive behavioral therapy and family-based treatment are also evidence-based treatments that have been shown to decrease substance use and related problems.[37] For youth with SUDs and co-occurring mental health diagnoses, integrated treatment of both disorders has been shown to result in superior outcomes compared with separate treatment of each diagnosis.[38] The AAP has published policy statements recommending buprenorphine for the treatment of OUD in adolescents and nicotine replacement therapy for adolescents with moderate or severe tobacco use disorder.[39,40] Although there has been limited research specifically examining the impact

of harm reduction interventions such as naloxone and syringe exchange programs on opioid-related harms in adolescents and young adults,[41] evidence has shown that these programs reduce risk of overdose as well as HIV and hepatitis C infection among people who inject drugs.[42-44]

REVIEW OF POLICIES THAT AFFECT THE CARE OF CHILDREN, ADOLESCENTS, AND YOUNG ADULTS AFFECTED BY SUBSTANCE USE

Several health care policies address the known financing barriers to receiving substance use services. The Mental Health Parity and Addiction Equity Act of 2008 (MHPAEA) is a federal law that requires health insurance issuers that provide SUD or other mental health benefits to provide this coverage on par with medical/surgical benefits. For example, if a person's health insurance plan allows unlimited medical appointments for conditions such as diabetes mellitus, then the plan must also allow for unlimited medical visits for a substance use condition such as alcohol use disorder. The MHPAEA does not require that substance use services be included as part of the scope of benefits within all health insurance plans, nor does it ensure the quality, availability, or timeliness of treatment services. Individual states can enact additional laws to further require private insurers to cover SUD treatment. State-level parity laws have been shown to be associated with a 26% increase in the number of adolescents with SUD in treatment.[45]

The 2010 Patient Protection and Affordable Care Act (ACA) gave all 50 states the opportunity to extend Medicaid eligibility to adults who are not pregnant or disabled, increase income-based eligibility to all households with income less than

138% of the federal poverty level, and include coverage of adult dependent children until 26 years of age. The law also required state Medicaid programs to cover tobacco cessation counseling and medications for pregnant women. Medicaid expansion to adults has been demonstrated to have positive effects on children's coverage and care.[46] As of February 2021, 38 states and the District of Columbia have accepted these federal funds to expand their Medicaid population.[47] The ACA also mandated that individually purchased health insurance plans and insurance plans in small group markets cover a list of "essential health benefits," which include substance use treatment and other mental health treatment services.

The 2016 Comprehensive Addiction and Recovery Act was undertaken in response to the opioid crisis and provides grant support for programs that expand education, prevention, treatment, or recovery services. Initiatives within the legislation that affect pediatric populations include those that support opioid misuse prevention programs for youth, access to OUD medications for adolescents and young adults, and treatment strategies for pregnant and postpartum women with OUD. The 2018 Substance Use disorder Prevention that Promotes Opioid Recovery and Treatment for Patients and Communities Act also includes provisions to improve access to evidence-based SUD prevention and treatment services, including medications for the treatment of OUD. In response to lawsuits filed by cities and states against opioid drug manufacturers and prescribers, public health experts have also identified opioid settlement funds as a potential source of revenue to support increased local access to care among those affected by OUD.[48]

FINANCING CHALLENGES FOR CHILDREN, ADOLESCENTS, AND YOUNG ADULTS AFFECTED BY SUBSTANCE USE

As of 2019, 5.1% of children younger than 18 years were uninsured, 41.4% had public insurance coverage, and 55.2% had private health insurance coverage.[49] Among young adults, 15.1% were uninsured, 20.3% had public insurance coverage, and 65.8% had private health insurance.[49] With the MHPAEA and the ACA in place, both public and private insurance plans (excluding those plans that are exempt from the ACA requirements) that choose to provide coverage for substance use and other mental health treatment should cover these services at a level comparable to medical or surgical diagnoses. This coverage should be available for children, adolescents, and young adults up to 26 years of age or until 18 years of age in states that did not expand their Medicaid programs with federal support.[50]

Despite these legislative milestones, continued lack of insurance coverage (uninsurance) and inadequate coverage (underinsurance) leave a substantial number of children, adolescents, and young adults without sufficient insurance coverage to access and pay for prevention, assessment, and treatment services for substance use.[51] Despite reduced disparities in uninsurance since the passage of the ACA, as of 2018, Hispanic and American Indian/Alaska Native children were still significantly more likely than White children to lack insurance coverage.[52] Undocumented immigrant children continue to lack eligibility for insurance coverage in many states.[53] Many individuals without insurance rely on a "safety net" system of care, such as federally qualified health centers, "free" clinics, emergency departments, and Hill-Burton facilities and hospitals. Compared

with care for insured patients, care for uninsured patients tends to be more limited, episodic, and without the benefits of a patient-centered medical home.[54]

Discontinuity of insurance disproportionately affects the ability of specific populations, such as adolescents exiting foster care or juvenile detention, to access timely prevention and treatment services.[55,56] Although Medicaid is the largest source of publicly funded insurance in the United States, eligibility requirements vary from state to state, leading to varying insurance coverage for children between states and systematic geographic inequities in access to substance use treatment. To address these systematic inequities, the AAP has published policy statements on the provision and funding of health care services for children, adolescents, and young adults from birth to the age of 26 years.[57,58]

Among those who are insured, limitations in the scope of benefits, high out-of-pocket costs, and inadequate payments create barriers to substance use care for children, adolescents, and young adults. When substance use or other mental health services are provided at a health maintenance visit or along with other medical services, insurers frequently do not pay separately for each of these services when provided on the same date. Even if substance use services are included as a covered benefit, the coverage may not be "sufficient in the type, amount, frequency, duration, setting, and scope to enable care that achieves the best clinical outcome."[58,59] In other words, optimal treatment of SUDs may require a greater number of outpatient visits and/or inpatient days than are specified within the patient's health insurance plan. Optimal treatment may also include prevention services, assessment,

early intervention, relapse prevention, crisis intervention, group therapy, family therapy, partial hospitalization or day treatment, or residential care, which may not be included as a covered benefit. Limitations on the number of follow-up visits or inpatient hospital days may interfere with access to high-quality care that may be needed for complete treatment and recovery. In the case of OUD, high out-of-pocket costs for medications, such as buprenorphine, may deter some adolescents from adequately accessing this evidence-based form of medication treatment.

Both private and public health insurance plans "carve out" benefits related to substance use via contracts between the health plans and third-party providers of these services. When the primary insurer carves out these services, contracting entities may not always have sufficient numbers of specialty physicians, nonphysician clinicians, psychologists, social workers, or counselors in their networks to provide the needed care for pediatric populations.

Suboptimal payment rates and funding also serve as a barrier to achieving optimal substance use screening, prevention, and treatment services.[50,59,60] Substance use services are medically necessary; therefore, payment for these services and payment should be sufficient to appropriately compensate physicians and nonphysician clinicians for these services. Although Medicaid benefits include coverage of substance use services, payment rates have been very low and, as a result, serve as a disincentive to provide pediatric substance use services.[61,62] Publicly supported substance use services are often underfunded and typically available only for youth with serious emotional disturbances.[63] Many young people, particularly those who are just beginning to use substances, may not qualify for Medicaid-funded services. Moreover, children who are privately insured but without adequate substance use and other mental health benefits are seldom eligible for Medicaid-funded services.

Assessment and treatment of SUDs often involves a team, including primary care physicians, psychologists, psychiatrists, addiction specialists, clinical social workers, drug and alcohol counselors, and community- and hospital-based programs. In the primary care setting, pediatricians are seldom able to receive adequate payment for providing counseling and education services for substance use. Insurance plans may require 15 to 30 minutes of counseling time to pay pediatricians for SBIRT or other services related to counseling and early intervention; lack of adequate payment for the time needed to appropriately perform the service is a barrier to SBIRT implementation in busy primary care settings.[64,65] Integrated behavioral health models, which encompass consultation, care coordination, and colocation of behavioral health clinicians in primary care, are difficult to implement because of lack of payment for collaborative care services, behavioral health "carve-out" contracts not allowing clinicians to bill for certain services in primary care, and lack of payment for medical and behavioral health visits provided on the same day.[66]

Compounding these difficulties is the overall shortage of ambulatory and inpatient substance use services for children, adolescents, and young adults. In the hospital setting, limited availability of ambulatory and inpatient substance use services contributes to increased emergency department visits for nonurgent substance use-related concerns and lengthened hospital stays for youth

with SUDs admitted for medical and psychiatric stabilization.[67]

Finally, difficulty in maintaining confidentiality in billing and referral processes adds another barrier for many youth seeking substance use services.[68] The primary care pediatrician can screen for substance use, provide assessment, initiate treatment, and refer to other specialists for further assessment and/or treatment. The confidentiality of these data are protected under the Health Insurance Portability and Accountability Act of 1996 Privacy Rule and state-specific privacy laws.[69] Patients receiving care within federally assisted SUD treatment programs are further protected by 42 CFR Part 2 regulations, which prohibit unauthorized disclosures of SUD-related patient records, except in limited circumstances.[69] Details on health care billing and insurance claims, such as the explanation of benefits, may disclose sensitive and confidential information to the parent as the policy holder of the insurance plan and therefore serve as a barrier to seeking services.[70,71]

Alternative payment models, such as value-based payment models, may offer a cost-effective approach to financing substance use services in the future.[72,73] A systematic review of 27 studies published between 1997 and 2019 showed that alternative payment models were associated with improvements in behavioral health process-of-care outcomes (eg, treatment initiation) and lower spending; however, very few payment models focused on pediatric populations.[74] These data support the need for further research to determine how to optimally design and implement pediatric-specific alternative payment models that target substance use services for children, adolescents, and young adults.

FINANCING RECOMMENDATIONS

Many changes need to be made to the financing and delivery of substance use care to improve the availability of services for all children, adolescents, and young adults. These changes are critical for advancing health equity and improving outcomes related to substance use. The AAP supports the following recommendations that address the needs of all children, adolescents, and young adults, regardless of insurance status, as well as specific recommendations that apply to those with private insurance, those with Medicaid or Children's Health Insurance Program (CHIP) coverage, and those who are uninsured.

Recommendations for National and State Policy Makers

To Improve Coverage of Substance Use Services:

- Enact and enforce additional laws, in addition to the Mental Health Parity and Addiction Equity Act of 2008, that promote full parity between medical services and substance use services so that coverage of the management of substance use and SUDs is equal to the coverage of other chronic conditions.
- Expand the eligibility criteria of states' substance use programs to include children with all levels of substance use and other mental health risk.
- Earmark a reasonable share of state block grants for prevention, assessment, and treatment services for children and adolescents.
- Identify and use new revenue sources, such as taxes on state legalized cannabis or opioid settlement funds obtained by states and local governments, to directly address the public health issues posed by SUDs, such as the need for harm reduction services.

To Improve Payment for Substance Use Services:

- Work with payers to ensure that separate payments are made for all covered services, including preventive, medical, substance use, and other mental health services, including those that are provided on the same day.
- Create financial incentives for coordination of substance use treatment between primary care and behavioral health care (eg, transferring some behavioral health dollars into primary care). For children who are underinsured and uninsured, create mechanisms for cost sharing between public and private insurers.
- Support payment mechanisms that incentivize the development and use of integrated behavioral health models within pediatric primary care.
- Continue to study the use of alternative payment models and encourage implementation of such models if appropriate.

To Improve Access and Availability of Services and Reduce Health Care Inequities:

- Create an integrated system of referral and treatment of substance use that is consistent with the referral and treatment process of other chronic diseases and includes gender-, language-, and culturally appropriate care.
- Expand Medicaid and CHIP eligibility and enrollment to reduce the rate of uninsured and ensure adequacy and equity in coverage of substance use benefits from state to state. Expansion of eligibility and benefits will require advocacy at the state and federal levels.
- Expand public insurance coverage that includes substance use services as a covered benefit to children and youth who have undocumented immigration status.

- Increase funding of state substance use and mental health programs for children and adolescents on the basis of comprehensive needs assessment within local communities.
- Establish clear delineation of responsibilities for children involved with multiple state agencies (eg, child protective services, juvenile justice system) who require court-ordered treatment.
- Require public and private payers to support the development and use of telemedicine through equitable payment and coverage for substance use prevention, assessment, and treatment services for children, adolescents, and young adults.
- Require payers to provide adequate payment for language interpretation services for spoken languages and American Sign Language provided during substance use-related health care.
- Expand access to naloxone by requiring insurers to include low- or no-cost naloxone as a pharmacy benefit with minimal out-of-pocket costs and no requirement for prior authorization.
- Support the funding of research that examines how health care financing systems can mitigate racial/ethnic, gender, socioeconomic, and geographic disparities in substance use prevention, assessment, and treatment services among children, adolescents, and young adults.

Recommendations for Public and Private Payers

To Improve Coverage of Substance Use Services:

- Offer substance use benefits sufficient in amount, duration, and scope to reasonably achieve their purpose.
- Extend private insurance benefits to include a broader array of

substance use prevention, assessment, and treatment services.
- Reduce cost-sharing requirements for substance use services to encourage their use.
- Provide comprehensive coverage and remove prior authorization for all evidence-based pharmacologic and nonpharmacologic treatment approaches for nicotine, alcohol, cannabis, and opioid use disorders in adolescents and young adults.

To Improve Payment for Substance Use Services:

- Provide reasonable payment for counseling, coordination, and consultation procedure codes to enable primary care pediatricians to provide evidence-based prevention services for substance use.
- Adjust capitation rates to consider substance use service needs and recommended clinical guidelines for length of care for children and adolescents rather than relying on historic use rates to establish capitation amounts.
- Provide payment for screening and brief intervention practices incorporated into medical home health maintenance appointments.

To Improve Access and Availability of Services:

- Improve preauthorization and utilization review criteria to be consistent with national standards on the treatment of substance use among youth developed by the AAP, the Substance Use and Mental Health Services Administration, the National Institute on Alcohol Use and Alcoholism, and the American Society of Addiction Medicine.
- Offer the continuum of substance use services, from prevention to treatment, for children and adolescents in state Medicaid plans and contracts using a variety of benefit categories, including Early and Periodic Screening, Diagnosis, and Treatment expanded services.

- In CHIP programs, offer wrap-around benefits, such as intensive, individualized care management benefits, to allow expanded behavioral health coverage for those who meet certain risk criteria.
- Simplify and coordinate processes for families attempting to access substance use and other mental health services for their children across public and private insurance plans and programs.
- Encourage the use of a primary care medical home for patients in which health maintenance and substance use screening can be accomplished.
- Guarantee that public and private health insurance networks include pediatricians and safety net nonphysician clinicians trained or experienced in child and adolescent substance use prevention, assessment, evaluation, and management services.
- Adopt medical record and billing procedures to protect the confidentiality of children and adolescents.
- Target outreach efforts to ensure that Medicaid- and CHIP-eligible adolescents are able to access care using their insurance coverage.

LEAD AUTHORS

Deepa R. Camenga, MD, MHS, FAAP
Lawrence D. Hammer, MD, FAAP

COMMITTEE ON SUBSTANCE USE AND PREVENTION, 2020–2021

Lucien Gonzalez, MD, MS, FAAP, Chairperson
Deepa R. Camenga, MD, MHS, FAAP
Stacey Engster, MD, MS, FAAP
Stephen W. Patrick, MD, MPH, MS, FAAP
Joanna Quigley, MD, FAAP
Leslie Walker-Harding, MD, FAAP

LIAISONS

Jennifer A. Ross, MD, MPH, FAAP – Section on Pediatric Trainees
Rebecca Ba'Gah, MD, FAAP – American Academy of Child and Adolescent Psychiatry

STAFF

Renee Jarrett, MPH

COMMITTEE ON CHILD HEALTH FINANCING, 2020–2021

Jonathan Price, MD, FAAP, Chairperson
Sandy Chung, MD, FAAP
Alison A. Galbraith, MD, FAAP
Angelo Giardino, MD, PhD, FAAP

William Moskowitz, MD, FAAP
Stephen A. Pearlman, MD, MS, FAAP
Renee Turchi, MD, MPH, FAAP

FORMER COMMITTEE MEMBER

Lawrence D. Hammer, MD, FAAP

LIAISONS

Kimberly Heggen, MD, FAAP – Section on Administration and Practice Management
Mike Chen, MD, FAAP – Section on Surgery

STAFF

Teresa Salaway, MHA

ABBREVIATIONS

AAP: American Academy of Pediatrics
ACA: Patient Protection and Affordable Care Act
CHIP: State Children's Health Insurance Program
MHPAEA: Mental Health Parity and Addiction Equity Act of 2008
OUD: opioid use disorder
SBIRT: screening, brief intervention, and referral to treatment
SUD: substance use disorder

All policy statements from the American Academy of Pediatrics automatically expire 5 years after publication unless reaffirmed, revised, or retired at or before that time.

DOI: https://doi.org/10.1542/peds.2022-057992

Address correspondence to: Deepa R. Camenga, MD. E-mail: deepa.camenga@yale.edu

PEDIATRICS (ISSN Numbers: Print, 0031-4005; Online, 1098-4275).

Copyright © 2022 by the American Academy of Pediatrics

FUNDING: No external funding.

CONFLICT OF INTEREST/FINANCIAL DISCLOSURES: The authors have indicated they have no potential conflicts of interest to disclose.

REFERENCES

1. US Department of Health & Human Services (HHS). *Facing Addiction in America: The Surgeon General's Report on Alcohol, Drugs, and Health.* Washington, DC: HHS; 2016

2. Straussner SLA, Fewell CH. A review of recent literature on the impact of parental substance use disorders on children and the provision of effective services. *Curr Opin Psychiatry.* 2018;31(4):363–367

3. Substance Abuse and Mental Health Services Administration. *Key Substance Use and Mental Health Indicators in the United States: Results From the 2019 National Survey on Drug Use and Health.* HHS publication no. PEP20-07-01-001, NSDUH Series H-55. Rockville, MD: Center for Behavioral Health Statistics and Quality, Substance Abuse and Mental Health Services Administration; 2020

4. National Academies of Sciences E. *Medicine. Ending Discrimination Against People with Mental and Substance Use Disorders: The Evidence for Stigma Change.* Washington, DC: The National Academies Press; 2016:170

5. Marrast L, Himmelstein DU, Woolhandler S. Racial and ethnic disparities in mental health care for children and young adults: a national study. *Int J Health Serv.* 2016;46(4):810–824

6. Jordan A, Mathis ML, Isom J. Achieving mental health equity: addictions. *Psychiatr Clin North Am.* 2020;43(3):487–500

7. Cummings JR, Wen H, Druss BG. Racial/ethnic differences in treatment for substance use disorders among U.S. adolescents. [Article] *J Am Acad Child Adolesc Psychiatry.* 2011;50(12):1265–1274

8. Pinedo M, Villatoro AP. The role of perceived treatment need in explaining racial/ethnic disparities in the use of substance abuse treatment services. *J Subst Abuse Treat.* 2020;118:108105

9. Hadland SE, Bagley SM, Rodean J, et al. Receipt of timely addiction treatment and association of early medication treatment with retention in care among youths with opioid use disorder. *JAMA Pediatr.* 2018;172(11):1029–1037

10. Alinsky RH, Zima BT, Rodean J, et al. Receipt of addiction treatment after opioid overdose among Medicaid-enrolled adolescents and young adults. *JAMA Pediatr.* 2020;174(3):e195183

11. Bagley SM, Larochelle MR, Xuan Z, et al. Characteristics and receipt of medication treatment among young adults who experience a nonfatal opioid-related overdose. *Ann Emerg Med.* 2020;75(1):29–38

12. Hadland SE, Bagley SM, Rodean J, Levy S, Zima BT. Use of evidence-based medication treatment among medicaid-enrolled youth with opioid use disorder, 2014-2015. *J Adolesc Health.* 2018;62(2 suppl 1):S16

13. Hadland SE, Wharam JF, Schuster MA, Zhang F, Samet JH, Larochelle MR. Trends in receipt of buprenorphine and naltrexone for opioid use disorder among adolescents and young adults, 2001-2014. *JAMA Pediatr.* 2017;171(8):747–755

14. Lipari RN, Van Horn SL. Children living with parents who have a substance use disorder. *The CBHSQ Report.* Rockville, MD: Substance Abuse and Mental Health Services Administration; 2017

15. Johnston LD, Miech RA, O'Malley PM, Bahman JG, Schulenberg JE, Patrick ME. 1975-2021 Data for In-School Surveys of 8th, 10th, and 12th Grade Students. Ann Arbor, MI: Institute of Social Research, University of Michigan. Available at: http://monitoringthefuture.org/data/21data.htm. Accessed January 7, 2022

16. US Department of Health and Human Services. Early intervention, treatment, and management of substance use disorders. *Facing Addiction in America: The Surgeon General's Report on Alcohol, Drugs, and Health.* Washington, DC: HHS; 2016

17. Amaro H, Sanchez M, Bautista T, Cox R. Social vulnerabilities for substance use: Stressors, socially toxic environments, and discrimination and racism. *Neuropharmacology.* 2021;188:108518

18. Cave L, Cooper MN, Zubrick SR, Shepherd CCJ. Racial discrimination and child and adolescent health in longitudinal studies: a systematic review. *Soc Sci Med.* 2020;250:112864

19. Mereish EH. Substance use and misuse among sexual and gender minority youth. *Curr Opin Psychol.* 2019;30:123–127

20. Stanley LR, Crabtree MA, Swaim RC. Opioid misuse among American Indian adolescents. *Am J Public Health.* 2021;111(3):471–474

21. Swaim RC, Stanley LR. Substance use among American Indian youths on reservations compared with a national sample of US adolescents. *JAMA Netw Open.* 2018;1(1):e180382

22. Jones CM, Clayton HB, Deputy NP, et al. Prescription opioid misuse and use of alcohol and other substances among high school students - Youth Risk Behavior Survey, United States, 2019. *MMWR Suppl.* 2020;69(1):38–46

23. Banks DE, Zapolski TCB. The crossover effect: a review of racial/ethnic variations in risk for substance use and substance use disorder across development. *Curr Addict Rep.* 2018;5(3):386–395

24. Crenshaw K. Demarginalizing the intersection of race and sex: a black feminist critique of antidiscrimination doctrine, feminist theory and antiracist politics. *University of Chicago Legal Forum.* 1989(1):139–167. Available at: https://chicagounbound.uchicago.edu/cgi/viewcontent.cgi?article=1052&context=uclf. Accessed May 13, 2022

25. Welsh JW, Knight JR, Hou SS-Y, et al. Association between substance use diagnoses and psychiatric disorders in an adolescent and young adult clinic-based population. *J Adolesc Health.* 2017;60(6):648–652

26. Chan Y-F, Dennis ML, Funk RR. Prevalence and comorbidity of major internalizing and externalizing problems among adolescents and adults presenting to substance abuse treatment. *J Subst Abuse Treat.* 2008;34(1):14–24

27. Mason MJ, Aplasca A, Morales-Theodore R, Zaharakis N, Linker J. Psychiatric comorbidity and complications. *Child Adolesc Psychiatr Clin N Am.* 2016;25(3):521–532

28. Rowe CL, Liddle HA, Greenbaum PE, Henderson CE. Impact of psychiatric comorbidity on treatment of adolescent drug abusers. *J Subst Abuse Treat.* 2004;26(2):129–140

29. Compton WM, Jones CM, Baldwin GT, Harding FM, Blanco C, Wargo EM. Targeting youth to prevent later substance use disorder: an underutilized response to the US opioid crisis. *Am J Public Health.* 2019;109(S3):S185–S189

30. Mihalic SF, Elliott DS. Evidence-based programs registry: blueprints for

Healthy Youth Development. *Eval Program Plann*. 2015;48:124–131

31. Perrin EC, Sheldrick RC, McMenamy JM, Henson BS, Carter AS. Improving parenting skills for families of young children in pediatric settings: a randomized clinical trial. *JAMA Pediatr*. 2014; 168(1):16–24

32. McCormick E, Kerns SEU, McPhillips H, Wright J, Christakis DA, Rivara FP. Training pediatric residents to provide parent education: a randomized controlled trial. *Acad Pediatr*. 2014;14(4):353–360

33. Levy SJL, Williams JF; AAP Committee on Substance Use and Prevention. Substance use screening, brief intervention, and referral to treatment. *Pediatrics*. 2016;138(1):e20161211

34. Asarnow JR, Rozenman M, Wiblin J, Zeltzer L. Integrated medical-behavioral care compared with usual primary care for child and adolescent behavioral health: a meta-analysis. *JAMA Pediatr*. 2015;169(10):929–937

35. Sterling S, Kline-Simon AH, Jones A, Satre DD, Parthasarathy S, Weisner C. Specialty addiction and psychiatry treatment initiation and engagement: results from an SBIRT randomized trial in pediatrics. *J Subst Abuse Treat*. 2017;82:48–54

36. Parthasarathy S, Kline-Simon AH, Jones A, et al. Three-year outcomes after brief treatment of substance use and mood symptoms. *Pediatrics*. 2021;147(1):e2020009191

37. Hogue A, Henderson CE, Becker SJ, Knight DK. Evidence base on outpatient behavioral treatments for adolescent substance use, 2014-2017: outcomes, treatment delivery, and promising horizons. *J Clin Child Adolesc Psychol*. 2018;47(4):499–526

38. Brewer S, Godley MD, Hulvershorn LA. Treating mental health and substance use disorders in adolescents: what is on the menu? *Curr Psychiatry Rep*. 2017;19(1):5

39. Committee on Substance Use and Prevention. Medication-assisted treatment of adolescents with opioid use disorders. *Pediatrics*. 2016;138(3):e20161893

40. Farber HJ, Walley SC, Groner JA, Nelson KE; Section on Tobacco Control. Clinical Practice Policy to Protect Children From Tobacco, Nicotine, and Tobacco Smoke. *Pediatrics*. 2015;136(5):1008–1017

41. Stockings E, Hall WD, Lynskey M, et al. Prevention, early intervention, harm reduction, and treatment of substance use in young people. *Lancet Psychiatry*. 2016;3(3):280–296

42. Platt L, Minozzi S, Reed J, et al. Needle and syringe programmes and opioid substitution therapy for preventing HCV transmission among people who inject drugs: findings from a Cochrane review and meta-analysis. *Addiction*. 2018;113(3):545–563

43. Fernandes RM, Cary M, Duarte G, et al. Effectiveness of needle and syringe programmes in people who inject drugs – an overview of systematic reviews. *BMC Public Health*. 2017;17(1):309

44. American Academy of Pediatrics. Preventing needlestick injuries. In: Kimberlin DW, Barnett ED, Lynfield R, Sawyer MH, eds. *Red Book: 2021 Report of the Committee on Infectious Diseases*. Itasca, IL: American Academy of Pediatrics; 2021:169

45. Hamersma S, Maclean JC. Insurance expansions and adolescent use of substance use disorder treatment. *Health Serv Res*. 2021;56(2):256–267

46. Hudson JL, Moriya AS. Medicaid expansion for adults had measurable 'welcome mat' effects on their children. *Health Aff (Millwood)*. 2017;36(9):1643–1651

47. Kaiser Family Foundation. Status of state Medicaid expansion decisions: interactive map. Available at: https://www.kff.org/medicaid/issue-brief/status-of-state-medicaid-expansion-decisions-interactive-map/ Accessed February 16, 2021

48. Sharfstein JM, Olsen Y. How not to spend an opioid settlement. *JAMA*. 2020;323(11):1031–1032 10.1001/jama.2020.1371

49. Cohen RACA, Martinez ME, Terlizzi EP. Health insurance coverage: Early release of estimates from the National Health Interview Survey, 2019. Atlanta, GA: Centers for Disease Control and Prevention; 2020. Available at: https://www.cdc.gov/nchs/nhis/health insurancecoverage.htm. Accessed July 26, 2019

50. Marcell AV, Breuner CC, Hammer L, Hudak ML; Committee on Adolescence; Committee on Child Health Financing. Targeted reforms in health care financing to improve the care of adolescents and young adults. *Pediatrics*. 2018; 142(6):e20182998

51. Substance Abuse and Mental Health Services Administration. 2018 NSDUH Detailed Tables. Rockville, MD: Substance Abuse and Mental Health Service Administration; 2019. Available at: https://www.samhsa.gov/data/report/2018-nsduh-detailed-tables. Accessed May 13, 2022

52. Artiga S, Orgera K, Damico A. Changes in health coverage by race and ethnicity since the ACA, 2010-2018. San Francisco, CA: Kaiser Family Foundation; 2020. Available at: https://files.kff.org/attachment/Issue-Brief-Changes-in-Health-Coverage-by-Race-and-Ethnicity-since-the-ACA-2010-2018.pdf. Accessed May 31, 2021

53. Artiga S, Diaz M. Health coverage and care of undocumented immigrants. Available at: https://files.kff.org/attachment/Issue-Brief-Health-Coverage-and-Care-of-Undocumented-Immigrants. Accessed May 31, 2021

54. Flores G, Lin H, Walker C, et al. The health and healthcare impact of providing insurance coverage to uninsured children: A prospective observational study. *BMC Public Health*. 2017;17(1):553

55. Raghavan R, Shi P, Aarons GA, Roesch SC, McMillen JC. Health insurance discontinuities among adolescents leaving foster care. *J Adolesc Health*. 2009;44(1):41–47

56. Acoca L, Stephens J, Van Vleet A. *Health coverage and care for youth in the juvenile justice system: the role of Medicaid and CHIP*. Menlo Park, CA: The Kaiser Family Foundation; 2014

57. Committee on Child Health Financing. Medicaid Policy Statement. *Pediatrics*. 2013;131(5):e1697

58. Hudak ML, Helm ME, White PH; Committee on Child Health Financing. Principles of child health care financing. *Pediatrics*. 2017;140(3):e20172098 10.1542/peds.2017-2098

59. Acevedo A, Harvey N, Kamanu M, Tendulkar S, Fleary S. Barriers, facilitators, and disparities in retention for

adolescents in treatment for substance use disorders: a qualitative study with treatment providers. *Subst Abuse Treat Prev Policy.* 2020;15(1):42 10.1186/s13011-020-00284-4

60. Palmer A, Karakus M, Mark T. Barriers faced by physicians in screening for substance use disorders among adolescents. *Psychiatr Serv.* 2019;70(5):409–412 10.1176/appi.ps.201800427

61. American Academy of Pediatrics. Advocacy: State Advocacy. Medicaid Payment. Available at: https://www.aap.org/en/advocacy/state-advocacy/medicaid-payment/. Accessed May 30, 2022

62. Tang SS, Hudak ML, Cooley DM, Shenkin BN, Racine AD. Increased Medicaid payment and participation by office-based primary care pediatricians. *Pediatrics.* 2018;141(1):e20172570

63. Grace AM, Noonan KG, Cheng TL, et al. The ACA's pediatric essential health benefit has resulted in a state-by-state patchwork of coverage with exclusions. *Health Aff (Millwood).* 2014;33(12):2136–2143

64. Ghitza UE, Tai B. Challenges and opportunities for integrating preventive substance-use-care services in primary care through the Affordable Care Act. *J Health Care Poor Underserved.* 2014;25(suppl 1):36–45

65. Nunes AP, Richmond MK, Marzano K, Swenson CJ, Lockhart J. Ten years of implementing screening, brief intervention, and referral to treatment (SBIRT): lessons learned. *Subst Abus.* 2017;38(4):508–512

66. Tyler ET, Hulkower RL, Kaminski JW. *Behavioral health integration in pediatric primary care: considerations and opportunities for policymakers, planners, and providers.* New York, NY: Milbank Memorial Fund; 2017:15

67. Lo CB, Bridge JA, Shi J, Ludwig L, Stanley RM. Children's mental health emergency department visits: 2007-2016. *Pediatrics.* 2020;145(6):e20191536

68. Wisk LE, Gray SH, Gooding HC. I thought you said this was confidential? Challenges to protecting privacy for teens and young adults. *JAMA Pediatr.* 2018;172(3):209–210

69. Code of Federal Regulations Part 2: Confidentiality of substance use disorder patient records. 82 FR 6115. Available at: https://www.ecfr.gov/current/title-42/chapter-I/subchapter-A/part-2. Accessed May 13, 2022

70. English A, Gold RB, Nash E, Levine JJNY. Confidentiality for individuals insured as dependents: a review of state laws and policies. Washington, DC: The Guttmacher Institute; 2012. Available at: https://www.guttmacher.org/sites/default/files/report_pdf/confidentiality-review.pdf. Accessed May 13, 2022

71. English A, Lewis J. Privacy protection in billing and health insurance communications. *AMA J Ethics.* 2016;18(3):279–287

72. Brykman KHR, Bailey M. Value-based payment to support children's health and wellness: shifting the focus from short-term to life course impact. Massachusetts Medicaid Policy Institute. Boston, MA: Blue Cross MA Foundation; 2021. Available at: https://www.bluecrossmafoundation.org/sites/g/files/csphws2101/files/2021-09/Value-Based%20Pmt_Childrens-Health_FINAL.pdf. Accessed January 3, 2022

73. Wong CA, Perrin JM, McClellan M. Making the case for value-based payment reform in children's health care. *JAMA Pediatr.* 2018;172(6):513–514

74. Carlo AD, Benson NM, Chu F, Busch AB. Association of alternative payment and delivery models with outcomes for mental health and substance use disorders: a systematic review. *JAMA Netw Open.* 2020;3(7):e207401

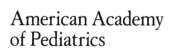

POLICY STATEMENT Organizational Principles to Guide and Define the Child Health Care System and/or Improve the Health of all Children

American Academy
of Pediatrics

DEDICATED TO THE HEALTH OF ALL CHILDREN™

Recommended Terminology for Substance Use Disorders in the Care of Children, Adolescents, Young Adults, and Families

Rachel H. Alinsky, MD, MPH, FAAP,[a] Scott E. Hadland, MD, MPH, MS, FAAP,[b] Joanna Quigley, MD, FAAP,[c] Stephen W. Patrick, MD, MPH, MS, FAAP,[d] COMMITTEE ON SUBSTANCE USE AND PREVENTION

Pediatricians across the United States encounter infants, children, adolescents, young adults, and families affected by substance use disorders in their daily practice. For much of history, substance use has been viewed as a moral failing for which individuals themselves are to blame; however, as addiction became understood as a medical disorder, clinical terminology has shifted along with a growing awareness of harm of stigmatizing language in medicine. In issuing this policy statement, the American Academy of Pediatrics (AAP) joins other large organizations in providing recommendations regarding medically accurate, person-first, and nonstigmatizing terminology. As the first pediatric society to offer guidance on preferred language regarding substance use to be used among pediatricians, media, policymakers, and government agencies and in its own peer-reviewed publications, the AAP aims to promote child health by highlighting the specific context of infants, children, adolescents, young adults, and families. In this policy statement, the AAP provides 3 specific recommendations, accompanied by a table that presents a summary of problematic language to be avoided, paired with the recommended more appropriate language and explanations for each. Pediatricians have an important role in advocating for the health of children and adolescents in the context of families affected by substance use and are optimally empowered to do so by avoiding the use of stigmatizing language in favor of medically accurate terminology that respects the dignity and personhood of individuals with substance use disorders and the children and adolescents raised in families affected by substance use.

abstract

[a]Division of Adolescent and Young Adult Medicine, Johns Hopkins School of Medicine, Baltimore, Maryland; [b]Division of Adolescent and Young Adult Medicine, Mass General Hospital for Children, Boston, Massachusetts; [c]Department of Psychiatry, University of Michigan, Ann Arbor, Michigan; and [d]Departments of Pediatrics and Health Policy, Vanderbilt Center for Child Health Policy, Vanderbilt University Medical Center, Nashville, Tennessee

Dr Alinsky conducted an extensive literature review, contributed to the development of the final recommendations, wrote the first draft of the manuscript, reviewed and revised the manuscript, and edited the final manuscript; Drs Hadland, Patrick, and Quigley contributed to the development of the final recommendations, reviewed and revised the manuscript, and edited the final manuscript; and all authors approved the final manuscript as submitted and agree to be accountable for all aspects of the work.

Address correspondence to Rachel H. Alinsky, MD, MPH. E-mail: Ralinsk1@jhmi.edu

To cite: Alinsky RH, Hadland SE, Quigley J, et al ; AAP COMMITTEE ON SUBSTANCE USE AND PREVENTION. Recommended Terminology for Substance Use Disorders in the Care of Children, Adolescents, Young Adults, and Families. Pediatrics. 2022;149(6):e2022057529

Pediatricians across the United States encounter infants, children, adolescents, and families affected by substance use disorders (SUDs) in their daily practice. Amid the national overdose crisis, the rise of widespread cannabis and e-cigarette availability, and persistently high prevalence of alcohol use, there is a renewed focus on recognition and treatment of SUDs. In previous policy statements, the American Academy of Pediatrics (AAP)[1] recognized the unique role of pediatricians in identifying and responding to familial substance use and has highlighted the importance of doing so in an empathetic, respectful, and supportive manner. Fundamental to this practice is an appreciation of the impact of language itself, with particular care paid to the terminology used in interactions with patients, family, and the public and in written materials.

A substantial hurdle to compassionately caring for patients and families affected by substance use is the widespread stigma against people with SUDs. For much of history, substance use has been viewed as a moral failing for which individuals themselves are to blame, particularly individuals of color.[2-6] Stigmatizing language reflecting this implicit bias and moralistic view, such as "substance abuse," "drug abuser," and "addict," have been commonplace not only in general conversation and the lay press[7] but also in medical literature.[8] Many of these pejorative terms have racist connotations, and derogatory terms like "crack babies" carry with them decades of legislation targeting communities of color with a carceral response to substance use, such as the War on Drugs.[5,6] In the face of the increasing prevalence of the use of opioids, marijuana, and novel psychoactive substances, the medical community has recognized

a great deal of scientific evidence revealing that addiction is a chronic illness that has the potential for recurrence similar to other medical conditions and is not a moral failing.[9]

As addiction became understood as a medical disorder, clinical terminology shifted, including that in the *Diagnostic and Statistical Manual of Mental Disorders* (DSM). Previous versions of the DSM used the phrase "substance abuse";[10] however, the DSM-5 uses the less stigmatizing term "substance use disorder," recognizing the chronic disease nature of addiction.[11] This shift in DSM nomenclature aligned with a growing awareness of the power of stigmatizing language in medicine. The use of derogatory terms such as "substance abuse" and "substance abuser" has been shown to negatively affect both lay community members' and health care providers' perceptions of individuals who use substances,[3,12-17] resulting in the view that these individuals need punishment as opposed to help or treatment. These internalized perceptions have tangible effects, as evidenced by a systematic review that found that health care providers' negatively biased views of individuals with SUDs result in worse health care delivery.[18]

In response to this evidence, the US government, as well as major scientific and journalism organizations, continue to issue statements guiding the use of appropriate language in the discussion of substance use and SUDs, including:

- The American Society of Addiction Medicine[19-21]
- Association for Multidisciplinary Education and Research in Substance Use and Addiction[22,23]
- American Medical Association[24]

- International Society for Addiction Journal Editors[25,26]
- The White House[27]
- National Institutes of Health[28]
- Associated Press[29]
- Columbia Journalism Review[30]
- National Academies of Science, Engineering, and Medicine[4,31]

THE PEDIATRIC CONTEXT

As the first pediatric society to offer guidance on preferred language regarding substance use to be used among pediatricians, media, policymakers, government agencies, and in its own peer-reviewed publications, the AAP aims to promote child health by highlighting the specific context of children, adolescents, and families. Pediatricians have an essential role in the prevention of, treatment of, and advocating for infants, children, adolescents, and young adults affected by substance use. They are empowered to do so by actively working to dismiss harmful stereotypes and avoiding the use of stigmatizing language in favor of medically accurate terminology that respects the dignity and personhood of individuals with substance use disorders and the children and adolescents raised in families affected by substance use.

Table 1 presents a summary of problematic language to be avoided, paired with the recommended more appropriate language and an explanation. The table is organized into 3 main topics. The first topic pertains to terminology regarding substance use, specifically covering the medically accurate diagnostic terminology for substance use disorders.

The second topic in the table relates to the use of "person-first" language that first and foremost acknowledges the innate personhood of an individual, rather than defining someone primarily on

TABLE 1 Recommended Terminology Regarding Substance Use

Say This:	Not This:	Here's Why:
Terminology regarding substance use		
◦ Substance use disorder; [insert specific substance: opioid, cocaine, alcohol, etc] use disorder ◦ Addiction	Drug abuse/dependence Substance abuse/dependence	The diagnostic terms "substance abuse" and "substance dependence" described in the DSM-IV have been combined in the DSM-5 into "substance use disorder." "Abuse" and "dependence" should only be used in specific reference to DSM-IV or earlier criteria or when using ICD-10 nomenclature, which still use the term "dependence;" "addiction" may also be used in conjunction with a severe substance use disorder.
◦ Substance use ◦ Hazardous substance use ◦ Unhealthy substance use ◦ Problematic substance use	Substance abuse Drug habit Vice	Substance use exists on a continuum, not all of which constitutes a diagnosable substance use disorder; therefore, these terms describe substance use that risks health consequences or is in excess of current safe use guidelines, without necessarily referencing or meeting criteria for a substance use disorder; it is more precise in describing health hazard than simply "misuse." Of note, any substance use in adolescents is considered unhealthy.
◦ Nonmedical prescription opioid use ◦ Nonmedical prescription drug use ◦ Nonmedical prescription medication use	Prescription opioid abuse Prescription drug abuse	Refers to using opioids or other prescription drugs in a way other than as prescribed or by a person to whom they were not prescribed.
◦ Intoxicated or in withdrawal	Strung out, tweaking, high, drunk (and other colloquial substance-specific terms)	Uses medically accurate language to describe the state of intoxication or withdrawal from a substance.
◦ Using ◦ Drinking	Getting high Getting drunk	Less stigmatizing way to describe the act of using a substance to reach intoxication.
Terminology regarding persons		
◦ Person with a substance use disorder	Substance/drug abuser, addict, junkie, druggie, stoner, alcoholic, drunk (and other colloquial substance-specific terms)	Uses person-first language, as individuals are not defined solely by their substance use. If unsure of whether the individual has a diagnosed disorder, then the description of "a person who uses [insert specific substance]" is most appropriate.
◦ Person who uses [insert specific substance: opioid, cocaine, alcohol, etc]	Drug user, heroin user, drinker, crackhead, pothead, drug-seeking (and other colloquial substance-specific terms)	
◦ Person who injects drugs (PWID)	Injection drug user	
◦ Treatment was not effective ◦ Patient in need of more support/ higher level of treatment	Patient who failed treatment Noncompliant, nonadherent	Referring to the treatment not meeting the needs of the patient or the patient needing a higher level of treatment, rather than the patient failing.
◦ Person with multiple recurrences ◦ Person with multiple treatment admissions	Frequent flyer Recidivist	Less stigmatizing way to denote someone with recurrence of substance use disorder, rather than referencing it as a criminal offense or a relapse, which is associated with the connotation of more blame.
◦ Infant/baby with neonatal withdrawal syndrome ◦ Infant/baby born substance-exposed ◦ Infant/baby with physiologic dependence/withdrawal	Addicted baby Born addicted Drug endangered Neonatal abstinence syndrome baby or NAS baby Crack baby	Substance use disorders, characterized by repeated use despite harmful consequences, cannot be diagnosed in an infant; an infant can develop physiologic dependence to a substance such as opioids, for which the medical term is neonatal opioid withdrawal syndrome or neonatal withdrawal.
◦ Concerned loved one	Enabler	Less stigmatizing way to describe a loved one who supports someone with a substance use disorder and at times may protect them from the negative consequences of their substance use.
Terminology regarding treatment		
◦ Treatment, pharmacotherapy ◦ Medication for addiction treatment (MAT) ◦ Medication for opioid use disorder (MOUD)	Medication-assisted treatment (MAT) Opioid substitution therapy Opioid replacement therapy	Medication *is* treatment and should not be referenced as "assisting" some other treatment, or as simply substituting one opioid for another; if use of acronym "MAT" is desired, recommend using it to refer to term "medication for addiction treatment."

TABLE 1 Continued

Say This:	Not This:	Here's Why:
○ In early remission ○ In sustained remission ○ In recovery ○ Entered recovery ○ Stopped using substances ○ Engaged in treatment	Clean Got clean	People with a history of substance use who are not currently using are deemed "in remission" or "in recovery," more neutral words than "clean" which implies that people actively using substances are "dirty."
○ Negative versus positive test result ○ [Insert substance] detected	Clean versus dirty test/urine	Refer to the actual results of the toxicology test, rather than "clean" and "dirty," which imply judgment.

ICD-10, *International Classification of Diseases and Related Health Problems, 10th Edition.*

the basis of a condition or characteristic (in this case, substance use). The use of person-first (or people-first) language is consistent with the standard set in previous AAP policy statements for describing individuals with other chronic medical conditions or disabilities, such as "a child with diabetes" rather than "a diabetic."[32] A special circumstance to highlight in this section is the problematic language that has been used to describe infants born substance-exposed who, in the lay press and elsewhere, have commonly and inappropriately been referred to as "born addicted." This language and the associated intense stigma surrounding SUDs in pregnant individuals can dissuade them from seeking treatment or cause them to abruptly end treatment, leading to worse outcomes for infants and families. The medically accurate terminology for infants who have withdrawal after birth is neonatal withdrawal.[33,34] This is in contrast to a substance use disorder, which, by definition, includes "a problematic pattern of substance use leading to clinically significant impairment or distress, as manifest by at least two [...maladaptive behaviors]."[11] On the basis of this medical definition, infants unequivocally cannot display the behavioral patterns necessary to be "addicted" to drugs, and the use of this terminology is highly stigmatizing to families.

The last topic in the table covers terminology for use in the discussion of the treatment of SUDs. Medication for opioid use disorder has been demonstrated to be safe and effective[31,35] and is recognized by the AAP, the Society for Adolescent Health and Medicine, the American Society of Addiction Medicine, and the American College of Obstetricians and Gynecologists as the recommended treatment for not only adults but also adolescents and pregnant people with an opioid use disorder.[36–40] For this reason, it is most accurate to refer to medication as treatment in and of itself, as opposed to "assisting" other treatment or being used as a "substitution" or "replacement" therapy. As of 2022, there are no data to suggest that the term nicotine replacement therapy is associated with stigma or that this terminology dissuades individuals from seeking medication treatment for nicotine use disorder; future studies could examine this question.

At times, patients may use some of these problematic terms to describe their own experiences. While allowing patients to choose their own language out of respect for their lived experience, pediatricians themselves should, nonetheless, continue to use the preferred terminology, because modeling accurate terminology remains valuable even in these circumstances so as not to

perpetuate the intense shame often associated with SUDs. Pediatricians can also use these opportunities as a catalyst for conversations with patients and parents about reducing stigma and why using nonstigmatizing language matters.

Lastly, individuals will undoubtedly encounter problematic terms in the existing literature and even in the *International Classification of Diseases and Related Health Problems, 10th Edition;*[41] when referencing or summarizing this literature, it is recommended to replace the problematic terms with the preferred terminology. If an exact citation is necessary, one can use quotations and the notation "[sic]," accompanied by an explanation of the outdated problematic terminology.

Recommendations

The AAP recommends the following:

1. Pediatricians, policymakers, government agencies, and media should use medically accurate terminology as opposed to stigmatizing jargon (see Table 1) in interactions with patients, families, and the public as well as in written materials including medical record documentation, correspondence, manuscripts, editorials and opinion articles, and news stories.
2. Pediatricians, health care facility spokespersons, policymakers,

government agencies, and media should use person-first language that respects the dignity of an individual first and foremost as a person (see Table 1) in interactions with patients, families, and the public, as well as in written materials, including medical record documentation, correspondence, manuscripts, editorials and opinion articles, and news stories.

3. Professional entities should encourage authors submitting manuscripts or materials for publication in their journals to use medically accurate and respectful person-first language (see Table 1).

Lead Authors

Rachel H. Alinsky, MD, MPH, FAAP
Scott E. Hadland, MD, MPH, MS, FAAP
Joanna Quigley, MD, FAAP
Stephen W. Patrick, MD, MPH, MS, FAAP

Committee on Substance Use and Prevention, 2020–2021

Lucien Gonzalez, MD, MS, FAAP, Chairperson
Deepa R. Camenga, MD, MHS, FAAP
Stacey Engster, MD, MS, FAAP
Stephen W. Patrick, MD, MPH, MS, FAAP

Joanna Quigley, MD, FAAP
Leslie Walker-Harding, MD, FAAP

Liaisons

Jennifer A. Ross, MD, MPH, FAAP –
Section on Pediatric Trainees
Rebecca Ba'Gah, MD, FAAP –
American Academy of Child and Adolescent Psychiatry

Staff

Renee Jarrett, MPH

DOI: https://doi.org/10.1542/peds.2022-057529

PEDIATRICS (ISSN Numbers: Print, 0031-4005; Online, 1098-4275).

CONFLICT OF INTEREST DISCLOSURES: The authors have indicated they have no potential conflicts of interest to disclose.

REFERENCES

1. Smith VC, Wilson CR; Committee on Substance Use and Prevention. Families affected by parental substance use. *Pediatrics.* 2016;138(2):e20161575

2. Botticelli MP, Koh HK. Changing the language of addiction. *JAMA.* 2016; 316(13):1361–1362

3. Kelly JF, Westerhoff CM. Does it matter how we refer to individuals with substance-related conditions? A randomized study of two commonly used terms. *Int J Drug Policy.* 2010;21(3):202–207

4. National Academies of Sciences Engineering and Medicine. *Ending Discrimination Against People with Mental and Substance Use Disorders: The Evidence for Stigma Change.* Washington, DC: National Academies Press; 2016

5. Netherland J, Hansen HB. The war on drugs that wasn't: wasted whiteness, "dirty doctors," and race in media coverage of prescription opioid misuse. *Cult Med Psychiatry.* 2016;40(4):664–686

6. James K, Jordan A. The opioid crisis in Black communities. *J Law Med Ethics.* 2018;46(2):404–421

7. McGinty EE, Stone EM, Kennedy-Hendricks A, Barry CL. Stigmatizing language in news media coverage of the opioid epidemic: implications for public health. *Prev Med.* 2019;124:110–114

8. Bailey NA, Diaz-Barbosa M. Effect of maternal substance abuse on the fetus, neonate, and child. *Pediatr Rev.* 2018;39(11):550–559

9. U.S. Department of Health and Human Services, Office of the Surgeon General. *Facing Addiction in America: The Surgeon General's Report on Alcohol, Drugs, and Health.* Washington, DC: CreateSpace Independent Publishing Platform; 2016

10. American Psychiatric Association. *Diagnostic and Statistical Manual of Mental Disorders.* 4th ed. Washington, DC: American Psychiatric Association; 1994

11. American Psychiatric Association. *Diagnostic and Statistical Manual of Mental Disorders.* 5th ed. Arlington, VA: American Psychiatric Association; 2013

12. Ashford RD, Brown AM, Curtis B. Substance use, recovery, and linguistics: the impact of word choice on explicit and implicit bias. *Drug Alcohol Depend.* 2018;189:131–138

13. Ashford RD, Brown AM, Curtis B. "Abusing addiction": our language still isn't good enough. *Alcohol Treat Q.* 2019;37(2):257–272

14. Ashford RD, Brown AM, McDaniel J, Curtis B. Biased labels: an experimental study of language and stigma among individuals in recovery and health professionals. *Subst Use Misuse.* 2019;54(8):1376–1384

15. Barry CL, McGinty EE, Pescosolido, BA, Goldman HH. Stigma, discrimination, treatment effectiveness and policy: public views about drug addiction and mental illness. *Psychiatr Serv.* 2014;65(10):1269–1272

16. Kelly JF, Dow SJ, Westerhoff C. Does our choice of substance-related terms influence perceptions of treatment need? An empirical investigation with two commonly used terms. *J Drug Issues.* 2010;40(4):805–818

17. McGinty EE, Goldman HH, Pescosolido B, Barry CL. Portraying mental illness and drug addiction as treatable health conditions: effects of a randomized experiment on stigma and discrimination. *Soc Sci Med.* 2015;126:73–85

18. van Boekel LC, Brouwers EPM, van Weeghel J, Garretsen HFL. Stigma among health professionals towards patients with substance use disorders and its

consequences for healthcare delivery: systematic review. *Drug Alcohol Depend.* 2013;131(1-2):23–35

19. American Society of Addiction Medicine. Terminology related to addiction, treatment, and recovery. Rockville, MD: American Society of Addiction Medicine; 2013. Available at: https://www.asam.org/advocacy/find-a-policy-statement/archived-public-policy-statements/public-policy-statements/2014/08/01/terminology-related-to-addiction-treatment-and-recovery. Accessed November 11, 2021

20. American Society of Addiction Medicine. Terminology related to the spectrum of unhealthy substance use. Rockville, MD: American Society of Addiction Medicine; 2013. Available at: https://www.asam.org/advocacy/find-a-policy-statement/archived-public-policy-statements/public-policy-statements/2014/08/01/terminology-related-to-the-spectrum-of-unhealthy-substance-use. Accessed November 11, 2021

21. American Society of Addiction Medicine. Language and terminology guidance for Journal of Addiction Medicine (JAM) manuscripts. Available at: https://journals.lww.com/journaladdictionmedicine/Pages/Instructions-and-Guidelines.aspx#languageandterminologyguidance. Accessed November 11, 2021

22. Association for Multidiscplinary Education and Research in Substance Use and Addiction. Interdisciplinary addiction strategies: discover, prevent, treat, teach. In: Program of the AMERSA 42nd Annual National Conference; November 8–10, 2018; San Francisco, CA.

23. Broyles LM, Binswanger IA, Jenkins JA, et al. Confronting inadvertent stigma and pejorative language in addiction scholarship: a recognition and response. *Subst Abus.* 2014;35(3):217–221

24. American Medical Association. Language matters to the American

Medical Association. Available at: https://end-overdose-epidemic.org/wp-content/uploads/2020/07/Language-Matters_Template-1.pdf. Accessed June 30, 2021

25. Saitz R. International statement recommending against the use of terminology that can stigmatize people. *J Addict Med.* 2016;10(1):1–2

26. Stenius K, Nesvåg S. ISAJE terminology statement. *Nordic Stud Alcohol Drugs.* 2015;32(5):539–540

27. Botticelli M. The White House. Changing the language of addiction. Washington, DC: The White House; January 13, 2017. Available at: https://obamawhitehouse.archives.gov/blog/2017/01/13/changing-language-addiction. Accessed November 11, 2021

28. National Institute on Drug Abuse. Words matter: terms to use and avoid when talking about addiction. Available at: https://d14rmgtrwzf5a.cloudfront.net/sites/default/files/nidamed_wordsmatter3_508.pdf. Accessed November 11, 2021

29. The Associated Press. *The Associated Press Stylebook 2017 and Briefing on Media Law.* 52nd ed. New York, NY: Basic Books; 2017

30. Feder KA, Krawczyk N. Columbia Journalism Review. Four facts every journalist should know when covering the opioid epidemic. *Columbia Journalism Review.* Published online August 15, 2017 Available at: https://www.cjr.org/united_states_project/opioid-journalist-advice.php. Accessed October 17, 2020

31. National Academies of Sciences Engineering and Medicine. *Medications for Opioid Use Disorder Save Lives.* Washington, DC: National Academies Press; 2019

32. Pont SJ, Puhl R, Cook SR, Slusser W; Section on Obesity; Obesity Society. Stigma experienced by children and adolescents with obesity. *Pediatrics.* 2017;140(6):e20173034

33. Hudak ML, Tan RC; Committee on Drugs; Committee on Fetus and Newborn; American Academy of Pediatrics. Neonatal drug withdrawal. *Pediatrics.* 2012;129(2):e540–e560

34. Patrick SW, Barfield WD, Poindexter BB; Committee on Fetus and Newborn, Committee on Substance Use and Prevention. Neonatal opioid withdrawal syndrome. *Pediatrics.* 2020;146(5):e2020029074

35. Murthy VH. Surgeon General's report on alcohol, drugs, and health. *JAMA.* 2017;317(2):133–134

36. Committee on Substance Use and Prevention. Medication-assisted treatment of adolescents with opioid use disorders. *Pediatrics.* 2016;138(3):e20161893

37. American College of Obstetricians and Gynecologists. Opioid use and opioid use disorder in pregnancy. *Obstet Gynecol.* 2017;130(2):e81–e94

38. American Society of Addiction Medicine. National practice guideline for the treatment of opioid use disorder. Available at: https://www.asam.org/Quality-Science/quality/2020-national-practice-guideline. Accessed November 11, 2021

39. Patrick SW, Schiff DM; Committee on Substance Use and Prevention. A public health response to opioid use in pregnancy. *Pediatrics.* 2017;139(3):e20164070

40. Society for Adolescent Health and Medicine. Medication for adolescents and young adults with opioid use disorder. *J Adolesc Health.* 2021;68(3):632–636

41. World Health Organization. The ICD-10 classification of mental and behavioural disorders: clinical descriptions and diagnostic guidelines. F10-F19: mental and behavioral disorders due to psychoactive substance use. Available at: https://www.who.int/substance_abuse/terminology/ICD10ClinicalDiagnosis.pdf. Accessed November 11, 2021

CLINICAL REPORT   Guidance for the Clinician in Rendering Pediatric Care

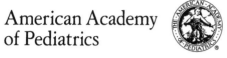

American Academy
of Pediatrics

DEDICATED TO THE HEALTH OF ALL CHILDREN®

Neonatal Opioid Withdrawal Syndrome

Stephen W. Patrick, MD, MPH, MS, FAAP,[a] Wanda D. Barfield, MD, MPH, FAAP,[b] Brenda B. Poindexter, MD, MS, FAAP,[c] COMMITTEE ON FETUS AND NEWBORN, COMMITTEE ON SUBSTANCE USE AND PREVENTION

abstract

The opioid crisis has grown to affect pregnant women and infants across the United States, as evidenced by rising rates of opioid use disorder among pregnant women and neonatal opioid withdrawal syndrome among infants. Across the country, pregnant women lack access to evidence-based therapies, including medications for opioid use disorder, and infants with opioid exposure frequently receive variable care. In addition, public systems, such as child welfare and early intervention, are increasingly stretched by increasing numbers of children affected by the crisis. Systematic, enduring, coordinated, and holistic approaches are needed to improve care for the mother-infant dyad. In this statement, we provide an overview of the effect of the opioid crisis on the mother-infant dyad and provide recommendations for management of the infant with opioid exposure, including clinical presentation, assessment, treatment, and discharge.

[a]Division of Neonatology, Department of Pediatrics and Health Policy, School of Medicine, Vanderbilt University and Vanderbilt Center for Child Health Policy, Vanderbilt University Medical Center, Nashville, Tennessee; [b]Centers for Disease Control and Prevention, Atlanta, Georgia; and [c]Department of Pediatrics, College of Medicine, University of Cincinnati and Cincinnati Children's Medical Hospital Center, Cincinnati, Ohio

Clinical reports from the American Academy of Pediatrics benefit from expertise and resources of liaisons and internal (AAP) and external reviewers. However, clinical reports from the American Academy of Pediatrics may not reflect the views of the liaisons or the organizations or government agencies that they represent.

Drs Patrick, Barfield, and Poindexter were directly involved in the planning, researching, and writing of this report and approved the final manuscript as submitted.

The guidance in this report does not indicate an exclusive course of treatment or serve as a standard of medical care. Variations, taking into account individual circumstances, may be appropriate.

All clinical reports from the American Academy of Pediatrics automatically expire 5 years after publication unless reaffirmed, revised, or retired at or before that time.

The findings and conclusions in this report are those of the authors and do not necessarily represent the views of the US Centers for Disease Control and Prevention.

This document is copyrighted and is property of the American Academy of Pediatrics and its Board of Directors. All authors have filed conflict of interest statements with the American Academy of Pediatrics. Any conflicts have been resolved through a process approved by the Board of Directors. The American Academy of Pediatrics has neither solicited nor accepted any commercial involvement in the development of the content of this publication.

DOI: https://doi.org/10.1542/peds.2020-029074

Address correspondence to Stephen W. Patrick, MD, MPH, MS, FAAP. E-mail: stephen.patrick@vanderbilt.edu

To cite: Patrick SW, Barfield WD, Poindexter BB, AAP COMMITTEE ON FETUS AND NEWBORN, COMMITTEE ON SUBSTANCE USE AND PREVENTION. Neonatal Opioid Withdrawal Syndrome. Pediatrics. 2020;146(5):e2020029074

INTRODUCTION

The United States has experienced a surge in opioid use and opioid-related complications. From 1999 to 2009, there was a quadrupling of opioid pain reliever prescription sales nationwide.[1] By 2015, 3 times as many prescriptions for opioid pain relievers were filled than in 1999,[2] reaching >37% of US adults using opioid pain relievers in 2015.[3] The rapid increase in opioid pain reliever use in the early 2000s was associated with a parallel increase in opioid pain reliever–related treatment facility admissions and overdose deaths.[1] Since 2011, however, deaths from opioid pain relievers have plateaued, whereas deaths from heroin and fentanyl have grown exponentially.[4] In 2017, >47 600 Americans died of opioid-related overdoses (including opioid pain relievers, heroin, and fentanyl), outnumbering deaths from car crashes and firearms.[5]

As the opioid crisis grew in scope and complexity in the population at large, opioid use[6] and opioid use disorder (OUD)[7–9] among pregnant women also increased. Opioid use in pregnancy can lead to a withdrawal syndrome in the newborn shortly after birth. The syndrome has been traditionally called neonatal abstinence syndrome but more recently has been called neonatal opioid withdrawal syndrome (NOWS) by federal

POLICY STATEMENT Organizational Principles to Guide and Define the Child Health
Care System and/or Improve the Health of all Children

American Academy
of Pediatrics

DEDICATED TO THE HEALTH OF ALL CHILDREN™

A Public Health Response to Opioid Use in Pregnancy

Stephen W. Patrick, MD, MPH, MS, FAAP,[a,b,c,d,e] Davida M. Schiff, MD, FAAP,[f] COMMITTEE ON SUBSTANCE USE AND PREVENTION

abstract

The use of opioids during pregnancy has grown rapidly in the past decade.
As opioid use during pregnancy increased, so did complications from their
use, including neonatal abstinence syndrome. Several state governments
responded to this increase by prosecuting and incarcerating pregnant
women with substance use disorders; however, this approach has no proven
benefits for maternal or infant health and may lead to avoidance of prenatal
care and a decreased willingness to engage in substance use disorder
treatment programs. A public health response, rather than a punitive
approach to the opioid epidemic and substance use during pregnancy,
is critical, including the following: a focus on preventing unintended
pregnancies and improving access to contraception; universal screening
for alcohol and other drug use in women of childbearing age; knowledge
and informed consent of maternal drug testing and reporting practices;
improved access to comprehensive obstetric care, including opioid-
replacement therapy; gender-specific substance use treatment programs;
and improved funding for social services and child welfare systems. The
American College of Obstetricians and Gynecologists supports the value of
this clinical document as an educational tool (December 2016).

[a]Departments of Pediatrics and [b]Health Policy, [c]Mildred Stahlman
Division of Neonatology, [d]Vanderbilt Center for Health Services
Research, and [e]Vanderbilt Center for Addiction Research, Vanderbilt
University, Nashville, Tennessee; and [f]Department of Pediatrics, Boston
Medical Center and Boston University School of Medicine, Boston,
Massachusetts

Dr Schiff conceptualized and drafted the initial manuscript and
critically reviewed the revised manuscript; Dr Patrick conceptualized
the manuscript and critically reviewed and revised the manuscript;
and both authors approved the final manuscript as submitted.

DOI: 10.1542/peds.2016-4070

Address correspondence to Stephen W. Patrick, MD, MPH, MS, FAAP.
E-mail: stephen.patrick@vanderbilt.edu

PEDIATRICS (ISSN Numbers: Print, 0031-4005; Online, 1098-4275).

To cite: Patrick SW, Schiff DM, AAP COMMITTEE ON SUBSTANCE
USE AND PREVENTION. A Public Health Response to Opioid Use
in Pregnancy. Pediatrics. 2017;139(3):e20164070

INTRODUCTION

Substance use during pregnancy occurs commonly in the United
States. In 2009, the Substance Abuse and Mental Health Administration
estimated that 400 000 infants each year are exposed to alcohol or illicit
drugs in utero.[1] Although concern regarding substance use in pregnancy
is not new, it has recently increased among health care providers, the
public, and policy makers as the opioid epidemic's impact reached an
increasing portion of the US population, including pregnant women
and their infants.[2,3] Several recent studies highlighted an increase in
prescription opioid use among women of childbearing age[4] and among
pregnant women.[5,6] As opioid use among pregnant women increased, the
rate of infants in the United States experiencing opioid withdrawal after

POLICY STATEMENT Organizational Principles to Guide and Define the Child Health Care System and/or Improve the Health of all Children

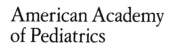

American Academy of Pediatrics

DEDICATED TO THE HEALTH OF ALL CHILDREN™

Medication-Assisted Treatment of Adolescents With Opioid Use Disorders

COMMITTEE ON SUBSTANCE USE AND PREVENTION

Opioid use disorder is a leading cause of morbidity and mortality among US youth. Effective treatments, both medications and substance use disorder counseling, are available but underused, and access to developmentally appropriate treatment is severely restricted for adolescents and young adults. Resources to disseminate available therapies and to develop new treatments specifically for this age group are needed to save and improve lives of youth with opioid addiction.

abstract

BACKGROUND

With a renewed emphasis on treating pain directed by the US Department of Health and Human Services in 1992[1] and institutionalized by the Joint Commission on Accreditation of Hospitals in 2001,[2] combined with the development of potent oral opioid pain medications, exponential increases in the annual number of opioid prescriptions written by US physicians have occurred over the past 2 decades.[3] Between 1991 and 2012, the rate of "nonmedical use" (ie, use without a prescription or more than prescribed) of opioid medication by adolescents (12–17 years of age) and young adults (18–25 years of age) more than doubled,[4,5] and the rate of opioid use disorders, including heroin addiction, increased in parallel.[6] The rate of fatal opioid overdose more than doubled between 2000 and 2013.[7] In 2008, more than 16 000 people died of opioid pain reliever overdose.[7] Other serious adverse health outcomes result from intravenous drug use and include endocarditis,[8] abscesses,[9] and infection with hepatitis C.[10]

Severe opioid use disorder is a chronic condition in which neurologic changes in the reward center of the brain are responsible for cravings and compulsive substance use.[11] The associated behavioral disruptions and change in functioning range from modest to severe; remarkably, some adolescents may continue to do well in school and in other areas of life despite severe opioid use disorder. The rate of spontaneous remission is low; however, patients can recover. Three medications are currently indicated for treating severe opioid use disorder: methadone,

This document is copyrighted and is property of the American Academy of Pediatrics and its Board of Directors. All authors have filed conflict of interest statements with the American Academy of Pediatrics. Any conflicts have been resolved through a process approved by the Board of Directors. The American Academy of Pediatrics has neither solicited nor accepted any commercial involvement in the development of the content of this publication.

Policy statements from the American Academy of Pediatrics benefit from expertise and resources of liaisons and internal (AAP) and external reviewers. However, policy statements from the American Academy of Pediatrics may not reflect the views of the liaisons or the organizations or government agencies that they represent.

The guidance in this statement does not indicate an exclusive course of treatment or serve as a standard of medical care. Variations, taking into account individual circumstances, may be appropriate.

All policy statements from the American Academy of Pediatrics automatically expire 5 years after publication unless reaffirmed, revised, or retired at or before that time.

DOI: 10.1542/peds.2016-1893

PEDIATRICS (ISSN Numbers: Print, 0031-4005; Online, 1098-4275).

FINANCIAL DISCLOSURE: The authors have indicated they do not have a financial relationship relevant to this article to disclose.

FUNDING: No external funding.

POTENTIAL CONFLICT OF INTEREST: The authors have indicated they have no potential conflicts of interest to disclose.

To cite: AAP COMMITTEE ON SUBSTANCE USE AND PREVENTION. Medication-Assisted Treatment of Adolescents With Opioid Use Disorders. *Pediatrics.* 2016;138(3):e20161893

CLINICAL REPORT Guidance for the Clinician in Rendering Pediatric Care

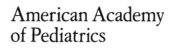

American Academy
of Pediatrics
DEDICATED TO THE HEALTH OF ALL CHILDREN™

This Clinical Report was reaffirmed September 2022.

Families Affected by Parental Substance Use

Vincent C. Smith, MD, MPH, FAAP, Celeste R. Wilson, MD, FAAP, COMMITTEE ON SUBSTANCE USE AND PREVENTION

abstract

Children whose parents or caregivers use drugs or alcohol are at increased risk of short- and long-term sequelae ranging from medical problems to psychosocial and behavioral challenges. In the course of providing health care services to children, pediatricians are likely to encounter families affected by parental substance use and are in a unique position to intervene. Therefore, pediatricians need to know how to assess a child's risk in the context of a parent's substance use. The purposes of this clinical report are to review some of the short-term effects of maternal substance use during pregnancy and long-term implications of fetal exposure; describe typical medical, psychiatric, and behavioral symptoms of children and adolescents in families affected by substance use; and suggest proficiencies for pediatricians involved in the care of children and adolescents of families affected by substance use, including screening families, mandated reporting requirements, and directing families to community, regional, and state resources that can address needs and problems.

This document is copyrighted and is property of the American Academy of Pediatrics and its Board of Directors. All authors have filed conflict of interest statements with the American Academy of Pediatrics. Any conflicts have been resolved through a process approved by the Board of Directors. The American Academy of Pediatrics has neither solicited nor accepted any commercial involvement in the development of the content of this publication.

Clinical reports from the American Academy of Pediatrics benefit from expertise and resources of liaisons and internal (AAP) and external reviewers. However, clinical reports from the American Academy of Pediatrics may not reflect the views of the liaisons or the organizations or government agencies that they represent.

The guidance in this report does not indicate an exclusive course of treatment or serve as a standard of medical care. Variations, taking into account individual circumstances, may be appropriate.

All clinical reports from the American Academy of Pediatrics automatically expire 5 years after publication unless reaffirmed, revised, or retired at or before that time.

DOI: 10.1542/peds.2016-1575

PEDIATRICS (ISSN Numbers: Print, 0031-4005; Online, 1098-4275).

Copyright © 2016 by the American Academy of Pediatrics

FINANCIAL DISCLOSURE: The authors have indicated they have no financial relationships relevant to this article to disclose.

FUNDING: No external funding.

POTENTIAL CONFLICT OF INTEREST: The authors have indicated they have no potential conflicts of interest to disclose.

To cite: Smith VC, Wilson CR, AAP COMMITTEE ON SUBSTANCE USE AND PREVENTION. Families Affected by Parental Substance Use. *Pediatrics.* 2016;138(2):e20161575

INTRODUCTION

In the course of providing health care services to children, pediatricians often encounter families affected by substance use, distribution, manufacturing, or cultivation that ultimately places parents and their children at risk. Substance use can include illicit substances such as marijuana, heroin, cocaine, and methamphetamine (eg, crystal meth), as well as misuse of alcohol and prescription medications. As defined by the National Alliance for Drug Endangered Children, drug-endangered children are those who are at risk for suffering physical or emotional harm as a result of their caregiver's substance use, possession, manufacturing, cultivation, or distribution.[1,2] Children also may be endangered when parents' substance use interferes with their ability to raise their children and provide a safe, nurturing environment.[1] Parents' substance use may affect their ability to consistently prioritize the child's basic physical and emotional needs over their own need for substances. Cigarette smoking often accompanies substance use and can

CLINICAL REPORT   Guidance for the Clinician in Rendering Pediatric Care

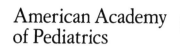

American Academy
of Pediatrics

DEDICATED TO THE HEALTH OF ALL CHILDREN™

Substance Use Screening, Brief Intervention, and Referral to Treatment

Sharon J.L. Levy, MD, MPH, FAAP, Janet F. Williams, MD, FAAP, COMMITTEE ON SUBSTANCE USE AND PREVENTION

abstract

The enormous public health impact of adolescent substance use and its preventable morbidity and mortality highlight the need for the health care sector, including pediatricians and the medical home, to increase its capacity regarding adolescent substance use screening, brief intervention, and referral to treatment (SBIRT). The American Academy of Pediatrics first published a policy statement on SBIRT and adolescents in 2011 to introduce SBIRT concepts and terminology and to offer clinical guidance about available substance use screening tools and intervention procedures. This clinical report provides a simplified adolescent SBIRT clinical approach that, in combination with the accompanying updated policy statement, guides pediatricians in implementing substance use prevention, detection, assessment, and intervention practices across the varied clinical settings in which adolescents receive health care.

Clinical reports from the American Academy of Pediatrics benefit from expertise and resources of liaisons and internal (AAP) and external reviewers. However, clinical reports from the American Academy of Pediatrics may not reflect the views of the liaisons or the organizations or government agencies that they represent.

The guidance in this report does not indicate an exclusive course of treatment or serve as a standard of medical care. Variations, taking into account individual circumstances, may be appropriate.

All clinical reports from the American Academy of Pediatrics automatically expire 5 years after publication unless reaffirmed, revised, or retired at or before that time.

DOI: 10.1542/peds.2016-1211

PEDIATRICS (ISSN Numbers: Print, 0031-4005; Online, 1098-4275).

Copyright © 2016 by the American Academy of Pediatrics

FINANCIAL DISCLOSURE: The authors have indicated they do not have a financial relationship relevant to this article to disclose.

FUNDING: No external funding.

POTENTIAL CONFLICT OF INTEREST: Dr. Levy has indicated she has a copyright relationship with Boston's Children's Hospital.

To cite: Levy SJ, Williams JF, AAP COMMITTEE ON SUBSTANCE USE AND PREVENTION. Substance Use Screening, Brief Intervention, and Referral to Treatment. *Pediatrics.* 2016;138(1): e20161211

INTRODUCTION

Adolescent substance use is an issue of critical importance to the American public. In 2011, a nationally representative household survey found that adults rated drug abuse as the number one health concern for adolescents.[1] These concerns are reflected in the *Healthy People 2020* objectives, which call for reducing teen substance use.[2] Alcohol, tobacco, and marijuana are the substances most often used by children and adolescents in the United States. Twenty-eight percent of students have tried alcohol by eighth grade, and 68.2% have tried alcohol by 12th grade. Twelve percent of eighth-graders and more than half of 12th-graders have been drunk at least once in their life.[3] Rates of marijuana use have increased substantially in recent years; in 2012, 45% of ninth- through 12th-graders reported ever using marijuana, and 24% reported marijuana use in the past 30 days.[4] Eight percent of teenagers reported using marijuana nearly every day, an increase of approximately 60% from 2008.[4] Decreases in tobacco use by high school students have plateaued since 2007; 41% of ninth- through 12th-graders reported having tried cigarettes and nearly one-quarter (22.4%)

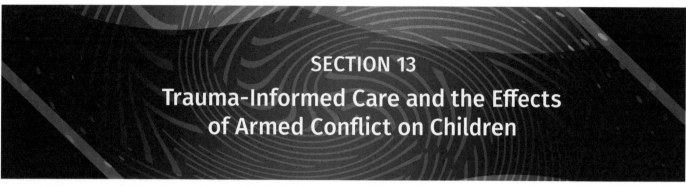

SECTION 13
Trauma-Informed Care and the Effects of Armed Conflict on Children

Some articles are available online only; scan the QR code to access online content.

POLICY STATEMENT Guidance for the Clinician in Rendering Pediatric Care

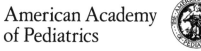

American Academy
of Pediatrics

DEDICATED TO THE HEALTH OF ALL CHILDREN™

Trauma-Informed Care in Child Health Systems

James Duffee, MD, MPH, FAAP,[a] Moira Szilagyi, MD, PhD, FAAP,[b] Heather Forkey, MD, FAAP,[c] Erin T. Kelly, MD, FAAP, FACP,[d] COUNCIL ON COMMUNITY PEDIATRICS, COUNCIL ON FOSTER CARE, ADOPTION, AND KINSHIP CARE, COUNCIL ON CHILD ABUSE AND NEGLECT, COMMITTEE ON PSYCHOSOCIAL ASPECTS OF CHILD AND FAMILY HEALTH

Recent progress in understanding the lifelong effects of early childhood adversities has clarified the need for an organized strategy to identify and intervene with children, adolescents, and families who may be at risk for maladaptive responses. Trauma-informed care (TIC) in child health care operationalizes the biological evidence of toxic stress with the insights of attachment and resilience to enhance health care delivery to mitigate the effects of trauma. The resulting pediatric health care delivery strategy promotes and restores resilience in children and adolescents, partners with families to support relational health, and reduces secondary trauma among pediatric health care clinicians. This policy statement summarizes what policy makers, legislators, and health care organizations need to consider in terms of infrastructure, resources, and financial support to facilitate the integration of TIC principles into all pediatric points of care. The accompanying clinical report describes the elements of TIC in the direct care of children, adolescents, and families and covers the spectrum from prevention to treatment. The recommendations in this statement and the clinical report build on other American Academy of Pediatrics policies that address the needs of special populations (such as children and adolescents in foster or kinship care, in immigrant and refugee families, or in poor or homeless families) and are congruent with American Academy of Pediatrics policies and technical reports concerning the role of pediatric clinicians in the promotion of lifelong health.

INTRODUCTION

Over the past 2 decades, basic science has explained how cumulative adverse childhood experiences in the relative absence of safe, stable, nurturing relationships (SSNRs)[1] alter neurohormonal stress responses, gene expression, telomere length, brain development, and immunity, enabling researchers to elucidate how the body biologically embeds

[a]Departments of Pediatrics and Psychiatry, Boonshoft School of Medicine, Wright State University, Dayton, Ohio; [b]Divisions of General and Developmental-Behavioral Pediatrics, Department of Pediatrics, University of California, Los Angeles, Los Angeles, California; [c]Department of Pediatrics, University of Massachusetts Medical School, Worcester, Massachusetts; and [d]Ambulatory Health Services, Philadelphia Department of Public Health, Philadelphia, Pennsylvania

Drs Duffee, Szilagyi, Forkey, and Kelly were equally responsible for conceptualizing, writing, and revising the manuscript and considering input from all reviewers and the Board of Directors; and all authors approved the final manuscript as submitted.

DOI: https://doi.org/10.1542/peds.2021-052579

Address correspondence to James Duffee, MD, MPH. E-mail: james.duffee@wright.edu

PEDIATRICS (ISSN Numbers: Print, 0031-4005; Online, 1098-4275).

To cite: Duffee J, Szilagyi M, Forkey H, et al. Trauma-Informed Care in Child Health Systems. *Pediatrics.* 2021;148(2):e2021052579

childhood trauma. Recent studies of toxic stress support assertions that the origins of lifelong health are in early childhood and that chronic stress in childhood strongly predicts adult health status.[2,3] In the context of expanding evidence, pediatricians and others involved in community-based early childhood systems need strategies to mitigate the damaging effects of early childhood trauma and to promote resilience in children and families. Trauma-informed care (TIC) offers an organizing principle for pediatric practice that improves awareness of the spectrum of trauma-related symptoms, promotes an emotionally safe environment of care, and provides specific interventions to mitigate the effects of trauma exposure.[4,5] This policy statement presents recommendations for policy makers, legislators, and health care organizations for implementation of TIC into pediatric health systems. The accompanying clinical report[6] presents best-practice guidance for TIC in the direct care of children and adolescents.

BACKGROUND

TIC is defined by the National Child Traumatic Stress Network as medical care in which all parties involved assess, recognize, and respond to the effects of traumatic stress on children, caregivers, and health care providers. TIC also includes attention to secondary traumatic stress (STS), the emotional strain that results when an individual, whether a health care worker or parent, hears about or witnesses the traumatic experiences, past or present, of children.

TIC Promotes Relational Health and Resilience

Every pediatric encounter presents opportunities to promote family resilience and relational health.[7] Informed by research in infant

mental health and neurodevelopment, early relational health refers to the establishment of foundational relationships during the first 3 years of life that are central to successful physiologic, emotional, and moral development of the young child.[8] Relational health, in a more general sense, is applicable to all age groups, is dyadic, and includes the capacity of both the child and caregiver to enter into a safe, secure, nurturing relationship allowing both to thrive.[1,9,10] Strong foundational relationships support resilience and buffer stress in children, so they can be considered primary prevention of stress-related disturbance. Trauma-informed practices also support relational health and family resilience as important protective factors for those who have been exposed to persistent adversity or potentially traumatic events (see Fig 1).

Human neuroendocrine–immune networks respond to internal and external sensors that identify danger and safety by activating in dangerous circumstances and deactivating when danger has subsided.[11] Toxic stress responses occur with prolonged activation of the neuroendocrine–immune system and dysregulation of homeostasis (or allostasis if multiple systems are involved)[12] in the absence of buffering by SSNRs. Toxic stress responses can result in lifelong impairments in physical, mental, and relational health.[13]

The concept of toxic stress adds an important physiologic basis to the study of attachment and our understanding of trauma. Trauma is defined as an event, series of events, or circumstances experienced by a person as physically or emotionally harmful that can have long-lasting adverse effects on the person's functioning and well-being (emotional, physical, or spiritual).[14] Attachment theory describes the

deep and enduring relationship between a child and adult caregiver that ideally provides a secure base from which the child can develop and explore the world.[15]

Resilience is the dynamic process of adaptation to or despite significant adversity by using protective factors and learned skills to manage stressful circumstances.[16] Resilience may allow a person to experience tolerable rather than toxic stress in response to adversity. Some characteristics of resilient children include strong executive functions (self-control of attention and impulses) and a strong personal identity, often related to a cultural or faith tradition.[17] However, most important to both resilience and relational health is the capacity for young children to form at least one stable, caring, and supportive relationship.[9,18]

Exposure to Trauma Is Common

Almost half of American children, or 34 million younger than 18 years, have faced at least one potentially traumatic early childhood experience.[19] More than 1 in 7 adults report exposure during childhood to 4 or more adverse childhood experiences such as abuse, neglect, or other household adversity,[20] including intimate partner violence or parental incarceration. Certain populations are at higher risk for trauma exposure, both physical and emotional. In surveys, poverty or financial stress is the most commonly reported childhood adversity, second only to loss of a parent.[21,22] Exposure to divorce, child maltreatment, sexual abuse, intimate partner violence, bullying, parental mental illness, parental substance use problems, and community violence are also common.[21] Specific populations at high risk for trauma include children and adolescents who

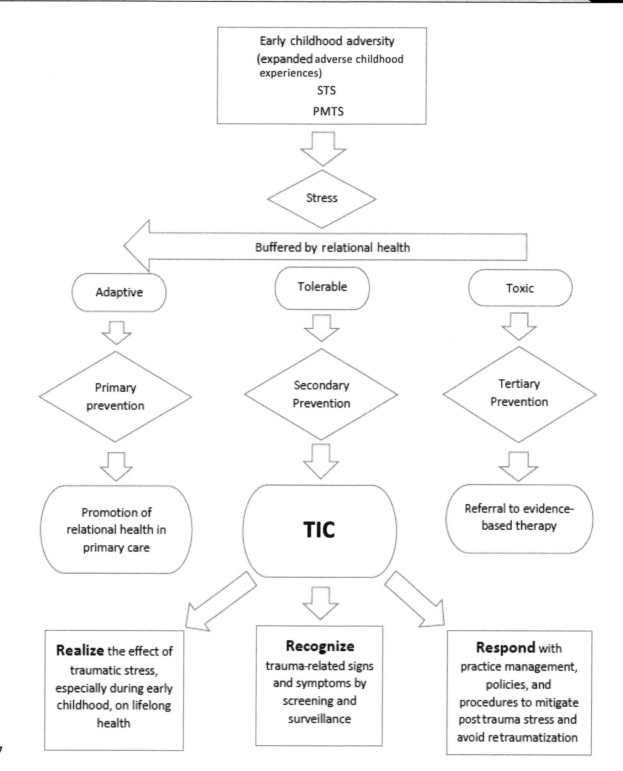

397

FIGURE 1 Pediatric approach to TIC.

identify as LGBTQ, have developmental or behavioral problems,[23-25] are in foster or kinship care, are incarcerated, are living in deep poverty, or are immigrants. Potentially traumatic environmental and community-level conditions include economic stress, school or community violence, adverse experiences during and after immigration, natural disasters, pandemics, and mass-casualty events such as shootings or bombings.

Racism is a common cross-cutting risk factor. Racial, ethnic, or religious bigotry magnifies the risk inherent to other special populations.[26] Experiences ranging from hate crimes, police profiling, bullying, or microaggressions to covert discrimination are traumatic events and may be internalized as trauma by those who are victims, indirectly or directly, of the events.[27,28] Historical trauma refers to the collective, transgenerational emotional and psychological injury of specific ethnic, racial, or cultural groups and their descendants who have experienced major events of oppression such as genocide, forced displacement, or slavery.[29,30] Originally applied to children of the Holocaust, the concept is now applied to American Indian and Alaskan native people, African American people, Mexican American people, Japanese American people, and other groups of people who have experienced mass trauma.[30] Investigators link historical "soul wounding" to current health and behavioral disorders including substance use disorder, domestic violence, and suicide, particularly in Indigenous communities.[29,31] Children separated from families during immigration and/or detained in group facilities overseen by the Office of Refugee Resettlement are a recent special population at severe risk for long-term sequelae resulting from forced family separation.[32,33]

The Effects of Early Life Trauma Are Felt Over the Life Course

In November 2019, the Centers for Disease Control and Prevention reviewed the emerging literature linking early childhood adversity with adult illnesses[20,34] and analyzed survey data from 25 states over 2 years.[3,35] Researchers concluded that reducing exposure to early childhood trauma and mitigating posttrauma effects would generally and significantly reduce adult morbidity and mortality. Using logistic regression modeling, they estimated potential reductions in incidence from low for obesity (1.7%) to high for heavy drinking, chronic obstructive pulmonary disease, and depression (23.9%, 27.0%, and 44.1%, respectively). Recommendations included creating healthy communities, supporting SSNRs, and developing programs that apply primary (reducing exposure to childhood adversity) and secondary prevention (mitigating the effects of exposure) on the basis of principles of TIC.

There Is Need for a Child-Specific Trauma Nosology

The *Diagnostic and Statistical Manual of Mental Disorders, Fifth Edition* (DSM-5) presents a list of trauma-related disorders ranging from mild (adjustment disorder) to severe (posttraumatic stress disorder [PTSD]).[36] Two additional categories, reactive attachment disorder and disinhibited social engagement disorder, are specific to young children (please see the DSM-5 for complete diagnostic criteria). This nosology can be expanded to describe other presentations common in pediatric health care settings: developmental trauma disorder (DTD), pediatric medical traumatic stress (PMTS), and STS, the last being most relevant for health care workers, family members, and caregivers.

DTD

The diagnosis of PTSD, as outlined in the current DSM-5, does not adequately describe the variable presentations of trauma manifestations in children across developmental stages.[37] Children with complex trauma histories often exhibit heterogeneous developmental symptoms as well as difficulties with intimate relationships and with regulation of attention and impulse control.[38] DTD is a proposed new diagnostic category that incorporates these differences and attempts to better describe the disturbances that occur in multiple developmental domains.[39] The omission of DTD in the DSM-5 has been controversial,[40] and the search for a better nosology of trauma, including DTD, is ongoing.[41]

PMTS

PMTS refers to the distress that patients and family members experience during hospitalization for a perceived life-threatening diagnosis or while living with or caring for individuals with life-altering chronic conditions.[42] PMTS is underrecognized and rarely addressed despite its high prevalence.[43,44] Up to 80% of ill or injured children and their families may have traumatic stress reactions after a life-threatening illness, injury, or procedure.[45] In some surveys, up to 20% of parents of children admitted to a PICU develop PTSD within a few months.[45] The suffering of family members and caregivers is often not addressed because of existing structural and reimbursement obstacles for multigenerational care.

Although research on PMTS (and on pediatric postintensive care syndrome)[46,47] is ongoing, researchers in 1 study found that approximately 10% of children developed PTSD 3 to 5 months after major surgery, and 28% developed posttraumatic stress symptoms (PTSS) resulting in functional disability by parent report.[48] PTSS can also occur after a severe injury or diagnosis of an illness such as cancer. In another family study, more than 10% of children had persistent functional impairment from PTSS at 6 weeks and 1 year after a potentially life-threatening injury or diagnosis, and 15% of mothers and 8% of fathers met criteria for PTSD at 1 year.[49]

STS

As described earlier, STS may occur in parents, other family members, and health care workers such as physicians, nurses, other hospital staff, first responders, and therapists. STS may have many of the same long-term effects on health that affect children exposed to trauma.[50] Some health care workers may also develop disabling posttrauma symptoms that can interfere with quality of life both at work and home. Health care workers may have their own trauma histories that contribute to their reactions when exposed to the suffering of others. Nonclinical staff may also experience STS triggered by their own trauma histories, especially if the health care facility is located in an area with high adversity and nonclinical staff live in the vicinity.

Burnout and STS

Preliminary evidence exists of a synergistic effect among STS, depression, and burnout in affected health care workers.[51] STS in combination with burnout has been associated with a significant increase in the frequency of medical errors.[52,53] Depression, anxiety, and suicide are greater risks for physicians than for the general population. In the United States, the rate of suicide among female physicians is 130% higher than among women who are not physicians; the rate for male physicians is 40% higher than for men who are not physicians.[51] Burnout includes a spectrum of pathologic conditions that develop in the context of occupational stress

and is almost twice as prevalent among physicians. The risk among nurses for burnout, depression, and STS is even higher. More than half of nurses reported suboptimal mental or physical health,[54] approximately 35% reported a high degree of emotional exhaustion,[55] and 18% reported depression in national surveys. Reports of posttraumatic stress among health care workers related to the coronavirus disease 2019 pandemic prompted worldwide concern for increased awareness and trauma-informed support for the mental health of all involved.[56]

CORE ELEMENTS OF TRAUMA-INFORMED SYSTEMS

Core principles that can be helpful for policy development, outlined by the National Council on Behavioral Health (2019)[57] are outlined in the following sections. Implementation of TIC at a practice level is described in detail in the accompanying clinical report.[6]

Safe Physical and Emotional Environment

The health care organization, workspace, and every encounter should be characterized by compassion, cultural humility, equity, collaboration, and safety for families and employees. An emotionally safe workplace includes acknowledgment of and particular attention to racial and gender discrimination, including implicit bias both in rendering care and workplace human relations. A review of health care settings from the viewpoints of patients, families, and staff can uncover practices, processes, or details in the environment that are potentially traumatizing.

Leadership Commitment to TIC

Hospital and health system leadership can annually review policies and procedures to ensure a

safe work environment and setting to provide TIC, to reduce STS and burnout, and to promote sensitivity to the needs of trauma survivors.[58] The alignment of financial and human capital resources to support an optimal health environment in all levels and locations of care is extremely important. Surveys designed to assess system readiness for implementation are available and can be adapted for pediatric health care settings.

Surveillance and standardized screening to assess staff and patients for trauma exposure, symptoms, and strengths are important components of trauma-informed pediatric care. Universal screening, when implemented within the larger context of trauma-informed approaches and endorsed and supported by administrative leadership, reduces stigma and allows standardized responses such as time off or referral to an employee assistance program. Families and youth may be queried at the point of care, such as at the time of hospital admission. Formal screening should always be for the benefit of children and adolescents, avoid retraumatization, and identify protective as well as risk factors.[59] More specific information about screening is included in the accompanying clinical report.[6]

Patient and Family Empowerment

Involvement of families and youth in the development of TIC policies and practices, particularly regarding cultural, historical, and gender issues, is essential to building an environment of support and mutuality.[14] Both formal and informal structures, such as Family Advisory Councils and family-centered rounds,[60] create a cultural expectation of collaboration and enable the health care team to understand the strengths and vulnerabilities of individual families and of the populations served. When appropriate, tribal elders, traditional healers, and other faith community leaders can be included in developing individual care plans or institutional quality-improvement efforts. A whole-person, whole-family, whole-community perspective promotes improved awareness of how cultural backgrounds affect the perception of trauma, safety, and privacy.[61,62]

TIC Continuous Through the Health Care System

TIC, from a public health perspective, includes primary, secondary, and tertiary prevention strategies. Primary prevention is a comprehensive approach that addresses social determinants of health (such as structural racism, poverty, and violence) that are often root causes of community trauma.[63] Promotion of relational health and other resilience factors (such as strong executive function and self-efficacy) may be considered primary prevention.[64] Following the fourth edition of *Bright Futures: Guidelines for Health Supervision of Infants, Children, and Adolescents*, promotion of early childhood relational health is a core purpose of both pediatric primary care and early childhood education.[65]

The National Child Traumatic Stress Network includes the promotion of child and family resilience, enhancement of protective factors, awareness of parent or caregiver trauma, and involvement of families in program development and evaluation as secondary prevention.[66] Trauma-informed therapies (eg, trauma-focused cognitive behavioral therapy) for symptomatic children and youth are considered tertiary prevention. These therapies are especially important for high-risk populations as identified earlier.[67-70]

Attachment-based dyadic therapies, such as parent–child interaction therapy, may serve to prevent development of persistent traumatic stress symptoms in high-risk families[71] and may be considered both secondary and tertiary prevention.

Recruitment and Training of a Trauma-Informed and Compassionate Workforce

Recruitment and pre-employment practices may help discern the capacity for empathy among prospective employees.[72] Training and education of all administrators, clinicians, and staff, both clinical and nonclinical, can promote the appreciation of the lifelong effects of trauma on child and adolescent development and family resilience and the implementation of trauma-aware practices. Continuous quality-improvement programs translate new knowledge and skills about childhood trauma into supervision, training, and patient care.

Prevention of STS requires specific training of all staff to raise awareness, promote resilience, and explore the interaction among STS, burnout, depression, substance use, and professional quality of life. Supportive supervision and peer mentoring offer opportunities for all employees to reflect on their own trauma histories and to promote compassion, nonjudgmental attitudes and collaboration.[73]

Coordination of Care Across Family-Serving Systems in the Community

Trauma-informed health care systems establish and support collaborative, interdisciplinary relationships among community and public health agencies that serve children and adolescents to coordinate care for children, adolescents, and families exposed to trauma. Schools,[74] juvenile justice

programs,[75] mental health professionals,[76] home visiting services, child welfare systems,[76] and foster care agencies[77] are natural partners for pediatric health organizations in promoting community resilience. Many have established TIC programs. Community early intervention programs can help prevent and mitigate adversity and often have the advantage of caring for young children in their natural environment as home visitors.[78-80]

RECOMMENDATIONS FOR SYSTEM-LEVEL IMPLEMENTATION

Federal and State Funding

Federal agencies such as the Centers for Disease Control and Prevention can continue and expand research to improve understanding of the developmental effects of trauma and the efficacy of specific interventions for historically resilient populations. Urgently needed are successful strategies to interrupt the intergenerational transfer of family violence. Strategies are also crucial to blunt the impact of historical trauma in communities of color and in American Indian and Alaskan native populations in the United States.[30] It is particularly important to identify the origins of and successfully mitigate community violence, including racism, misogyny, and religious, ethnic, and cultural bias.

State-level resources can be directed to implementation, dissemination, and evaluation of trauma-informed community programs, such as interagency and multigenerational strategies for opioid dependency. One example of a state interagency, multigenerational treatment program is Ohio START (Sobriety, Treatment and Reducing Trauma).[81] States could develop a communication infrastructure to facilitate data sharing, improve interdisciplinary/interagency cooperation, and engage community partners including foundations and academic institutions.

Federal guidelines can require that state Medicaid programs ensure comprehensive coverage for all children and adolescents and pregnant mothers without regard for legal or immigration status and mandate that coverage include mental health and substance use disorder services. Financing that increases access to high-quality, comprehensive, coordinated, culturally competent health care for high-risk populations is a high priority. Federal and state regulations can require all insurers, including Medicaid and private health insurers, to include coverage for TIC elements, including surveillance, screening, diagnosis, counseling, case management, follow-up, community collaboration, mental health care, and home visiting.

Large Health Systems, Insurers, and Managed Care Organizations

In large health systems, leadership can align its mission and financing with the core elements of trauma-informed systems.[82] Supporting TIC includes payment for trauma-informed, integrated mental health services, care coordination, rigorous case management, and seamless referral networks for intensive treatment. Prevention of secondary trauma, including care of affected health care workers, should be built into the mission of the health system.

Academic Centers and Children's Hospitals

Academic health centers train and educate the next generation of physicians, nurses, and ancillary health personnel and can promote the transformation to TIC in all health settings through education, research, and advocacy. Children's hospitals and health systems can model mental health integration[83] and trauma-informed practices throughout all service lines.[84] Because children's hospitals embrace population health management and community advocacy, they may serve as the anchor institution collaborating with community agencies to address social adversity at the neighborhood level while promoting TIC services.[85] Together with community pediatric care systems, academic health centers and children's hospitals can integrate core elements of education into workforce training for health care workers and community partners such as first responders, child welfare workers, teachers, and juvenile justice personnel.[86,87]

SUMMARY OF RECOMMENDATIONS

Federal and State Government

- Continue and expand research funding for the National Institutes of Health, Centers for Disease Control and Prevention, Substance Abuse and Mental Health Services Administration, and other federal agencies to improve the understanding of the root causes and developmental effects of trauma and effective interventions.
- Support epidemiological research of at-risk populations emphasizing prevention, early identification, and mitigation of the effects of community trauma.
- Facilitate interdisciplinary and interagency cooperation and data sharing to promote seamless care, research data collection, and amplification of promising practices in TIC.
- Engage national partners, foundations, and academic institutions in cross-systems planning to support early relational health.
- Support curriculum development and implementation through mechanisms such as the Agency for Healthcare Research and Quality.
- Expand health care coverage and payment for enhanced services such as integrated mental and social care.
- Mandate coverage for TIC services by government and private payers, including screening, diagnosis, office-based management, counseling, case management, community collaboration, and home visiting.

Large Health Systems and Managed Care Organizations

- Commit to becoming a trauma-informed system of care and integrate clinical practice of TIC into all services.
- Recruit, retain, and train a trauma-informed workforce.
- Expand and improve system-wide strategies for identification and treatment of all children and adolescents affected by traumatizing experiences.
- Build seamless referral networks for intensive treatment when indicated.
- Develop care models and fair payment mechanisms to promote implementation of TIC, including practice-level case management.
- Promote system-wide trauma-informed quality-improvement programs.
- Support engagement by including family advisors and employees in service planning and quality improvement, with particular emphasis on cultural, ethnic, gender, and racial concerns.

- Develop, implement, and evaluate policies and procedures to reduce retraumatization and STS and to identify, support, and refer for treatment health care workers who are symptomatic from traumatic stress.

American Academy of Pediatrics, American Academy of Pediatrics Chapters, and Academic Institutions

- Develop curricula on trauma and resilience for trainees, practicing pediatricians, and their teams.
- Support community collaboration with agencies that serve children and adolescents to create a seamless trauma-informed system of care.
- Develop and share quality improvement and maintenance of certification modules at state, chapter, and national levels.
- Develop a comprehensive research agenda for TIC in pediatric health systems.
- Partner with organizations such as the National Child Traumatic Stress Network to investigate new models of integrated care including pediatric and psychiatric telenetworks.
- Include questions about TIC in periodic surveys of pediatricians.
- Evaluate intervention and treatment strategies in collaboration with federal and state initiatives and mental health partners.
- Provide workshops, seminars, or online modules to train cross-system professionals about childhood trauma and resilience.

LEAD AUTHORS

James Duffee, MD, MPH, FAAP
Moira Szilagyi, MD, PhD, FAAP
Heather Forkey, MD, FAAP
Erin T. Kelly, MD, FAAP

COUNCIL ON COMMUNITY PEDIATRICS, 2019–2021

James Duffee, MD, MPH, FAAP, Chairperson

Kimberly G. Montez, MD, FAAP, Vice Chairperson
Kimberley J. Dilley, MD, MPH, FAAP
Andrea E. Green, MD, FAAP
Joyce Javier, MD, MPH, MS, FAAP
Madhulika Mathur, MD, MPH, FAAP
Gerri Mattson, MD, FAAP
Jacqueline L. Nelson, MD, FAAP
Mikah Owen, MD, MPH, FAAP
Kenya Parks, MD, MPH, FAAP
Christopher B. Peltier, MD, FAAP

LIAISONS

Donene Feist – *Family Voices*
Rachel Nash, MD, MPH – *Section on Pediatric Trainees*
Judith Thierry, DO, MPH, FAAP - *Committee on Native American Child Health*

STAFF

Dana Bennett-Tejes, MA, MNM

COUNCIL ON FOSTER CARE, ADOPTION, AND KINSHIP CARE EXECUTIVE COMMITTEE, 2019–2021

Sarah H. Springer, MD, FAAP, Chairperson
Moira Ann Szilagyi, MD, PhD, FAAP, Past Chairperson
Heather C. Forkey, MD, FAAP
Kristine Fortin, MD, MPH, FAAP
Mary Booth Vaden Greiner, MD, MS, FAAP
Todd J. Ochs, MD, FAAP
Anu N. Partap, MD, MPH, FAAP
Linda Davidson Sagor, MD, MPH, FAAP
Deborah L. Shropshire, MD, FAAP
Jonathan David Thackeray, MD, FAAP
Douglas Waite, MD, FAAP
Lisa Weber Zetley, MD, FAAP

LIAISONS

Jeremy Harvey – *Foster Care Alumni of America*
Wynne Shepard Morgan, MD – *American Academy of Child and Adolescent Psychiatry*

Camille Robinson, MD, FAAP – *Section on Pediatric Trainees*

STAFF

Tammy Piazza Hurley
Mary Crane, PhD, LSW
Müge Chavdar, MPH

COUNCIL ON CHILD ABUSE AND NEGLECT, 2019–2021

Suzanne B. Haney, MD, MS, FAAP, Chairperson
Andrew P. Sirotnak, MD, FAAP, Immediate Past-Chairperson
Andrea Gottsegen Asnes, MD, FAAP
Amy R. Gavril, MD, MSCI, FAAP
Rebecca Greenlee Girardet, MD, FAAP
Amanda Bird Hoffert Gilmartin, MD, FAAP
Nancy D. Heavilin, MD, FAAP
Sheila M. Idzerda, MD, FAAP
Antoinette Laskey, MD, MPH, MBA, FAAP
Lori A. Legano, MD, FAAP
Stephen A. Messner, MD, FAAP
Bethany A. Mohr, MD, FAAP
Shalon Marie Nienow, MD, FAAP
Norell Rosado, MD, FAAP

LIAISONS

Heather C. Forkey, MD, FAAP – *Council on Foster Care, Adoption, and Kinship Care*
Brooks Keeshin, MD, FAAP – *American Academy of Child and Adolescent Psychiatry*
Jennifer Matjasko, PhD – *Centers for Disease Control and Prevention*
Anish Raj, MD – *Section on Pediatric Trainees*
Elaine Stedt, MSW, ACSW – *Administration for Children, Youth and Families, Office on Child Abuse and Neglect*

STAFF

Tammy Piazza Hurley
Müge Chavdar, MPH

COMMITTEE ON PSYCHOSOCIAL ASPECTS OF CHILD AND FAMILY HEALTH, 2019–2021

Arthur Lavin, MD, FAAP, Chairperson
George L. Askew, MD, FAAP
Rebecca Baum, MD, FAAP
Evelyn Berger-Jenkins, MD, FAAP
Tiffani J. Johnson, MD, MSc, FAAP
Douglas Jutte, MD, MPH, FAAP
Arwa Abdulhaq Nasir, MBBS, MSc, MPH, FAAP

LIAISONS

Sharon Berry, PhD, ABPP, LP – *Society of Pediatric Psychology*

Edward R. Christophersen, PhD, FAAP – *Society of Pediatric Psychology*
Kathleen Hobson Davis, LSW – *Family Liaison*
Norah L. Johnson, PhD, RN, CPNP-BC – *National Association of Pediatric Nurse Practitioners*
Abigail Boden Schlesinger, MD – *American Academy of Child and Adolescent Psychiatry*
Rachel Segal, MD – *Section on Pediatric Trainees*
Amy Starin, PhD, LCSW – *National Association of Social Workers*

STAFF

Carolyn Lullo McCarty, PhD

ABBREVIATIONS

DSM-5: *Diagnostic and Statistical Manual of Mental Disorders, Fifth Edition*
DTD: developmental trauma disorder
PMTS: pediatric medical traumatic stress
PTSD: posttraumatic stress disorder
PTSS: posttraumatic stress symptoms
SSNR: safe, stable, nurturing relationship
STS: secondary traumatic stress
TIC: trauma-informed care

FINANCIAL DISCLOSURE: The authors have indicated they have no financial relationships relevant to this article to disclose.

FUNDING: No external funding.

POTENTIAL CONFLICT OF INTEREST: The authors have indicated they have no potential conflicts of interest to disclose.

REFERENCES

1. Centers for Disease Control and Prevention. Essentials for childhood: creating safe, stable, nurturing relationships and environments. Available at: https://www.cdc.gov/violenceprevention/childabuseandneglect/essentials.html. Accessed January 11, 2021

2. Center on the Developing Child. The Foundations of Lifelong Health Are Built in Early Childhood. Cambridge, MA: Center on the Developing Child at Harvard University; 2010. Available at: www.developingchild.harvard.edu. Accessed June 24, 2021

3. Merrick MT, Ford DC, Ports KA, et al. Vital signs: estimated proportion of adult health problems attributable to adverse childhood experiences and implications for prevention - 25 states, 2015–2017. *MMWR Morb Mortal Wkly Rep.* 2019;68(44):999–1005

4. Substance Abuse and Mental Health Services Administration. National Child Traumatic Stress Initiative. Available at: https://www.samhsa.gov/child-trauma. Accessed January 11, 2021

5. National Child Traumatic Stress Network. Interventions. Available at: https://www.nctsn.org/treatments-and-practices/trauma-treatments/interventions. Accessed January 11, 2021

6. Forkey H, Szilagyi M, Kelly ET, Duffee J; American Academy of Pediatrics, Council on Foster Care, Adoption, and Kinship Care, Council on Community Pediatrics, Council on Child Abuse and Neglect, and Committee on Psychosocial Aspects of Child and Family Health. Trauma-informed care. *Pediatrics.* 2021;148(2):e2021052580

7. Oral R, Ramirez M, Coohey C, et al. Adverse childhood experiences and trauma informed care: the future of health care. *Pediatr Res.* 2016;79(1–2):227–233

8. FrameWorks Institute. *Building Relationships: Framing Early Relational Health.* Washington, DC: FrameWorks Institute; 2020. Available at: https://www.frameworksinstitute.org/wp-content/uploads/2020/06/FRAJ8069-Early-Relational-Health-paper-200526-WEB.pdf. Accessed January 11, 2021

9. National Scientific Council on the Developing Child. *Supportive Relationships and Active Skill-Building Strengthen the Foundations of Resilience: Working Paper 13.* Cambridge, MA: Center for the Developing Child, Harvard University; 2015. Available at: https://developingchild.harvard.edu/resources/supportive-relationships-and-active-skill-building-strengthen-the-foundations-of-resilience/. Accessed January 11, 2021

10. Centers for Disease Control and Prevention. *Preventing Adverse Childhood Experiences: Leveraging the Best Available Evidence.* Atlanta, GA: National Center for Injury Prevention and Control, Centers for Disease Control and Prevention; 2019. Available at: https://www.cdc.gov/violenceprevention/pdf/preventingACES.pdf. Accessed January 11, 2021

11. Johnson SB, Riley AW, Granger DA, Riis J. The science of early life toxic stress for pediatric practice and advocacy. *Pediatrics.* 2013;131(2):319–327

12. McEwen BS. Stressed or stressed out: what is the difference? *J Psychiatry Neurosci.* 2005;30(5):315–318

13. Shonkoff JP, Garner AS; Committee on Psychosocial Aspects of Child and Family Health; Committee on Early Childhood, Adoption, and Dependent Care; Section on Developmental and Behavioral Pediatrics. The lifelong effects of early childhood adversity and toxic stress. *Pediatrics.* 2012;129(1). Available at: www.pediatrics.org/cgi/content/full/129/1/e232

14. Substance Abuse and Mental Health Services Administration. *SAMHSA's Concept of Trauma and Guidance for a Trauma-Informed Approach.* Rockville, MD: Substance Abuse and Mental Health Services Administration; 2014

15. Bowlby J. *A Secure Base: Parent-Child Attachment and Healthy Human Development.* New York, NY: Basic Books; 1988

16. Masten AS. Resilience theory and research on children and families: past, present and future. *J Fam Theory Rev.* 2018;10(1):12–31

17. Chen Y, VanderWeele TJ. Associations of religious upbringing with subsequent health and well-being from adolescence to young adulthood: an outcome-wide analysis. *Am J Epidemiol.* 2018;187(11):2355–2364

18. Sege R, Linkenbach J. Essentials for childhood: promoting healthy outcomes from positive experiences. *Pediatrics.* 2014;133(6) Available at: www.pediatrics.org/cgi/content/full/133/6/e1489

19. Bethell C, Davis MB, Gombojav N, Stumbo S, Powers K. *A National and Across State Profile on Adverse Childhood Experiences Among Children and Possibilities to Heal and Thrive: Issue Brief October 2017.* Baltimore, MD: Johns Hopkins Bloomberg School of Public Health; 2017

20. Felitti VJ, Anda RF, Nordenberg D, et al. Relationship of childhood abuse and household dysfunction to many of the leading causes of death in adults. The Adverse Childhood Experiences (ACE) Study. *Am J Prev Med.* 1998;14(4):245–258

21. Cronholm PF, Forke CM, Wade R, et al. Adverse childhood experiences: expanding the concept of adversity. *Am J Prev Med.* 2015;49(3):354–361

22. Sacks V, Murphey D. The prevalence of adverse childhood experiences, nationally, by state, and by race/ethnicity. 2018. Available at: https://www.childtrends.org/wp-content/uploads/2018/02/ACESBriefUpdatedFinal_ChildTrends_February2018.pdf. Accessed January 11, 2021

23. Berg KL, Shiu CS, Feinstein RT, Acharya K, MeDrano J, Msall ME. Children with developmental disabilities experience higher levels of adversity. *Res Dev Disabil.* 2019;89:105–113

24. Schüssler-Fiorenza Rose SM, Xie D, Stineman M. Adverse childhood experiences and disability in U.S. adults. *PM R.* 2014;6(8):670–680

25. Hoover DW, Kaufman J. Adverse childhood experiences in children with autism spectrum disorder. *Curr Opin Psychiatry.* 2018;31(2):128–132

26. Trent M, Dooley DG, Dougé J; Section on Adolescent Health; Council on Community Pediatrics; Committee on Adolescence; Council on Community Pediatrics; Committee on Adolescence. The impact of racism on child and adolescent health. *Pediatrics.* 2019;144(2):e20191765

27. Huynh VW. Ethnic microaggressions and the depressive and somatic symptoms of Latino and Asian American adolescents. *J Youth Adolesc.* 2012;41(7):831–846

28. Heard-Garris NJ, Cale M, Camaj L, Hamati MC, Dominguez TP. Transmitting trauma: a systematic review of vicarious racism and child health. *Soc Sci Med.* 2018;199:230–240

29. Mohatt NV, Thompson AB, Thai ND, Tebes JK. Historical trauma as public narrative: a conceptual review of how history impacts present-day health. *Soc Sci Med.* 2014;106:128–136

30. Sotero MM. A conceptual model of historical trauma: implications for public health, practice and research. *J Health Dispar Res Pract.* 2006;1(1):93–108

31. Brave Heart MYH. The historical trauma response among natives and its relationship with substance abuse: a Lakota illustration. *J Psychoactive Drugs.* 2003;35(1):7–13

32. Linton JM, Griffin M, Shapiro AJ; Council on Community Pediatrics. Detention of immigrant children. *Pediatrics.* 2017;139(5):e20170483

33. Wood LCN. Impact of punitive immigration policies, parent-child separation and child detention on the mental health and development of children. *BMJ Paediatr Open.* 2018;2(1):e000338

34. Bellis MA, Hughes K, Ford K, Ramos Rodriguez G, Sethi D, Passmore J. Life course health consequences and associated annual costs of adverse childhood experiences across Europe and North America: a systematic review and meta-analysis. *Lancet Public Health.* 2019;4(10):e517–e528

35. Jones CM, Merrick MT, Houry DE. Identifying and preventing adverse childhood experiences: implications for clinical practice. *JAMA.* 2020;323(1):25–26

36. American Psychiatric Association. *Diagnostic and Statistical Manual of Mental Disorders,* 5th ed. Washington, DC: American Psychiatric Publishing; 2013

37. D'Andrea W, Ford J, Stolbach B, Spinazzola J, van der Kolk BA. Understanding interpersonal trauma in children: why we need a developmentally appropriate trauma diagnosis. *Am J Orthopsychiatry.* 2012;82(2):187–200

38. Rahim M. Developmental trauma disorder: an attachment-based perspective. *Clin Child Psychol Psychiatry.* 2014;19(4):548–560

39. van der Kolk BA. Developmental trauma disorder. *Psychiatr Ann.* 2005;35(5):401

40. Bremness A, Polzin W. Commentary: developmental trauma disorder: a missed opportunity in DSM V. *J Can Acad Child Adolesc Psychiatry.* 2014;23(2):142–145

41. Schmid M, Petermann F, Fegert JM. Developmental trauma disorder: pros and cons of including formal criteria in the psychiatric diagnostic systems. *BMC Psychiatry.* 2013;13:3

42. Kazak AE, Kassam-Adams N, Schneider S, Zelikovsky N, Alderfer MA, Rourke M. An integrative model of pediatric medical traumatic stress. *J Pediatr Psychol.* 2006;31(4):343–355

43. Shah AN, Jerardi KE, Auger KA, Beck AF. Can hospitalization precipitate toxic

stress? *Pediatrics*. 2016;137(5):e20160204

44. Rzucidlo SE, Campbell M. Beyond the physical injuries: child and parent coping with medical traumatic stress after pediatric trauma. *J Trauma Nurs*. 2009; 16(3):130–135

45. National Child Traumatic Stress Network. Medical trauma: effects. Available at: https://www.nctsn.org/ what-is-child-trauma/trauma-types/ medical-trauma/effects. Accessed January 11, 2021

46. Watson RS, Choong K, Colville G, et al. Life after critical illness in children-toward and understanding of pediatric post-intensive care syndrome. *J Pediatr*. 2018;198:16–24

47. Goldberg R, Mays M, Halpern NA. Mitigating post-intensive care syndrome-family: a new possibility. *Crit Care Med*. 2020;48(2):260–261

48. Ari AB, Peri T, Margalit D, Galili-Weisstub E, Udassin R, Benarroch F. Surgical procedures and pediatric medical traumatic stress (PMTS) syndrome: Assessment and future directions. *J Pediatr Surg*. 2018;53(8):1526–1531

49. Landolt MA, Ystrom E, Sennhauser FH, Gnehm HE, Vollrath ME. The mutual prospective influence of child and parental post-traumatic stress symptoms in pediatric patients. *J Child Psychol Psychiatry*. 2012;53(7):767–774

50. Administration for Children and Families. Secondary traumatic stress. Available at: https://www.acf.hhs.gov/ trauma-toolkit/ secondary-traumatic-stress. Accessed January 11, 2021

51. Dyrbye LN, Shanafelt TD, Sinsky CA, et al. *Burnout Among Health Care Professionals: A Call to Explore and Address This Underrecognized Threat to Safe, High-Quality Care: Discussion Paper*. Washington, DC: National Academy of Medicine; 2017

52. Melnyk BM, Orsolini L, Tan A, et al. A national study links nurses' physical and mental health to medical errors and perceived worksite wellness. *J Occup Environ Med*. 2018;60(2): 126–131

53. Shoji K, Lesnierowska M, Smoktunowicz E, et al. What comes first, job burnout or secondary traumatic stress? Findings from two longitudinal studies from the U.S. and Poland. *PLoS One*. 2015; 10(8):e0136730

54. Paton F. Depressed nurses more likely to make medical errors. *Nursing News*. October 31, 2017. Available at: https:// nurseslabs.com/depressed-nurses-likely-make-medical-errors. Accessed June 24, 2021

55. McHugh MD, Kutney-Lee A, Cimiotti JP, Sloane DM, Aiken LH. Nurses' widespread job dissatisfaction, burnout, and frustration with health benefits signal problems for patient care. *Health Aff (Millwood)*. 2011;30(2):202–210

56. Walton M, Murray E, Christian MD. Mental health care for medical staff and affiliated healthcare workers during the COVID-19 pandemic. *Eur Heart J Acute Cardiovasc Care*. 2020;9(3):241–247

57. National Council for Behavioral Health. *Fostering Resilience and Recover: A Change Package for Advancing Trauma-Informed Primary Care*. Washington, DC: National Council for Behavioral Health; 2019. Available at: https://www. thenationalcouncil.org/wp-content/ uploads/2019/12/FosteringResilience ChangePackage_Final.pdf?daf= 375ateTbd56. Accessed January 11, 2021

58. Fallot RD, Harris M. *Creating Cultures of Trauma-Informed Care (CCTIC): A Self-Assessment and Planning Protocol Community Connections*. Washington, DC: Trauma-Informed Care Project; 2009. Available at: https://www. theannainstitute.org/CCTICSELFASSPP. pdf. Accessed June 24, 2021

59. Garg A, Boynton-Jarrett R, Dworkin PH. Avoiding the unintended consequences of screening for social determinants of health. *JAMA*. 2016;316(8):813–814

60. National Institute for Children's Health Quality. Creating a patient and family advisory council: a toolkit for pediatric practices. 2012. Available at: https:// www.nichq.org/sites/default/files/ resource-file/PFAC%20Updated.pdf. Accessed June 24, 2021. Accessed January 11, 2021

61. Benner GJ. Comprehensive trauma-informed care for the whole community: the whole child initiative model. *Educational Considerations*. 2019;44(2):8

62. Center for Healthcare Strategies. Key ingredients for successful trauma-informed care implementation. 2016. Available at: www.chcs.org/media/ ATC_whitepaper_040616.pdf. Accessed January 11, 2021

63. Rawles PD. The link between poverty, the proliferation of violence and the development of traumatic stress among urban youth in the united states to school violence. 2010. Available at: http://forumonpublicpolicy.com/Vol2010. no4/archive.vol2010.no4/ rawles.pdf. Accessed January 11, 2021

64. Garner A, Yogman M; American Academy of Pediatrics, Committee on Psychosocial Aspects of Child and Family Health, Section on Developmental and Behavioral Pediatrics, Council on Early Childhood. Preventing childhood toxic stress: partnering with families and communities to promote relational health. *Pediatrics*. 2021;148(2): e2021052582

65. Hagan JF, Shaw JS, Duncan PM, eds. *Bright Futures: Guidelines for Health Supervision of Infants, Children, and Adolescents*. 4th ed. Itasca, IL: American Academy of Pediatrics; 2017

66. National Child Traumatic Stress Network. Essential elements. Available at: https://www.nctsn.org/ trauma-informed-care/ trauma-informed-systems/healthcare/ essential-elements. Accessed January 11, 2021

67. Gleason MM, Goldson E, Yogman MW; Council on Early Childhood; Committee on Psychosocial Aspects of Child and Family Health; Section on Developmental and Behavioral Pediatrics. Addressing early childhood emotional and behavioral problems. *Pediatrics*. 2016;138(6):e20163025

68. Council on Early Childhood; Committee on Psychosocial Aspects of Child and Family Health; Section on Developmental and Behavioral Pediatrics. Addressing early childhood emotional and behavioral problems. *Pediatrics*. 2016;138(6):e20163023

69. Machtinger EL, Cuca YP, Khanna N, Rose CD, Kimberg LS. From treatment to healing: the promise of trauma-

informed primary care. *Womens Health Issues.* 2015;25(3):193–197

70. Annie E. Casey Foundation. Trauma-informed practice with young people in foster care. Issue brief #5. 2012. Available at: www.aecf.org/resources/trauma-informed-practice-with-young-people-in-foster-care/. Accessed January 11, 2021

71. Allen B, Timmer SG, Urquiza AJ. Parent-child interaction therapy as an attachment-based intervention: theoretical rationale and pilot data with adoptive children. *Child Youth Serv Rev.* 2014;47(3):334–341

72. The Chadwick Trauma-Informed Systems Dissemination and Implementation Project. Secondary traumatic stress in child welfare practice. Trauma-informed guidelines for organizations. 2016. Available at: www.chadwickcenter.com/wp-content/uploads/2017/08/stsinchildwelfare practice-trauma-informedguidelinesfo rorganizations.pdf. Accessed January 11, 2021

73. Head Start. Reflective supervision. Available at: https://eclkc.ohs.acf.hhs.gov/family-engagement/building-partnerships -guide-developing-relationships-families/ reflective-supervision. Accessed January 11, 2021

74. Children's Defense Fund. Addressing children's trauma. A toolkit for Ohio's schools. 2015. Available at: https://www.cdfohio.org/wp-content/uploads/sites/6/2018/07/addressing-childrens-trauma-issue-brief-JULY2015.pdf. Accessed June 24, 2021

75. National Child Traumatic Stress Network. Essential elements of a trauma-informed juvenile justice system. Available at: https://www.nctsn.org/sites/default/files/resources//essential_elements_trauma_informed_juvenile_justice_system.pdf. Accessed January 11, 2021

76. Chadwick Trauma-Informed Systems Project. *Creating Trauma-Informed Child Welfare Systems: A Guide for Administrators*, 2nd ed. San Diego, CA: Chadwick Center for Children and Families; 2013

77. Schilling S, Fortin K, Forkey H. Medical management and trauma-informed care for children in foster care. *Curr Probl Pediatr Adolesc Health Care.* 2015;45(10):298–305

78. Beckmann KA. Mitigating adverse childhood experiences through investments in early childhood programs. *Acad Pediatr.* 2017;17(7, suppl):S28–S29

79. Center on the Developing Child. A science-based framework for early childhood policy. Available at: https://developingchild.harvard.edu/resources/a-science-based-framework-for-early-childhood-policy/. Accessed January 11, 2021

80. Duffee JH, Mendelsohn AL, Kuo AA, Legano LA, Earls MF; Council on Community Pediatrics; Council on Early Childhood; Committee on Child Abuse and Neglect. Early childhood home visiting. *Pediatrics.* 2017;140(3):e20172150

81. Ohio START. (Sobriety, Treatment and Reducing Trauma). Available at: https://

ohiostart.org/. Accessed January 11, 2021

82. Marsac ML, Kassam-Adams N, Hildenbrand AK, et al. Implementing a trauma-informed approach in pediatric health care networks. *JAMA Pediatr.* 2016;170(1):70–77

83. Dayton L, Agosti J, Bernard-Pearl D, et al. Integrating mental and physical health services using a socio-emotional trauma lens. *Curr Probl Pediatr Adolesc Health Care.* 2016;46(12):391–401

84. Wissow LS. Introducing psychosocial trauma-informed integrated care. *Curr Probl Pediatr Adolesc Health Care.* 2016;46(12):389–390

85. Zuckerman D, ed. *Hospitals Building Healthier Communities: Embracing the Anchor Mission.* College Park, MD: The Democracy Collaborative at the University of Maryland; 2013. Available at https://community-wealth.org/content/hospitals-building-healthier-communities-embracing-anchor-mission. Accessed January 11, 2021

86. Ko SJ, Ford JD, Kassam-Adams N, et al. Creating trauma-informed systems: child welfare, education, first responders, health care, juvenile justice. *Prof Psychol Res Pr.* 2008;39(4):396–404

87. Child Welfare Information Gateway. The importance of a trauma-informed children's welfare system. 2015. Available at: https://www.childwelfare.gov/pubs/issue-briefs/trauma-informed. Accessed January 11, 2021

CLINICAL REPORT Guidance for the Clinician in Rendering Pediatric Care

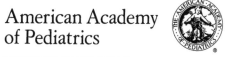

American Academy
of Pediatrics

DEDICATED TO THE HEALTH OF ALL CHILDREN™

Trauma-Informed Care

Heather Forkey, MD, FAAP,[a] Moira Szilagyi, MD, PhD, FAAP,[b] Erin T. Kelly, MD, FAAP, FACP,[c] James Duffee, MD, MPH, FAAP[d]
THE COUNCIL ON FOSTER CARE, ADOPTION, AND KINSHIP CARE, COUNCIL ON COMMUNITY PEDIATRICS, COUNCIL ON CHILD ABUSE
AND NEGLECT, COMMITTEE ON PSYCHOSOCIAL ASPECTS OF CHILD AND FAMILY HEALTH

abstract

Most children will experience some type of trauma during childhood, and many children suffer from significant adversities. Research in genetics, neuroscience, and epidemiology all provide evidence that these experiences have effects at the molecular, cellular, and organ level, with consequences on physical, emotional, developmental, and behavioral health across the life span. Trauma-informed care translates that science to inform and improve pediatric care and outcomes. To practically address trauma and promote resilience, pediatric clinicians need tools to assess childhood trauma and adversity experiences as well as practical guidance, resources, and interventions. In this clinical report, we summarize current, practical advice for rendering trauma-informed care across varied medical settings.

[a]Department of Pediatrics, University of Massachusetts, Worcester, Massachusetts; [b]Divisions of General and Developmental-Behavioral Pediatrics, Department of Pediatrics, University of California, Los Angeles, Los Angeles, California; [c]Ambulatory Health Services, Philadelphia Department of Public Health, Philadelphia, Pennsylvania; and [d]Departments of Pediatrics and Psychiatry, Boonshoft School of Medicine, Wright State University, Dayton, Ohio

Drs Forkey, Szilagyi, Kelly, and Duffee were equally responsible for conceptualizing, writing, and revising the manuscript and considering input from all reviewers and the Board of Directors; and all authors approved the final manuscript as submitted.

Clinical reports from the American Academy of Pediatrics benefit from expertise and resources of liaisons and internal (AAP) and external reviewers. However, clinical reports from the American Academy of Pediatrics may not reflect the views of the liaisons or the organizations or government agencies that they represent.

The guidance in this report does not indicate an exclusive course of treatment or serve as a standard of medical care. Variations, taking into account individual circumstances, may be appropriate.

All clinical reports from the American Academy of Pediatrics automatically expire 5 years after publication unless reaffirmed, revised, or retired at or before that time.

DOI: https://doi.org/10.1542/peds.2021-052580

Address correspondence to Heather Forkey, MD. E-mail: heather.forkey@umassmemorial.org

PEDIATRICS (ISSN Numbers: Print, 0031-4005; Online, 1098-4275).

To cite: Forkey H, Szilagyi M, Kelly ET, et al. AAP COUNCIL ON FOSTER CARE, ADOPTION, AND KINSHIP CARE, COUNCIL ON COMMUNITY PEDIATRICS, COUNCIL ON CHILD ABUSE AND NEGLECT, COMMITTEE ON PSYCHOSOCIAL ASPECTS OF CHILD AND FAMILY HEALTH. Trauma-Informed Care. Pediatrics. 2021;148(2):e2021052580

INTRODUCTION

Experiences in childhood, both positive and negative, have a significant effect on subsequent health, mental health, and developmental trajectories. For many children and adolescents, traumatic experiences are all too common. Almost one-half of American children, or 34 million younger than 18 years, have faced at least 1 potentially traumatic early childhood experience.[1-7] Such traumas may include those originating outside the home, such as community violence, natural disasters, unintentional injuries, terrorism, immigrant or refugee traumas (including detention, discrimination,[6,8,9] or racism), and/or those involving the caregiving relationship, such as intimate partner violence, parental substance use, parental mental illness, caregiver death, separation from a caregiver, neglect, or abuse, originally defined as adverse childhood experiences (ACEs).[10] For many children, medical events, such as injury, medical procedures, and/or invasive medical treatments, can be traumatic. Given the robust science explaining the physiologic consequences of accumulated trauma experiences on the brain and body,[11-14] there have been calls for pediatric clinicians to address childhood trauma and child traumatic stress.[10,14-16] However, practical guidance about how to consider, address, and operationalize this care, although necessary, has been insufficient.

Pediatric clinicians are on the front lines of caring for children and adolescents and, thus, have the greatest potential for early identification of and response to childhood trauma. Data indicate that, although pediatric providers intuitively understand the negative effects of trauma, they report a lack of knowledge, time, and resources as major barriers to providing trauma-informed care (TIC).[5,6] Yet, experts believe that the complete assessment of child and adolescent behavioral, developmental, emotional, and physical health requires consideration of trauma as part of the differential diagnosis to improve diagnostic accuracy and appropriateness of care.[17,18]

TIC is defined by the National Child Traumatic Stress Network as medical care in which all parties involved assess, recognize, and respond to the effects of traumatic stress on children, caregivers, and health care providers. This includes attention to secondary traumatic stress (STS), the emotional strain that results when an individual hears about the first-hand trauma experiences of another. In the clinical setting, TIC includes the prevention, identification, and assessment of trauma, response to trauma, and recovery from trauma as a focus of all

services. TIC can be conceptualized in a public health stratification, as summarized in Table 1:

- primary prevention of trauma and promotion of resilience;
- secondary prevention and intervention for those exposed to potentially traumatic experiences, including caregivers, siblings, guardians, and health care workers; and
- tertiary care for children who display symptoms related to traumatic experiences.

This clinical report and the accompanying policy statement[19] address secondary prevention and intervention: practical strategies for identifying children at risk for trauma and/or experiencing trauma symptoms. "Children," unless otherwise specified, refers to youth from birth to 21 years of age. These clinical strategies and skills include the following[16,20]:

- knowledge about trauma and its potential lifelong effects;
- support for the caregiver-child relationship to build resilience and prevent traumatic stress reactions;
- screening for trauma history and symptoms;
- recognition of cultural context of trauma experiences, response, and recovery;
- anticipatory guidance for families and health care workers;
- avoidance of retraumatization;

- processes for referral to counseling with evidence-based therapies when indicated; and
- attention to the prevention and treatment of STS and associated sequelae.

Pediatricians have a powerful voice and reach that could promote the policies and procedures necessary to transform pediatric health care into a TIC system. This guidance for pediatric clinicians is organized around 5 strategies for implementation to become trauma informed: awareness, readiness, detection and assessment, management, and integration. The companion policy statement[19] outlines broad recommendations for implementing TIC in child health systems.

AWARENESS

Pediatric clinicians can promote resilience, identify adversity and trauma, and ameliorate the effects of adversity in their work with children and families. Although the epidemiology and physiology of trauma have been explored in the literature,[9,12,13,21,22] few concepts have been translated into the provision of practical TIC in pediatric settings.[6,16,23] Awareness of the science and epidemiology of trauma provides the scientific grounding for the practices of TIC.

TABLE 1 Range of Trauma Experiences, Symptoms, and Response

Potentially Traumatic Experiences	Trauma Symptoms (Table 5)	Office Response
None	None to some	Primary prevention: anticipatory guidance; resilience promotion
Single-incident or minor trauma	None or latent or mild	Secondary prevention: anticipatory guidance; resilience promotion; trauma-informed guidance; close monitoring: screen for trauma history and symptoms
Major event or cumulative	Mild to moderate	Secondary and tertiary prevention: anticipatory guidance; resilience promotion; psychoeducation; trauma-informed guidance, close monitoring, and follow-up; possible referrals to community services, mental health
Major event or cumulative	Moderate to severe	Tertiary prevention and treatment: anticipatory guidance; resilience promotion; psychoeducation; trauma-informed guidance, close monitoring, and follow-up; avoidance of retraumatization; referrals to community services; referral to evidence-based and evidence-informed trauma mental health services

Adapted from Forkey H, Griffin J, Szilagyi M. *Childhood Trauma and Resilience: A Practical Guide.* Itasca, IL: American Academy of Pediatrics; 2021.

Safe, Stable, and Nurturing Relationships

The most fundamental adaptational mechanism for any child is a secure relationship with a safe, stable, nurturing adult who is continuous over time in the child's life.[24] This is usually the child's parent or caregiver but can involve extended family and biological or fictive kin. It is in the protective context of this secure relationship that the child develops the varied resilience skills that will prevent or ameliorate the effects of cumulative adversities. The nurturing caregiver protects the child from harm, mediates the world for the child, and helps the child to develop the adaptive skills to manage stressful experiences. Physiology, in addition to psychology, is affected by protective relationships.[14,25–27]

Toxic Stress and Trauma

All children experience some stress and adversity at some point in life, but when it is managed within the context of these nurturing relationships, such events can be weathered and even used for growth. Adverse events that lead to the frequent or prolonged activation of the stress response (see Fig 1) in the relative absence of protective relationships has been termed "toxic stress" in the pediatric literature.[14] Toxic stress responses result from events that may be long lasting, severe in intensity, or frequent in occurrence. The available caregiver support is insufficient to turn off the body's stress response. It is critical to note that the toxic stress response has 2 components: the significant stressors and the relative insufficiency of protective relationships. In sum, there is a marked imbalance between stressors and protective factors.[28]

Toxic stress responses can result in potentially long-lasting or lifelong impairments in physical and mental health through biological processes that embed developmental, neurologic, epigenetic, and immunologic

	Stress Responses
Freeze	• Originates in central nucleus of the amygdala and mediated by hypothalamus and superior colliculus[222]
	• Typically brief response, forces the organism to alert to danger
	• Can be followed by the fight-or-flight responses
	• Parasympathetic and vagal response can lead to dissociation or faint
Fight or flight	• Results from adrenal release of epinephrine and cortisol that allow the threat to be addressed
	• Short term: physiological changes, including increased heart rate and blood pressure
	• Excess or frequent activation in childhood can result in long-term changes in HPA axis function, which leads to dysregulation of the neuroendocrine stress response and consequent physiologic changes (see Table 2)[12,223]
Affiliate (gather social support, "tend and befriend")	• Higher brain response mediated by oxytocin,[224,225] appears to mediate stress within the social context by promoting the ability to look to others in the environment for support in managing a threat (social salience)[70,226]
	• With the provision of support, stress response declines[70,227]
	• Having no support or a hostile environment leads to negative perceptions of others, induces less adaptive responses and antisocial behaviors, and leads to increased perception of stress and increased cortisol[70,228–230]
	• Emerging science underlying the affiliative response elucidates how safe, stable, nurturing relationships can buffer adversity and promote resilience

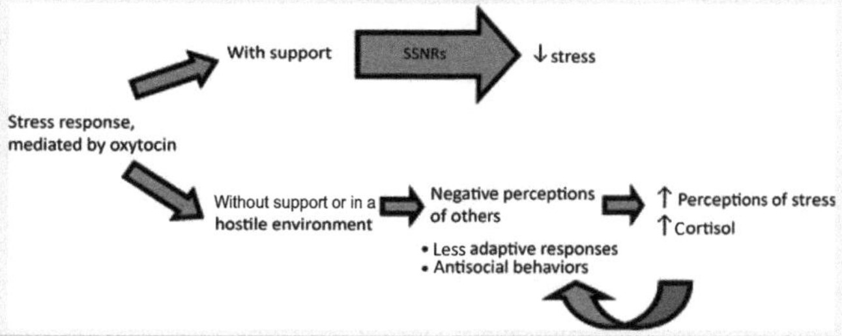

FIGURE 1 Stress responses. HPA, hypothalamic-pituitary-adrenal.

TABLE 2 Physiologic Effects of Trauma in Children

Area	Impact	Specifics	Implications and Associations
Brain connectivity[93]	Cortisol acts on rapidly developing brain structures	Amygdala overactive; hippocampus underactive; prefrontal cortex not accessible	Preliminary association with more severe clinical course in major depressive disorder
Epigenetic changes[21]	Methylation patterns impacted by threat, mediated by cortisol	Methyl groups attach to promoter region or come off promotor regions of genes, leading to the transcription or lack of transcription of genes	Adult stress and reactivity behavior[231,232]
Immune function[80]	Alteration of immune system in response to constant threat	Inflammatory system up-regulated; humoral immunity diminished; cytokine-induced "sickness behavior"[81] (feeling sick)	Symptoms including the following: decreased appetite, fatigue, mood changes including depression and irritability, poor cognitive function

changes.[12,14] The lifelong effects of toxic stress are statistically related to many adult illnesses, particularly those related to chronic inflammation, and causes for early mortality.[29] The robust literature on the physiologic effects of toxic stress is beyond the scope of this clinical report yet briefly summarized in Table 2.

Trauma is a broader term used to describe both a precipitant and a human response. The Substance Abuse and Mental Health Services Administration defines trauma as an event, series of events, or circumstances experienced by a person as physically or emotionally harmful that have long-lasting adverse effects on the person's functioning and well-being (emotional, physical, or spiritual).[16] This definition accounts for the fact that people may respond differently to potentially traumatic events and informs TIC with appreciation that the traumas people experience can result in behavioral changes that may allow them to manage the trauma in the short-term but can have lasting negative effects on conduct. These difficulties should not be viewed as malicious actions or even intentional but as consequences of adversity.[30]

Because these epidemiological and physiologic studies provide the background and impetus for TIC, understanding the terminology

derived from this literature is important in appreciating the scope, variety, and nuances of TIC and how to actualize them. These are summarized in Table 3.

High-risk Populations

It is important to be aware that the exposures of some child populations and their families put them at particular risk of experiencing trauma but also that the components of TIC can benefit these children and families.[31–34] More than 7.4 million children, or nearly 1 in 10 children, are reported as potential victims of child abuse and neglect annually.[35] In 2019, more than 670 000 children spent time in foster care.[36] Children who remain at home after child protective services investigation or are moved to kinship care resemble their peers in foster care in having an extremely high prevalence of significant childhood trauma.[37–39] Immigrant and refugee children may have left poverty, war, and violence, may have encountered abuse or separation from family members, and can be at risk for deportation, detention, and separation and discrimination.[6,40,41] Poverty, or near poverty, affects approximately 43% of US children, and both urban and rural poverty have been linked with multiple stressors and increased risk of trauma.[42–44] Children of underrepresented racial, ethnic, and religious groups are

more likely to be exposed to discrimination.[45,46] The psychological, interpersonal, and perhaps physiologic effects of trauma inflicted on a community (particularly because of race, identity, or ethnicity) may be passed to succeeding generations and is referred to as historical trauma.[47,48] Community violence and bullying, along with cyberbullying, are experienced by many children and recognized as traumatic exposures included in expanded definitions of ACEs.[49–51] Lesbian, gay, bisexual, transgender, and queer children and adolescents, children of color, American Indian and Alaskan native children, immigrant children, neurodiverse children and adolescents, and children and adolescents with overweight and obesity are all more likely to experience discrimination, both overt and as a series of microaggressions (small slights, insults, or indignities either intentional or unintentional) that accumulate over time.[52–54] Additionally, children of military families have a higher prevalence of trauma, abuse, grief, and loss.[55] Populations at higher risk for pediatric medical traumatic stress include preterm infants, children with complex and/or chronic medical conditions, and those suffering from serious injury or illness.[56] Up to 80% of children and family members experience trauma

TABLE 3 Definitions of Terminology in TIC

Terminology of Traumas	Definitions
Acute stress disorder and Post-traumatic stress disorder (PTSD)	Psychiatric diagnoses that include having experienced or witnessed a traumatic event and then having persistent symptoms that include the following: reexperiencing (intrusive thoughts, nightmares, or flashbacks); avoidance (feeling numb, refusing to talk about the event); hyperarousal (irritability, exaggerated startle response, always expecting danger); acute stress disorder: symptoms occur 3 d to 1 mo after traumatic exposure[81]; PTSD: symptoms must occur ≥3 mo after the trauma[233]
ACEs	Stressful or traumatic events, including child abuse and neglect, that occur within the primary caregiving relationship; often breach the parent-child relationship, which is fundamental to nurturing healthy development; linked in population studies to physiologic and behavioral changes impacting the health and well-being of patients over their life course with a wide array of health problems, including associations with substance misuse.[10,21,24,80] The original ACEs (from initial study published in 1998) are the following: physical abuse, sexual abuse, emotional abuse, physical neglect, emotional neglect, intimate partner violence, mother treated violently, substance misuse within household, household mental illness, parental separation or divorce, and incarcerated household member. Subsequent studies have expanded the original ACE panel to include other adversities,[9,234] including the following: experiencing racism, experiencing bullying, separation from caregiver (resulting from immigration, foster care, incarceration, death, or any other reason), witnessing violence, community violence,[49] adverse neighborhood experience,[235] and financial insecurity[236]
Complex childhood trauma (as defined by the National Child Traumatic Stress Network)	Encompasses both a child's exposure to multiple interpersonal traumatic events, including maltreatment and household dysfunction, and the broad, pervasive, and predictable impact this exposure has on the individual child[83,237]; can disrupt a child's attachment with caregivers, development, and sense of self
Developmental trauma disorder (DTD)	A proposed diagnosis based on evidence that children exposed to complex trauma are at risk for severe pervasive disruptions in their development in the domains of emotional health, physical health, attention, cognition, learning, behavior, interpersonal relationships, and sense of self; sometimes used interchangeably with complex childhood trauma; describes problems in affect dysregulation, negative self-concept, and difficulty with relationships that occur as a result of trauma-related developmental impairments; symptoms overlap or co-occur with several PTSD symptoms, but DTD includes a fuller spectrum of dysregulation resulting from the insults to multiple pathways in the developing brain when nurturing and is seen as a result of complex childhood trauma; more accurately describes the outcomes of such trauma in children than does the diagnosis PTSD[158,238]
Pediatric medical traumatic stress (PMTS)	The distress that children and family members experience during hospitalization for a perceived life-threatening diagnosis or while living with or caring for someone with life-altering chronic conditions[239–241]; often related to the person's subjective experience of the medical event rather than its objective severity and is mitigated by SSNRs that promote resilience
Secondary traumatic stress (STS)	A response that may occur in parents, other family members, and health care workers such as physicians, nurses, other hospital staff (including nonclinical staff), first responders, and therapists who are exposed to the suffering of others, particularly children[242]; may have many of the same long-term effects on health that affect children exposed to trauma; individual trauma histories can contribute to the reaction
Social determinants of health (SDoHs)	Conditions of the greater ecology or environment, occurring where people live, learn, work and play, which affect the neuroendocrine stress response and affect a wide range of health risks and outcomes[8,22]; can be mitigated by an SSNR and other protective factors and exacerbated by ACEs and intrafamilial and interpersonal traumas; examples include: poverty, food insecurity, homelessness, and lack of access to health care; examples that also overlap with the expanded ACEs include racism, discrimination, and community violence
Trauma	An event, series of events, or set of circumstances an individual experiences as physically or emotionally harmful that can have lasting adverse effects on the person's functioning and mental, physical, emotional, or spiritual well-being[14]; can occur outside caregiving relationships (eg, dog bites, natural disasters), within the context of the caregiving relationship (eg, exposure to domestic violence, various forms of abuse or disordered caregiving because of parental mental illness or substance use disorder), or in the context of relationships outside the family (racism, bias, discrimination, bullying)

symptoms after a life-threatening illness, injury, or painful medical procedure.[57]

READINESS

TIC transforms the fundamental questions in medical care from "What is wrong with you?" to "What happened to you?" and, finally, to "What's strong with you?" A trauma-informed approach acknowledges the biological effects of adversity without suggesting that childhood adversity is destiny. It requires a compassionate approach that does not suggest blame. It requires pediatric health care workers at every level to understand the context of a child's relationships, especially within the family, and ask, "What are the caregiver's strengths and challenges?" "What are the child's strengths and challenges?" and "Who supports you?" This changes the pediatric role from "I must fix you" to "I must understand you (and the relationships that created you and can help you heal)."[25,58] Thus, readiness includes an understanding of what provides resilience and how to promote it.

Relational Health Care

TIC is fundamentally relational health care, the ability to form and maintain safe, stable, and nurturing relationships (SSNRs). Pediatricians are able to support the caregiver-child relationship, the context in which there can be recovery from trauma and the restoration of resilience. Fundamental to these concepts is an understanding of attachment.

Attachment

Attachment describes the emotionally attuned give-and-take between caregiver and child and the trust, safety, and security provided to the child[59] that promotes healthy brain growth, development of accurate mental maps of self and others, development of resilience, and protection from trauma.[60] Fundamentally, the predictable compassionate availability of the caregiver promotes the secure attachment of the child.[61,62] Recent studies show attachment remains malleable beyond infancy, even into adolescence and adulthood, to some extent.[63,64]

Effective Parenting

Effective parenting encompasses the skills that caregivers bring to the task of parenting and is the context in which secure attachment develops and is relied on during and after traumatic experiences. Although caregivers approach parenting with a range of skills, attitudes, and beliefs rooted in their cultural and family contexts, studies have shown that effective or positive parenting has some universal features.[65–67]

It is through secure attachment with a predictably empathic caregiver that children learn to regulate their emotions. Children start by turning to a caregiver when upset. The caregiver comforts the child by touch, words, and compassion, which shuts down the stress response and restores emotional regulation. Secure attachment happens as a child predictably receives this sympathetic support from the caregiver when the child is distressed and the child comes to confidently anticipate that support. This relationship becomes a reliable source of safety, and the caregiver is a secure base from which the child can explore their environment.[62] Multiple studies have shown that a secure attachment relationship is the best means for building or rebuilding resilience in children; it is also the context for promoting healthy brain growth and development.[62,65,68,69] With these positive affiliative experiences, modulation of the stress response begins and includes the release of oxytocin, a potent hormone regulator of the sense of safety and well-being.[68,70]

Thus, the first step of TIC is to assess this aspect of the relationship, observing the child-caregiver interaction, including the caregiver's attention to the child, the caregiver's ability to read and respond to the child in developmentally appropriate ways, and the child's ease, comfort, and response to the caregiver. Discussion can begin by focusing on the caregiver's and child's strengths and noting the constructive aspects of the relationship while providing the caregiver with empathy. When attachment is strained, caregivers have often lost empathy for the child. The positive regard and attuned attentive listening provided before and while raising concerns supports the caregiver. The empathy provided to the caregiver thus allows the opportunity for them to reattune to the child.[62]

Resilience

Resilience is defined as a dynamic process of positive adaptation to or despite significant adversities.[71] This is not a static or innate quality but includes skills children can learn over time with reliable support from attachment figures. The development of resilience includes aptitudes that are attained through play, exploration, and exposure to a variety of normal activities and resources. Studies have shown that development can be robust, even in the face of severe adversity, if certain basic adaptational mechanisms of human development (resilience factors) are protected and in good working order. These mechanisms include attachment to a competent caregiver, cognitive development with opportunity for continued growth, mastery of age-salient developmental tasks, self-control or self-regulation, belief that life has meaning, hope for the future, a sense of self-efficacy, and a network of supportive relationships.[71] On the other hand, if those basic adaptational mechanisms or protective factors are absent or impaired before, during, or after the adversity, then the outcomes for children tend to be poorer[71] (see Table 4).

TABLE 4 Adaptational Mechanisms of Resilience

T	Thinking and learning brain, with opportunity for continued growth; cognitive development
H	Hope, optimism, faith, belief in a future for oneself
R	Regulation (self-regulation, self-control of emotions, behaviors, attention, and impulses)
E	Efficacy (self-efficacy) or sense that one can impact their environment or outcomes
A	Attachment, secure attachment relationship with safe, stable, and nurturing caregiver or competent caregiver
D	Development, mastery of age-salient developmental tasks
S	Social context, or the larger network of healthy relationships in which one lives and learns

Adapted from Masten AS. Ordinary magic. Resilience processes in development. *Am Psychol.* 2001;56(3)227–238; Forkey H, Griffin J, Szilagyi M. *Childhood Trauma and Resilience: A Practical Guide.* Itasca, IL: American Academy of Pediatrics; 2021.

Robust implementation of TIC is strength-based, building on family protective factors rather than emphasizing deficits. At almost every encounter, from early childhood through adolescence, pediatric care can include resilience promotion, building on identified strengths. Because resilience is a dynamic process of positive adaptation, routine anticipatory guidance about development or safety can be used to promote relational health and positive childhood experiences, including achievements at home, at school, and in neighborhoods, which enhance resilience.[72] When addressing adversities or concerns about development, surmounting the challenges can be framed with resilience and positive experiences as the goal.[73] For example, when speaking with a caregiver about a child learning to fall asleep on their own, sleep skills can be framed as building resilience by supporting self-regulation and self-efficacy. Alternatively, when a caregiver expresses concern about a child or teenager who had been sleeping until experiencing a traumatic event, the discussion can be framed around what resilience factors are being challenged (developmental skill mastery, self-efficacy, self-regulation) and which ones can be used to support the child's recovery (attachment and thinking).

DETECTION AND ASSESSMENT

Detection involves both surveillance and formal screening to identify children and families with the history of exposure to potentially traumatic experiences as well as those who exhibit signs and symptoms of trauma. Although TIC is common in social services and other mental health settings, in a health care environment, TIC can be conceptualized by using a medical model. Similar to other medical conditions, TIC includes purposeful triage, engagement, history-taking, surveillance and screening, examination, differential diagnosis, sharing of the diagnosis, and management, which may include office-based anticipatory guidance, referral, psychopharmacology, and/or follow-up or recommendations.

Surveillance for maladaptation after experiencing trauma includes consideration of all those who may be affected by exposure to the direct suffering of the child. Health care workers, such as first responders, nurses, social workers, trainees, physicians, and nonclinical hospital or clinic employees, may be deeply affected by witnessing or hearing about the traumatic experiences of children. Parents (biological, foster, kinship, or adoptive) are particularly at risk for prolonged trauma reactions that may impair their ability to care for and comfort their children. Siblings may also be affected, particularly when there is complex trauma or exposure to suffering, such as having a sibling with cancer or another life-altering disease that involves chronic pain.

Peri-trauma

Peri-trauma refers to situations in which medical providers are caring for children as the traumatic events are unfolding. One example is pediatric medical traumatic stress. Pediatric medical traumatic stress is a situation in which children experience medical procedures or other aspects of medical care as traumatic events. The effects of such trauma can be mitigated by attending to the child's and family's experience of medical care and reducing (as much as possible) frightening or painful aspects of necessary care and procedures. This mitigation can include asking children (and caregivers) about their fears and worries, optimizing pain management and comfort measures, and working with caregivers to increase their ability to provide effective support for their child. The Healthcare Toolbox includes a number of specific suggestions, including assessing distress (D), providing emotional support (E), and addressing the family needs (F)—a D, E, F protocol to follow the A, B, Cs of resuscitation.[74]

Another comprehensive strategy used by schools and community agencies when a mass trauma or disaster occurs is Psychological First Aid (PFA).[75] Developed by the National Child Traumatic Stress Network, PFA is an evidence-informed program that is designed to help children, families, adults, and other witnesses in the immediate aftermath of a disaster or terror event. Core skills for implementation of PFA are identical to TIC: establish an emotionally safe environment, connect with primary support persons (relational health), link to community resources, and provide psychoeducational materials to help understand the potential responses of children to the exposure.

Triage

The first step in medical care is to identify an emergency versus nonemergency situation. When dealing with trauma, its causes, or its consequences, consideration of whether a child may be emergently at risk requires assessment and response as a top priority. In practicing TIC, protocols and practices to identify and address child or family safety issues, both physical and psychological, are integral to care.

Trauma may result from children being in unsafe settings because of abuse, neglect, or impaired caregiving. When the practitioner suspects maltreatment or failure of the caregiver to protect a child at any point in a health encounter, referral to child protective services is necessary and mandated. These issues need to be considered even before screening and addressed with standard protocols to respond to identified risks.[76–78]

Other immediate safety issues may arise when a consequence of trauma is self-harm or intent to injure others. Screening for suicidality, self-injury, or intent to harm others is included in TIC along with clear protocols for how to address positive endorsement of these issues.

Engagement

TIC creates a respectful and emotionally safe space in which to engage children, adolescents, and families around the discussion and management of these issues and to prevent retraumatization. Discussion of trauma may raise stress levels, and appropriate engagement reassures the child and family that the setting is safe. Culture can also affect how trauma is experienced and understood by families, and cultural awareness can ease the conversation. Engaging children and families begins with greeting the patient and family and being fully present in the moment while maintaining a balance between professionalism and friendliness. It involves initially asking open-ended questions, followed by more specific and probing questions as needed and that are elicited by caregiver and child or adolescent responses. It involves listening in an active, nonjudgmental, attuned way, reflecting back to the family what is heard for clarification and confirmation, seeking clarification when necessary, paraphrasing, attending to and reflecting on the emotions that accompany the information, and summarizing what is discussed. Implicit bias can affect the provider's ability to be nonjudgmental in these conversations.[46,79] Acceptance,

curiosity, and empathy are conveyed to the patient or caregiver in the process of attentive listening.[61] Engagement also involves mutual regard between the provider and family. Adolescents and capable children bring their own perspective. Each brings expertise to the TIC of the child or adolescent. The provider has expertise in medicine, whereas the patient and family have expertise about the child, what happened, and their situation, beliefs, strengths, and culture.

When working with families and patients who have experienced trauma, the provider's body language, affect, and tone of voice can promote or inhibit care. Affect describes the facial and body expressions that reflect our emotional state. Individuals who have experienced trauma are more sensitive to body language, facial expressions, and tone of voice.[70] Approaching children slowly and calmly or letting them sit with a caregiver and using higher pitched, more musical speech may ease a child's tension because these sounds are associated with the release of oxytocin in the amygdala, resulting in calming of this threat-sensitive brain area. A shift to low tones during a discussion may alert a child or caregiver to potential danger and stimulate defensive responses.[61]

History

Much of the information needed to integrate TIC into practice may be obtained as part of the routine health evaluation. Social, developmental, and medical history are all opportunities to identify risks, stressors, and strengths. The health history provides an opportunity to assess child and family resilience factors, social connectedness, parenting attitudes, and skills. The review of systems allows the medical provider to

collect symptoms of trauma that may not have been identified in the chief complaint but that can offer valuable insight into the current impact of trauma on the patient.[80,81] Symptoms may be functional, neurodevelopmental, or related to immune function.

1. Functional symptoms: Manifestation of the symptoms of trauma may evolve over time. Functional complaints can result after single-incident traumas (eg, automobile crash, hurricane) or may be early manifestations of complex trauma.[82–84] Sleep difficulty, changes in appetite, toileting concerns (eg, constipation, abdominal pain or enuresis), and challenges with school functioning (eg, poor attention or attendance) may be the early presentation of ongoing trauma.[84,85] Diagnostic criteria for attention-deficit/hyperactivity disorder and adjustment disorder overlap with some of these functional symptoms. When these signs and symptoms are noted, it can be useful to include trauma in the differential diagnosis.[17,86,87]

2. Neurodevelopmental symptoms: Some of the most recognizable manifestations of early trauma result from the effect on areas of the rapidly developing brain of young children. Developmental skill acquisition (higher brain) can be hindered as recognition of and response to threat is prioritized (lower brain).[88,89] Specific areas of the brain affected are the limbic system, hippocampus, and prefrontal cortex.[12,13,90–92] The prefrontal cortex is involved in cognition, emotional regulation, attention, impulse control, and executive function. Consequently, children may have developmental delay and behave as if they are younger than their actual age[89,93] (see Table 5 for an easy way to remember these effects). Other

TABLE 5 Most Common Symptoms of Trauma Exposure

F	Frets (anxiety and worry) and fears
R	Regulation difficulties (disorders of behaviors or emotions; hyperactive, impulsive, easily becomes aggressive or emotional; inattentive)
A	Attachment challenges (insecure attachment relationships with caregivers); poor peer relationships
Y	Yawning (sleep problems) and yelling (aggression, impulsivity)
E	Educational and developmental delays (especially cognitive, social-emotional, and communication)
D	Defeated (hopeless), depressed, or dissociated (separated from reality of moment, lives in own head)

Adapted from Forkey H, Griffin J, Szilagyi M. *Childhood Trauma and Resilience: A Practical Guide*. Itasca, IL: American Academy of Pediatrics; 2021.

observed symptoms may include the following:

- rapid, reflexive response to stimuli, reminders, or triggers[93,94];
- inattention, poor focus, hyperactivity, and difficulty completing tasks[86,95];
- difficulty tolerating negative mood so the child seeks ways to defuse the tension through hyperactivity, impulsive behaviors, aggression, self-harm, such as cutting and suicidality, or engagement in health risk behaviors (substance use, sexual activity)[89,95,96];
- reactions to stimuli, triggers, or reminders can be transient and flip suddenly back to "normal"; this appears to the observer as emotional lability[88,92]; and
- negative world view and self-narrative; flat affect; difficulty engaging socially or viewing themselves as worthless.[88,92,97]

3. Immune function symptoms: When a child is exposed to early, severe, or prolonged trauma, the immune system is chronically pressed into action, and, over time, changes can occur in the inflammatory system and humoral immunity.[80,89] A persistent inflammatory response can leave children vulnerable to diseases, such as asthma and metabolic syndrome.[80,98,99] Humoral immunity may be impaired so that children are more susceptible to infection. Additionally, immune system stimulation may result in the "sick syndrome," which is a perception of feeling unwell that can include headaches, stomachaches, and lethargy.[80,81]

Surveillance

Surveillance or monitoring is the process of recognizing children who might be at risk for being affected by trauma and is modeled after developmental surveillance. Surveillance is less formal than screening and can be conducted at every visit. Asking about caregivers' concerns, obtaining a trauma history, observing the child, and identifying risk and protective factors provides information about resilience supports and trauma exposure.[100] Surveillance requires attention to relationships and engagement. Questions such as "Has anything scary or concerning happened to you or your child since the last visit?" are a way to more specifically explore the possibility of adverse experiences.[85] Recognizing that certain symptoms may indicate exposure to childhood adversities, we can ask, "What has happened to you (or your family)?" For adolescents, these questions can be asked as part of the HEADSSS (questions about Home environment, Education and employment, Eating, peer-related Activities, Drugs, Sexuality, Suicide/depression, and Safety) psychosocial interview.[101,102] Questions that are considered less threatening are asked first and followed with questions that may be perceived as more intrusive.[101] Providers may be concerned that asking questions about a family's needs, a child's trauma history, or a child's symptoms may distress the child or caregiver, but studies in which this topic has been explored indicate that, when the topic is raised, families respond well to having the issues acknowledged and addressed in a supportive setting.[85,103,104]

Children only heal from trauma in the context of SSNRs, so it is also necessary to ask about the strengths that are already present in the family. Starting these conversations with questions about child, adolescent, or family strengths frames the conversation in a positive and resilience-focused way.[105,106] For instance, a clinician may ask how the child, adolescent, or family copes with stress, what a teenager does well, whether they have frequent family meetings to talk about solving problems, and whether each member of the family has someone to turn to for safety and comfort when they are upset. Trauma that occurs because of problems in the primary attachment relationship represents the greatest threat to the child or adolescent and may be the most challenging for providers to explore. Caregivers may have their own trauma histories or mental health struggles, substance use issues, and/or multiple stressors related to social determinants of health (SDoHs), including poverty, housing instability, and violence exposure that affect their parenting. Exploring parenting stressors, strengths, and attitudes in conversation can help the provider to pinpoint specific leverage points to help children but may also create an opportunity for the caregiver to reflect about the effects of their parenting or stressors on the child. TIC is compassionate and assumes that all caregivers love their children and are doing the best they can. It also assumes that children are doing the best they can.[107,108] Adolescents should be included in these conversations and have a role in identifying strengths and challenges. Pediatricians who have cared for a family over time may already have considerable insight into the family's dynamics and be able to engage the caregivers in an empathic yet open conversation. Furthermore, compassionate surveillance can be combined with use of screeners or questionnaires to elicit more information.

Screening

Validated screeners used at preventive health care visits can provide valuable information about child development, mental health, and behavior.[109] They can be reassuring when normal or alert the pediatric provider to symptoms or risks when borderline or abnormal. Commonly used tools, such as the Ages and Stages Questionnaire,[110] the Pediatric Symptom Checklist,[111] the Strengths and Difficulties Questionnaire,[112] and the Patient Health Questionnaire-9[113] may elicit symptoms that are the possible result of trauma (developmental delays, social-emotional problems, anxiety, etc). Perinatal depression screening may not only identify symptoms of this illness but provide opportunities to explore maternal stressors and strengths.[114] Those exposed to known traumas can be evaluated by using standardized posttraumatic stress disorder (PTSD) screening tools such as the PTSD Reaction Index Brief Form,[115] and those exposed to medical traumas can be evaluated by using a tool such as the Psychosocial Assessment Tool.[116,117] The Pediatric Traumatic Stress Screening Tool in the Intermountain Care Process Model has been recently developed to screen for pediatric traumatic stress in the primary care setting, either as a universal screen or with targeted screening when

traumas are known.[118] These tools effectively help identify the diagnostic criteria for PTSD, although they are not designed to identify the full spectrum of symptoms of complex trauma (developmental trauma disorder [DTD]).

Screening, per American Academy of Pediatrics (AAP) guidelines, suggests using instruments that are standardized and validated and have defined psychometric properties (sensitivity, specificity, positive predictive value). By that definition, there are currently no screening tools for ACEs and only a few validated screening tools for SDoHs. However, standardized (but not validated) tools are being used in some pediatric settings to assess ACEs and SDoHs and are using aggregate risk scoring to target providing increased support.[119–121] Many of the available screening tools expanded on the domains included in the original Centers for Disease Control and Prevention/ Kaiser ACE study to include additional items applicable to urban and minority populations, including witnessing neighborhood violence and experiencing bullying or discrimination.[9] Parental ACE screening may offer the opportunity to align with caregivers and build a partnership to explore issues that may be affecting their parenting. Indeed, several recent studies suggest that parental ACEs can be linked with concerning outcomes for children.[122–125] Concurrent resilience screening offers the opportunity to identify protective factors that can buffer identified stressors, thus providing more nuanced understanding of a child's risk. Screening also offers the opportunity to then frame the discussion around promoting strengths in the caregiver-child relationship to protect a child from toxic stress and build adaptive

skills.[107] Similar to ACE screening, there are few available standardized validated resilience screening tools, although the Connor-Davidson Resilience Scale[126] and Brief Resilience Scale[127] assess caregiver resilience.[128] (Readers are referred to the AAP Screening Technical Assistance Web site at https://www.aap.org/en-us/ advocacy-and-policy/ aap-health-initiatives/Screening/ Pages/About-Us.aspx for developmental and SDoH screening tools.)

A limitation of ACE and SDoH screening tools is their lack of nuance: they identify risk factors that have been derived from epidemiological studies, not outcomes at the individual level.[129,130] Those outcomes are the result of the physiologic response to adversities. Although currently only available in the research setting, biomarkers of this physiologic response have the potential to be more accurate measures of the effects of adversity at the individual level.[131–133] Eventually, clinic-friendly, noninvasive biomarkers could also be used to identify patient-specific response to both stressors and therapeutic interventions.[134,135]

Screening health care workers for the effects of hearing about and addressing the trauma experiences of others is most commonly achieved with informal self-assessment strategies to identify symptoms or experiences that may be associated with burnout or STS.[136] Substance use disorder, depression, and suicidality may be associated with exposure to secondary trauma, and there appears to be overlap between burnout and STS.[137–144] An example of a screening tool for health care workers is the Professional Quality of Life Scale,[145] which includes subscales for compassion satisfaction, burnout, and STS.

Cultural considerations affect all aspects of TIC, including screening. Instruments that are not normed for the population or translated and validated in the language of the patient and family can result in misleading results. Thus, it is important to consider screening results cautiously with consideration of the family's culture and ethnicity in relation to the screening tool being used.[146]

Examination

Blood pressure measurement at preventive health visits or when stress is a potential etiologic factor for concerns is indicated.[147] Elevated blood pressure may be the first symptom of childhood traumatic stress, especially as youth age.[148,149] Abnormalities in hearing, vision, and growth parameters can be clues to adversities.[150,151] Overweight and obesity have been associated with ACEs.[152-154] Physical examination may reveal signs of neglect or abuse. The immunologic effect of trauma may result in inflammatory or infectious consequences identifiable on examination.[1,80,99,155,156] Children who have sustained cumulative ACEs and traumas may exhibit certain common behaviors the provider may witness during physical and mental health evaluation (refer to history and symptoms described earlier).

Differential Diagnosis Considerations and Comorbidities

The provider is encouraged to consider trauma as a possible etiology in the assessment of developmental, mental health, behavioral, and physical symptoms in all pediatric encounters because of the following: (1) the experience of adversity is so common; (2) the symptoms of trauma overlap with the symptoms of other common pediatric conditions[87,95]; and (3) failure to do so might lead to an

incorrect or incomplete diagnosis and treatment, enabling the effects of trauma to further embed.[17,157,158] Trauma may be mistaken for other conditions, such as attention-deficit/hyperactivity disorder, and includes symptoms that overlap with other diagnostic categories, such as anxiety and depression.[86,87,159] It has been proposed that trauma may result in a different "ecophenotype" of common conditions that have a different trajectory and different response to common treatments.[93] Children may also have comorbid conditions, such as ADHD, anxiety, depression, or developmental and learning issues, because they frequently accompany childhood trauma. A more detailed description of diagnoses that are commonly confused with trauma or comorbid with it are covered in the AAP clinical report "Children Exposed to Maltreatment: Assessment and the Role of Psychotropic Medication."[87]

Diagnostic Continuum

Pediatric providers may encounter children with a wide range of symptoms resulting from trauma. As noted, trauma can result in short-term changes in behavior or have a more lasting impact depending on the child, the trauma itself, and the supports or emotional buffers in a child's life. When traumatic events are more severe, prolonged, or less buffered by a caregiver, effects on various aspects of functioning can be more severe.[1,160-163] Children exposed to chaotic households, abuse, or neglect, especially in the early years of life, may have more severe symptoms and symptoms that evolve over time.[94,159,164,165] Diagnostically, this may result in children who have functional symptoms (short-term problems with sleeping, eating, toileting), adjustment disorder, PTSD, or complex trauma symptoms.[163,166,167]

MANAGEMENT

Sharing the Diagnosis With Children and Caregivers

Some parents and caregivers may come to understand the role of adversities in their child's symptoms through discussion of the trauma history and symptoms, and others will require the provider to explain this connection before they can appreciate the provider's advice and recommendations. Psychoeducation is the first step in management of childhood trauma and includes empathic, nonjudgmental sharing of diagnostic information and provider concerns about the etiology of a child's symptoms The provider's role is to integrate the child or adolescent and caregiver's concerns, the child or adolescent's symptoms, and elements of a thorough history and examination into an explanation of why this raises a concern about trauma exposure or why trauma may be the underlying cause or one of the causes of a child's symptoms, much as is done for any diagnosis. A simple explanation of the pathophysiology of trauma may help the caregiver to move from frustration with the child or adolescent's behaviors or symptoms to empathy. In some situations, the explanation may also provide the caregiver with insight into their own history of trauma and its impact on their parenting behaviors or responses to their child's behaviors, or how an event that affected their child may have traumatized the caregiver as well.

Psychoeducation includes acknowledging that a trauma history can affect behavior and thoughts, with some discussion of how that happens. Table 6 has information on specific psychoeducation. The variable responses of children to trauma can be frustrating or confusing. Discussion of the emerging data on the biological sensitivity to context may be useful

TABLE 6 Responses to Trauma to Explain to Caregivers: Psychoeducation

Impacts of Trauma on Function and Behavior	Clinical Presentation
Changes in auditory processing	Children may lose the ability to hear sounds of safety (musical high-pitched voice) and be preferentially attuned to low-pitched sounds that warn of caregiver depression and anger.[247]
Changes in how children interpret facial expressions	Children may misinterpret the affects and emotions of others, particularly confusing anger and fear.[93]
Limited vocabulary for emotions	Children may also not accurately recognize or express their own emotions, leading them to act out or respond in ways that seem "off." What a child (or caregiver) identifies as "anger" may be disappointment, frustration, fear, grief, or anxiety.[88]
Negativity	Trauma results in children having overactive limbic systems with a focus on safety and a presumption of danger. This can result in strong negative reactions as the first response to a stimulus that might be benign or ambiguous.[61]
Triggers	Triggers can be physical (smells or sounds that recall details of the trauma) or emotional (feeling embarrassed or shamed, recalling how child felt during abuse). Prevention of exposures to reminders or triggers is the best approach. Triggers may be subtle, so educating and assisting caregivers with their identification is key. This helps caregivers understand a child's response.[167]
Learned Behavior	Behaviors that were adaptive for a child in a previous environment may be maladaptive in their current environment. These behaviors can evoke some of the same reactions from caregivers that the child experienced with other adults, reinforcing a familiar pattern of interactions that may not be productive in the new setting.[61]

Adapted from the National Child Traumatic Stress Network. Families and caregivers. Available at: https://www.nctsn.org/audiences/families-and-caregivers. Accessed January 11, 2021;[243] US Department of Health and Human Services, Administration for Children and Families. Resources on trauma for caregivers and families. Available at: https://www.childwelfare.gov/topics/responding/trauma/caregivers/. Accessed January 11, 2021[244]; and American Academy of Pediatrics. Parenting After Trauma: Understanding Your Child's Needs. Available at: https://www.aap.org/en-us/advocacy-and-policy/aap-health-initiatives/healthy-foster-care-america/Documents/FamilyHandout.pdf. Accessed June 24, 2021[245].

to caregivers.[168,169] Genetic variations in how a person responds to stress may contribute to a child's sensitivity to adversity.[170] Yet, those with high reactivity who are supported and learn to channel that reactivity to positive activities and passions may have the greatest potential.[168] This information, along with specific suggestions about how to support children, can address some of the consternation of caregivers regarding children's heterogeneous responses to both adversity and interventions.

Office-Based Anticipatory Guidance and Management

Trauma-informed anticipatory guidance provided by pediatricians can help families promote resilience and begin to address the effects of trauma. If screening for SDoHs is being conducted and/or social needs are identified, referral to applicable community-based services is indicated (eg, food bank, pro bono legal aid, etc). Having a list of community providers, such as Early Head Start, Head Start, evidence-based maternal, infant, and early childhood home visiting programs,

state Maternal Child Health Title V programs, and Family to Family Health Information Centers ready for distribution, directly contacting the referral provider with the patient present, or providing formal care coordination all facilitate family engagement and help families connect to needed community resources. For older children and adolescents, trauma-informed schools and teenager crisis centers may be available in the community. In trauma-informed schools, personnel at all levels have a basic realization about trauma and an understanding of how trauma affects student learning and behavior in the school environment.[171,172]

Every encounter in an office setting, from those with young children to those with adolescents, is an opportunity to strengthen the attachment between a child and caregiver.[173] Through techniques such as reinforcing positive back-and-forth interactions between a parent and a child (serve and return), helping the caregiver to understand the child's experience (keeping the child's mind in mind),

helping the children to learn words to describe a variety of emotions, and promoting self-reflection concerning the caregiver's own trauma history, the pediatric clinician can render primary prevention against the development of anxious and maladaptive attachment patterns and promote regulation.[82,174] Examples of relevant anticipatory guidance include advice, resources, or referrals to community programs, including Reach Out and Read[175–177]; developmentally appropriate play with others[178–180]; promoting positive, authoritative (in contrast to punitive or authoritarian) parenting styles[181–183]; and mindfulness.[184–186] Table 7 includes specific advice to promote regulation after trauma.

Referral for Treatment

The presence of complex symptoms, mental health diagnoses, substance abuse, and/or a significant trauma history are indications for referral to evidence-based trauma-informed mental health services.

TABLE 7 Anticipatory Guidance

	Office-Based Guidance to Promote Regulation After Trauma
Restoring safety	To reduce the stress response after trauma, caregivers can: repeatedly assure a child or teenager that they are safe now; allow the youth to express how they feel and listen attentively; provide extra physical contact (if appropriate) with hugs, touch, and rocking for younger children.
Routines	Routines or rituals also help reduce the stress response after the unpredictability and chaos of trauma by restoring a sense of order. Caregivers can use visual (pictorial schedule or charts) and verbal cues for well-defined mealtimes, sleep times, and rituals ("Before bed, we are going to brush teeth, read a story, sing a song, and then turn lights out"). Preparing children for changes in routines, or, for the child in foster care or the child of separated or divorced parents, for visitation, can reduce stress responses.
Relaxation techniques	Provide information verbally, with printed instructions or on phone apps that guide relaxation, meditation, and mindfulness. Refer to community programs that provide training in belly breathing, guided imagery, meditation, mindfulness, yoga, stretching, and massage, which can help to reduce the fight-or-flight responses and symptoms.[247]
Time-in or special time	Dedicated, child-chosen or child-directed play with a caregiver. Caregiver chooses a time that works for them and plans to spend 10 to 30 min with the child in fun activity of child's choosing. For infant or toddler, reading time is a good example of "time-in." Recommended for children from early childhood through adolescence.
Small successes	Children who experience trauma may have delays in skill development. Expectations may need to be tailored to the child's developmental level rather than actual age. It may take lots of repetition and practice before a skill or behavior is learned, so it is useful to celebrate and reward small steps toward desired behaviors.
Emotional container	Child may have strong emotions if reminded of trauma, and the emotions may be directed at the caregiver, although they are usually not about the caregiver. Caregiver needs to remain calm to model self-regulation and avoid retraumatizing the child.
Cognitive triangle	Thoughts impact feelings, which then impact behavior, which then reimpacts thoughts. For example, if children worry they cannot fall asleep, they will then feel nervous and stressed, and then not be able to fall asleep, reinforcing their cognitive belief that they cannot fall asleep. Similarly, if children think no one likes them, they will feel rejected and may lash out at another child, leading to rejection by that child and reinforcing their belief that they are not liked. It can help to identify this triangle and break the link between thoughts and emotions (through new experiences that link thought with different emotions) and/or the link between the emotions and the behavior ("It is ok to feel ___, but it is better to do ___ than to do ___." This technique involves labeling the emotions and teaching an alternative behavior.)
Distraction	Children who are dysregulating may benefit from distraction from the traumatic thoughts by suggesting a game, music, calling a friend, or deep breathing in a calm environment.
Positive parenting techniques	Positive parenting techniques have to be adapted to the age and developmental stage of the child, but they are principles that are known to work: (1) helping children identify and name their emotions; the next step for the child is to understand the emotion and then to learn healthy ways to express the emotion and build regulation skills; (2) reassuring safety and keeping the child safe both emotionally and physically; (3) attuned, attentive listening, which starts in infancy with "serve and return" but evolves into conversational exchanges over time; (4) setting appropriate boundaries and providing guidance through connecting and listening with children; it is best to teach rather than tell or command; for example, "We draw on paper, not on walls, because it is hard to wash markers off the walls"; (5) catching the child being good and offering the child positive, specific praise for good behaviors; (6) implementing rewards and privileges to create opportunities to develop skills; start small so the child can earn a reward quickly and then build up; (7) using positive language instead of "no" commands: for example, "We color on paper, not on the table," is a better way to approach a child who is drawing on the table than, "Stop that," Or, "we use gentle hands—we don't hit others"; (8) being a good role model as child mimics what they see rather than what they are told; (9) having some fun together as a family (time-in): read, talk, sing, play; (10) reinforcing positive skills as they develop: cooperation, politeness, appropriate assertiveness, kindness, etc; and (11) the law of natural consequences: sometimes the best lesson is letting the consequences play out (not cleaning your room means it will be a mess when your friends come over).

Adapted from Camoirano A. Mentalizing makes parenting work: a review about parental reflective functioning and clinical interventions to improve it. *Front Psychol.* 2017;8:14; Zuckerman B, Augustyn M. Books and reading: evidence-based standard of care whose time has come. *Acad Pediatr.* 2011;11(1)11–17; Zuckerman B, Khandekar, A. Reach Out and Read: evidence based approach to promoting early child development. *Curr Opin Pediatr.* 2010;22(4):539–544; Needlman R, Toker KH, Dreyer BP, Klass P, Medelsohn AL. Effectiveness of a primary care intervention to support reading aloud: a multicenter evaluation. *Ambul Pediatr.* 2005;5(4)209–215; Mendelsohn AL, Cates CB, Weisleder A, et al. Reading aloud, play, and social-emotional development. *Pediatrics.* 2018;141(5):e20173393; Shah R, DeFrino D, Kim Y, Atkins M. Sit Down and Play: a preventive primary care-based program to enhance parenting practices. *J Child Fam Stud.* 2017;26(2):540–547; Chang SM, Grantham-McGregor SM, Powell CA, et al. Integrating a parenting intervention with routine primary health care: a cluster randomized trial. *Pediatrics.* 2015;136(2)272–280; Girard LC, Doyle O, Tremblay RE. Maternal warmth and toddler development support for transactional models in disadvantaged families. *Eur Child Adolesc Psychiatry.* 2017;26(4):497–507; Weisleder A, Cates CB, Dreyer BP, et al. Promotion of positive parenting and prevention of socioemotional disparities. *Pediatrics.* 2016;137(2):e20153239; Shah R, Kennedy S, Clark MD, Bauer SC, Schwartz A. Primary care-based interventions to promote positive parenting behaviors: a meta-analysis. *Pediatrics.* 2016;137(5)e20153250; Perry-Parrish C, Copeland-Linder N, Webb L, Sibinga EMS. Mindfulness-based approaches for children and youth. *Curr Probl Pediatr Adolesc Health Care.* 2016;46(6):172–178; Bauer CCC, Caballero C, Scherer E, et al. Mindfulness training reduces stress and amygdala reactivity to fearful faces in middle-school children. *Behav Neurosci.* 2019;133(6):569–585; Ortiz R, Sibinga EM. The role of mindfulness in reducing the adverse effects of childhood stress and trauma. *Children (Basel).* 2017;4(3):16; Forkey H, Griffin J, Szilagyi M. Childhood Trauma and Resilience: A Practical Guide. Itasca, IL: American Academy of Pediatrics; 2021.

The most effective therapies are evidence-based treatments (EBTs) with demonstrated efficacy for children who have experienced trauma.[85,187,188] Treatments that are designated as evidence based have had the most rigorous evaluation, whereas evidence-informed treatments range from newly emerging practices that are building evidence support to less rigorously studied tools. Sege et al[189] published an overview of evidence-based individual and family-based psychotherapeutic interventions. Gleason et al[190] specifically outlined services for the treatment of young children. Having these services available on-site or through direct communication with colleagues in mental health (a "warm handoff") has been revealed to be the most effective approach.[191] It is important for caregivers who have their own history of trauma to seek individual therapy, and the pediatric provider may find it useful to have a list of adult mental health providers who address trauma. As research continues to elucidate the neurocognitive basis of trauma symptoms and methods to address those effects, new treatment modalities are being developed and may offer increased therapeutic resources for both adults and children.[192–194]

Even if therapies are not available on-site, it is useful to familiarize self and staff with evidence-based trauma therapies, how they work, how to refer locally and how to incorporate principals of treatment into pediatric anticipatory guidance. A quick reference for EBTs that includes a brief description of each and the level of evidence can be found on the California Evidence-Based Clearinghouse for Child Welfare (http://www.cebc4cw.org/). Some EBTs have been successfully adapted for telehealth,[195,196] and, in the wake of the coronavirus disease

2019 pandemic, opportunities for EBT via telehealth have expanded.[197] Telehealth is a mechanism to provide EBT in rural and other underresourced communities.[196]

Psychopharmacology

No medication, to date, is approved by the US Food and Drug Administration for trauma-specific symptoms or PTSD in children and adolescents. Medications may be judiciously considered for specific symptoms that are interfering with a child's ability to function normatively in specific ways.[72] Readers are referred to the AAP clinical report "Children Exposed to Maltreatment: Assessment and the Role of Psychotropic Medication" for discussion of medication use in identified comorbid mental health conditions.[87]

Role of Close Follow-up and Support

A commitment to working with the family over time may prevent or reduce feelings of abandonment or rejection, especially when community and mental health resources are in short supply. The pediatric provider who is continuous over time can continue to listen attentively and offer practical trauma-informed advice that reinforces resilience building and healing. Obtaining consent to share information with a mental health provider may also be reassuring to the caregiver or patient even after a referral and linkage to mental health care is established.

Integration

Once these aspects of care are part of a provider's repertoire of care, integrating knowledge about trauma into policies and procedures and daily practice are the next steps in creating a trauma-informed medical setting.[198,199]

Train All Staff in TIC

All staff, from schedulers to billers to nurses and care coordinators, can benefit from training in TIC that is thorough and discipline specific and includes information about physiology, presentation, recognition, and response.[15,200,201] This training would ideally promote patient empowerment and include caregiver and patient perspectives.

Implementing TIC in any setting is effective when there is consideration of clinic workflow to maintain efficiency. Specific strategies can include a warm and welcoming waiting room, clear communication of expectations and procedures, and providing choices when possible (eg, do you want blood pressure taken on right arm or left?).[201] As noted earlier, the care of a child who has experienced trauma requires an approach that is similar to addressing other health concerns. TIC can include members of the staff, all aware of and empowered to emphasize safety, patient self-efficacy, and a trauma-informed approach.[15,201] Use of formalized training in TIC for all staff has been found to be effective in changing staff-reported beliefs and behaviors for caregivers of children in residential care[202,203,204] and in improving child functioning and behavioral regulation.[204] In pediatrics, training of pediatrics residents caring for substance-exposed infants in TIC was effective at changing attitudes and improving therapeutic relationships.[205]

Office personnel may engage with caregivers and patients in ways that trigger strong emotions, especially if they themselves have experienced adversity or trauma. Financial considerations, scheduling, and conflict in the small spaces of an office can also be explored from a TIC perspective. Personnel would ideally engage in some planning about how to handle a crisis or difficult situations that occasionally arise, such as the following: patients or caregivers who are indifferent or shut down, demanding, provocative, rejecting or hostile, or inattentive and distracted; or a child who is out of control and threatening to elope from the office. It is helpful to monitor one's own response when difficult situations arise and resist the urge to be angry or retaliate. It is less provocative to focus or comment on the emotion than the behavior: "I can see that you are angry, worried, sad, upset, etc," or "You probably don't want to be here right now." These responses are more affiliative and can help to shut down the stress response of the patient or caregiver whose fight-or-flight response may have been triggered by the health care setting, the interaction, or the medical stressor.

Integrated Health Care

Many providers find that the most efficient TIC can be provided by integrating physical and mental health services and social supports. Integrated care has been found to increase social-emotional screening rates[206] through colocation of services with clear strategies for medical provider introduction of the patient to the behavioral health consultant in real-time (warm handoff), by reducing the stigma of a mental health referral, or through facilitated or prearranged referral protocols.[191,207] Financial and staffing resource issues vary significantly by region, but investigating opportunities for primary care and mental health integration, social work, and/or formal engagement of referral sources and partnering organizations may increase the efficiencies of TIC. Providing case management to address the social modifiers of health (eg, referral to food bank, legal aid) can help to increase family resilience and

prevent the consequences of trauma. Referring to resources has been revealed to be associated with increased employment, use of child care, and a decrease in the use of homeless shelters.[208]

Two-Generation Approach

Growing evidence has linked increasing parental ACE scores and negative effects on child health and development,[122,123,125,209] providing compelling evidence that taking a 2-generation approach is important. Families may customarily live in multigenerational family units, and this is a cultural norm for some. The opioid crisis has produced many kinship and grand-families, emphasizing the need for multigenerational care because both children and caregivers have suffered traumatic losses and may be influenced by their own trauma histories.[210] Addressing how adversity experienced by a caregiver in childhood may affect their parenting and resilience can have profound effects on a child's health and outcomes. This approach can include asking these questions in engagement, surveillance, and screening; careful consideration of how the provider or practice can and will respond to elicited issues is important before integrating this into practice flow.

Community Partnerships

Pediatric offices can develop methods to coordinate trauma-related care with schools, child care, early educators, courts, legal supports, child welfare services, and other community partners (see policy statement[19]).

Staff and Provider Support

Addressing the trauma experiences of others can have significant consequences for health providers and staff. Per the National Child Traumatic Stress Network, STS is the emotional distress that results

when an individual hears about the first-hand trauma experiences of another.[136] The essential act of listening to trauma stories may take an emotional toll that compromises professional functioning and diminishes quality of life. Burnout is a syndrome characterized by a high degree of emotional exhaustion and depersonalization (ie, cynicism) and a low sense of personal accomplishment from work. Burnout refers more to general occupational stress and is not used to describe the effects of indirect trauma exposure specifically.[136] At least one meta-analysis concluded that job burnout contributes to, or at least increases the risk of, STS.[142] Recent surveys of medical students and residents reveal a high rate of depression (Patient Health Questionnaire-9 score >10) of 25% to 30%.[139,211] Some data indicate that more than 50% of the physician workforce in the United States suffers from burnout related to their profession.[212-214] For the individual physician, burnout can result in increased rates of apathy, depression, substance abuse, and suicide and can affect personal relationships.[139,212] STS similarly affects providers, although it is more often discussed in the mental health and child welfare literature rather than the medical literature.[144]

Detailed discussion of the response to burnout and STS is beyond the scope of this clinical report. However, effective TIC includes recognition of the effect of indirect trauma exposure on the workforce and safeguards to protect those caring for children and caregivers.[136,143] Acknowledgment that these are issues and providing resources to address them, with attention to leadership and supervision, have been cited as the most important first steps.[143,212,215] For both burnout and STS, support from the immediate supervisor and organizational leadership have been demonstrated to be effective ways to combat the effects of trauma.[143,209] Team-based care, efficiencies in practice, and opportunities to share successes and frustrations with peers can all be helpful.[216-218] Promoting self-care remains an important part of TIC, with adequate time for rest, distance from the office or hospital, exercise, healthy diet, and prayer, meditation, or mindfulness shown to reduce symptoms of burnout and STS.[143,219,220] Such interventions are integral to developing and sustaining a trauma-informed practice and include all members of the health care team.

SUMMARY

TIC recognizes that exposure to adversities is common to many, if not most, children and that the developmental, behavioral, and health consequences can be profound and long lasting. Pediatric clinicians with an understanding of the physiology of both resilience and trauma are in a position to promote resilience, recognize and respond to traumas, and promote recovery.

Key Points

1. TIC is fundamentally relational health care, the ability to form and maintain SSNRs. Pediatric clinicians are well positioned to use a 2-generation approach, evaluate attachment relationships, and harness these attachments to encourage the caregiver's role in promoting regulation and resilience.

2. Providing TIC is achieved through common pediatric practices, starting with engagement and providing a safe setting for patients and families. Obtaining history, using surveillance or screening tools appropriate to the pediatric setting and clinical need, and effecting a response involving the pediatric provider and other

community resources is consistent with addressing most health-related issues.

3. Trauma symptoms can vary, from changes in eating and sleeping to severe physical and mental health effects requiring extensive treatment. Individual differences in trauma symptoms relate to the interplay of exposures and buffering from SSNRs as well as genetic variations impacted by the early environment (biological differential sensitivity to context).

4. Treatment can begin in the office setting with psychoeducation and brief guidance for caregivers. Facilitating linkages to community resources for families to programs that promote positive parenting skills, regulation, and self-efficacy; address the SDoHs (poverty, housing, food insecurity, etc); or provide EBT further supports those at risk and can effectively treat those who are symptomatic.

5. Integrating this relational model of care to prevent and mitigate the impact of trauma so that all members of the care team feel supported and valued is integral to TIC. Addressing safety and supporting relationships that promote affiliative responses, decrease stress responses, and promote building resilience are principles of TIC for children, caregivers, and health care personnel.

Lead Authors

Heather Forkey, MD, FAAP
Moira Szilagyi, MD, PhD, FAAP
Erin T. Kelly, MD, FAAP, FACP
James Duffee, MD, MPH, FAAP

Council on Foster Care, Adoption, and Kinship Care Executive Committee, 2019–2021

Sarah H. Springer, MD, FAAP, Chairperson
Moira Szilagyi, MD, PhD, FAAP, Immediate Past Chairperson

Heather Forkey, MD, FAAP
Kristine Fortin, MD, MPH, FAAP
Mary Booth Vaden Greiner, MD, MS, FAAP
Todd J. Ochs, MD, FAAP
Anu N. Partap, MD, MPH, FAAP
Linda Davidson Sagor, MD, MPH, FAAP
Deborah L. Shropshire, MD, FAAP
Jonathan D. Thackeray, MD, FAAP
Douglas Waite, MD, FAAP
Lisa Weber Zetley, MD, FAAP

Liaisons

Jeremy Harvey – *Foster Care Alumni of America*
Wynne Shepard Morgan, MD – *American Academy of Child and Adolescent Psychiatry*
Camille Robinson, MD, FAAP – *Section on Pediatric Trainees*

Staff

Tammy Piazza Hurley
Mary Crane, PhD, LSW
Müge Chavdar, MPH

Council on Community Pediatrics Executive Committee, 2019–2021

James Duffee, MD, MPH, FAAP, Chairperson
Kimberly G. Montez, MD, MPH, FAAP, Vice Chairperson
Kimberley J. Dilley, MD, MPH, FAAP
Andrea E. Green, MD, FAAP
Joyce Javier, MD, MPH, MS, FAAP
Madhulika Mathur, MD, MPH, FAAP
Gerri Mattson, MD, FAAP
Kimberly Montez, MD, MPH, FAAP
Jacqueline L. Nelson, MD, FAAP
Mikah Owen, MD, MPH, FAAP
Kenya Parks, MD, MPH, FAAP
Christopher B. Peltier, MD, FAAP

Liaisons

Donene Feist – *Family Voices*
Rachel Nash, MD, MPH, MD – *Section on Pediatric Trainees*
Judith Thierry, DO, MPH, FAAP – *Committee on Native American Child Health*

Staff

Dana Bennett-Tejes, MA, MNM

Council on Child Abuse and Neglect Executive Committee, 2019–2021

Suzanne B. Haney, MD, MS, FAAP, Chairperson
Andrew P. Sirotnak, MD, FAAP, Immediate Past Chairperson
Andrea Gottsegen Asnes, MD, FAAP
Amy R. Gavril, MD, MSCI, FAAP
Amanda Bird Hoffert Gilmartin, MD, FAAP
Rebecca Greenlee Girardet, MD, FAAP
Nancy D. Heavilin, MD, FAAP
Sheila M. Idzerda, MD, FAAP
Antoinette Laskey, MD, MPH, MBA, FAAP
Lori A. Legano, MD, FAAP
Stephen A. Messner, MD, FAAP
Bethany A. Mohr, MD, FAAP
Shalon Marie Nienow, MD, FAAP
Norell Rosado, MD, FAAP

Liaisons

Heather Forkey, MD, FAAP – *Council on Foster Care, Adoption, and Kinship Care*
Brooks Keeshin, MD, FAAP – *American Academy of Child and Adolescent Psychiatry*
Jennifer Matjasko, PhD – *Centers for Disease Control and Prevention*

Anish Raj, MD – *Section on Pediatric Trainees*
Elaine Stedt, MSW, ACSW – *Administration for Children, Youth and Families, Office on Child Abuse and Neglect*

Staff

Tammy Piazza Hurley
Müge Chavdar, MPH

Committee on Psychosocial Aspects of Child and Family Health, 2019–2020

Arthur Lavin, MD, FAAP, Chairperson
George L. Askew, MD, FAAP
Rebecca Baum, MD, FAAP
Evelyn Berger-Jenkins, MD, FAAP
Tiffani J. Johnson, MD, MSc, FAAP
Douglas Jutte, MD, MPH, FAAP
Arwa Abdulhaq Nasir, MBBS, MSc, MPH, FAAP

Liaisons

Sharon Berry, PhD, ABPP, LP – *Society of Pediatric Psychology*
Edward R. Christophersen, PhD, FAAP – *Society of Pediatric Psychology*
Kathleen Hobson Davis, LSW – *Family Liaison*
Norah L. Johnson, PhD, RN, CPNP-BC – *National Association of Pediatric Nurse Practitioners*

Abigail Boden Schlesinger, MD – *American Academy of Child and Adolescent Psychiatry*
Rachel Segal, MD, FAAP – *Section on Pediatric Trainees*
Amy Starin, PhD, LCSW – *National Association of Social Workers*

Staff

Carolyn Lullo McCarty, PhD

ABBREVIATIONS

ACE: adverse childhood experience
DTD: developmental trauma disorder
EBT: evidence-based treatment
PFA: Psychological First Aid
PTSD: posttraumatic stress disorder
SDoH: social determinant of health
SSNR: safe, stable, and nurturing relationship
STS: secondary traumatic stress
TIC: trauma-informed care

FINANCIAL DISCLOSURE: The authors have indicated they have no financial relationships relevant to this article to disclose.

FUNDING: No external funding.

POTENTIAL CONFLICT OF INTEREST: The authors have indicated they have no potential conflicts of interest to disclose.

REFERENCES

1. Copeland WE, Keeler G, Angold A, Costello EJ. Traumatic events and posttraumatic stress in childhood. *Arch Gen Psychiatry.* 2007;64(5):577–584

2. Schilling EA, Aseltine RH Jr, Gore S. Adverse childhood experiences and mental health in young adults: a longitudinal survey. *BMC Public Health.* 2007;7:30

3. Burke NJ, Hellman JL, Scott BG, Weems CF, Carrion VG. The impact of adverse childhood experiences on an urban pediatric population. *Child Abuse Negl.* 2011;35(6):408–413

4. Lipschitz DS, Rasmusson AM, Anyan W, Cromwell P, Southwick SM. Clinical and functional correlates of posttraumatic stress disorder in urban adolescent girls at a primary care clinic. *J Am Acad Child Adolesc Psychiatry.* 2000;39(9):1104–1111

5. Suicide Prevention Resource Center; Substance Abuse and Mental Health Services Administration. Fact sheet: trauma among American Indians and Alaska natives. Missoula, MT: National Native Children's Trauma Center; 2016. Available at: https://www.sprc.org/resources-programs/fact-sheet-trauma-among-american-indians-alaska-natives. Accessed January 11, 2021

6. Miller KK, Brown CR, Shramko M, Svetaz MV. Applying trauma-informed practices to the care of refugee and immigrant youth: 10 clinical pearls. *Children (Basel).* 2019;6(8):94

7. Bethell C, Davis MB, Gombojav N, Stumbo S, Powers K. Issue brief: a national and across-state profile on adverse childhood experiences among children and possibilities to heal and thrive. 2017. Available at: https://www.cahmi.org/wp-content/uploads/2018/05/aces_brief_final.pdf. Accessed January 11, 2021

8. Ellis WR, Dietz WH. A new framework for addressing adverse childhood and community experiences: the building community resilience model. *Acad Pediatr.* 2017;17(7S):S86–S93

9. Cronholm PF, Forke CM, Wade R, et al. Adverse childhood experiences: expanding the concept of adversity. *Am J Prev Med.* 2015;49(3):354–361

10. Garner AS, Shonkoff JP; Committee on Psychosocial Aspects of Child and Family Health; Committee on Early Childhood, Adoption, and Dependent Care; Section on Developmental and Behavioral Pediatrics. Early childhood adversity, toxic stress, and the role of the pediatrician: translating developmental science into lifelong health. *Pediatrics.* 2012;129(1):e224–e231

11. American Academy of Pediatrics. *Adverse Childhood Experiences and the Lifelong Consequences of Trauma.* Elk Grove Village, IL: American Academy of Pediatrics; 2014. Available at: https://www.aap.org/en-us/documents/ttb_aces_consequences.pdf. Accessed January 11, 2021

12. Anda RF, Felitti VJ, Bremner JD, et al. The enduring effects of abuse and related adverse experiences in childhood. A convergence of evidence from neurobiology and epidemiology. *Eur Arch Psychiatry Clin Neurosci.* 2006;256(3):174–186

13. Heim C, Shugart M, Craighead WE, Nemeroff CB. Neurobiological and psychiatric consequences of child abuse and neglect. *Dev Psychobiol.* 2010;52(7):671–690

14. Shonkoff JP, Garner AS; Committee on Psychosocial Aspects of Child and Family Health; Committee on Early Childhood, Adoption, and Dependent Care; Section on Developmental and Behavioral Pediatrics. The lifelong effects of early childhood adversity and toxic stress. *Pediatrics.* 2012;129(1):e232–e246

15. Marsac ML, Kassam-Adams N, Hildenbrand AK, et al. Implementing a trauma-informed approach in pediatric health care networks. *JAMA Pediatr.* 2016;170(1):70–77

16. Substance Abuse and Mental Health Services Administration. *SAMHSA's Concept of Trauma and Guidance for a Trauma-Informed Approach.* Rockville, MD: Substance Abuse and Mental Health Services Administration; 2014

17. Stein REK, Storfer-Isser A, Kerker BD, et al. Beyond ADHD: how well are we doing? *Acad Pediatr.* 2016;16(2):115–121

18. Horwitz SM, Storfer-Isser A, Kerker BD, et al. Barriers to the identification and management of psychosocial problems: changes from 2004 to 2013. *Acad Pediatr.* 2015;15(6):613–620

19. Duffee J, Szilagyi M, Forkey H, Kelly ET; American Academy of Pediatrics, Council on Community Pediatrics, Council on Foster Care, Adoption, and Kinship Care, Council on Child Abuse and Neglect, Committee on Psychosocial Aspects of Child and Family Health. Policy statement: trauma-informed care in child health systems. *Pediatrics.* 2021;148(2):e2021052579

20. National Child Traumatic Stress Network. *The 12 Core Concepts: Concepts for Understanding Traumatic Stress Responses in Children and Families.* Los Angeles, CA: National Child Traumatic Stress Network; 2007. Available at: https://www.nctsn.org/resources/12-core-concepts-concepts-understanding-traumatic-stress-responses-children-and-families. Accessed January 11, 2021

21. Houtepen LC, Vinkers CH, Carrillo-Roa T, et al. Genome-wide DNA methylation levels and altered cortisol stress reactivity following childhood trauma in humans. *Nat Commun.* 2016;7:10967

22. Felitti VJ, Anda RF, Nordenberg D, et al. Relationship of childhood abuse and household dysfunction to many of the leading causes of death in adults. The Adverse Childhood Experiences (ACE) Study. *Am J Prev Med.* 1998;14(4):245–258

23. Flynn AB, Fothergill KE, Wilcox HC, et al. Primary care interventions to prevent or treat traumatic stress in childhood: a systematic review. *Acad Pediatr.* 2015;15(5):480–492

24. Centers for Disease Control and Prevention. Essentials for childhood: creating Safe, stable, nurturing relationships and environments. Available at: https://www.cdc.gov/violenceprevention/childabuseandneglect/essentials.html. Accessed January 11, 2021

25. Garner AS, Forkey H, Szilagyi M. Translating developmental science to address childhood adversity. *Acad Pediatr.* 2015;15(5):493–502

26. Lahey BB, Rathouz PJ, Lee SS, et al. Interactions between early parenting and a polymorphism of the child's dopamine transporter gene in predicting future child conduct disorder symptoms. *J Abnorm Psychol.* 2011;120(1):33–45

27. Whittle S, Simmons JG, Dennison M, et al. Positive parenting predicts the development of adolescent brain structure: a longitudinal study. *Dev Cogn Neurosci.* 2014;8:7–17

28. McEwen BS, Gianaros PJ. Central role of the brain in stress and adaptation: links to socioeconomic status, health, and disease. *Ann N Y Acad Sci.* 2010;1186:190–222

29. Merrick MT, Ford DC, Ports KA, et al. Vital Signs: estimated proportion of adult health problems attributable to adverse childhood experiences and implications for prevention - 25 states, 2015–2017. *MMWR Morb Mortal Wkly Rep.* 2019;68(44):999–1005

30. Center for the Developing Child. ACEs and toxic stress: frequently asked questions. Available at: https://developingchild.harvard.edu/resources/aces-and-toxic-stress-frequently-asked-questions/. Accessed January 11, 2021

31. McHugo GJ, Kammerer N, Jackson EW, et al. Women, co-occurring disorders, and violence study: evaluation design and study population. *J Subst Abuse Treat.* 2005;28(2):91–107

32. Bethell C, Jones J, Gombojav N, Linkenbach J, Sege R. Positive childhood experiences and adult mental and relational health in a statewide sample: associations across adverse childhood experiences levels. *JAMA Pediatr.* 2019;173(11):e193007

33. Bethell CD, Gombojav N, Whitaker RC. Family resilience and connection promote flourishing among US children, even amid adversity. *Health Aff (Millwood)*. 2019;38(5):729–737

34. Zeanah P, Burstein K, Cartier J. Addressing Adverse childhood experiences: it's all about relationships. *Societies*. 2018;8(4):115

35. US Department of Health and Human Services, Administration for Children and Families, Administration on Children, Youth and Families, Children's Bureau. *Child Maltreatment*. Washington, DC: US Department of Health and Human Services; 2017. Available at: www.acf.hhs.gov/programs/cb/research-data-technology/statistics-research/child-maltreatment. Accessed January 11, 2021

36. Child Welfare Information Gateway. *Foster Care Statistics 2019*. Washington, DC: US Department of Health and Human Services, Children's Bureau; 2019. Available at: https://www.acf.hhs.gov/cb/report/afcars-report-27. Accessed January 11, 2021

37. Burgess AL, Borowsky IW. Health and home environments of caregivers of children investigated by child protective services. *Pediatrics*. 2010;125(2):273–281

38. Campbell KA, Thomas AM, Cook LJ, Keenan HT. Longitudinal experiences of children remaining at home after a first-time investigation for suspected maltreatment. *J Pediatr*. 2012;161(2):340–347

39. Horwitz SM, Hurlburt MS, Cohen SD, Zhang J, Landsverk J. Predictors of placement for children who initially remained in their homes after an investigation for abuse or neglect. *Child Abuse Negl*. 2011;35(3):188–198

40. Perez D, Sribney WM, Rodríguez MA. Perceived discrimination and self-reported quality of care among Latinos in the United States. *J Gen Intern Med*. 2009;24(Suppl 3):548–554

41. Wood LCN. Impact of punitive immigration policies, parent-child separation and child detention on the mental health and development of children. *BMJ Paediatr Open*. 2018;2(1):e000338

42. Johnson SB, Riis JL, Noble KG. State of the art review: poverty and the developing brain. *Pediatrics*. 2016;137(4):e20153075

43. National Advisory Committee on Rural Health and Human Services. *Exploring the Rural Context For Adverse Childhood Experiences: Policy Brief and Recommendations*. Washington, DC: US Department of Health and Human Services; 2018

44. Evans GW, English K. The environment of poverty: multiple stressor exposure, psychophysiological stress, and socioemotional adjustment. *Child Dev*. 2002;73(4):1238–1248

45. Hackman DA, Farah MJ. Socioeconomic status and the developing brain. *Trends Cogn Sci*. 2009;13(2):65–73

46. Trent M, Dooley DG, Dougé J; Section on Adolescent Health; Council on Community Pediatrics; Committee on Adolescence. Council on Community Pediatrics; Committee on Adolescence. The impact of racism on child and adolescent health. *Pediatrics*. 2019;144(2):e20191765

47. Heard-Garris NJ, Cale M, Camaj L, Hamati MC, Dominguez TP. Transmitting trauma: a systematic review of vicarious racism and child health. *Soc Sci Med*. 2018;199:230–240

48. Mohatt NV, Thompson AB, Thai ND, Tebes JK. Historical trauma as public narrative: a conceptual review of how history impacts present-day health. *Soc Sci Med*. 2014;106:128–136

49. Wade R Jr, Shea JA, Rubin D, Wood J. Adverse childhood experiences of low-income urban youth. *Pediatrics*. 2014;134(1):e13–e20

50. Nixon CL. Current perspectives: the impact of cyberbullying on adolescent health. *Adolesc Health Med Ther*. 2014;5:143–158

51. Finkelhor D, Turner HA, Shattuck A, Hamby SL. Violence, crime, and abuse exposure in a national sample of children and youth: an update. [published correction appears in JAMA Pediatr. 2014;168(3):286]. *JAMA Pediatr*. 2013;167(7):614–621

52. Roberts AL, Austin SB, Corliss HL, Vandermorris AK, Koenen KC. Pervasive trauma exposure among US sexual orientation minority adults and risk of posttraumatic stress disorder. *Am J Public Health*. 2010;100(12):2433–2441

53. Carroll G. Mundane extreme environmental stress and African American families: a case for recognizing different realities. *J Comp Fam Stud*. 1998;29(2):271–284

54. Huynh VW. Ethnic microaggressions and the depressive and somatic symptoms of Latino and Asian American adolescents. *J Youth Adolesc*. 2012;41(7):831–846

55. Siegel BS, Davis BE; Committee on Psychosocial Aspects of Child and Family Health and Section on Uniformed Services. Health and mental health needs of children in US military families. *Pediatrics*. 2013;131(6):e2002–e2015

56. Marsac ML, Kassam-Adams N, Delahanty DL, Widaman KF, Barakat LP. Posttraumatic stress following acute medical trauma in children: a proposed model of bio-psycho-social processes during the peri-trauma period. *Clin Child Fam Psychol Rev*. 2014;17(4):399–411

57. Brosbe MS, Hoefling K, Faust J. Predicting posttraumatic stress following pediatric injury: a systematic review. *J Pediatr Psychol*. 2011;36(6):718–729

58. Garner AS. Thinking developmentally: the next evolution in models of health. *J Dev Behav Pediatr*. 2016;37(7):579–584

59. Bretherton I. The origins of attachment theory: John Bowlby and Mary Ainsworth. *Dev Psychol*. 1992;28(5):759–775

60. Feldman R. The adaptive human parental brain: implications for children's social development. *Trends Neurosci*. 2015;38(6):387–399

61. Hughes DA, Baylin J. *The Neurobiology of Attachment-Focused Therapy: Enhancing Connection and Trust in the Treatment of Children and Adolescents*. New York, NY: W.W. Norton and Co; 2016

62. Allen JG. *Restoring Mentalizing in Attachment Relationships: Treating Trauma with Plain Old Therapy*. Arlington, VA: American Psychiatric Publishing; 2013

63. Cantor P, Osher D, Berg J, Steyer L, Rose T. Malleability, plasticity, and individuality: how children learn and develop in context. *Appl Dev Sci*. 2019;23(4):307–337

64. Ainsworth MD. Attachments beyond infancy. *Am Psychol*. 1989;44(4):709–716

65. Perry RE, Blair C, Sullivan RM. Neurobiology of infant attachment: attachment despite adversity and parental programming of emotionality. *Curr Opin Psychol*. 2017;17:1–6

66. Hoghughi M, Speight AN. Good enough parenting for all children—a strategy for a healthier society. *Arch Dis Child*. 1998;78(4):293–296

67. Winnicott DW. *The Maturational Process and the Facilitative Environment*. New York, NY: International Universities Press; 1965

68. Porges SW. Social engagement and attachment: a phylogenetic perspective. *Ann N Y Acad Sci*. 2003;1008: 31–47

69. Benoit D. Infant-parent attachment: definition, types, antecedents, measurement and outcome. *Paediatr Child Health*. 2004;9(8):541–545

70. Olff M, Frijling JL, Kubzansky LD, et al. The role of oxytocin in social bonding, stress regulation and mental health: an update on the moderating effects of context and interindividual differences. *Psychoneuroendocrinology*. 2013;38(9):1883–1894

71. Masten AS. Ordinary magic. Resilience processes in development. *Am Psychol*. 2001;56(3):227–238

72. Sege RD, Harper Browne C. Responding to ACEs With HOPE: health outcomes from positive experiences. *Acad Pediatr*. 2017;17(7S):S79–S85

73. Garner A, Yogman M; American Academy of Pediatrics, Committee on Psychosocial Aspects of Child and Family Health, Section on Developmental and Behavioral Pediatrics, Council on Early Childhood. Preventing childhood toxic stress: partnering with families and communities to promote relational health. *Pediatrics*. 2021;148(2):e2021052582

74. Children's Hospital of Philadelphia Research Institute. Basics of trauma-informed care. Available at: https://www.healthcaretoolbox.org/. Accessed January 11, 2021

75. Brymer M, Jacobs A, Layne C, et al. *Psychological First Aid Field Operations Guide*. 2nd ed. Los Angeles, CA: National Child Traumatic Stress Network and National Center for Posttraumatic Stress Disorder; 2006

76. Finkelhor D. Screening for adverse childhood experiences (ACEs): cautions and suggestions. *Child Abuse Negl*. 2018;85:174–179

77. Flaherty E, Legano L, Idzerda S; Council on Child Abuse and Neglect. Ongoing pediatric health care for the child who has been maltreated. *Pediatrics*. 2019;143(4):e20190284

78. Flaherty EG, Stirling J Jr; American Academy of Pediatrics. Committee on Child Abuse and Neglect. Clinical report—the pediatrician's role in child maltreatment prevention. *Pediatrics*. 2010;126(4):833–841

79. Schnierle J, Christian-Brathwaite N, Louisias M. Implicit bias: what every pediatrician should know about the effect of bias on health and future directions. *Curr Probl Pediatr Adolesc Health Care*. 2019;49(2):34–44

80. Johnson SB, Riley AW, Granger DA, Riis J. The science of early life toxic stress for pediatric practice and advocacy. *Pediatrics*. 2013;131(2):319–327

81. Dantzer R, O'Connor JC, Freund GG, Johnson RW, Kelley KW. From inflammation to sickness and depression: when the immune system subjugates the brain. *Nat Rev Neurosci*. 2008;9(1): 46–56

82. Jonson-Reid M, Wideman E. Trauma and very young children. *Child Adolesc Psychiatr Clin N Am*. 2017;26(3): 477–490

83. Cook A, Spinazzola J, Ford J, et al. Complex trauma in children and adolescents. *Psychiatr Ann*. 2005;35(5): 390–398

84. Substance Abuse and Mental Health Services Administration. *Recognizing and Treating Child Traumatic Stress*. Washington, DC: Substance Abuse and Mental Health Services Administration; 2004. Available at: https://www.samhsa.gov/child-trauma/recognizing-and-treating-child-traumatic-stress#signs. Accessed January 11, 2021

85. Cohen JA, Kelleher KJ, Mannarino AP. Identifying, treating, and referring traumatized children: the role of pediatric providers. *Arch Pediatr Adolesc Med*. 2008;162(5):447–452

86. Siegfried CB, Blackhear K; National Child Traumatic Stress Network and National Resource Center on ADHD. *Is it ADHD or Child Traumatic Stress? A Guide for Clinicians*. Los Angeles, CA, and Durham. NC: National Center for Child Traumatic Stress; 2016

87. Keeshin B, Forkey HC, Fouras G, MacMillan HL; American Academy of Pediatrics, Council on Child Abuse and Neglect, Council on Foster Care, Adoption, and Kinship Care, American Academy of Child and Adolescent Psychiatry, Committee on Child Maltreatment and Vioence, Committee on Adoption and Foster Care.. Children exposed to maltreatment: assessment and the role of psychotropic medication. *Pediatrics*. 2020;145(2):e20193751

88. Blaustein M, Kinniburgh K. *Treating Traumatic Stress in Children and Adolescents: How to Foster Resilience Through Attachment, Self-Regulation and Competency*, 2nd ed. New York, NY: The Guilford Press; 2019

89. De Bellis MD, Zisk A. The biological effects of childhood trauma. *Child Adolesc Psychiatr Clin N Am*. 2014;23(2): 185–222, vii

90. Bremner JD. Traumatic stress: effects on the brain. *Dialogues Clin Neurosci*. 2006;8(4):445–461

91. Lupien SJ, McEwen BS, Gunnar MR, Heim C. Effects of stress throughout the lifespan on the brain, behaviour and cognition. *Nat Rev Neurosci*. 2009;10(6):434–445

92. Penza KM, Heim C, Nemeroff CB. Neurobiological effects of childhood abuse: implications for the pathophysiology of depression and anxiety. *Arch Women Ment Health*. 2003;6(1):15–22

93. Teicher MH, Samson JA, Anderson CM, Ohashi K. The effects of childhood maltreatment on brain structure, function and connectivity. *Nat Rev Neurosci*. 2016;17(10):652–666

94. Miller LE. Perceived threat in childhood: a review of research and implications for children living in violent households. *Trauma Violence Abuse*. 2015;16(2):153–168

95. Teicher MH, Samson JA. Childhood maltreatment and psychopathology: a case for ecophenotypic variants as clinically and neurobiologically distinct subtypes. *Am J Psychiatry*. 2013; 170(10):1114–1133

96. Birn RM, Roeber BJ, Pollak SD. Early childhood stress exposure, reward pathways, and adult decision making. *Proc Natl Acad Sci USA.* 2017;114(51):13549–13554

97. Syed SA, Nemeroff CB. Early life stress, mood, and anxiety disorders. *Chronic Stress (Thousand Oaks).* 2017;1:2470547017694461

98. Ringeisen H, Casanueva C, Urato M, Cross T. Special health care needs among children in the child welfare system. *Pediatrics.* 2008;122(1):e232–e241

99. Clougherty JE, Levy JI, Kubzansky LD, et al. Synergistic effects of traffic-related air pollution and exposure to violence on urban asthma etiology. *Environ Health Perspect.* 2007;115(8):1140–1146

100. Centers for Disease Control and Prevention. Developmental monitoring and screening for health professionals. Available at: https://www.cdc.gov/ncbddd/childdevelopment/screening-hcp.html. Accessed January 11, 2021

101. Klein D, Goldenring JM, Adelman WP. HEEADSSS 3.0: the psychosocial interview for adolescents updated for a new century fueled by media. *Contemp Pediatr.* 2014;31(1):16–28

102. Goldenring JM, Rosen DS. Getting into adolescent heads: an essential update. *Contemp Pediatr.* 2004;21(1):64–90

103. Conn AM, Szilagyi MA, Jee SH, Manly JT, Briggs R, Szilagyi PG. Parental perspectives of screening for adverse childhood experiences in pediatric primary care. *Fam Syst Health.* 2018;36(1):62–72

104. Colvin JD, Bettenhausen JL, Anderson-Carpenter KD, Collie-Akers V, Chung PJ. Caregiver opinion of in-hospital screening for unmet social needs by pediatric residents. *Acad Pediatr.* 2016;16(2):161–167

105. Wissow L, Anthony B, Brown J, et al. A common factors approach to improving the mental health capacity of pediatric primary care. *Adm Policy Ment Health.* 2008;35(4):305–318

106. Ginsburg K. Viewing our patients through a positive lens. *Contemp Pediatr.* 2007;24(1):65–76

107. Traub F, Boynton-Jarrett R. Modifiable resilience factors to childhood adversity for clinical pediatric practice. *Pediatrics.* 2017;139(5):e20162569

108. Greene R, Winkler J. Collaborative and Proactive Solutions (CPS): a review of research findings in families, schools, and treatment facilities. *Clin Child Fam Psychol Rev.* 2019;22(4):549–561

109. Lipkin PH, Macias MM; Council on Children With Disabilities, Section on Developmental and Behavioral Pediatrics. Promoting optimal development: identifying infants and young children with developmental disorders through developmental surveillance and screening. *Pediatrics.* 2020;145(1):e20193449

110. Squires J, Potter L, Bricker D. *The ASQ User's Guide,* 3rd ed. Baltimore, MD: Paul H. Brookes Publishing Co; 2009

111. Jellinek MS, Murphy JM, Little M, Pagano ME, Comer DM, Kelleher KJ. Use of the Pediatric Symptom Checklist to screen for psychosocial problems in pediatric primary care: a national feasibility study. *Arch Pediatr Adolesc Med.* 1999;153(3):254–260

112. Stone LL, Otten R, Engels RCME, Vermulst AA, Janssens JM. Psychometric properties of the parent and teacher versions of the strengths and difficulties questionnaire for 4- to 12-year-olds: a review. *Clin Child Fam Psychol Rev.* 2010;13(3):254–274

113. Richardson LP, McCauley E, Grossman DC, et al. Evaluation of the Patient Health Questionnaire-9 Item for detecting major depression among adolescents. *Pediatrics.* 2010;126(6):1117–1123

114. Earls MF, Yogman MW, Mattson G, Rafferty J; Committee on Psychosocial Aspects of Child and Family Health. Incorporating recognition and management of perinatal depression into pediatric practice. *Pediatrics.* 2019;143(1):e20183259

115. Rolon-Arroyo B, Oosterhoff B, Layne CM, Steinberg AM, Pynoos RS, Kaplow JB. The UCLA PTSD Reaction Index for DSM-5 Brief Form: a screening tool for trauma-exposed youths. *J Am Acad Child Adolesc Psychiatry.* 2020;59(3):434–443

116. Kazak A, Schneider S, Didonato S, Pai ALH. Family psychosocial risk screening guided by the Pediatric Preventative Psychosocial Health Model (PPPHM) using the Psychosocial Assessment Tool (PAT). *Acta Oncol.* 2015;54(5):574–580

117. Kazak AE, Hwang WT, Chen FF, et al. Screening for family psychosocial risk in pediatric cancer: validation of the Psychosocial Assessment Tool (PAT) Version 3. *J Pediatr Psychol.* 2018;43(7):737–748

118. Keeshin B, Byrne K, Thorn B, Shepard L. Screening for trauma in pediatric primary care. *Curr Psychiatry Rep.* 2020;22(11):60

119. Bethell CD, Carle A, Hudziak J, et al. Methods to assess adverse childhood experiences of children and families: toward approaches to promote child well-being in policy and practice. *Acad Pediatr.* 2017;17(7S):S51–S69

120. Purewal SK, Bucci M, Gutiérrez Wang L, et al. Screening for adverse childhood experiences (ACEs) in an integrated pediatric care model. *Zero Three.* 2016;36(3):10–17

121. Colvin JD, Bettenhausen JL, Anderson-Carpenter KD, et al. Multiple behavior change intervention to improve detection of unmet social needs and resulting resource referrals. *Acad Pediatr.* 2016;16(2):168–174

122. Shah AN, Beck AF, Sucharew HJ, et al; H2O Study Group. Parental adverse childhood experiences and resilience on coping after discharge. *Pediatrics.* 2018;141(4):e20172127

123. Folger AT, Eismann EA, Stephenson NB, et al. Parental adverse childhood experiences and offspring development at 2 years of age. *Pediatrics.* 2018;141(4):e20172826

124. Schickedanz A, Halfon N, Sastry N, Chung PJ. Parents' adverse childhood experiences and their children's behavioral health problems. *Pediatrics.* 2018;142(2):e20180023

125. Lê-Scherban F, Wang X, Boyle-Steed KH, Pachter LM. Intergenerational associations of parent adverse childhood experiences and child health outcomes. *Pediatrics.* 2018;141(6):e20174274

126. Connor KM, Davidson JRT. Development of a new resilience scale: the Connor-Davidson Resilience Scale (CD-

RISC). *Depress Anxiety.* 2003;18(2): 76–82

127. Smith BW, Dalen J, Wiggins K, Tooley E, Christopher P, Bernard J. The brief resilience scale: assessing the ability to bounce back. *Int J Behav Med.* 2008;15(3):194–200

128. Windle G, Bennett KM, Noyes J. A methodological review of resilience measurement scales. *Health Qual Life Outcomes.* 2011;9:8

129. Anda RF, Porter LE, Brown DW. Inside the Adverse Childhood Experience Score: strengths, limitations, and misapplications. *Am J Prev Med.* 2020;59(2):293–295

130. Dube SR. Continuing conversations about adverse childhood experiences (ACEs) screening: a public health perspective. *Child Abuse Negl.* 2018;85: 180–184

131. Shonkoff JP. Capitalizing on advances in science to reduce the health consequences of early childhood adversity. *JAMA Pediatr.* 2016;170(10):1003–1007

132. Boyce WT, Levitt P, Martinez FD, McEwen BS, Shonkoff JP. Genes, environments and time: the biology of adversity and resilience. *Pediatrics.* 2020;147(2):e20201651

133. Shonkoff JP, Boyce WT, Levitt P, Martinez F, McEwen B. Leveraging the biology of adversity and resilience to transform pediatric practice. *Pediatrics.* 2020;147(2):e20193845

134. Slopen N, McLaughlin KA, Shonkoff JP. Interventions to improve cortisol regulation in children: a systematic review. *Pediatrics.* 2014;133(2):312–326

135. Le-Niculescu H, Roseberry K, Levey DF, et al. Towards precision medicine for stress disorders: diagnostic biomarkers and targeted drugs. *Mol Psychiatry.* 2020;25(5):918–938

136. National Child Traumatic Stress Network. *Secondary Traumatic Stress: A Fact Sheet for Child-Serving Professionals.* Los Angeles, CA: National Child Traumatic Stress Network; 2011. Available at: https://www.nctsn.org/resources/secondary-traumatic-stress-fact-sheet-child-serving-professionals. Accessed January 11, 2021

137. Cieslak R, Shoji K, Douglas A, Melville E, Luszczynska A, Benight CC. A meta-analysis of the relationship between job burnout and secondary traumatic stress among workers with indirect exposure to trauma. *Psychol Serv.* 2014;11(1):75–86

138. Cocker F, Joss N. Compassion fatigue among healthcare, emergency and community service workers: a systematic review. *Int J Environ Res Public Health.* 2016;13(6):618

139. Dyrbye LN, Thomas MR, Massie FS, et al. Burnout and suicidal ideation among U.S. medical students. *Ann Intern Med.* 2008;149(5):334–341

140. Oreskovich MR, Shanafelt T, Dyrbye LN, et al. The prevalence of substance use disorders in American physicians. *Am J Addict.* 2015;24(1):30–38

141. Robins PM, Meltzer L, Zelikovsky N. The experience of secondary traumatic stress upon care providers working within a children's hospital. *J Pediatr Nurs.* 2009;24(4):270–279

142. Shoji K, Lesnierowska M, Smoktunowicz E, et al. What comes first, job burnout or secondary traumatic stress? Findings from two longitudinal studies from the U.S. and Poland. *PLoS One.* 2015;10(8):e0136730

143. Sprang G, Craig C, Clark J. Secondary traumatic stress and burnout in child welfare workers: a comparative analysis of occupational distress across professional groups. *Child Welfare.* 2011;90(6):149–168

144. van Mol MMC, Kompanje EJ, Benoit DD, Bakker J, Nijkamp MD. The prevalence of compassion fatigue and burnout among healthcare professionals in intensive care units: a systematic review. *PLoS One.* 2015;10(8):e0136955

145. The Center for Victims of Torture. Professional quality of life: elements, theory, and measurement. 2019. Available at: https://proqol.org/. Accessed January 11, 2021

146. Wilson JP, So-Kum Tang CC. *Cross-Cultural Assessment of Psychological Trauma and PTSD.* New York, NY: Springer Publishing; 2007

147. Flynn JT, Kaelber DC, Baker-Smith CM, et al; Subcommittee on Screening and Management of High Blood Pressure in Children. Clinical practice guideline for screening and management of high blood pressure in children and adolescents. *Pediatrics.* 2017;140(3): e20171904

148. Gooding HC, Milliren CE, Austin SB, Sheridan MA, McLaughlin KA. Child abuse, resting blood pressure, and blood pressure reactivity to psychosocial stress. *J Pediatr Psychol.* 2016;41(1):5–14

149. Su S, Wang X, Pollock JS, et al. Adverse childhood experiences and blood pressure trajectories from childhood to young adulthood: the Georgia stress and Heart study. *Circulation.* 2015;131(19):1674–1681

150. Szilagyi MA, Rosen DS, Rubin D, Zlotnik S; Council on Foster Care, Adoption, and Kinship Care; Committee on Adolescence; Council on Early Childhood. Health care issues for children and adolescents in foster care and kinship care. *Pediatrics.* 2015;136(4): e1142–e1166

151. Davis L, Barnes AJ, Gross AC, Ryder JR, Shlafer RJ. Adverse childhood experiences and weight status among adolescents. *J Pediatr.* 2019;204: 71–76.e1

152. Javier JR, Hoffman LR, Shah SI; Pediatric Policy Council. Making the case for ACEs: adverse childhood experiences, obesity, and long-term health. *Pediatr Res.* 2019;86(4):420–422

153. Purswani P, Marsicek SM, Amankwah EK. Association between cumulative exposure to adverse childhood experiences and childhood obesity. *PLoS One.* 2020;15(9):e0239940

154. Heerman WJ, Krishnaswami S, Barkin SL, McPheeters M. Adverse family experiences during childhood and adolescent obesity. *Obesity (Silver Spring).* 2016;24(3):696–702

155. Exley D, Norman A, Hyland M. Adverse childhood experience and asthma onset: a systematic review. *Eur Respir Rev.* 2015;24(136):299–305

156. Gilbert LK, Breiding MJ, Merrick MT, et al. Childhood adversity and adult chronic disease: an update from ten states and the District of Columbia, 2010. *Am J Prev Med.* 2015;48(3): 345–349

157. Heneghan A, Stein RE, Hurlburt MS, et al. Mental health problems in teens investigated by U.S. child welfare

agencies. *J Adolesc Health.* 2013;52(5): 634–640

158. Ford JD, Grasso D, Greene C, Levine J, Spinazzola J, van der Kolk B. Clinical significance of a proposed developmental trauma disorder diagnosis: results of an international survey of clinicians. *J Clin Psychiatry.* 2013;74(8):841–849

159. Keeshin BR, Strawn JR. Psychological and pharmacologic treatment of youth with posttraumatic stress disorder: an evidence-based review. *Child Adolesc Psychiatr Clin N Am.* 2014;23(2): 399–411, x

160. Carrion VG, Weems CF, Reiss AL. Stress predicts brain changes in children: a pilot longitudinal study on youth stress, posttraumatic stress disorder, and the hippocampus. *Pediatrics.* 2007;119(3):509–516

161. Gunnar M, Quevedo K. The neurobiology of stress and development. *Annu Rev Psychol.* 2007;58:145–173

162. McDonald MK, Borntrager CF, Rostad W. Measuring trauma: considerations for assessing complex and non-PTSD Criterion A childhood trauma. *J Trauma Dissociation.* 2014;15(2):184–203

163. van der Kolk B. Developmental trauma disorder. *Psychiatr Ann.* 2005;35(5): 401–409

164. Ogle CM, Rubin DC, Siegler IC. The impact of the developmental timing of trauma exposure on PTSD symptoms and psychosocial functioning among older adults. *Dev Psychol.* 2013;49(11): 2191–2200

165. Perry BD, Pollard RA, Blakley TL, Baker WL, Vigilante D. Childhood trauma, the neurobiology of adaptation, and "use-dependent" development of the brain: how "states" become "traits.". *Infant Ment Health J.* 1995;16(4):271–291

166. Scheeringa MS. Developmental considerations for diagnosing PTSD and acute stress disorder in preschool and school-age children. *Am J Psychiatry.* 2008;165(10):1237–1239

167. Treisman K. *Working with Relational and Developmental Trauma in Children and Adolescents.* New York, NY: Routledge; 2017

168. Obradović J, Bush NR, Stamperdahl J, Adler NE, Boyce WT. Biological

sensitivity to context: the interactive effects of stress reactivity and family adversity on socioemotional behavior and school readiness. *Child Dev.* 2010;81(1):270–289

169. Boyce WT, Ellis BJ. Biological sensitivity to context: I. An evolutionary-developmental theory of the origins and functions of stress reactivity. *Dev Psychopathol.* 2005;17(2):271–301

170. Kennedy E. Orchids and dandelions: how some children are more susceptible to environmental influences for better or worse and the implications for child development. *Clin Child Psychol Psychiatry.* 2013;18(3):319–321

171. Cole SF, Eisner A, Gregory M, Ristuccia J. *Creating and Advocating for Trauma-Sensitive Schools.* Cambridge, MA: Trauma and Learning Policy Initiative; 2013

172. Overstreet S, Chafouleas SM. Trauma-informed schools: introduction to the special issue. *School Ment Health.* 2016;8(1):1–6

173. Allen B, Timmer SG, Urquiza AJ. Parent–child interaction therapy as an attachment-based intervention: theoretical rationale and pilot data with adopted children. *Child Youth Serv Rev.* 2014;47(Part 3):334–341

174. Camoirano A. Mentalizing makes parenting work: a review about parental reflective functioning and clinical interventions to improve it. *Front Psychol.* 2017;8:14

175. Zuckerman B, Augustyn M. Books and reading: evidence-based standard of care whose time has come. *Acad Pediatr.* 2011;11(1):11–17

176. Zuckerman B, Khandekar A. Reach Out and Read: evidence based approach to promoting early child development. *Curr Opin Pediatr.* 2010;22(4):539–544

177. Needlman R, Toker KH, Dreyer BP, Klass P, Mendelsohn AL. Effectiveness of a primary care intervention to support reading aloud: a multicenter evaluation. *Ambul Pediatr.* 2005;5(4):209–215

178. Mendelsohn AL, Cates CB, Weisleder A, et al. Reading aloud, play, and social-emotional development. *Pediatrics.* 2018;141(5):e20173393

179. Shah R, DeFrino D, Kim Y, Atkins M. Sit Down and Play: a preventive primary

care-based program to enhance parenting practices. *J Child Fam Stud.* 2017;26(2):540–547

180. Chang SM, Grantham-McGregor SM, Powell CA, et al. Integrating a parenting intervention with routine primary health care: a cluster randomized trial. *Pediatrics.* 2015;136(2):272–280

181. Girard LC, Doyle O, Tremblay RE. Maternal warmth and toddler development: support for transactional models in disadvantaged families. *Eur Child Adolesc Psychiatry.* 2017;26(4):497–507

182. Weisleder A, Cates CB, Dreyer BP, et al. Promotion of positive parenting and prevention of socioemotional disparities. *Pediatrics.* 2016;137(2):e20153239

183. Shah R, Kennedy S, Clark MD, Bauer SC, Schwartz A. Primary care-based interventions to promote positive parenting behaviors: a meta-analysis. *Pediatrics.* 2016;137(5):e20153393

184. Perry-Parrish C, Copeland-Linder N, Webb L, Sibinga EMS. Mindfulness-based approaches for children and youth. *Curr Probl Pediatr Adolesc Health Care.* 2016;46(6):172–178

185. Bauer CCC, Caballero C, Scherer E, et al. Mindfulness training reduces stress and amygdala reactivity to fearful faces in middle-school children. *Behav Neurosci.* 2019;133(6):569–585

186. Ortiz R, Sibinga EM. The role of mindfulness in reducing the adverse effects of childhood stress and trauma. *Children (Basel).* 2017;4(3):16

187. Foa EBKT, Friedman MJ, Cohen JA. *Effective Treatments for Posttraumatic Stress Disorder: Practice Guidelines From the International Society for Traumatic Stress Studies,* 2nd ed. New York, NY: Guilford Press; 2008

188. Dorsey S, McLaughlin KA, Kerns SEU, et al. Evidence base update for psychosocial treatments for children and adolescents exposed to traumatic events. *J Clin Child Adolesc Psychol.* 2017;46(3):303–330

189. Sege RD, Amaya-Jackson L; American Academy of Pediatrics Committee on Child Abuse and Neglect, Council on Foster Care, Adoption, and Kinship Care; American Academy of Child and Adolescent Psychiatry Committee on Child Maltreatment and Violence; National Center for Child Traumatic

Stress. Clinical considerations related to the behavioral manifestations of child maltreatment. *Pediatrics.* 2017;139(4):e20170100

190. Gleason MM, Goldson E, Yogman MW; Council on Early Childhood; Committee on Pyschosocial Aspects of Child and Family Health; Section on Developmental and Behavioral Pediatrics. Addressing early childhood emotional and behavioral problems. *Pediatrics.* 2016;138(6):e20163025

191. Asarnow JR, Rozenman M, Wiblin J, Zeltzer L. Integrated medical-behavioral care compared with usual primary care for child and adolescent behavioral health: a meta-analysis. *JAMA Pediatr.* 2015;169(10):929–937

192. Dunsmoor JE, Kroes MCW, Li J, Daw ND, Simpson HB, Phelps EA. Role of human ventromedial prefrontal cortex in learning and recall of enhanced extinction. *J Neurosci.* 2019;39(17): 3264–3276

193. Giustino TF, Fitzgerald PJ, Ressler RL, Maren S. Locus coeruleus toggles reciprocal prefrontal firing to reinstate fear. *Proc Natl Acad Sci USA.* 2019;116(17):8570–8575

194. Sloan DM, Marx BP, Lee DJ, Resick PA. A brief exposure-based treatment vs cognitive processing therapy for posttraumatic stress disorder: a randomized noninferiority clinical trial. *JAMA Psychiatry.* 2018;75(3):233–239

195. Jones AM, Shealy KM, Reid-Quiñones K, et al. Guidelines for establishing a telemental health program to provide evidence-based therapy for trauma-exposed children and families. *Psychol Serv.* 2014;11(4):398–409

196. Bashshur RL, Shannon GW, Bashshur N, Yellowlees PM. The empirical evidence for telemedicine interventions in mental disorders. *Telemed J E Health.* 2016;22(2):87–113

197. Conrad R, Rayala H, Diamon R, Busch B, Kramer N. Expanding telemental health in response to the COVID-19 pandemic. 2020. Available at: https://www.psychiatrictimes.com/view/expanding-telemental-health-response-covid-19-pandemic. Accessed January 11, 2021

198. Menschner C, Maul A, Center for Health Care Strategies. *Key Ingredients for Successful Trauma-Informed Care*

Implementation. Hamilton, NJ: Center for Health Care Strategies; 2016, Available at https://www.chcs.org/resource/key-ingredients-for-successful-trauma-informed-care-implementation/. Accessed January 11, 2021

199. Schulman M, Menschner C. *Laying the Groundwork for Trauma Informed Care.* Hamilton, NJ: Center for Health Care Strategies; 2018. Available at https://www.chcs.org/resource/laying-groundwork-trauma-informed-care/. Accessed January 11, 2021

200. American Academy of Pediatrics. *Trauma Toolbox for Primary Care.* Elk Grove Village, IL: American Academy of Pediatrics; 2014. Available at: www.aap.org/en-us/advocacy-and-policy/aap-health-initiatives/healthy-foster-care-america/Pages/Trauma-Guide.aspx. Accessed January 11, 2021

201. Pediatric Integrated Care Collaborative. *Improving the Capacity of Primary Care to Serve Children and Families Experiencing Trauma and Chronic Stress: A Toolkit.* Baltimore, MD: Pediatric Integrated Care Collaborative; 2016. Available at: https://picc.jhu.edu/the-toolkit.html. Accessed January 11, 2021

202. Brown SM, Baker CN, Wilcox P. Risking connection trauma training: a pathway toward trauma-informed care in child congregate care settings. *Psychol Trauma.* 2012;4(5):507–515

203. Bryson SA, Gauvin E, Jamieson A, et al. What are effective strategies for implementing trauma-informed care in youth inpatient psychiatric and residential treatment settings? A realist systematic review. *Int J Ment Health Syst.* 2017;11:36

204. Murphy K, Moore KA, Redd Z, Malm K. Trauma-informed child welfare systems and children's well-being: a longitudinal evaluation of KVC's bridging the way home initiative. *Child Youth Serv Rev.* 2017;75:23–34

205. Schiff DM, Zuckerman B, Hutton E, Genatossio C, Michelson C, Bair-Merritt M. Development and pilot implementation of a trauma-informed care curriculum for pediatric residents. *Acad Pediatr.* 2017;17(7):794–796

206. Substance Abuse and Mental Health Services Administration. *The*

Integration of Behavioral Health into Pediatric Primary Care Settings. Washington, DC: Substance Abuse and Mental Health Services Administration; 2017

207. Kolko DJ, Perrin E. The integration of behavioral health interventions in children's health care: services, science, and suggestions. *J Clin Child Adolesc Psychol.* 2014;43(2):216–228

208. Garg A, Toy S, Tripodis Y, Silverstein M, Freeman E. Addressing social determinants of health at well child care visits: a cluster RCT. *Pediatrics.* 2015;135(2):e296–e304

209. Sun J, Patel F, Rose-Jacobs R, Frank DA, Black MM, Chilton M. Mothers' adverse childhood experiences and their young children's development. *Am J Prev Med.* 2017;53(6):882–891

210. Feder KA, Letourneau EJ, Brook J. Children in the opioid epidemic: addressing the next generation's public health crisis. *Pediatrics.* 2019;143(1): e20181656

211. West CP, Tan AD, Habermann TM, Sloan JA, Shanafelt TD. Association of resident fatigue and distress with perceived medical errors. *JAMA.* 2009;302(12):1294–1300

212. Shanafelt TD, Noseworthy JH. Executive leadership and physician well-being: nine organizational strategies to promote engagement and reduce burnout. *Mayo Clin Proc.* 2017;92(1): 129–146

213. Shanafelt TD, Boone S, Tan L, et al. Burnout and satisfaction with work-life balance among US physicians relative to the general US population. *Arch Intern Med.* 2012;172(18):1377–1385

214. Shanafelt TD, Hasan O, Dyrbye LN, et al. Changes in burnout and satisfaction with work-life balance in physicians and the general US working population between 2011 and 2014 [published correction appears in *Mayo Clin Proc.* 2016;91(2):276]. *Mayo Clin Proc.* 2015;90(12):1600–1613

215. Shanafelt TD, Gorringe G, Menaker R, et al. Impact of organizational leadership on physician burnout and satisfaction. *Mayo Clin Proc.* 2015;90(4): 432–440

216. Shanafelt TD, Dyrbye LN, Sinsky C, et al. Relationship between clerical

burden and characteristics of the electronic environment with physician burnout and professional satisfaction. *Mayo Clin Proc.* 2016;91(7):836–848

217. Sinsky CA, Willard-Grace R, Schutzbank AM, Sinsky TA, Margolius D, Bodenheimer T. In search of joy in practice: a report of 23 high-functioning primary care practices. *Ann Fam Med.* 2013;11(3):272–278

218. Wallace JE, Lemaire J. On physician well being-you'll get by with a little help from your friends. *Soc Sci Med.* 2007;64(12):2565–2577

219. Horn DJ, Johnston CB. Burnout and self care for palliative care practitioners. *Med Clin North Am.* 2020;104(3):561–572

220. Ofei-Dodoo S, Cleland-Leighton A, Nilsen K, Cloward JL, Casey E. Impact of a mindfulness-based, workplace group yoga intervention on burnout, self-care, and compassion in health care professionals: a pilot study. *J Occup Environ Med.* 2020;62(8):581–587

221. Forkey H, Griffin J, Szilagyi M. *Childhood Trauma and Resilience: A Practical Guide.* Itasca, IL: American Academy of Pediatrics; 2021

222. Roelofs K. Freeze for action: neurobiological mechanisms in animal and human freezing. *Philos Trans R Soc Lond B Biol Sci.* 2017;372(1718):20160206

223. Shonkoff JP, Boyce WT, McEwen BS. Neuroscience, molecular biology, and the childhood roots of health disparities: building a new framework for health promotion and disease prevention. *JAMA.* 2009;301(21):2252–2259

224. Taylor SE, Klein LC, Lewis BP, Gruenewald TL, Gurung RA, Updegraff JA. Biobehavioral responses to stress in females: tend-and-befriend, not fight-or-flight. *Psychol Rev.* 2000;107(3):411–429

225. Taylor SE. Tend and befriend: biobehavioral bases of affiliation under stress. *Curr Dir Psychol Sci.* 2006;15(6):273–277

226. Bartz JA, Zaki J, Bolger N, Ochsner KN. Social effects of oxytocin in humans: context and person matter. *Trends Cogn Sci.* 2011;15(7):301–309

227. Romano A, Tempesta B, Micioni Di Bonaventura MV, Gaetani S. From autism to eating disorders and more: the role

of oxytocin in neuropsychiatric disorders. *Front Neurosci.* 2016;9:497

228. Cardoso C, Valkanas H, Serravalle L, Ellenbogen MA. Oxytocin and social context moderate social support seeking in women during negative memory recall. *Psychoneuroendocrinology.* 2016;70:63–69

229. Shamay-Tsoory SG, Abu-Akel A. The social salience hypothesis of oxytocin. *Biol Psychiatry.* 2016;79(3):194–202

230. Bethlehem RAI, Baron-Cohen S, van Honk J, Auyeung B, Bos PA. The oxytocin paradox. *Front Behav Neurosci.* 2014;8:48

231. Chen J, Evans AN, Liu Y, Honda M, Saavedra JM, Aguilera G. Maternal deprivation in rats is associated with corticotrophin-releasing hormone (CRH) promoter hypomethylation and enhances CRH transcriptional responses to stress in adulthood. *J Neuroendocrinol.* 2012;24(7):1055–1064

232. Weaver ICG, Cervoni N, Champagne FA, et al. Epigenetic programming by maternal behavior. *Nat Neurosci.* 2004;7(8):847–854

233. American Psychiatric Association. *Diagnostic and Statistical Manual of Mental Disorders,* 5th ed. Washington, DC: American Psychiatric Publishing; 2013

234. Koita K, Long D, Hessler D, et al. Development and implementation of a pediatric adverse childhood experiences (ACEs) and other determinants of health questionnaire in the pediatric medical home: a pilot study. *PLoS One.* 2018;13(12):e0208088

235. Wade R Jr, Cronholm PF, Fein JA, et al. Household and community-level adverse childhood experiences and adult health outcomes in a diverse urban population. *Child Abuse Negl.* 2016;52:135–145

236. Child and Adolescent Health Measurement Initiative. 2019 National Survey of Children's Health: guide to topics and questions. Data Resource Center for Child and Adolescent Health supported by the US Department of Health and Human Services, Health Resources and Services Administration, Maternal and Child Health Bureau. 2020. Available at: https://

www.childhealthdata.org/learn-about-the-nsch/topics_questions. Accessed April 21, 2021

237. National Child Traumatic Stress Network. Complex trauma. Available at: www.nctsn.org/trauma-types/complex-trauma. Accessed January 11, 2021

238. Schmid M, Petermann F, Fegert JM. Developmental trauma disorder: pros and cons of including formal criteria in the psychiatric diagnostic systems. *BMC Psychiatry.* 2013;13:3. DOI: https://doi.org/10.1186/1471-244X-13-3

239. Shah AN, Jerardi KE, Auger KA, Beck AF. Can hospitalization precipitate toxic stress? *Pediatrics.* 2016;137(5):e20160204

240. Rzucidlo SE, Campbell M. Beyond the physical injuries: child and parent coping with medical traumatic stress after pediatric trauma. *J Trauma Nurs.* 2009;16(3):130–135

241. National Child Traumatic Stress Network. Effects. Available at: https://www.nctsn.org/what-is-child-trauma/trauma-types/medical-trauma/effects. Accessed January 11, 2021

242. US Department of Health and Human Services, Administration for Children and Families. Secondary traumatic stress. Available at: https://www.acf.hhs.gov/trauma-toolkit/secondary-traumatic-stress. Accessed January 11, 2021

243. The National Child Traumatic Stress Network. Families and caregivers. Available at: https://www.nctsn.org/audiences/families-and-caregivers. Accessed January 11, 2021

244. US Department of Health and Human Services, Administration for Children and Families. Resources on trauma for caregivers and families. Available at: https://www.childwelfare.gov/topics/responding/trauma/caregivers/. Accessed January 11, 2021

245. American Academy of Pediatrics. Parenting After Trauma: Understanding Your Child's NeedsAvailable at: https://www.aap.org/en-us/advocacy-and-policy/aap-health-initiatives/healthy-foster-care-america/Documents/Family Handout.pdf. Accessed June 24, 2021

246. Porges S, Lewis GF. The polyvagal hypothesis: common mechanisms mediating autonomic regulation, vocalizations and listening. In: Brudzynski SM, ed. *Handbook of Mammalian Vocalization: An Integrative Neuroscience Approach*. New York, NY: Elsevier; 2009:255–264

247. Bethell C, Gombojav N, Solloway M, Wissow L. Adverse childhood experiences, resilience and mindfulness-based approaches: common denominator issues for children with emotional, mental, or behavioral problems. *Child Adolesc Psychiatr Clin N Am*. 2016;25(2):139–156

POLICY STATEMENT Organizational Principles to Guide and Define the Child Health Care System and/or Improve the Health of all Children

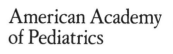

American Academy
of Pediatrics

DEDICATED TO THE HEALTH OF ALL CHILDREN™

This Policy Statement was reaffirmed December 2023.

The Effects of Armed Conflict on Children

Sherry Shenoda, MD, FAAP,[a] Ayesha Kadir, MD, MSc, FAAP,[b] Shelly Pitterman, PhD,[c] Jeffrey Goldhagen, MD, MPH, FAAP,[a] SECTION ON INTERNATIONAL CHILD HEALTH

abstract

Children are increasingly exposed to armed conflict and targeted by governmental and nongovernmental combatants. Armed conflict directly and indirectly affects children's physical, mental, and behavioral health. It can affect every organ system, and its impact can persist throughout the life course. In addition, children are disproportionately impacted by morbidity and mortality associated with armed conflict. A children's rights–based approach provides a framework for collaboration by the American Academy of Pediatrics, child health professionals, and national and international partners to respond in the domains of clinical care, systems development, and policy formulation. The American Academy of Pediatrics and child health professionals have critical and synergistic roles to play in the global response to the impact of armed conflict on children.

If we are to reach real peace in this world, and if we are to carry on a real war against war, we shall have to begin with the children.

Mahatma Gandhi

BACKGROUND

The acute and chronic effects of armed conflict on child health and well-being are among the greatest children's rights violations of the 21st century. For the purpose of this policy statement and the associated technical report,[1] armed conflict is defined as any organized dispute that involves the use of weapons, violence, or force, whether within national borders or beyond and whether involving state actors or nongovernmental entities (Table 1). Examples include international wars, civil wars, and conflicts between other kinds of groups, such as ethnic conflicts and violence associated with narcotics trafficking and gang violence involving narcotics. Civilian casualties have increased such that 90% of deaths from armed conflicts in the first decade of the 21st century were civilians,[2] a significant number of whom were children.[3–5] Children

[a]Division of Community and Societal Pediatrics, University of Florida College of Medicine—Jacksonville, Jacksonville, Florida; [b]Centre for Social Paediatrics, Herlev Hospital, Herlev, Denmark; and [c]United Nations High Commissioner for Refugees, Washington, District of Columbia

Dr Shenoda identified the need to write this policy statement, conducted the supporting literature review, and wrote the first draft of the manuscript; Dr Goldhagen identified the need to write this policy statement and wrote the first draft of the manuscript; Dr Kadir and Mr Pitterman contributed to revisions; and all authors approved the final manuscript as submitted.

DOI: https://doi.org/10.1542/peds.2018-2585

Address correspondence to Sherry Shenoda, MD, FAAP. E-mail: sshenoda@thechildrensclinic.org.

To cite: Shenoda S, Kadir A, Pitterman S, et al. The Effects of Armed Conflict on Children. *Pediatrics.* 2018;142(6): e20182585

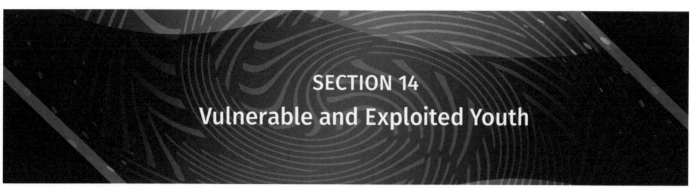

SECTION 14
Vulnerable and Exploited Youth

Some articles are available online only; scan the QR code to access online content.

CLINICAL REPORT Guidance for the Clinician in Rendering Pediatric Care

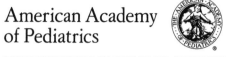

American Academy
of Pediatrics

DEDICATED TO THE HEALTH OF ALL CHILDREN™

Exploitation, Labor and Sex Trafficking of Children and Adolescents: Health Care Needs of Patients

Jordan Greenbaum, MD,[a] Dana Kaplan, MD, FAAP,[b,d] Janine Young, MD, FAAP,[c]
COUNCIL ON CHILD ABUSE AND NEGLECT, COUNCIL ON IMMIGRANT CHILD AND FAMILY HEALTH

abstract

Exploitation and labor and sex trafficking of children and adolescents is a major public health problem in the United States and throughout the world. Significant numbers of US and non-US–born children and adolescents (including unaccompanied immigrant minors) are affected by this growing concern and may experience a range of serious physical and mental health problems associated with human trafficking and exploitation (T/E). Despite these considerations, there is limited information available for health care providers regarding the nature and scope of T/E and how providers may help recognize and protect children and adolescents. Knowledge of risk factors, recruitment practices, possible indicators of T/E, and common medical, mental, and emotional health problems experienced by affected individuals will assist health care providers in recognizing vulnerable children and adolescents and responding appropriately. A trauma-informed, rights-based, culturally sensitive approach helps providers identify and treat patients who have experienced or are at risk for T/E. As health care providers, educators, and leaders in child advocacy and development, pediatricians play an important role in addressing the public health issues faced by children and adolescents who experience exploitation and trafficking. Working across disciplines with professionals in the community, health care providers can offer evidence-based medical screening, treatment, and holistic services to individuals who have experienced T/E and assist vulnerable patients and families in recognizing signs of T/E.

[a]International Centre for Missing and Exploited Children, Alexandria, Virginia; [b]Department of Pediatrics, Staten Island University Hospital, Northwell Health Physician Partners, Staten Island, New York; [c]Department of Pediatrics, University of California, San Diego, California; and [d]The Barbara and Donald Zucker School of Medicine at Hofstra/Northwell, Hempstead, New York

Each author contributed to report design, literature review, manuscript development, and editing.

Clinical reports from the American Academy of Pediatrics benefit from expertise and resources of liaisons and internal (AAP) and external reviewers. However, clinical reports from the American Academy of Pediatrics may not reflect the views of the liaisons or the organizations or government agencies that they represent.

The guidance in this report does not indicate an exclusive course of treatment or serve as a standard of medical care. Variations, taking into account individual circumstances, may be appropriate.

All clinical reports from the American Academy of Pediatrics automatically expire 5 years after publication unless reaffirmed, revised, or retired at or before that time.

DOI: https://doi.org/10.1542/peds.2022-060416

Address correspondence to Jordan Greenbaum, MD. E-mail: jgreenbaum@icmec.org

To cite: Greenbaum J, Kaplan D, Young J, et al; AAP Council on Child Abuse and Neglect, AAP Council on Immigrant Child and Family Health. Exploitation, Labor and Sex Trafficking of Children and Adolescents: Health Care Needs of Patients. *Pediatrics.* 2023;151(1):e2022060416

This clinical report targets primary care and specialty pediatric providers working in private and public clinics, hospitals, emergency departments, and urgent care centers. Research demonstrates that children and youth who experience sex and labor trafficking and exploitation (T/E) may seek health care in a variety of settings,[1-3] making it essential that pediatric providers anywhere are equipped to recognize potential T/E and respond appropriately. The guidance offered here is aimed to assist health care professionals in recognizing previously unidentified T/E, as well as in providing a basic initial response to suspected and confirmed cases of exploitation. Referrals for higher-level care may be indicated and are discussed. Providers and all of their staff need to adopt a trauma-informed, rights-based, culturally responsive approach to care of patients suspected of experiencing T/E, although these skills are relevant to care of any patient who may have experienced significant trauma. That is, the skills are generalizable and highly relevant to daily clinical practice. Creating a trauma-informed workspace and providing care to patients who have experienced T/E and other major traumatic experiences is, admittedly, time-consuming and poorly reimbursed by payers. However, having basic skills in rights-based practices and a protocol summarizing staff roles and responsibilities for managing suspected T/E will significantly reduce the time expenditure and very likely improve outcomes for vulnerable patients. Ample resources for training staff on trauma-informed care and creating a clinic or hospital protocol are available in this document and elsewhere.[4-8]

Human sex and labor trafficking and exploitation (T/E) are significant global health issues involving egregious violations of an individual's fundamental dignity and human rights.[9] However, many who experience T/E do not perceive themselves as being exploited, which makes identification and assistance challenging. Per the International Labor Organization, child sex trafficking is considered a subset of forced labor, with global estimates of

approximately 3.3 million children and adolescents experiencing forced labor in 2021, of whom approximately 1.7 million were subjected to commercial sexual exploitation.[10] Reliable national prevalence data for child labor and sex T/E in the United States are not yet available. Violence and psychological manipulation are common in both types of T/E, and affected individuals are at increased risk of inflicted and work-related injury, sexual assault, infectious diseases, substance use disorders, untreated chronic medical conditions, malnutrition, toxic exposures, posttraumatic stress disorder (PTSD), complex PTSD, major depression, anxiety disorders, and other mental health diagnoses.[3,11-20] Given the large number of children and adolescents involved and the numerous adverse effects on physical and mental health, pediatricians and pediatric health care providers are in a unique position to identify and assist those who experience labor and/or sex T/E.[21]

When labor or sex trafficking occurs in a person's home country, it is termed domestic trafficking; when international boundaries are crossed, it is termed transnational trafficking.[22] In fiscal year 2018 (the most recent federal data available), the top 3 countries of origin of persons experiencing trafficking in the United States were the United States, Mexico, and the Philippines.[23] However, few data are available on the prevalence of transnational trafficking of both accompanied and unaccompanied children and adolescents immigrating to the United States or of domestic trafficking once these individuals have settled in the United States.[24] Available data from the Unaccompanied Refugee Minor Program of the Office of Refugee Resettlement demonstrates that the number of children and adolescents experiencing labor and sex trafficking

has significantly increased in recent years.[25]

According to US federal laws, child sex trafficking occurs when a minor (<18 years) exchanges a sex act for something of perceived value. Unlike adult sex trafficking (persons over age 18), sex trafficking involving a minor does not require demonstration of force, fraud, or coercion, although these are often present. Child labor trafficking occurs when someone compels a minor to perform forced labor.[26,27] Given that minors may work legally and willingly (as a general rule, the Federal Labor Standards Act sets 14 years as the minimum age for employment[28]), force, fraud, or coercion are necessary to constitute child labor trafficking. Individual state laws vary somewhat but generally resemble the federal definition.

Smuggling differs from trafficking in that it represents a crime against a country (illegally crossing a border), rather than a person (exploitation), and by definition, requires transportation.[29] Trafficking may occur in the absence of victim transport. Although smuggling may be transformed into trafficking through fraud and deceit, the former typically involves a limited and voluntary business agreement between smuggler (often called a coyote) and client that ends after border crossing, whereas human trafficking involves force, fraud, or coercion or exploitation of a minor and an indefinite period of exploitation. Smuggling across the US-Mexico border has increased significantly in recent years and crossing to the US side without detection has become more difficult. As such, smugglers may charge immigrant families upwards of $10 000 with children and adolescents. Furthermore, families may be subsequently forced to work to pay off these inordinate debts.[30]

It is important to note the spectrum of terminology surrounding human T/E. Specific terms being used in legal and other settings have implications for children and adolescents, themselves, in addition to influencing public perception. Commercial sexual exploitation of children is closely related to sex trafficking and involves online or offline "crimes of a sexual nature committed against juvenile victims for financial or other economic reasons. ..."[31] These crimes include sex trafficking, "prostitution" (a term no longer being used when referring to children and adolescents,[32] given the psychosocial implications of this term), the mail-order-bride trade, underage marriage, the production and/or viewing of child sexual abuse materials (formerly termed "child pornography"), stripping, online sexual exploitation, and performing in sexual venues such as "peep shows" or "clubs." Many also include "survival sex" in this definition (exchange of sexual activity for basic necessities, such as shelter, food, or money), a practice common among homeless and runaway youth.[33–36] This report addresses both trafficking and exploitation (T/E).

Child marriage is common in many areas of the world[10,37,38–40]; the International Labor Organization estimated that approximately 40% of the 22 million people involved in a forced marriage in 2021 were married when they were younger than 18 years.[10] One example of forced underage marriage involves immigrant youth, including US-born individuals of immigrant parents who are sent to the parental country of origin to be married to a relative or family acquaintance. The marriage partner may be decades older than the child. It is unknown how many children and adolescents residing in the United States are at risk for forced underage marriage. In some situations, child marriage may involve slavery-like conditions, including coercion, force, and sexual and labor exploitation, consistent with human trafficking.[40] Globally, forced underage marriage may increase significantly with pandemics such as the coronavirus disease 2019 (COVID-19) pandemic[10] and with other natural disasters or public health crises as in some cultures, female children and adolescents are considered a "burden" economically, with significant cultural restrictions in education and opportunities for financial independence. Rates of child marriage may increase in response to extreme economic and/or social conditions, such as during the mass migration related to the Syrian crisis.[41]

RISK FACTORS FOR LABOR AND SEX TRAFFICKING AND EXPLOITATION

Studies generally indicate that the typical age of entrance into sex T/E is 11 to 17 years, although much younger individuals may be involved, especially in intrafamilial cases (eg, situations in which a family member is involved in the exploitation).[12,22,29,42,43] Labor T/E in the United States tends to focus on adults and adolescents rather than young children;[36,44–46] whether this reflects true disparities among age groups or a bias in recognition and reporting (perhaps young children are harder to identify) is unclear. Certainly, forced labor involving young children is a major global problem and is well-documented.[47–51]

By virtue of their young age, children and adolescents are vulnerable to manipulation and exploitation, because they have limited life experiences, a need for attachment and acceptance, an immature prefrontal cortex (with limited ability to control impulses, think critically about alternative actions, and analyze risks and benefits of situations), and limited options for action. Adolescents are learning about their own sexuality and adjusting to physical changes associated with puberty. However, some children and adolescents are at further risk because of individual, relationship, and community factors.[52] Extreme poverty may drive children, adolescents, and caregivers to migrate to large cities or immigrate to other countries and accept high-risk proposals for jobs that involve exploitative conditions. Early childhood adversity, including child abuse and neglect, is common,[53] especially among those in foster care. These traumatic experiences may drive children and adolescents to run away from home or custodial care.[54] Other risk factors are listed in Table 1.

In the United States, societal attitudes of gender bias and discrimination, sexualization of females, exoticism of American Indian and Alaskan Native (AI/AN) and Asian females, and glorification of the "pimp" in US popular culture, add to the vulnerability of children and adolescents.[23] In addition to the vulnerability associated with young age, many groups including lesbian, gay, bisexual, transgender, and queer or questioning (LGBTQ+) (particularly Black trans "womyn/gurls") and AI/AN youth are at high risk of T/E, not because of individual or group characteristics that render them vulnerable but because of the very history of US systematic enslavement, colonization, forced migration, marginalization, and discrimination against Black, Indigenous, and people of color over centuries. This systematic, often codified marginalization and discrimination has led to a loss of cultural identity, language, family ties (through US forced separation of enslaved children and adolescents and AI/AN minors from their parents), community, and means for advancement and prosperity.[55] In the case of the LGBTQ+ community, this

TABLE 1 Risk Factors for Labor and Sex T/E[22,36,53,81,90,99,181–189]

Individual	Relationship	Community	Societal
History of maltreatment	Family violence and/or dysfunction	Tolerance of sexual exploitation	Gender-based violence and discrimination
Homeless or runaway	Family poverty	High crime rate, lack of law enforcement	Cultural attitudes or beliefs (eg, homophobia, transphobia, xenophobia)
Substance misuse	Forced migration	Lack of community resources or support	Systemic and historical racism or discrimination
History with juvenile justice	Intolerance of gender identity and/or sexual orientation	Transient male populations	Natural disasters
History with child protective services			Political or social upheaval
Unaccompanied immigrant minor or undocumented immigrant status			
Exposure of children and adolescents to sexual abuse material or violent pornography			
High number of adverse childhood experiences (ACEs)			
Mental illness			

marginalization, including by family members, may lead to increased rates of running away from home, limited job opportunities, substance use, and social isolation. All of these factors play a part in increasing the risk of T/E.[56–60]

There are global concerns that vulnerability to T/E has increased during the COVID-19 pandemic, although it is too early in the pandemic to obtain a strong evidence base to confirm these concerns.[61–69] Evidence suggests that the pandemic has disproportionately impacted minority communities within the United States, consistent with global reports that stress the particularly heavy impact on marginalized groups.[63,65,68,70,71] Some of this disparity may be related to differences in prevalence and severity of pre-existing chronic disease among population groups and to variations in social determinants of health.[71] Although measures undertaken to control viral spread are critical for public health, unintended negative consequences may increase the risk of T/E. For example, closures of businesses and schools, lockdowns (which vary in severity by country), travel restrictions, and border closures have led to (a) increased isolation of persons at risk for exploitation; (b) increased exposure to abusers and traffickers (eg, intrafamilial traffickers and exploiters of domestic workers); (c) loss of income (particularly impacting those working in low-paying jobs and the informal sector); (d) increased vulnerability to unscrupulous money lenders and to debt bondage; (e) limited access of mandatory reporters to children and adolescents at risk for T/E; and (f) limited services to individuals who have experienced, or are at risk for T/E (eg, immigrants, street-based children and adolescents, AI/AN communities).[61,67,68,72–74] School closures, increased poverty, and lack of access to social support during a crisis exacerbate these conditions.[60,75] COVID-19–related anxiety and stress may increase the risk for T/E by exacerbating mental health issues in parents, children and adolescents, and individuals who have experienced exploitation. Substance use, exposure of minors to violence in the home, and unsupervised online screen time also may have increased during the COVID-19 pandemic.[76–79]

The ratio of female-to-male children and adolescents experiencing T/E is unclear, because reliable estimates of the prevalence of human trafficking are difficult to obtain.[80] Much more attention has been paid to affected females, and this may be related to a number of factors, including a true higher proportion of females identified in large-scale studies,[9] evidence to suggest that females are more likely than males to be controlled by third-party traffickers,[81,82] that females present for health care more often because of T/E-related pregnancy and/or pelvic inflammatory disease, public discomfort with the idea of males having sex with men, public and media misperception that males cannot be subjected to sex T/E, objectified, or coerced,[83] and a general lack of screening of males for possible commercial sexual activity.[84] Sex trafficking also tends to dominate the public interest at the expense of attention to labor T/E, where males are frequently identified.[9] It is likely that the number of males experiencing T/E is grossly underestimated, because males may be less likely to be seen as "victims" by themselves[82] or by others.[14,85]

Individuals identifying as LGTBQ+ are at elevated risk of running away from home, being told to leave home, and of homelessness, and further, of engaging in transactional sex.[81,86–88] In a study of homeless youth in New York City, transgender youth were nearly 7 times more likely to engage in transactional sex than were nontransgender youth, and homosexual and bisexual youth were 6.6 times more likely than their heterosexual counterparts to engage in transactional sex.[89]

Individuals experiencing labor and/ or sex T/E may be recruited by peers, relatives, community members, or strangers.[12,90–92] They may be seduced by promises of love, money, attention, assistance, or acceptance.[42] They may be induced (by force, coercion, or lack of options) to exchange sex or engage in exploitative labor to obtain drugs, meet survival needs, or help their family's extreme poverty.[47,50,93] Fraudulent employment agencies may promise lucrative jobs, only to involve the children and adolescents in debt bondage.[94] Smugglers may decide to traffic immigrant youth after crossing a border.[19] Parental authority may be used in cases of intrafamilial T/E.[4,12]

Recruitment may begin over the Internet, often through use of social media, or it may involve face-to-face encounters. The process may be abrupt or prolonged. Once recruited into labor and/or sex T/E, many children and adolescents may be controlled by traffickers through use of psychological manipulation, false information (eg, labor rights, immigrant rights, deportation policies), fulfillment of an individual's need for attention and love, or threats of harm to the youth or their family. Traffickers may exert control through blackmail, fraud or deception, and/or violence.[42,45,92,95] By alternating acts of violence and cruelty with acts of kindness and "love," a trafficker may build strong bonds with children and adolescents, making it very difficult for youth to leave the situation.[22] Individuals experiencing labor or sex T/E may not recognize their situation as exploitative, instead feeling that they "owe" their traffickers obedience because of previous kind behaviors or because of an exorbitant debt. They may feel that engaging in commercial sex or submitting to exploitative work conditions is "voluntary," or that their actions demonstrate their love for an intimate partner or family member.[42,96,97] Immigrant children and adolescents exploited in a new country may feel they have no rights to better treatment and are often unfamiliar with local labor laws. They may lack familiarity with a new culture or may hold cultural views that condone inequality and discrimination.[98,99] Individuals may remain in exploitative conditions for extended periods and may return to a trafficking relationship 1 or more times before final extrication.[92]

As a result of the intense and prolonged psychological and physical trauma experienced by children and adolescents during their periods of forced labor or sexual T/E, many develop medical and mental health issues (Table 2). Some may have preexisting physical and mental health diagnoses. A history of prior sexual abuse and other adverse childhood experiences may be associated with subsequent health problems that are exacerbated by exploitation.[100,101–104]

IDENTIFICATION AND EVALUATION

Health care providers may encounter children and adolescents with a history of T/E in emergency departments, family planning clinics (including Title X clinics), tribal clinics, child abuse or foster care clinics, public clinics or private offices, school-based health centers, urgent care centers, inpatient hospital wards, pediatric intensive care units, or institutional settings.[1,3,16,57,105,106] Care may be sought for routine health maintenance, child abuse, sexual assault, or any of the conditions listed in Table 2.[1,3,105,107] Clinicians may provide care to children and adolescents whose parent has experienced T/A for labor or sex. In these cases, it is essential for providers to determine current risk to the patient as well as to the parent or guardian and intervene for both patient and guardian, as relevant.

It is critically important for health care facilities to have guidelines or protocols in place to assist providers in identifying patients at risk for labor and sex T/E and to offer optimal, patient-centered, trauma-informed, rights-based, and culturally sensitive care to the patient and caregivers.[108] The patient's best interest should guide all decisions, as should respect for basic child rights, such as the need for information, privacy, and the right to consent or provide assent.[109] There are resources to assist in the development of such guidelines (https://training.icmec. org/courses/course-v1:icmec+ ICMEC103 + 2021/about).[7,8,110] It is also feasible to incorporate T/E information into guidelines originally created for related conditions, such as child sexual abuse,[6] and into protocols for the medical care of immigrant children and adolescents and patients in foster care.[111]

Although many individuals experiencing T/E have access to medical facilities for primary, reproductive, mental health, or emergency care,[112] others experience significant barriers related to transportation, inability to miss work, lack of knowledge of health care services, insurance issues, lack of identification, language barriers, fear of deportation because of immigration status, fear of stigma or shame, or the need to care for

TABLE 2 Health Conditions Associated with Labor and Sex T/E[11,14–16,18–20,47–49,52,59,98,120,146,190–194,195–197]

Health Condition
Physical
Traumatic injury (work-related; assault)
Sexually transmitted infections (STIs)
Other communicable diseases (eg, tuberculosis,[2] scabies)
Unwanted pregnancy and associated complications
HIV or AIDS
Malnutrition, weight loss, or stunting
Dehydration
Exposure (heat or cold)
Toxic exposures (eg, lead, chemicals, dust, silica, mercury)
Over-use injuries; scarring; loss of function
Chronic pain
Fatigue
Dizziness
Untreated or late-presenting acute or chronic conditions
Mental or emotional health
Post-traumatic stress disorder (PTSD)
Complex PTSD
Major depression
Suicidality
Anxiety disorders
Substance use disorders
Behavioral problems (eg, opposition, aggression, antisocial behavior)
Somatization
Memory problems
Attention deficit, hyperactivity
Self-harm behaviors

others.[57,107] Minors may seek care without parental consent for certain conditions (ie, reproductive health, substance use, mental health, and sexual assault). However, if care is sought for other conditions, parental consent may be necessary, unless the clinician determines that emergency care is required. In these cases, the need for parental consent may prevent children and adolescents from seeking health services.

Some individuals may access care but experience significant barriers to disclosing their exploitation.[91,113–115] Fear of involvement of police or child protective services, deportation, breaches in patient confidentiality, or repercussions by the trafficker may inhibit children and adolescents from openly discussing their situation with clinicians. Some individuals may be told to provide false information to health care staff and may be closely monitored by their trafficker (who may accompany the child or track

the health visit through a cell phone).[107] Others may not perceive their situation as exploitative, as described previously. Mistrust of health professionals and the health system may be associated with deep roots in systemic racism, historical trauma, discrimination (eg, homophobia and transphobia), and expectations of and/or prior direct experience of implicit or explicit bias by medical staff.[57,116]

Barriers to patient disclosure of victimization originate with health care providers and health facilities as well. Lack of labor and sex T/E staff training is a major problem. In 1 study of health care professionals working in outpatient and inpatient settings, 75.9% reported no prior training related to human trafficking.[117] Provider discomfort with asking sensitive questions, provider bias, and lack of knowledge of resources may prevent clinicians from broaching the subject of T/E; limited time, use of

family members as interpreters rather than certified medical interpreters, and lack of space for private conversations may present additional challenges.[107,112,118,119]

Given the numerous barriers to patient disclosure of T/E, health care providers must remain alert for the possibility of exploitation. "Red flags" for potential labor or sexual T/E may be associated with the circumstances around the patient's presentation for care (eg, delayed presentation for a significant medical condition; domineering companion), historical factors identified during the medical history (eg, prior work-related trauma; multiple sexually transmitted infections [STIs]), or findings noted on physical examination (eg, evidence to suggest inflicted injury). Some red flag signs and symptoms are listed in Table 3. However, it is important to keep in mind that patients who have experienced T/E may exhibit none of these characteristics, and the presence of such conditions is not specific for trafficking and exploitation. In addition, strong empirical data are lacking for many of the red flags listed in Table 3, especially for specific populations such as AI/AN and immigrant children and adolescents.

Screening Tools

Screening tools to identify people who may be experiencing T/E designed for a busy health care setting are emerging.[120,105,121–123] The goal of a screen is not to obtain a patient's definitive disclosure of T/E but to determine which patients are at particularly high risk and what major factors may be contributing to that risk to inform medical intervention. For example, the Short Screen for Child Sex Trafficking[120,105,124] includes questions about risk factors (eg, substance use, involvement with law enforcement, number of sex partners, and history of STIs) rather than

TABLE 3 Potential "Red Flags" for Labor or Sex T/E

Initial presentation
    Accompanied by domineering adult who does not allow child to answer questions
    Accompanied by unrelated adult
    Accompanied by peers and only 1 other adult
    Inconsistent information provided by patient or companion
    Delay in seeking medical care
    Patient is poor historian (from sleep deprivation or drug intoxication)
Chief complaint involves:
    • Acute assault (sexual or physical)
    • Work-related trauma or toxic exposure
    • Mental and emotional health issues
    • Genitourinary symptoms or signs
    • Substance use or ingestion
Historical factors
    Multiple sexually transmitted infections
    Previous pregnancy or termination
    Frequent visits for emergency contraception
    Frequent substance use
    Prior sexual abuse, assault, or other maltreatment
    Recent immigration; does not speak local language; undocumented immigrant status
Physical findings
    Withdrawn, fearful, hostile, or suspicious demeanor
    Evidence of malnutrition
    Untreated chronic disease or injury
Evidence suggestive of inflicted injury
Signs of substance use or abuse (eg, nonmedical use)
Dental trauma or evidence of neglect
In possession of expensive items, such as clothing, inconsistent with rest of presentation
Constantly checking phone, appears anxious or afraid

specific questions about T/E. A positive screen should prompt follow-up questions to assess the level of risk and to determine patient needs. This focus on risk allows for a tailored approach to intervention and emphasizes patient needs over law enforcement response. Furthermore, most health care providers are not in a position to discern the nuances of legal definitions (eg, between child labor exploitation and labor trafficking).

The screen may be performed verbally using pen and paper or via electronic devices. If administered in a language other than English, certified medical interpretation or translation should be used. A review of psychosocial assessment tools found that adolescents demonstrated higher disclosure rates with written or online instruments compared with verbal administration of the tool.[106,] [125] A study using the Short Screen for Child Sex Trafficking administered in English and Spanish

via electronic tablet showed high rates of disclosure of sensitive information, suggesting that patients are comfortable sharing this type of information with health professionals.[122]

If screen results indicate features of concern for possible T/E, further assessment with open-ended questions about the positive screen items is indicated. Depending on patient comfort level, more direct questions about T/E may be asked as well. Examples include:

1. "You indicated in your questionnaire that you have run away from home in the past. Can you tell me about the last time this happened?"
2. "Sometimes kids are in a position where they really need food, clothing, a place to stay, or they want to buy something for themselves or someone else, but they don't have money, so they have to consider trading sex for

what they need. Have you ever been in a position where you've had to consider doing this?" (Note: A positive answer does NOT indicate sex T/E actually occurred [children and adolescents may have decided not to engage in transactional sex] but likely indicates a high-risk situation warranting intervention on the part of the provider. This may involve a discussion of possible community services to address underlying needs, and potentially a report to authorities about suspected trafficking.)
3. "I have heard that sometimes people are asked if they would have sex in exchange for something. Has that ever happened to you?"
4. "Have you ever been forced to do things for someone to pay off a debt, or make money for that person? Do you feel comfortable telling me about that?"

These questions should be asked sensitively, using a conversational approach rather than reading, verbatim, from a checklist. For example, the clinician may engage the patient in a general discussion about sexual practices, sexual identity, and sexual preference, including some of these questions in the conversation.

Pediatric T/E screening tools designed for health settings are limited and are not validated for preadolescents, children, and adolescents with significant cognitive disabilities, immigrant populations, or AI/AN patients. They do not screen for labor T/E. In these situations, the health care provider may choose to "screen" for T/E by asking general, open-ended questions about risk factors, such as early childhood abuse and neglect as well as about living and working conditions. For example, the clinician might begin with: "My next question is about work. The words, 'work' and 'job' can mean lots of things, from formal jobs in areas like construction or restaurant work, to informal arrangements to clean someone's home, take care of children, or to help a relative with their job. Sometimes 'work' involves selling drugs, stealing or some other activity that a person does for someone else. Have you ever had a job or done work for someone else?" With an affirmative answer, the clinician might continue with, "Can you tell me something about it? What did your work involve? Did you have specific work hours? Did you wear any safety equipment (if appropriate)?" Then, move on to more specific questions about possible exploitation, "Have you ever had a job, only to find that the work you are doing, or the conditions of your work are not what you were promised? Has anyone associated with your work ever made you feel scared?"

Helpful information may be gained from detailed social histories. As an example, AI/AN children and adolescents are at high risk for homelessness, family violence, sexual abuse or assault, poverty, and severe systemic racism and discrimination, all of which render them at risk for T/E.[57-60] Undocumented immigrant children and adolescents (especially those who are unaccompanied) are very vulnerable to T/E because of their age and dependence on others, their unfamiliarity with new culture and laws, difficulty accessing resources, widespread xenophobia and adjustment challenges with family reunification, or placement with a nonparent sponsor.[126-128] Some of these risk factors may be identified through use of the HEADSSS assessment (home, education or employment, activities, drugs, sexuality, suicide or depression, and safety),[125] especially if questions about family conflict and living and work conditions are incorporated. If during the HEADSSS questions, a patient mentions something that may raise concern for sex and/or

labor T/E, this should be explored in more detail to better assess risk. HEADSSS questions focusing on the child's feelings regarding their sexuality, school experiences of bullying and discrimination, and potential familial tension over the child's gender identity or sexual orientation may reveal evidence of significant social rejection and ostracism. Such rejection may increase the risk of running away from home and experiencing sex or labor T/E.[35,129]

Whether formal screening is conducted, it is very helpful to offer patients education about healthy relationships and the impact of violence on health, with an offer of relevant resources.[130] Such "universal education and resources" have been shown to be helpful for women experiencing intimate partner violence.[130,131] Other topics of education may also be relevant, including basic worker rights for youth who have a job,[132] common exploitative work practices, STI prevention, and harm reduction techniques for those experiencing high-risk situations such as homelessness. Examples of the latter include strategies to minimize risk of assault when sleeping at night or having a companion present if the individual will be engaging in high-risk activities (eg, getting into a car with a stranger).

Screening, education, and provision of resources are unlikely to be fruitful if not provided in a trauma-informed, rights-based, and culturally appropriate manner and in the patient's primary language.[5,108,109] These strategies should be employed by all staff interacting with the patient, from those in charge of scheduling, to interpreters, clinicians, and support staff. Multigenerational, historical trauma, and other forms of chronic, repeated, and severe trauma experienced before and during a period of T/E may cause an individual

to adopt feelings, beliefs, attitudes, and behaviors that help them to survive a dangerous world but that seem maladaptive in nonthreatening situations.[133] Examples may include hostility toward health professionals or others in positions of perceived authority, marked withdrawal, very low self-esteem, self-medication through substance use, or engagement in high-risk sexual behavior. Considering the impact of trauma on a patient's thoughts, emotions, behaviors, and development and making appropriate accommodations in response are hallmarks of a trauma-informed approach.[4,5] Building a sense of trust and safety is a critical first step in enabling a patient to discuss their needs and concerns.[134] To further establish trust and foster a supportive clinical relationship, the health care provider needs to promptly address the chief complaint and other immediate concerns that are voiced so that children and adolescents feel their needs are being taken seriously.[135] Table 4 outlines practical strategies for a trauma-informed approach to patient interaction.[5]

Individuals who experience T/E may be subjected to bias and discrimination on multiple levels related to stigma against homelessness, poverty, immigration status, systemic racism, and historical domination (Fig 1).[136] Cultural sensitivity must extend beyond the individual practitioner to the health care organization,[137] with policies and practices in place to foster a sense of cultural safety ("an environment which is safe for people; where there is no ... challenge or denial of their identity, of who they are and what they need. It is about shared respect, shared meaning, shared knowledge and experience, of learning together with dignity, and truly listening").[138,139] Cultural sensitivity includes zero tolerance policies for bias and

TABLE 4 Practical Strategies for a Trauma-Informed, Rights-Based Approach to Patient Care[5,108,109,137,140–142,156,198–201]

Concept	Strategies
Safety and trust	(1) Have a discussion with the patient without the companion present, to promote sharing of sensitive information. Separating the child or adolescent from the companion may be facilitated by explaining that it is organizational practice to spend some time alone with patients. Once alone with the patient, the provider can ask if the child or adolescent feels comfortable or if they wish the companion to be present. If the child does not feel safe speaking to the provider alone, sensitive questions should NOT be asked in the presence of the companion.
	(2) Take time to build rapport.
	(3) Attend to basic physical needs ("Are you warm enough?")
	(4) Avoid any suggestion of blame or shame.
	(5) Have a chaperone in the room (preferably of a gender of patient's choosing).
	(6) Promptly address the patient's chief complaint(s).
Privacy and confidentiality	(1) Ensure the room is quiet and staff interruptions are minimized (eg, put a sign on the door).
	(2) Discuss limits of confidentiality involving:
	• Mandatory reporting
	• Access to electronic health record (EHR) by others
Respect	(1) Use a calm, nonjudgmental, open, and empathic manner.
	(2) Actively listen, maintain good eye contact, acknowledge patient's views, and accept their perspective.
	(3) Listen more than speak. Ask questions to demonstrate caring and involvement.
	(4) Recognize the strengths and resilience of your patient and remind them of these strengths.
Transparency	(1) Explain your role, and review all steps of visit, including the reasons for each step (eg, reason for asking sensitive questions, performing physical and anogenital examination, obtaining forensic evidence kit and diagnostic tests, and offering specific treatments).
Empowerment and collaboration	(1) After explaining each portion of the medical visit, ask "What questions do you have?" Invite patient to share their concerns.
	(2) Ask permission to perform each of the steps of the medical visit; respect patient wishes to decline steps whenever safe and feasible. Make sure the patient understands that they can refuse components of the health visit.
	(3) Offer choices whenever possible (eg, "Would you like to sit in the chair or on the exam table while we chat?")
	(4) Ask for the individual's opinion, acknowledging their role as an expert on themselves.
	(5) Before offering services and resources yourself, ask the patient what they feel would be helpful to them after they leave the health facility. Then ask them if they would like to hear some ideas you have for possible resources.
	(6) Encourage shared decision-making throughout all steps of the visit, and when discussing potential referrals and resources.
	(7) Recognize circumstances that require patient consent, parent consent and/or patient assent when proceeding with medical intervention (must be familiar with adolescent rights in the state you practice).
Sensitivity to culture, gender, and historical issues as well as systemic racism and discrimination	(1) Be aware of potential cultural differences involving gender roles; views of sex, sexuality, and virginity; mental health disorders and treatment; social hierarchies; communication styles; causes of health problems; and philosophies of life.
	(2) Avoid assumptions about gender identity, sexual orientation; use gender-neutral language; clarify preferred pronouns.
	(3) Consider your own biases that may influence your interaction with the patient; take steps to monitor yourself to avoid engaging in discriminatory or stigmatizing behavior.
	(4) Be aware of bias and discrimination in the workplace and actively address issues that arise.
	(5) Use professional medical interpreters in all cases and not patient companions. Ensure that the patient and family do not know the interpreter or come from the same community.
	(6) Take time to learn about beliefs and practices within the cultures often encountered in your health care setting; learn from interpreters, staff at refugee organizations, and other experts in the community.
Minimize retraumatization	(1) Be aware of conditions in the health setting that may mimic adverse experiences related to trafficking, including situations in which the patient feels out of control, uncertain about what will happen next, threatened, shamed, coerced, or vulnerable. Many of these situations may be prevented by demonstrating respect, providing explanations, obtaining permission, and maintaining transparency.
	(2) Monitor the patient for signs of distress while obtaining the history and conducting the examination. Take steps to diffuse the anxiety (eg, pause, acknowledge distress, allow the patient control over whether to continue or stop the activity [if feasible]; provide support and reassurance).
	(3) Do not label or judge the patient; use language the patient is using so as to avoid making assumptions or being perceived as judgmental or biased, though that may not be the intention of the provider. Give the patient the power to ask the provider to stop or indicate (verbally or nonverbally) when something makes them uncomfortable.

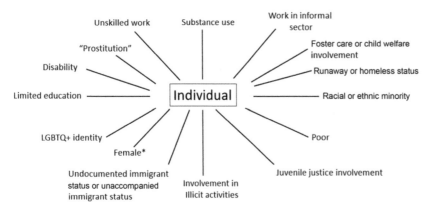

FIGURE 1

Intersectionality of bias and stigma with trafficking and exploitation. *Male status may also lead to stigma in situations involving sexual exploitation.

discrimination by staff, strategies for patients, families, and staff to report experiences of discrimination, and encouragement of staff to appropriately respond to discriminatory behavior observed in the practice (active bystander approach). Resources to assist health care providers and facilities in developing culturally sensitive strategies for patient interaction are available.[108,138,140,141,142,143–145]

MEDICAL HISTORY AND EVALUATION

In addition to obtaining details of the chief complaint and addressing the typical elements of a medical history, information may be sought regarding whether children and adolescents have a regular source of medical care or a medical home, their immunization status, reproductive history (eg, STIs, pregnancy or abortions, use of emergency contraception, anogenital trauma, number and gender of sexual partners, types of sexual activity, age at first intercourse, condom use), history of work-related injuries, physical abuse and assault or dating violence, substance use, and history of mental health signs or symptoms. Such information should be obtained using an open and nonjudgmental approach, with the goal of informing recommendations for testing and

referrals and opening the door to anticipatory guidance. Questions regarding current housing and the youth's feelings of safety in that housing also may be enlightening. A brief mental health assessment may be especially important because many patients who experience labor or sex T/E develop mental and emotional health conditions listed in Table 1, some of which may present as acute psychiatric emergencies.[11,13,16–19,20,60,146,147,148] The provider may ask about past thoughts or actions related to self-harm, current suicidal ideation, and current symptoms, such as intrusive thoughts, nightmares, dissociation, and panic attacks.

For migrant children, it is important to obtain travel and detailed social histories. These histories may include questions regarding how and with whom the child came to the United States (or other destination country), their current living situation, immigration status, possible child or family debt, school enrollment and attendance, and employment or work status. Also important is information about prior abuse, assault, T/E, or persecution in the child's home country and during their journey. It is essential to explain that legal status (or lack thereof) will not be documented in the patient's chart and

will not affect patient care and that the reason these questions are asked is to determine the potential need for confidential referrals to immigration legal support services.

Each step of the medical examination and diagnostic evaluation should be explained to children and adolescents and permission sought to proceed, as developmentally appropriate. A patient's refusal of aspects of the examination or diagnostic evaluation should be respected, if at all possible. In some cases, an individual may refuse 1 step of the evaluation (eg, STI testing), but agree to have it completed at the follow-up visit. The evaluation focuses on:

- Assessing and treating acute and chronic medical conditions, including documentation of late-presenting conditions, and evidence of toxic exposures.
- Assessing overall health, nutritional status (including iron and other micronutrient deficiencies), hydration, growth, and development.
- Assessing dental health and care.
- Referring to an appropriate sexual assault response team, if indicated, with potential forensic evidence collection. Health care providers should work collaboratively with law enforcement investigators to refer the patient to the medical provider in the community who provides such services, and keep in mind that people who have experienced labor T/E may also have experienced sexual exploitation. When these resources are not available locally, care may be obtained via telemedicine, either as a real-time consultation or a delayed review of examination photographs or video by a professional with expertise in T/E and sexual abuse or assault.[9]
- Documenting acute or remote injuries, genital and extragenital

(ie, cutaneous, oral, closed head, neck, thoracoabdominal injuries, and skeletal fractures); sequelae of old injuries, including functional impairment, permanent injury, and scarring.

- Documenting tattoos, especially those signifying gang affiliation, those with sexual connotations, or symbols of money or wealth and those suggesting that a patient is someone's property.[149]
- Assessing for mental health issues, especially acute emergencies.[150]
- Testing for pregnancy, STIs (ie, gonorrhea and/or *Chlamydia* infection, trichomoniasis, syphilis, hepatitis B and C, and HIV), and repeat testing for syphilis, HIV, hepatitis B and C at 6 weeks and 3 months after last known exposure; if an immigrant child, testing also for possibly vertically transmitted infections (eg, HIV, hepatitis B and C, and syphilis).[151] Sites of STI testing will depend on history of contact and may include the pharynx, vagina, cervix, urethra, and anus. Urine and serum specimens may be obtained.
- Urine and/or serum screening for alcohol and substance use, as clinically indicated (eg, if the patient gives a history of unexplained lapses of time and drug-facilitated sexual assault is suspected). Testing should only occur with the patient's permission and only after explaining how the results will be used.[150]
- Laboratory testing for micronutrient deficiencies (eg, iron, vitamins A, E, and B_{12}, folate), toxin exposure (eg, lead, mercury, nicotine, depending on occupational sector involved), communicable diseases related to crowded living conditions (eg, tuberculosis), COVID-19, or for infectious diseases endemic in the country where the child lived or traveled, as indicated (eg,

strongyloidiasis, schistosomiasis, hepatitis B and C, soil-transmitted helminth infections) (https://www.cdc.gov/immigrantrefugeehealth/guidelines/domestic-guidelines.html).[151]

- Offering contraceptive options, with particular focus on long-acting reversible contraception. Given that this population can be medically transient, efforts should be made to address this concern at the time of evaluation, when able, given that this is 1 of the most frequent reasons for seeking health care in this population. Referral for a later visit may not be possible, given the patient's circumstance.
- Offering prophylaxis for STIs and emergency contraception and postexposure prophylaxis, and preexposure prophylaxis for HIV, as appropriate.
- Offering immunizations as needed.

Health care providers who do not routinely provide gynecologic services for children and adolescents, forensic examinations in cases of sexual assault or abuse, health care for transgender patients, or medical evaluations for immigrant populations are encouraged to familiarize themselves with the resources available in their communities, including child abuse pediatricians or hospital child protection teams, child advocacy centers, sexual assault nurse examiner programs, adolescent medicine specialists or gynecologists, immigrant or refugee clinics, legal clinics for undocumented immigrants, and federally qualified health centers. The National Children's Alliance (https://www.nationalchildrensalliance.org/cac-coverage-maps/) provides links to local child advocacy centers throughout the United States. In addition, American Academy of Pediatrics (AAP) resources are available, such as the Immigrant Health Toolkit (https://www.aap.org/en-us/

advocacy-and-policy/aap-health-initiatives/Immigrant-Child-Health-Toolkit/Pages/Immigrant-Child-Health-Toolkit.aspx), as are resources from the Centers for Disease Control and Prevention (CDC [https://www.cdc.gov/]), particularly the CDC Domestic Refugee Screening Guidelines (https://www.cdc.gov/immigrantrefugeehealth/guidelines/domestic-guidelines.html), CareRef (https://careref.web.health.state.mn.us/), and the World Health Organization (http://www.who.int/en/). The clinician should be aware of state laws on conducting medical evaluations (including sexual assault evidence kits) without guardian consent.[152,153] In many cases, the guardian does not accompany the trafficked patient, and laws regarding consent to examination, photography, testing, treatment, and obtaining forensic evidence are complex. Clarification and recommendations are available.[154,155]

The trauma-informed, victim-centered, culturally sensitive approach extends to the examination. A staff chaperone (of the gender preferred by the patient, if available) should be present during the examination, and the patient may want the person accompanying them to be present as well. If that person is a suspected exploiter, their presence should be avoided if at all possible and if exclusion is not likely to prompt retaliation toward the patient.[156] It is helpful to carefully explain each step to the patient and monitor for signs of distress.[157] Routine aspects of the examination may trigger traumatic memories; this often involves the anogenital examination or photography of injuries.

Documentation of acute and healed anogenital, oral, and cutaneous injuries is best accomplished with photography and detailed written description of the size, shape, color, location, and other notable characteristics of each mark.[158] Photographs should be stored on a secure electronic platform; if this is not available, other security measures should be taken to protect privacy and confidentiality. Inflicted trauma may be suspected when injuries are noted in protected areas of the body (ie, torso, genitals, neck, medial thighs),[159] when they have a patterned appearance, or when the explanation provided by the patient is incongruous with the injury.[158] Laboratory testing and diagnostic imaging for possible internal injury may be indicated.

The anogenital examination is best performed with the aid of a colposcope, digital camera, or camcorder so that if a provider with specific training in child sexual abuse or assault (eg, child abuse pediatrician or sexual assault nurse examiner) or a pediatric gynecologist is not available to perform the examination, photographs or videos can later be submitted to an expert for evaluation (see above). The assistance of a child life specialist may help reduce patient anxiety. Complete visualization of the external genitalia and perianal area is necessary. Typically, a speculum exam is not necessary unless there is bleeding and internal injury is suspected;[160] a bimanual examination is helpful to assess for pelvic inflammatory disease in adolescent females. If speculum examination is required, pubertal status as well as patient discomfort must be considered and an examination under anesthesia (EUA) may be necessary. The provider should consider the potential for patient distress associated with an EUA, related to the child's loss of control and/or pain or disorientation experienced during recovery of full consciousness. Although visible injury may be present, it is not unusual to have a normal or nonspecific anogenital examination in cases of sexual abuse even with repeat anogenital penetration.[161,162] Injuries that do occur typically heal quickly,

within days to a few weeks, and scarring is very unusual.[163]

With the patient's informed consent, a sexual assault evidence kit may be obtained up to 120 hours after an assault (according to patient age and law enforcement jurisdictions).[164] Time must be taken to explain the purpose of the sexual assault evidence kit to clarify that it may be used in a law enforcement investigation. This explanation requires an open discussion about whether the patient may choose to proceed with speaking to law enforcement to file a formal complaint.

Pregnancy testing and baseline testing for STIs may be offered and performed, as described previously. Other testing may be considered (eg, hepatitis D in addition to HBV; herpes simplex virus). The F has issued guidelines for testing and treatment of STIs in cases of acute sexual assault.[165] Because follow-up of patients is not guaranteed, the health care provider should consider offering the patient prophylaxis for gonorrhea, *Chlamydia*, and trichomoniasis as well as hepatitis B vaccination or hepatitis B immune globulin if the child has not been vaccinated previously. For females, emergency contraception may be offered as appropriate. In addition, human papillomavirus vaccination may be offered to a patient 9 years or older who has not yet been immunized. Postexposure prophylaxis for HIV should be considered and discussed with the patient and nonoffending caregiver, because multiple HIV risk factors are frequently present (eg, multiple sexual partners of unknown HIV status; potential anal intercourse; inconsistent condom use; potential mucosal injury at time of intercourse). The health care provider may want to consult with an infectious disease specialist or refer to CDC guidelines.[165] Tetanus boosters may be considered if

patients have open wounds without confirmation of up-to-date tetanus immunizations. Many patients, especially those from resource-limited countries, may have had limited access to health care and need other immunizations.

DOCUMENTATION

Documentation of sensitive information regarding risk factors for T/E and details of exploitation should be approached with careful consideration for patient privacy and confidentiality. Patients may fear that information in their medical record will become accessible to those who may cause them harm (eg, angry caregiver, trafficker, Immigration and Customs Enforcement), that medical staff will stigmatize and judge them, or that sensitive information may be used against them in court proceedings (eg, criminal, immigration, or civil cases). Guardian access to an electronic patient portal increases the ease with which parents may access health information on a minor.

The health care professional should explain to the patient (as developmentally appropriate) and nonoffending caregiver that although health facilities go to great lengths to protect patient privacy and confidentiality, others outside the care team may gain access to the record (eg, law enforcement and child protective services in cases involving mandatory reporting, legal officials, health care administrative staff, payer of claims staff, guardian, etc). Before broaching sensitive topics of the medical history, it is important for the clinician to discuss with the patient and nonoffending caregiver these limitations and those associated with mandatory reporting. It is helpful to discuss changes to information available in the electronic patient portal associated with the 21st Century Cures Act.[166] This should include a description of strategies used by the health facility to protect access to sensitive information (eg, "confidential notes"). If the guardian is present, it is preferable to obtain verbal consent to speak with the patient alone and include disclosed information in a confidential note, as appropriate.

Providing clear information on the limits of confidentiality allows the patient to determine what information they choose to disclose, consistent with their basic human rights. The level of detail of this conversation will vary according to the circumstances of the visit and the developmental capabilities of the patient. For undocumented immigrant individuals, expert opinion suggests that legal status not be documented in a patient record per standard practice.

At the end of the visit, the clinician should discuss what information a patient wants included in the health record. The goal is to include information that is critical to the continuity of patient care yet respects the individual's desires for confidentiality, excluding nonessential information, and taking steps to phrase relevant information in a way that does not result in patient shame, distress, or retraumatization. Decisions about information to be included in the record must be subject to legal and administrative policies. Additional discussion of documentation of sensitive health information is available.[167,168]

REFERRALS, RESOURCES, AND MULTIDISCIPLINARY INTERVENTION

As with all aspects of the patient interaction, the discussion about reports and referrals should be trauma informed. It is important to engage the patient (and caregiver as appropriate) in this process, seeking their active input and opinions about suggested resources. The health care provider may empower their patient by beginning the discussion of potential referrals by asking what children and adolescents think would be most beneficial after discharge and if they have ideas for resources. Any referrals should be consistent with patient and family cultural practices and beliefs.[57,141] The latter may influence the way the patient views their condition, their health, and their desired treatment. Cultural practices and traditions may be empowering to children and adolescents and assist in building resilience. When making referrals for services, the health care provider should strive for a "warm handoff" to the referring agency. That is, the provider should offer to contact the referral agency while the patient and family are present or allow the patient or family to make the call while still in the health care setting. This helps to ensure that appointments for follow-up are made.

Individuals who have experienced sex or labor T/E have a variety of immediate needs (eg, shelter, food, clothing, materials and resources to address menstrual needs, interpretation services, emotional support, health and mental health care, and treatment of substance use disorders) and long-term needs (eg, housing, education, life skills and job training, victim advocacy, family services, immigrant legal services, a medical home, and mental health resources).[169] Undocumented immigrant children and adolescents who may have been trafficked, abused, neglected, and/or abandoned need prompt referral to a pro bono immigration attorney or other qualified professional who can assist in addressing immigration issues and in applying for federal assistance through the Trafficking Victims Protection Act. They may also qualify for asylum or other legal status protections. A Department of Health and Human Services (DHHS) Interim Assistance and Eligibility Letter will allow children and adolescents access to federal programs typically available to asylees and refugees, including food stamps, public housing, Medicaid, medical and mental health services, Temporary Assistance for Needy Families (TANF), and employment opportunities through Job Corps.[170]

Providing for the many needs of patients with a history of T/E requires health care providers to work with law enforcement, social services, mental health professionals, immigration lawyers, and service organizations. It is important for the medical provider to identify available community resources and if possible, to establish relationships with agency representatives to ensure that referrals are appropriate for patient needs. Cultivating these relationships before encountering a patient is paramount. To identify local, state, and federal resources, health care providers may:

- Conduct a community mapping exercise: Engage with community partners and other health professionals with expertise in child abuse or human T/E for assistance in creating a directory of available services to address the needs of patients who have experienced T/E or who are at risk.
- Request assistance from the National Human Trafficking Resource Center Hotline (1-888-3737-888), which offers information in more than 200 languages and operates 24 hours per day.
- Contact the US Department of Health and Human Services, which has comprehensive information about services available to trafficked persons who may or may not have legal status in the United States.[145,169]
- Obtain information and resources for homeless and runaway youth from the National Network for Youth (http://www.nn4youth.org; 1-202-783-7949).

It is helpful for health care providers to be aware of policies that may or may not allow organizations to provide shelter and support for a period of time before disclosing a patient's whereabouts to family or authorities.

Health care providers need to consider and discuss with the patient potential referrals for easily accessible healthcare, including primary care, reproductive health care (with HIV pre and postexposure prophylaxis monitoring), family planning, prenatal care (as indicated), and substance use disorder treatment with access to addiction pharmacotherapy when indicated. Patients may need nutritional guidance and treatment of malnutrition. Children and adolescents in foster care may benefit from referrals to clinics specializing in the needs of these patients. Chronic medical conditions may require subspecialty care. Members of special populations, such as those within the LGBTQ+ community, may require additional subspecialty care, such as referral to a health care provider who is well versed in working with transgender youth. Dental care may be required for acute problems related to trauma or infection or for treatment of long-standing issues related to lack of care. Referral to a plastic surgeon may also be warranted, given that a patient may wish to remove marks or brands related to the trafficking experience.

Referrals to trauma-trained mental health professionals familiar with T/E issues may be extremely beneficial to patients. There may be untreated, undertreated, or misdiagnosed mental health issues related to complex trauma occurring before and during the period of T/E. Local child advocacy centers (eg, organizations serving children, adolescents and families experiencing child maltreatment; child advocacy centers) may provide many helpful services, including mental health assessment and treatment,

forensic interviews, and in some cases, second-opinion anogenital examinations. Such centers are available throughout the United States (National Child Advocacy Center: https://www.nationalcac.org/find-a-cac/; National Children's Alliance: https://www.nationalchildrensalliance.org/), and similar programs exist in Europe (Barnahus: https://www.barnahus.eu/en/). However, for patients who have not yet made a disclosure of involvement in labor or sex T/E, child advocacy centers may not be an available resource because of restrictions on patient population, by age, and because of the need for involvement of child protective services and/or law enforcement. This reinforces the need for the health care provider to be aware of other local resources for vulnerable youth.

Health care providers also need to be acutely aware of risk factors and potential indicators of exploitation that migrant children and youth may have experienced in their home country, during migration, while in US custody, or after release to guardians. Clinically validated screening tools designed for the health care setting are not yet available for this population, but open-ended questions about living, working, and traveling experiences; sensitive discussions about potential trauma experiences; and universal education about T/E and basic human and worker rights may set the stage for vulnerable patients and caregivers to seek help. Offering referrals to pro bono immigration attorneys and legal clinics and culturally sensitive mental health organizations is recommended.

The myriad of needs for patients with a history of T/E require a medical home with clinicians well-versed in trauma-informed care. Ideally, multidisciplinary services are integrated into a single-site program, allowing patients increased accessibility to varied services that

may improve health outcomes. Across the United States, special clinics are being developed for adults and/or youth with a history of or ongoing involvement in labor and/or sex T/E.[171,172] Such clinics strive to provide services that meet the unique needs of traumatized individuals who may have difficulty accessing health services that use standard operating procedures for clinic hours, no-show rules, and cancellation policies. A youth-serving approach emphasizes recognizing and addressing patient needs promptly, building trusting relationships with patients who respect agency and choice, improving accessibility with 24-hour clinical coverage, and free or sliding scale care.[135] Other clinics that serve vulnerable populations, such as immigrant health clinics, tribal clinics, and teen clinics, may also be appropriate sources of ongoing integrated medical and mental health care. Finally, telehealth services may provide access to a range of care options when on-site care is unavailable; however, clinicians must be aware that exploiters may be monitoring telehealth interactions, out of view of the camera; in these cases, safety issues become ever more important to consider. Although there may be limitations, there may be benefits as well; the provision of telehealth is an area of continued expansion and research.

Health care providers must comply with existing child abuse mandatory reporting laws.[173] In May 2015, the federal Child Abuse Prevention and Treatment Act was amended by adding human trafficking and child sexual abuse materials as forms of child abuse, regardless of parent or caregiver involvement.[26] However, this definition has not been adopted by each state at this time, making it imperative for clinicians to be familiar with the state mandates in their area. Patients currently involved in the child welfare system, even those with an active child abuse investigation underway, require a new report to be made when trafficking is suspected. It should be noted that mandatory reporting for suspected child labor trafficking is not present in most states. Clinicians should refer to their state social services law for further direction or reach out to state child protective services. The AAP supports chapter advocacy efforts to classify child trafficking as a form of child maltreatment.

It is critical for health care providers to remember that most mandated reporter laws require only that a "reasonable suspicion" of maltreatment (eg, trafficking) is necessary to make a report in good faith; definitive evidence of exploitation (such as a disclosure from the patient) is not required. However, clinical suspicion and reasonable suspicion (for reporting) may not be synonymous. Regardless, the most important action to be taken is to offer resources to the patient according to needs identified during the visit. In many cases, individuals who are deemed at risk for T/E will have needs very similar to those whose trafficking status is confirmed. Health care providers need to consult relevant law and health administrators to determine whether to contact law enforcement, child protective services (CPS), or other agencies in any given case. For assistance in determining how to proceed with a suspected labor and/or sex trafficking case before initiating a report and to obtain information on relevant laws and reporting recommendations, health care providers may contact national trafficking organizations, such as:

- National Human Trafficking Resource Center Hotline (1-888-3737-888)
- Polaris Project (www. polarisproject.org) (sponsors the hotline above)

- Shared Hope International (sharedhope.org)
- National Center for Missing and Exploited Youth (www. missingkids.com)

Other helpful sources of guidance include:

- Staff from state law enforcement task forces on child trafficking
- State or local law enforcement
- CPS agencies
- Local child advocacy centers (see above)
- Immigration relief clinics that provide medical and mental health forensic evaluations (see the Society of Asylum Medicine, https://asylummedicine.com/ and Physicians for Human Rights https://phr.org/ for details).

In cases involving undocumented immigrants, when a formal or informal screen identifies labor conditions that are potentially exploitative or there are concerns for sex trafficking, the health care provider should contact local authorities. In turn, local, state, and federal officials are required to report suspected labor and/or sex trafficking to the Office of Trafficking in Persons (OTIP) within 24 hours of receiving the information. Prompt reporting is very important, because OTIP may be able to facilitate federal assistance to individuals with a history of trafficking, including those with undocumented status. It is also possible for the health care provider to contact OTIP on their own to make the request for assistance. In addition, it is important to link the patient to free legal services (through government legal aid and nongovernmental organizations) or a pro bono immigration attorney who is part of a local nonprofit legal aid program. This will allow the individual's T/E status to be more fully assessed and options for legal aid initiated (see Resources). The availability of immigration legal assistance varies with geographic

region, and clinicians may well lack knowledge of available attorneys within their area. In such cases, referrals may be obtained by contacting a local refugee to immigrant service organization or the National Human Trafficking Hotline (888-373-7888 or text 233733), or visiting the Web site of Kids In Need of Defense. The health care provider should be sure to explain to the individual and caregiver the importance of contacting a legal professional and the need to act promptly. Ideally, the clinician provides a "warm handoff" by calling the referral agency from their office before the patient leaves (or assists the patient or caregiver in making the call). Follow-up at the next patient visit may be very helpful to ensure that contact has been made with the legal professional or to provide further assistance in making the connection.

As has been stressed, mandatory reporting laws and policies must be followed. However, providers should be aware of the potential issues related to reporting to authorities so that they can help minimize potential harm to the patient. Depending on the degree of understanding by child protective services workers regarding the unique issues facing children and adolescents who experience T/E (which generally extend beyond those related to the home environment and caregiver behavior), making a report may not lead to positive intervention for the patient, and the response to the report may be "uncertain and potentially ineffective or even harmful."[31] In addition, although federal antitrafficking laws clearly indicate that a minor cannot consent to engage in commercial sex acts and must be considered a victim,[27] in some cases children and adolescents may be treated as offenders (eg, charged with "prostitution").[12,14,83,85] Involvement in the juvenile justice system as an offender decreases the likelihood that an individual with a history of T/E will receive critical services and protection and may lead to further trauma, including reentry into T/E and involvement in other high-risk behaviors. A cogent discussion of the ethical issues related to reporting of child trafficking may be found in a report from the Institute of Medicine,[31] and information regarding individual state laws regarding child trafficking and commercial sexual exploitation may prove helpful to health care providers.[174]

To help minimize potential harm associated with mandatory reporting of suspected child T/E, it is important for health care providers to emphasize to authorities that the patient is a victim of exploitation who needs services rather than a juvenile offender. Describing a child or adolescent's limited ability to understand sophisticated psychological manipulation practiced by traffickers and the lack of brain maturation, which limits their ability to weigh risks and benefits of various behaviors, may help investigators understand the patient's status. Similarly, the health care provider may stress the particular vulnerabilities identified in the individual which have made him or her susceptible to T/E.

In responding to cases of suspected labor or sex T/E, a health care provider should be transparent about the need for mandatory reports and explain to their patient the reason for the actions. Child and adolescent concerns should be explored, even if their requests cannot be fulfilled. If a report to authorities is not mandated, the clinician should seek caregiver and patient consent before reaching out to law enforcement or child protective services.

Recognizing and responding to suspected child labor and/or sex T/E is complex. Health care organizations should develop a set of guidelines for staff to follow when working with a patient who may have experienced T/E, or who is at

risk. Resources for guideline development include:

- The AAP patient care webpage on child trafficking (https:// www.aap.org/en/patient-care/ child-trafficking-and-exploitation)
- International Centre for Missing and Exploited Children's "A 'How-To' Guide to Develop a Healthcare Protocol for Responding to Child Trafficking and Exploitation"
- Dignity Health's "Human Trafficking Response Program Shared Learning Manual"[175]
- HEAL Trafficking and Hope for Justice's "Protocol Toolkit for Developing a Response to Victims of Human Trafficking in Health Care Settings"[7]
- International Centre for Missing and Exploited Children's "Improving Physical and Mental Health Care for Those at Risk of, or Experiencing Human Trafficking and Exploitation: The Complete Toolkit, 2nd Edition,"[8] (https://www.icmec.org/ healthportal-resources/topic/ human-trafficking-toolkit/).

A patient who has experienced labor and/or sex T/E faces numerous challenges to exiting their exploitative situation, including emotional bonds with the exploiter, fear of retribution, reluctance to return to a dysfunctional home, ostracism by family or community, debt bondage, fear of deportation, and other difficulties. It is not unusual for patients to return to the T/E environment, sometimes several times, before final extrication.[176]

SELF-CARE FOR THE CLINICIAN

Those caring for patients who have experienced T/E are at risk themselves for secondary traumatic stress (STS), a syndrome with symptoms similar to those of PTSD experienced by those learning about others' trauma.[177] A health care provider may experience emotional, physical, and mental exhaustion

attributable to excessive and prolonged stress as a result of too many demands and too few resources. As such, for those working with patients experiencing T/E, self-care is a high priority. The first step in mitigating secondary STS is to identify its signs and symptoms (eg, irritability, hopelessness, intrusive thoughts). Support from others and a work environment that acknowledges and seeks to minimize secondary trauma help combat STS. Resources addressing STS are available.[178]

CONCLUSIONS AND GUIDANCE FOR HEALTH CARE PROVIDERS

1. Individuals who identify as male, female, or any gender identity and who have experienced labor and/ or sex T/E may present for health care related to trauma, infection, reproductive issues, mental health concerns (including severe intoxication and overdose from substance use) and other concerns.
2. Patients with a history of T/E rarely spontaneously disclose their situation. Although some individuals have no obvious risk factors or red flags, many have 1 or more vulnerabilities at the individual, relationship, community, and/or societal levels.
3. Screening and/or universal education with resources are helpful strategies for identifying and assisting high-risk patients. Health care providers should use clinically validated screening tools whenever possible. The goal of screening is not to obtain a disclosure of T/E, but instead, to assess the level of risk and identify patient vulnerabilities that may be addressed with community services.
4. To increase patient and family awareness of child T/E, health care providers may display posters translated into multiple languages, including the National Human Trafficking Hotline (1-888-

3737-888), in waiting rooms, examination rooms, or restrooms, and make brochures and other resources regarding healthy relationships readily available.

5. Evaluation of patients who have, or who are at risk for experiencing T/E is best completed using a trauma-informed,[5] culturally sensitive, rights-based[109] approach that emphasizes support, acceptance, transparency, safety, and patient empowerment.

6. Medical evaluation of a patient who has experienced labor or sex T/E involves addressing acute medical or surgical issues (eg, injuries, toxic exposures, sexual assault), assessing nutrition and hydration status, evaluating possible chronic untreated health conditions, documenting acute or remote injuries, testing for and treating STIs, and obtaining a sexual assault evidence kit, as appropriate. Immigrant patients should be screened as outlined in the CDC "Domestic Refugee Screening Guidelines."[151] Steps of the evaluation should be explained to the patient and permission obtained before proceeding (except in cases of medical emergency).

7. Documentation of sensitive patient information related to T/E, to existing vulnerabilities to exploitation (eg, substance use), and to certain health conditions (eg, STIs, HIV or AIDS) should be undertaken with careful consideration regarding who may access the information in the health record, and under what circumstances. As appropriate, providers should discuss documentation options with patients, working to ensure safety and to respect the individual's wishes for privacy while at the same time preserving continuity of care and complying with relevant laws and policies.

8. Patients who have experienced T/E have many and varied needs, and meeting these needs requires a multidisciplinary, holistic approach (eg, one that addresses all of the needs of the individual, including physical and mental health, as well as social, legal, and immigration needs). The health care provider has an opportunity to work collaboratively as part of a team of community professionals from a number of disciplines. Increasingly, T/E clinics are being developed to provide integrated and comprehensive, multidisciplinary health and mental health care for vulnerable patients.

9. Providers may advocate for patients at risk for and experiencing T/E by educating child-serving professionals and families regarding labor and sexual exploitation and offering anticipatory guidance to parents and children and adolescents regarding internet safety, common trafficking recruitment scenarios, healthy versus unhealthy relationships, and basic labor rights. They may help to prevent T/E by offering high-risk patients and families community and national resources to address vulnerabilities.[179] Finally, health care providers may advocate for victim services at the community, state, and national levels. The AAP has published a policy statement on child trafficking, with recommendations for advocacy measures.[180]

10. Health care providers are mandated reporters of suspected child abuse and neglect. In states where sex trafficking is considered a form of abuse, the provider must make a formal report of suspected T/E to law enforcement and to CPS.

11. Clinic and hospital guidelines for the recognition and response to suspected human labor and sex T/E are necessary so that all staff members are aware of their roles and responsibilities and vulnerable patients may be identified and offered resources. Guidelines should be supplemented with staff training on T/E as well as trauma-informed care, cultural sensitivity and awareness, and management of implicit and explicit biases.

12. Self-care for the clinician is critical in preventing and addressing secondary traumatic stress. A work environment that fosters peer support, encourages open discussion of work-related stress, and implements reasonable work-life balance policies can help protect providers from secondary stress and its consequences.

13. The financial impact and management implications for a clinical practice may be significant, and there is a need for advocacy to ensure fair and equitable resourcing. Staff training, screening of patients, assessment, and provision of services require time and resources for which practices need support.

RESOURCES

- National Human Trafficking Resource Center and Hotline (1-888- 3737-888); https://humantraffickinghotline.org/
- Administration of Children and Families, Office of Trafficking in Persons (https://www.acf.hhs.gov/otip/victim-assistance/services-available-victims-trafficking)
- HEAL Trafficking: An organization of professionals addressing human trafficking through a public health lens; numerous resources for health professionals available on Web site (www.healtrafficking.org)
- Polaris Project: A national resource for human trafficking: https://polarisproject.org/
- Office of Refugee Resettlement release of information: https://

- www.acf.hhs.gov/orr/policy-guidance/requests-uac-case-file-information
- CDC Domestic Refugee Screening Guidelines: Information on approach to medical and mental health screening of immigrants and refugees. https://www.cdc.gov/immigrantrefugeehealth/guidelines/domestic-guidelines.html
- CareRef: In-office tool for medical screening of immigrants and refugees https://careref.web.health.state.mn.us/
- The Society for Asylum Medicine https://asylummedicine.com/
- National Immigration Legal Services Directory: https://www.immigrationadvocates.org/nonprofit/legaldirectory/
- Federally funded mental health counseling for immigrant youth and parents separated by ICE in the US: https://www.senecafoa.org/todopormifamilia/

LEAD AUTHORS

Jordan Greenbaum, MD
Dana Kaplan, MD, FAAP
Janine Young, MD, FAAP

COUNCIL ON CHILD ABUSE AND NEGLECT (COCAN) EXECUTIVE COMMITTEE, 2021–2022

Suzanne B. Haney, MD, MS, FAAP, Chairperson
Andrew P. Sirotnak, MD, FAAP, Immediate Past Chairperson
Andrea Gottsegen Asnes, MD, FAAP
Amy R. Gavril, MD, MSCI, FAAP
Amanda Bird Hoffert Gilmartin, MD, FAAP
Rebecca Greenlee Girardet, MD, FAAP
Nancy D. Heavilin, MD, FAAP
Antoinette Laskey, MD, MPH, MBA, FAAP
Stephen A. Messner, MD, FAAP
Bethany A. Mohr, MD, FAAP
Shalon Marie Nienow, MD, FAAP
Norell Rosado, MD, FAAP

COCAN LIAISONS

Heather Forkey, MD, FAAP – Council on Foster Care, Adoption, and Kinship Care
Rachael Keefe, MD, MPH, FAAP – Council on Foster Care, Adoption, and Kinship Care
Brooks Keeshin, MD, FAAP – American Academy of Child and Adolescent Psychiatry
Jennifer Matjasko, PhD – Centers for Disease Control and Prevention
Heather Edward, MD – Section on Pediatric Trainees
Elaine Stedt, MSW, ACSW – Administration for Children, Youth and Families, Office on Child Abuse and Neglect

STAFF

Tammy Piazza Hurley

COUNCIL ON IMMIGRANT CHILD AND FAMILY HEALTH EXECUTIVE COMMITTEE, 2021–2022

Julie Linton, MD, FAAP, *Co-Chairperson*
Raul Gutierrez, MD, FAAP, *Co-Chairperson*
Tania Caballero, MD, FAAP
Olanrewaju "Lanre" Omojokun Falusi, MD, FAAP
Minal Giri, MD, FAAP
Marsha Griffin, MD, FAAP
Anisa Ibrahim, MD, FAAP
Kimberly Mukerjee, MD, FAAP
Sural Shah, MD, FAAP
Alan Shapiro, MD, PhD, FAAP
Janine Young, MD, FAAP

STAFF

Ngozi Onyema-Melton, MPH

ABBREVIATIONS

AAP: American Academy of Pediatrics
CPS: child protective services
PTSD: posttraumatic stress disorder
STS: secondary traumatic stress
T/E: trafficking and exploitation

PEDIATRICS (ISSN Numbers: Print, 0031-4005; Online, 1098-4275).

Copyright © 2023 by the American Academy of Pediatrics

FUNDING: No external funding.

FINANCIAL/CONFLICT OF INTEREST DISCLOSURES: The authors have indicated they have no potential conflicts of interest to disclose.

REFERENCES

1. Hornor G, Sherfield J. Commercial sexual exploitation of children: health care use and case characteristics. *J Pediatr Health Care.* 2018;32(3):250–262

2. Hornor G, Hollar J, Landers T, Sherfield J. Healthcare use and case characteristics of commercial sexual exploitation of children: teen victims versus high-risk teens [published online ahead of print August 5, 2022]. *J Forensic Nurs.* doi: 10.1097/JFN.0000000000000402

3. Lederer L, Wetzel C. The health consequences of sex trafficking and their implications for identifying victims in healthcare facilities. *Ann Health Law.* 2014;23(1):61–91

4. Forkey H, Szilagyi M, Kelly ET, Duffee J; Council on Foster Care, Adoption, and Kinship Care, Council on Community Pediatrics, Council on Child Abuse and Neglect, Committee on Psychosocial

Aspects of Child and Family Health. Trauma-informed care. *Pediatrics.* 2021;148(2):e2021052580

5. Substance Abuse and Mental Health Services Administration. *SAMHSA's Concept of Trauma and Guidance for a Trauma-Informed Approach.* Rockville, MD: Substance Abuse and Mental Health Services Administration; 2014

6. World Health Organization. Responding to children and adolescents who have been sexually abused: WHO clinical guidelines. Available at: https://apps. who.int/iris/bitstream/handle/10665/ 259270/9789241550147-eng.pdf; jsessionid=37ADD6616474C995A 0D79A2EE83BC1DD?sequence=1. Accessed May 12, 2020

7. HEAL Trafficking, Hope for Justice. HEAL Trafficking and Hope for Justice's protocol toolkit for developing a response to victims of human trafficking in health care settings. Available at: https://healtraffickingorg/ 2017/06/new-heal-trafficking-and-hope-for-justices-protocol-toolkit-for-developing-a-response-to-victims-of-human-trafficking-in-health-care-settings/. Accessed Mar 8, 2022

8. International Centre for Missing and Exploited Children. Improving physical and mental health care for those at risk of, or experiencing human trafficking and exploitation: the complete toolkit, 2nd edition. Available at https://www.icmec.org/ healthportal-resources/topic/ human-trafficking-toolkit/. Accessed September 18, 2022

9. United Nations Office on Drugs and Crime. Global report on trafficking in persons 2020. Available at https://www. unodc.org/unodc/data-and-analysis/ glotip.html. Accessed February 6,21

10. International Labour Organization, Walk Free, International Organization for Migration. *Global Estimates of Modern Slavery: Forced Labour and Forced Marriage.* Geneva, Switzerland: International Labour Organization, Walk Free, International Organization for Migration; 2022

11. Ottisova L, Smith P, Oram S. Psychological consequences of human trafficking: complex posttraumatic stress disorder in trafficked children. *Behav Med.* 2018;44(3):234–241

12. Sprang G, Cole J. Familial sex trafficking of minors: trafficking conditions, clinical presentation, and system involvement. *J Fam Violence.* 2018;33(3):185–195

13. Le PD, Ryan N, Rosenstock Y, Goldmann E. Health issues associated with commercial sexual exploitation and sex trafficking of children in the United States: a systematic review. *Behav Med.* 2018;44(3):219–233

14. Moynihan M, Mitchell K, Pitcher C, Havaei F, Ferguson M, Saewyc E. A systematic review of the state of the literature on sexually exploited boys internationally. *Child Abuse Negl.* 2018;76:440–451

15. Barnert ES, Godoy SM, Hammond I, et al. Pregnancy outcomes among girls impacted by commercial sexual exploitation. *Acad Pediatr.* 2020; 20(4):455–459

16. Ertl S, Bokor B, Tuchman L, Miller E, Kappel R, Deye K. Healthcare needs and utilization patterns of sex-trafficked youth: missed opportunities at a children's hospital. *Child Care Health Dev.* 2020;46(4):422–428

17. Ottisova L, Hemmings S, Howard LM, Zimmerman C, Oram S. Prevalence and risk of violence and the mental, physical and sexual health problems associated with human trafficking: an updated systematic review. *Epidemiol Psychiatr Sci.* 2016;25(4):317–341

18. Bath E, Barnert E, Godoy S, et al. Substance use, mental health, and child welfare profiles of juvenile Justice-involved commercially sexually exploited youth. *J Child Adolesc Psychopharmacol.* 2020;30(6):389–397

19. Hopper EK, Gonzalez LD. A comparison of psychological symptoms in survivors of sex and labor trafficking. *Behav Med.* 2018;44(3):177–188

20. Palines PA, Rabbitt AL, Pan AY, Nugent ML, Ehrman WG. Comparing mental health disorders among sex trafficked children and three groups of youth at high-risk for trafficking: a dual retrospective cohort and scoping review. *Child Abuse Negl.* 2020;100:104196

21. Chaffee T, English A. Sex trafficking of adolescents and young adults in the United States: healthcare provider's role. *Curr Opin Obstet Gynecol.* 2015;27(5):339–344

22. Smith L, Vardaman S, Snow M. The national report on domestic minor sex trafficking: America's prostituted children. Available at http:// sharedhope.org/wp-content/uploads/ 2012/09/SHI_National_Report_ on_DMST_2009.pdf. Accessed October 28, 2019

23. United States Department of State. Trafficking in persons report. Available at: https://wwwstategov/wp-content/ uploads/2019/06/2019-Trafficking-in-Persons-Reportpdf. Accessed October 28, 2019

24. United States Senate PsoiCohsaga. Protecting unaccompanied alien children from trafficking and other abuses: the role of the Office of Refugee Resettlement. Available at: https://www.hsgac.senate.gov/imo/ media/doc/Majority%20&%20Minority% 20Staff%20Report%20-%20Protecting% 20Unaccompanied%20Alien%20Children %20from%20Trafficking%20and% 200ther%20Abuses%202016-01-282.pdf. Accessed May 17, 2021

25. US Department of Health and Human Services, Office of Refugee Resettlement. Unaccompanied refugee minors program. Available at: https://www.acf. hhs.gov/orr/programs/refugees/urm. Accessed November 17, 2022

26. United States Government. Justice for Victims of Trafficking Act of 2015. Available at: https://www.congress.gov/ 114/plaws/publ22/PLAW-114publ22.pdf. Accessed May 18, 2020

27. United States Government. Trafficking Victims Protection Act Pub L No 106-386 Division A 103(8) [USC02] 22 USC Ch 78. Available at: https://uscode. house.gov/view.xhtml?path=/prelim@ title22/chapter78&edition=prelim. Accessed December 30, 2019

28. United States Department of Labor. Fair Labor Standards Act of 1938 29 U.S.C. § 203. Available at https://www. dol.gov/agencies/whd/flsa. Accessed May 24, 2021

29. U.S. Immigration and Customs Enforcement. Human trafficking and smuggling. Available at: https://www.

ice.gov/factsheets/human-trafficking. Accessed July 25, 2017

30. Kristof N. What it costs to be smuggled across the US border. Available at: https://www.nytimes.com/interactive/2018/06/30/world/smuggling-illegal-immigration-costs.html. Accessed May 17, 2021

31. Institute of Medicine and National Research Council. *Confronting Commercial sexual Exploitation and Sex Trafficking of Minors in the United States*. Washington, D.C.: The National Academies Press; 2013

32. Greijer S, Doek J; Interagency Working Group on Sexual Exploitation of Children. Terminology guidelines for the protection of children from sexual exploitation and abuse. Available at: www.ilo.org/wcmsp5/groups/public/—ed_norm/—ipec/documents/instructionalmaterial/wcms_490167.pdf. Accessed May 7, 2018

33. Boyer CB, Greenberg L, Chutuape K, et al; Adolescent Medicine Trials Network. Exchange of sex for drugs or money in adolescents and young adults: an examination of sociodemographic factors, HIV-related risk, and community context. *J Community Health*. 2017;42(1):90–100

34. Greeson JKP, Treglia D, Wolfe DS, Wasch S. Prevalence and correlates of sex trafficking among homeless and runaway youths presenting for shelter services. *Soc Work Res*. 2019;43(2):91–100

35. Hogan KA, Roe-Sepowitz D. LGBTQ+ homeless young adults and sex trafficking vulnerability. *J Hum Traffick*. 2020:1–16

36. Murphy LT. Labor and sex trafficking among homeless youth: a ten-city study executive summary. Available at: https://covenanthousestudyorg/landing/trafficking/docs/Loyola-Research-Resultspdf. Accessed on August 8, 2018

37. El Arab R, Sagbakken M. Child marriage of female Syrian refugees in Jordan and Lebanon: a literature review. *Glob Health Action*. 2019;12(1):1585709

38. Hotchkiss DR, Godha D, Gage AJ, Cappa C. Risk factors associated with the practice of child marriage among

Roma girls in Serbia. *BMC Int Health Hum Rights*. 2016;16(6):6

39. Raj A, Saggurti N, Balaiah D, Silverman JG. Prevalence of child marriage and its effect on fertility and fertility-control outcomes of young women in India: a cross-sectional, observational study. *Lancet*. 2009;373(9678):1883–1889

40. Warria A. Forced child marriages as a form of child trafficking. *Child Youth Serv Rev*. 2017;79:274–279

41. International Centre for Migration Policy Development. Targeting vulnerabilities: the impact of the Syrian war and refugee situation on trafficking in persons: a study of Syria, Turkey, Lebanon, Jordan and Iraq. Available at: https://respect.international/wp-content/uploads/2021/07/Targeting-Vulnerabilities-The-Impact-of-the-Syrian-War-and-Refugee-Situation-on-Trafficking-in-Persons-Briefing-Paper.pdf. Accessed March 17, 2022

42. Reid JA. Entrapment and enmeshment schemes used by sex traffickers. *Sex Abuse*. 2016;28(6):491–511

43. Saewyc EM, Shankar S, Pearce LA, Smith A. Challenging the stereotypes: unexpected features of sexual exploitation among homeless and street-involved boys in Western Canada. *Int J Environ Res Public Health*. 2021;18(11):5898

44. Bracy K, Lul B, Roe-Sepowitz D. A four-year analysis of labor trafficking cases in the United States: exploring characteristics and labor trafficking patterns. *J Hum Traffick*. 2019;7(1):1–18

45. Walts KK. Child labor trafficking in the United States: a hidden crime. *Soc Incl (Lisboa)*. 2017;5(2):59–68

46. Polaris Project. The typology of modern slavery: defining sex and labor trafficking in the United States. Available at https://polarisproject.org/sites/default/files/Polaris-Typology-of-Modern-Slavery.pdf. Accessed December 18, 2019

47. Srivastava RN. Children at work, child labor and modern slavery in India: an overview. *Indian Pediatr*. 2019;56(8):633–638

48. International Labour Office. Global estimates of child labour: results and trends 2012-2016. Available at: https://www.ilo.org/global/publications/books/WCMS_575499/lang—en/index.htm. Accessed August 30, 2020

49. International Labour Organization. Towards the urgent elimination of hazardous child labour. Available at: https://wwwiloorg/ipec/Informationresources/WCMS_IPEC_PUB_30315/lang—en/indexhtm. Accessed December 18, 2019

50. International Labour Organization, Food and Agriculture Organization of the United Nations, Arab Councli for Childhood and Development. Child labour in the Arab region: a quantitative and qualitative analysis. Available at: https://wwwiloorg/beirut/publications/WCMS_675262/lang—en/indexhtm. Accessed December 19, 2019

51. International Programme on the Elimination of Child Labour. Children in hazardous labour: what we know, what we need to do. Available at: https://www.ilo.org/global/publications/ilo-bookstore/order-online/books/WCMS_155428/lang—en/index.htm. Accessed Sept 25, 2020

52. Wood LCN. Child modern slavery, trafficking and health: a practical review of factors contributing to children's vulnerability and the potential impacts of severe exploitation on health. *BMJ Paediatr Open*. 2020;4(1):e000327

53. Reid JA, Baglivio MT, Piquero AR, Greenwald MA, Epps N. Human trafficking of minors and childhood adversity in Florida. *Am J Public Health*. 2017;107(2):306–311

54. Greeson JKP, Treglia D, Wolfe DS, Wasch S, Gelles RJ. Child welfare characteristics in a sample of youth involved in commercial sex: an exploratory study. *Child Abuse Negl*. 2019;94:104038

55. Kendi IX. *Stamped From the Beginning: The Definitive History of Racist Ideas in America*. New York, NY: Bold Type Books; 2016

56. Wesche SD. Métis women at risk: health and service provision in urban British Columbia. *Pimatziwin*. 2013;11(2):187–196

57. Bell S, Deen JF, Fuentes M, Moore K; Committee on Native American Child Health. Caring for American Indian and Alaska Native children and adolescents. *Pediatrics.* 2021;147(4):e2021050498

58. Farley M, Deer S, Golding JM, et al. The prostitution and trafficking of American Indian/Alaska Native women in Minnesota. *Am Indian Alsk Native Ment Health Res.* 2016;23(1):65–104

59. Pierce AS. Shattered hearts (full report): the commercial sexual exploitation of American Indian women and girls in Minnesota. Available at: https://digitalcommons.unl.edu/humtraffconf/26/. Accessed February 25, 2020

60. Pierce AS. American Indian adolescent girls: vulnerability to sex trafficking, intervention strategies. *Am Indian Alsk Native Ment Health Res.* 2012; 19(1):37–56

61. Interpol. Threats and trends: child sexual exploitation and abuse: Covid-19 impact. Available at: ///C:/Users/riley/Downloads/COVID19%20-%20Child%20Sexual%20Exploitation%20and%20Abuse%20threats%20and%20trends%20(1).pdf. Accessed November 10, 2020

62. New Hampshire Department of Health and Human Services. Trending in DYF data during Covid 19. Available at: https://www.covid19.nh.gov/dashboard. Accessed November 17, 2022

63. Ratzan SC, Kimball S, Rauh L, Sommariva S. CUNY New York City Covid-19 survey week 2. Available at https://sph.cuny.edu/research/covid-19-tracking-survey/week-2/. Accessed August 28, 2020

64. Alliance for Child Protection in Humanitarian Action, End Violence Against Children, Unicef, World Health Organization. Covid 19: protecting children from violence, abuse and neglect in the home. Version 1. Available at https://www.unicef.org/documents/covid-19-protecting-children-violence-abuse-and-neglect-home. Accessed November 9, 2020

65. Fraser E. *Impact of Covid-19 Pandemic on Violence Against Women and Girls.* London, UK: UK Department for International Development; 2020

66. Migration IOo. Covid-19 analytical snapshot #14: human trafficking. Available at: https://healtraffickingorg/wp-content/uploads/2020/07/covid-19_analytical_snapshot_14_human_traffickingpdf. Accessed August 28, 2020

67. Unicef, WePROTECT Global Alliance, World Health Organization, United Nations Office on Drugs and Crime, World Childhood Foundation, et al. Covid-19 and its implications for protecting children online. Available at: https://www.unicef.org/sites/default/files/2020-04/COVID-19-and-Its-Implications-for-Protecting-Children-Online.pdf. Accessed August 28, 2020

68. United Nations Office on Drugs and Crime. Impact of the Covid-19 pandemic on trafficking in persons: preliminary findings and messaging based on rapid stocktaking. Available at: https://www.un.org/ruleoflaw/wp-content/uploads/2020/05/Thematic-Brief-on-COVID-19-EN-ver.21.pdf. Accessed December 21, 2020

69. Wagner L, Hoang T. Aggravating circumstances: how coronavirus impacts human trafficking. Available at: https://globalinitiative.net/analysis/human-trafficking-covid-impact/. Accessed December 21, 2020

70. Phiri P, Delanerolle G, Al-Sudani A, Rathod S. COVID-19 and Black, Asian, and minority ethnic communities: a complex relationship without just cause. *JMIR Public Health Surveill.* 2021;7(2):e22581

71. Tai DBG, Shah A, Doubeni CA, Sia IG, Wieland ML. The disproportionate impact of COVID-19 on racial and ethnic minorities in the United States. *Clin Infect Dis.* 2021;72(4):703–706

72. Todres J, Diaz A. COVID-19 and human trafficking-the amplified impact on vulnerable populations. *JAMA Pediatr.* 2020;175(2):123–124

73. Greenbaum J, Stoklosa H, Murphy L. The public health impact of coronavirus disease on human trafficking. *Front Public Health.* 2020;8:561184

74. Walk Free Foundation, Minderoo Foundation. Protecting people in a pandemic: Urgent collaboration is needed to protect vulnerable workers and prevent exploitation. Available at: https://wwwminderooorg/walk-free/reports/protecting-people-in-a-pandemic/. Accessed August 28, 2020

75. UNICEF. 10 million additional girls at risk of child marriage due to COVID-19. Available at: https://www.unicef.org/press-releases/10-million-additional-girls-risk-child-marriage-due-covid-19. Accessed November 17, 2022

76. Boserup B, McKenney M, Elkbuli A. Alarming trends in US domestic violence during the COVID-19 pandemic. *Am J Emerg Med.* 2020;38(12):2753–2755

77. Brewster T. Child sexual exploitation complaints rise 106% to hit 2 million in just one month: is Covid-19 to blame? Available at: https://www.forbes.com/sites/thomasbrewster/2020/04/24/child-exploitation-complaints-rise-106-to-hit-2-million-in-just-one-month-is-covid-19-to-blame/?sh=30697e2e4c9c. Accessed November 17, 2022

78. Czeisler ME, Lane RI, Petrosky E, et al. Mental health, substance use, and suicidal ideation during the COVID-19 pandemic: U.S., June 24-30, 2020. *MMWR Morb Mortal Wkly Rep.* 2020;69(32):1049–1057

79. Office for Democratic Institutions and Human Rights, UN Women. Guidance: addressing emerging human trafficking trends and consequences of the Covid-19 pandemic. Available at: https://wwwosceorg/files/f/documents/2/a/458434_3pdf. Accessed August 28, 2020

80. Stansky M, Finkelhor D. How many juveniles are involved in prostitution in the U.S.? Available at: www.unh.edu/ccrc/prostitution/Juvenile_Prostitution_factsheet.pdf. Accessed May 7, 2008

81. Dank M, Yahner J, Madden K, et al. *Surviving the Streets of New York: Experiences of LGBTQ Youth, YMSM, YWSW Engaged in Survival Sex.* Washington, D.C.: Urban Institute; 2015

82. Curtis R, Terry K, Dank M, Dombrowski K, Khan B. *The Commercial Sexual Exploitation of Children in New York City: Volume 1: The CSEC Population in New York City: Size, Characteristics and Needs.* New York, NY: Center for Court Innovation; 2008

83. Dennis J. Women are victims, men make choices: the invisibility of men and boys in the global sex trade. *Gend Issues.* 2008;25:11–25

84. ECPAT USA. And boys too: an ECPAT-USA discussion paper about the lack of recognition of the commercial sexual exploitation of boys in the United States. Available at: https://d1qkyo3pi1c9bxcloudfrontnet/00028B1B-B0DB-4FCD-A991-219527535DAB/1b1293ef-1524-4f2c-b148-91db11379d11pdf. Accessed on October 29, 2017

85. Josenhans V, Kavenagh M, Smith S, Wekerle C. Gender, rights and responsibilities: the need for a global analysis of the sexual exploitation of boys. *Child Abuse Negl.* 2020;110(Pt 1):104291

86. Choi SK, Wilson BDM, Shelton J, Gates G. *Serving Our Youth 2015: The Needs and Experiences of Lesbian, Gay, Bisexual, Transgender, and Questioning Youth Experiencing Homelessness.* Los Angeles, CA: The Williams Institute With True Colors Fund; 2015

87. Cochran BN, Stewart AJ, Ginzler JA, Cauce AM. Challenges faced by homeless sexual minorities: comparison of gay, lesbian, bisexual, and transgender homeless adolescents with their heterosexual counterparts. *Am J Public Health.* 2002;92(5):773–777

88. Morton MH, Dworsky A, Matjasko JL, et al. Prevalence and correlates of youth homelessness in the United States. *J Adolesc Health.* 2018;62(1):14–21

89. Freeman L, Hamilton D. A count of homeless youth in New York City. Available at: www.racismreview.com/downloads/HomelessYouth.pdf. Accessed May 19, 2019

90. Reed SM, Kennedy MA, Decker MR, Cimino AN. Friends, family, and boyfriends: an analysis of relationship pathways into commercial sexual exploitation. *Child Abuse Negl.* 2019;90:1–12

91. Mostajabian S, Santa Maria D, Wiemann C, Newlin E, Bocchini C. Identifying sexual and labor exploitation among sheltered youth experincing homelessness: a comparison of screening methods. *Int*

J Environ Res Public Health. 2019;16(3):363

92. Twis MK, Kirschner L, Greenwood D. Trafficked by a friend: a qualitative analysis of adolescent trafficking victims' archival case files. *Child Adolescent Social Work J.* 2021;38:611–620

93. Gibbs DA, Aboul-Hosn S, Kluckman MN. Child labor trafficking within the US: A first look at allegations investigated by Florida's child welfare agency. *J Human Trafficking.* 2019;6(6):1–15

94. United States Department of State. 2020 trafficking in persons report. Available at: https://www.state.gov/reports/2020-trafficking-in-persons-report/. Accessed April 30, 2021

95. Koegler E, Howland W, Gibbons P, Teti M, Stoklosa H. "When her visa expired, the family refused to renew it," intersections of human trafficking and domestic violence: qualitative document analysis of case examples from a major Midwest city. *J Interpers Violence.* 2022;37(7-8):NP4133–NP4159

96. Anderson PM, Coyle KK, Johnson A, Denner J. An exploratory study of adolescent pimping relationships. *J Prim Prev.* 2014;35(2):113–117

97. Edinburgh L, Pape-Blabolil J, Harpin SB, Saewyc E. Assessing exploitation experiences of girls and boys seen at a Child Advocacy Center. *Child Abuse Negl.* 2015;46:47–59

98. Buller AM, Vaca V, Stoklosa H, Borland R, Zimmerman C. Labour exploitation, trafficking and migrant health: multi-country findings on the health risks and consequences of migrant and trafficked workers. Available at: https://publications.iom.int/system/files/pdf/labour_exploitation_trafficking_en.pdf. Accessed February 11, 2019

99. Landers M, McGrath K, Johnson MH, Armstrong MI, Dollard N. Baseline characteristics of dependent youth who have been commercially sexually exploited: findings from a specialized treatment program. *J Child Sex Abuse.* 2017;26(6):692–709PubMed

100. Dhakal S, Niraula S, Sharma NP, et al. History of abuse and neglect and their associations with mental health in rescued child labourers in Nepal. *Aust*

N Z J Psychiatry. 2019;53(12):1199–1207

101. Hébert M, Amédée LM, Blais M, Gauthier-Duchesne A. Child sexual abuse among a representative sample of Quebec high school students: prevalence and association with mental health problems and health-risk behaviors. *Can J Psychiatry.* 2019;64(12):846–854

102. Hailes HP, Yu R, Danese A, Fazel S. Long-term outcomes of childhood sexual abuse: an umbrella review. *Lancet Psychiatry.* 2019;6(10):830–839

103. Easton SD, Kong J, Gregas MC, Shen C, Shafer K. Child sexual abuse and depression in late life for men: a population-based, longitudinal analysis. *J Gerontol B Psychol Sci Soc Sci.* 2019;74(5):842–852

104. Adams J, Mrug S, Knight DC. Characteristics of child physical and sexual abuse as predictors of psychopathology. *Child Abuse Negl.* 2018;86:167–177

105. Kaltiso SO, Greenbaum VJ, Agarwal M, et al. *Evaluation of a Screening Tool for Child Sex Trafficking Among Patients With High-Risk Chief Complaints in a Pediatric Emergency Department.* Des Plaines, IL: Society Academic Emergency Medicine; 2018

106. Jouk N, Capin I, Greenbaum J, Kaplan D. Recognizing suspected human trafficking in the pediatric intensive care unit. *J Hum Traffick.* 2021:1–4

107. Wallace C, Lavina I, Mollen C. Share our stories: an exploration of the healthcare experiences of child sex trafficking survivors. *Child Abuse Negl.* 2021;112:104896

108. National Human Trafficking Training and Technical Assistance Center, US Department of Health and Human Services OoTiP, US Department of Health and Human Services SCG, HEAL Trafficking, International Centre for Missing and Exploited Children, National Association of Pediatric Nurse Practitioners. Core competencies for human trafficking response in health care and behavioral health systems. Available at: https://nhttac.acf.hhs.gov/resource/report-core-competencies-human-trafficking-response-health-

care-and-behavioral-health. Accessed Mar 6, 2021

109. United Nations Human Rights, Office of the High Commissioner for Human Rights. Convention on the rights of the child. Available at: http://wwwohchrorg/EN/ProfessionalInterest/Pages/CRCaspx. Accessed July 23, 2022

110. Tiller J, Reynolds S. Human trafficking in the emergency department: improving our response to a vulnerable population. *West J Emerg Med.* 2020;21(3):549–554

111. American Academy of Pediatrics. Immigrant child health toolkit. Available at: https://www.aap.org/en-us/about-the-aap/Committees-Councils-Sections/Council-on-Community-Pediatrics/Pages/Section-1-Clinical-Care.aspx#q1. Accessed on September 20, 2020

112. Richie-Zavaleta AC, Villanueva A, Martinez-Donate A, Turchi RM, Ataiants J, Rhodes SM. Sex trafficking victims at their junction with the healthcare setting: a mixed-methods inquiry. *J Hum Traffick;* 2020;6(1):1–29

113. Barnert E, Kelly M, Godoy S, Abrams LS, Rasch M, Bath E. Understanding commercially sexually exploited young women's access to, utilization of, and engagement in health care: "Work around what I need". *Wommen's Health Issues.* 2019;29(4):315–324

114. Ijadi-Maghsoodi R, Bath E, Cook M, Textor L, Barnert E. Commercially sexually exploited youths' health care experiences, barriers, and recommendations: a qualitative analysis. *Child Abuse Negl.* 2018;76:334–341

115. Lavoie J, Dickerson KL, Redlich AD, Quas JA. Overcoming disclosure reluctance in youth victims of sex trafficking: new directions for research, policy, and practice. *Psychology.* 2019;25(4):225–238

116. Trent M, Dooley DG, Dougé J; Section on Adolescent Health, Council on Community Pediatrics, Committee on Adolescence. The impact of racism on child and adolescent health. *Pediatrics.* 2019;144(2):e20191765

117. Nordstrom BM. Multidisciplinary human trafficking education: Inpatient and outpatient healthcare settings. *J Human Trafficking.* 2020;8(2):184–194

118. Dols JD, Beckmann-Mendez D, McDow J, Walker K, Moon MD. Human trafficking victim identification, assessment, and intervention strategies in south Texas emergency departments. *J Emerg Nurs.* 2019;45(6):622–633

119. Macias Konstantopoulos W, Ahn R, Alpert EJ, et al. An international comparative public health analysis of sex trafficking of women and girls in eight cities: achieving a more effective health sector response. *J Urban Health.* 2013;90(6):1194–1204

120. Greenbaum VJ, Dodd M, McCracken C. A short screening tool to identify victims of child sex trafficking in the health care setting. *Pediatr Emerg Care.* 2018;34(1):33–37

121. Chang KSG, Lee K, Park T, Sy E, Quach T. Using a clinic-based screening tool for primary care providers to identify commercially sexually exploited children. *J Appl Res Child.* 2015;6(1). Available at: https://digitalcommons.library.tmc.edu/childrenatrisk/vol6/iss1/6. Accessed November 17, 2022

122. Hurst IA, Abdoo DC, Harpin S, Leonard J, Adelgais K. Confidential screening for sex trafficking among minors in a pediatric emergency department. *Pediatrics.* 2021;147(3):e2020013235

123. Chisolm-Straker M, Singer E, Rothman EF, et al. Building RAFT: trafficking screening tool derivation and validation methods. *Acad Emerg Med.* 2020;27(4):297–304

124. Greenbaum VJ, Livings MS, Lai BS, et al. Evaluation of a tool to identify child sex trafficking victims in multiple healthcare settings. *J Adolesc Health.* 2018;63(6):745–752

125. Cohen E, Mackenzie RG, Yates GL. HEADSS, a psychosocial risk assessment instrument: implications for designing effective intervention programs for runaway youth. *J Adolesc Health.* 1991;12(7):539–544

126 Sanchez M. Inside the lives of immigrant teens working dangerous night shifts in suburban factories. Available at: https://www.propublica.org/article/inside-the-lives-of-immigrant-teens-working-dangerous-night-shifts-in-suburban-factories?

token=G02S0YJIa4aG_YqTgzQclmtJNrT4JR6T. Accessed November 22, 2020

127. UNICEF. Harrowing journeys: children and youth on the move across the Mediterranean Sea, at risk of trafficking and exploitation. Available at: https://wwwuniceforg/publications/files/Harrowing_Journeys_Children_and_youth_on_the_move_across_the_Mediterraneanpdf. Accessed November 17, 2018

128. Cardoso JB, Brabeck K, Stinchcomb D, et al. Integration of unaccompanied migrant youth in the United States: a call for research. *J Ethn Migr Stud.* 2019;45(2):273–292

129. Corliss HL, Goodenow CS, Nichols L, Austin SB. High burden of homelessness among sexual-minority adolescents: findings from a representative Massachusetts high school sample. *Am J Public Health.* 2011;101(9):1683–1689

130. Futures Without Violence. *Prevent, Assess, and Respond: A Domestic Violence Toolkit for Health Centers and Domestic Violence Progams.* Washington, DC: National Health Resource Center on Domestic Violence; 2017

131. Bair-Merritt MH, Lewis-O'Connor A, Goel S, et al. Primary care-based interventions for intimate partner violence: a systematic review. *Am J Prev Med.* 2014;46(2):188–194

132. U.S. Equal Employment Opportunity Commission. Employee rights. Available at https://www.eeoc.gov/employers/small-business/employee-rights#:~:text=Employees%20have%20a%20right%20to,(including%20family%20medical%20history). Accessed March 8, 2021

133. National Child Traumatic Stress Network. The 12 core concepts: concepts for understanding traumatic stress responses in children and families. Available at: http://wwwnctsnorg/sites/default/files/assets/pdfs/ccct_12coreconceptspdf. Accessed May 17, 2020

134. Richie-Zavaleta AC, Villanueva AM, Homicile LM, Urada LA. Compassionate care: going the extra mile: sex trafficking survivors'

recommendations for healthcare best practices. *Sexes.* 2021;2(1):26–49

135. Einbond J, Diaz A, Cossette A, Scriven R, Blaustein S, Arden MR. Human trafficking in adolescents: adopting a youth-centered approach to identification and services. *Prim Care.* 2020; 47(2):307–319

136. Fukushima AI, Gonzalez-Pons K, Gezinski L, Clark L. Multiplicity of stigma: cultural barriers in anti-trafficking response. *Int J Hum Rights Healthc.* 2020;13:125–142

137. The Joint Commission. *The Joint Commission: Advancing Effective Communication, Cultural Competence, and Patient- and Family-Centered Care: A Roadmap for Hospitals.* IL, Oakbrook Terrace:The Joint Commission; 2010

138. Williams R. Cultural safety—what does it mean for our work practice? *Aust N Z J Public Health.* 1999;23(2):213–214

139. Eckermann AK, Dowd T, Chong E, et al. *Binan Goonj: Bridging Cultures in Aboriginal Health,* 3rd ed. Australia: Churchill Livingstone; 2010

140. Cross TL. Services to minority populations: what does it mean to be a culturally competent professional? *Focal Point.* 1988;2(4):1–5

141. National Committee for Quality Assurance. A practical guide to implementing the national CLAS standards: for racial, ethnic and linguistic minorities, people with disabilities and sexual and gender minorities. Available at: https://www.cms.gov/About-CMS/Agency-Information/OMH/Downloads/CLAS-Toolkit-12-7-16.pdf. Accessed on Novebmer 29, 2020

142. Engebretson J, Mahoney J, Carlson ED. Cultural competence in the era of evidence-based practice. *J Prof Nurs.* 2008;24(3):172–178

143. Bradford JB, Cahill S, Grasso C, Makadon HJ. Policy focus: how to gather data on sexual orientation and gender identity in clinical settings. Available at: https://www.lgbthealtheducation.org/wp-content/uploads/policy_brief_how_to_gather.pdf; Accessed May 1, 2020

144. Lewis-Fernández R, Aggarwal NK, Bäärnhielm S, et al. Culture and psychiatric evaluation: operationalizing cultural formulation for DSM-5. *Psychiatry.* 2014;77(2):130–154

145. Gay and Lesbian Medical Association. Guidelines for care of lesbian, gay, bisexual, and transgender patients. Available at: https://wwwrainbow welcomeorg/uploads/pdfs/GLMA%20guidelines%202006%20FINALpdf. Accessed November 27, 2019

146. Ibrahim A, Abdalla SM, Jafer M, Abdelgadir J, de Vries N. Child labor and health: a systematic literature review of the impacts of child labor on child's health in low- and middle-income countries. *J Public Health (Oxf).* 2019;41(1):18–26

147. Volgin RN, Shakespeare-Finch J, Shochet IM. Posttraumatic distress, hope, and growth in survivors of commercial sexual exploitation in Nepal. *Traumatology.* 2019;25(3): 181–188

148. Frey LM, Middleton J, Gattis MN, Fulginiti A. Suicidal ideation and behavior among youth victims of sex trafficking in Kentuckiana. *Crisis.* 2019;40(4):240–248

149. Fang S, Coverdale J, Nguyen P, Gordon M. Tattoo recognition in screening for victims of human trafficking. *J Nerv Ment Dis.* 2018;206(10):824–827

150. Levy SJL, Williams JF; Committee on Substance Use and Prevention. Substance use screening, brief intervention, and referral to treatment. *Pediatrics.* 2016;138(1):e20161211

151. Centers for Disease Control and Prevention. Guidance for the U.S. domestic medical examination for newly arriving refugees. Available at: https://www.cdc.gov/immigrantrefugeehealth/guidelines/domestic-guidelines.html. Accessed May 24, 2021

152. Guttmacher Institute. An Overview of Consent to Reproductive Health Services by Young People. 2022. Available at: https://www.guttmacher.org/state-policy/explore/overview-minors-consent-law. Accessed November 17, 2022

153. Lukefahr J, Narang S, Kellogg N. Medical Liability and Child Abuse. In: *Medicolegal Issues in Pediatrics,* 7th ed. Elk Grove Village, IL: American Academy of Pediatrics; 2012:255

154. Committee on Bioethics. Informed consent, parental permission, and assent in pediatric practice. Committee on Bioethics, American Academy of Pediatrics. *Pediatrics.* 1995;95(2): 314–317

155. Committee on Pediatric Emergency Medicine and Committee on Bioethics. Consent for emergency medical services for children and adolescents. *Pediatrics.* 2011;128(2):427–433

156. Zimmerman C, Watts C. World Health Organization ethical and safety recommendations for interviewing trafficked women. In: *Health Policy Unit.* London, UK: London School of Hygiene and Tropical Medicine; 2003

157. Kellogg ND. Medical care of the children of the night. In: Cooper SW, RJ E, Giardino AP, Kellogg ND, Vieth VI, eds. *Medical, Legal and Social Science Aspects of Child Sexual Exploitation: A Comprehensive Review of Child Pornography, Child Prostitution and Internet Crimes Against Children.* St. Louis, MO: GW Medical; 2005:349–368

158. Kellogg ND, Committee on Child Abuse and Neglect American Academy of Pediatrics. Evaluation of suspected child physical abuse. *Pediatrics.* 2007;119(6):1232–1241

159. Labbé J, Caouette G. Recent skin injuries in normal children. *Pediatrics.* 2001;108(2):271–276

160. Smith T, Chauvin-Kimoff L, Baird B, Ornstein A. The medical evaluation of prepubertal children with suspected sexual abuse. *Paediatr Child Health.* 2020;25(3):180–194

161. Chipler-Chico L. Assisting survivors of human trafficking: multicultural case studies. Available at: https://zxh3cbmyftpuploadcom/wp-content/uploads/2017/09/HTS-Assisting-Survivors-1pdf. Accessed September 26, 2020

162. Smith TD, Raman SR, Madigan S, Waldman J, Shouldice M. Anogenital findings in 3569 pediatric examinations for sexual abuse/assault. *J Pediatr Adolesc Gynecol.* 2018; 31(2):79–83

163. McCann J, Miyamoto S, Boyle C, Rogers K. Healing of hymenal injuries in prepubertal and adolescent girls: a

descriptive study. *Pediatrics.* 2007; 119(5):e1094–e1106

164. Jenny C, Crawford-Jakubiak JE; Committee on Child Abuse and Neglect; American Academy of Pediatrics. The evaluation of children in the primary care setting when sexual abuse is suspected. *Pediatrics.* 2013;132(2):e558–e567

165. Workowski KA, Bachmann LH, Chan PA, et al. Sexually transmitted infection treatment guidelines. *MMWR Recomm Rep.* 2021;70(4):1–187

166. Toney-Butler TJ, Mittel O. Human Trafficking. In: *StatPearls.* Treasure Island, FL: StatPearls Publishing; 2022

167. Gray SH, Pasternak RH, Gooding HC, et al; Society for Adolescent Health and Medicine. Recommendations for electronic health record use for delivery of adolescent health care. *J Adolesc Health.* 2014;54(4):487–490

168. Greenbaum J, McClure RC, Stare S, et al. Documenting ICD codes and other sensitive information in electronic health records: guidelines for healthcare professionals who encounter patients with a history of human trafficking or other forms of violence. Available at: https://www. icmec.org/healthportal-resources/ topic/research-and-resources- child-sexual-abuse-exploitation-and- trafficking/guidelines-protocols- for-child-sexual-abuse-exploitation- trafficking/. Accessed March 27, 2021

169. Department of Health and Human Services. Services available to victims of human trafficking: A resource guide for social service providers. Available at: https://freedomnetworkusa.org/ app/uploads/2018/11/HHS-OTIP- Services-Available-to-Victims-of- Human-Trafficking.pdf. Accessed May 1, 2021

170. Administration for Children and Families Office on Trafficking in Persons. Services available to survivors of trafficking. Available at https://www.acf.hhs.gov/otip/ victim-assistance/services-available- victims-trafficking. Accessed May 1, 2021

171. Recknor F, Gordon M, Coverdale J, Gardezi M, Nguyen PT. A descriptive study of United States-based human trafficking specialty clinics. *Psychiatr Q.* 2020;91(1):1–10

172. Chambers R. Caring for human trafficking victims: a description and rationale for the Medical Safe Haven model in family medicine residency clinics. *Int J Psychiatry Med.* 2019;54(4-5):344–351

173. Jones Day Legal Firm, HEAL Trafficking, American Hospital Association. Human trafficking and health care providers: legal requirements for reporting and education. Available at: https://www. jonesday.com/en/insights/2021/01/ human-trafficking-and-health-care- providers. Accessed on March 6, 2021

174. Shared Hope International. 2018 state report cards: protected innocence challenge. Available at: https://sharedhopeorg/what-we-do/ bring-justice/reportcards/ 2018-reportcards/. Accessed October 30, 2019

175. Dignity Health. Human trafficking response program shared learnings manual. Available at: https://www. dignityhealth.org/-/media/cm/media/ documents/Human-Trafficking/Dignity% 20Health_HTRP_SharedLearnings Manual_170512.ashx?la=en. Accessed June 16, 2019

176. McIntyre S. Under the radar: the sexual exploitation of young men- Western Canadian Edition. Available at: http://humanservices. alberta.ca/documents/child- sexual-exploitation-under-the-radar- western-canada.pdf. Accessed February 16, 2016

177. Passmore S, Hemming E, McIntosh HC, Hellman CM. The relationship between hope, meaning in work, secondary traumatic stress, and burnout among child abuse pediatric clinicians. *The Permanente Journal.* 2020;24:19.087

178. Tomlin AM, Weatherston DJ, Pavkov T. Critical components of reflective supervision: responses from expert supervisors in the field. *Infant Ment Health J.* 2014;35(1):70–80

179. Greenbaum VJ, Titchen K, Walker- Descartes I, Feifer A, Rood CJ, Fong HF. Multi-level prevention of human trafficking: the role of health care professionals. *Prev Med.* 2018; 114:164–167

180. Greenbaum J, Bodrick N; Committee on Child Abuse and Neglect, Section on International Child Health. Global human trafficking and child victimization. *Pediatrics.* 2017;140(6):e20173138

181. Bigelsen J, Vuotto S. Homelessness, survival sex and human trafficking: as experienced by the youth of Covenant House New York. Available at: https:// humantraffickinghotlineorg/sites/default/ files/Homelessness%2C%20Survival% 20Sex%2C%20and%20Human% 20Trafficking%20-%20Covenant%20House %20NYpdf. Accessed August 28, 2021. 2013

182. Fedina L, Williamson C, Perdue T. Risk factors for domestic child sex trafficking in the United States. *J Interpers Violence.* 2019;34(13): 2653–2673

183. Cole J, Sprang G. Sex trafficking of minors in metropolitan, micropolitan, and rural communities. *Child Abuse Negl.* 2015;40:113–123

184. Panlilio CC, Miyamoto S, Font SA, Schreier HMC. Assessing risk of commercial sexual exploitation among children involved in the child welfare system. *Child Abuse Negl.* 2019;87:88–99

185. Reid JA. Sex trafficking of girls with intellectual disabilities: an exploratory mixed methods study. *Sex Abuse.* 2018;30(2):107–131

186. Carey C, Peterson S. Trafficking people with disabilities: a legal analysis. *Cardozo J Equal Rts & Soc Just.* 2019;26:471–497

187. Shared Hope International. *Domestic Minor Sex Trafficking: Intervene: Resource Package.* Vancouver, Washington: Shared Hope International; 2013

188. United Nations Office on Drugs and Crime. *Global Report on Trafficking in Persons.* Vienna, Austria: United Nations;2018

189. Lewis H, Waite L. Asylum, immigration restrictions and exploitation: hyper-precarity as a lens for understanding and tackling forced labour. *Anti-Trafficking Review.* 2015;5:49-67. Available at: https://www. antitraffickingreview.org/index.php/ atrjournal/article/view/83. Accessed November 17, 2022

190. Kiss L, Pocock NS, Naisanguansri V, et al. Health of men, women, and children in post-trafficking services in Cambodia, Thailand, and Vietnam: an observational cross-sectional study. *Lancet Glob Health.* 2015;3(3): e154–e161

191. Pocock NS, Nguyen LH, Lucero-Prisno Iii DE, Zimmerman C, Oram S. Occupational, physical, sexual and mental health and violence among migrant and trafficked commercial fishers and seafarers from the Greater Mekong Subregion (GMS): systematic review. *Glob Health Res Policy.* 2018;3:28

192. Moore J, Fitzgerald M, Owens T, Slingsby B, Barron C, Goldberg A. Domestic minor sex trafficking: a case series of male pediatric patients. *J Interpers Violence.* 2020;36 (23-24):886260519900323

193. Moore JL, Goldberg AP, Barron C. Substance use in a domestic minor sex trafficking patient population. *Pediatr Emerg Care.* 2021;37(4): e159–e162

194. Varma S, Gillespie S, McCracken C, Greenbaum VJ. Characteristics of child commercial sexual exploitation and sex trafficking victims presenting for medical care in the United States. *Child Abuse Negl.* 2015;44:98–105

195. Jones A. Malnutrition, poverty, and climate change are also human rights issues in child labor. *Health Hum Rights.* 2018;20(2):249–251

196. International Labour Organization. The psychological health of children working in brick kilns: a classification tree analysis. Available at: https:// wwwiloorg/wcmsp5/groups/public/ —ed_norm/—ipec/documents/ publication/wcms_672539pdf. Accessed December 17, 2019

197. Iglesias-Rios L, Harlow SD, Burgard SA, Kiss L, Zimmerman C. Mental health, violence and psychological coercion among female and male trafficking survivors in the greater Mekong sub-region: a cross-sectional study. *BMC Psychol.* 2018;6(1):56

198. Lazarus L, Deering KN, Nabess R, Gibson K, Tyndall MW, Shannon K. Occupational stigma as a primary barrier to health care for street-based sex workers in Canada. *Cult Health Sex.* 2012;14(2): 139–150

199. Chung RC. Cultural perspectives on child trafficking, human rights and social justice: a model for psychologists. *Couns Psychol Q.* 2009;22(1):85–96

200. Hofstede G. Dimsensionalizing cultures: the Hofsteded model in context. *Online Read Psychol Cult.* 2011;2(1)

201. Meyer E. *The Culture Map: Breaking Through the Invisible Boundaries of Global Business.* New York: Public Affairs; 2014

CLINICAL REPORT Guidance for the Clinician in Rendering Pediatric Care

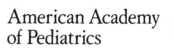

American Academy
of Pediatrics

DEDICATED TO THE HEALTH OF ALL CHILDREN™

Runaway Youth: Caring for the Nation's Largest Segment of Missing Children

Thresia B. Gambon, MD, MPH, MBA, FAAP,[a] Janna R. Gewirtz O'Brien, MD, FAAP,[b] COMMITTEE ON PSYCHOSOCIAL ASPECTS OF CHILD AND FAMILY HEALTH, COUNCIL ON COMMUNITY PEDIATRICS

abstract

The largest segment of missing children in the United States includes runaways, children who run away from home, and thrownaways, children who are told to leave or stay away from home by a household adult. Although estimates vary, as many as 1 in 20 youth run away from home annually. These unaccompanied youth have unique health needs, including high rates of trauma, mental illness, substance use, pregnancy, and sexually transmitted infections. While away, youth who run away are at high risk for additional trauma, victimization, and violence. Runaway and thrownaway youth have high unmet health care needs and limited access to care. Several populations are at particular high risk for runaway episodes, including victims of abuse and neglect; lesbian, gay, bisexual, transgender, and questioning youth; and youth in protective custody. Pediatricians and other health care professionals have a critical role to play in supporting runaway youth, addressing their unique health needs, fostering positive relationships within their families and with other supportive adults, and connecting them with available community resources. This report provides clinical guidance for pediatricians and other health care professionals regarding (1) the identification of adolescents who are at risk for running away or being thrown away and (2) the management of the unique medical, mental health, and social needs of these youth. In partnership with national, state, and local resources, pediatricians can significantly reduce risk and improve long-term outcomes for runaway youth.

[a]Citrus Health Network, Miami, Florida; and [b]Department of Pediatrics, University of Minnesota, Minneapolis, Minnesota

Clinical reports from the American Academy of Pediatrics benefit from expertise and resources of liaisons and internal (AAP) and external reviewers. However, clinical reports from the American Academy of Pediatrics may not reflect the views of the liaisons or the organizations or government agencies that they represent.

Drs Gambon and Gewirtz O'Brien drafted, reviewed, and revised the manuscript, approved the final manuscript as submitted, and agree to be accountable for all aspects of the work.

The guidance in this report does not indicate an exclusive course of treatment or serve as a standard of medical care. Variations, taking into account individual circumstances, may be appropriate.

All clinical reports from the American Academy of Pediatrics automatically expire 5 years after publication unless reaffirmed, revised, or retired at or before that time.

DOI: https://doi.org/10.1542/peds.2019-3752

Address correspondence to Thresia B. Gambon. E-mail: tbgambon@me.com

PEDIATRICS (ISSN Numbers: Print, 0031-4005; Online, 1098-4275).

Copyright © 2020 by the American Academy of Pediatrics

FINANCIAL DISCLOSURE: The authors have indicated they have no financial relationships relevant to this article to disclose.

To cite: Gambon TB, Gewirtz O'Brien JR, AAP COMMITTEE ON PSYCHOSOCIAL ASPECTS OF CHILD AND FAMILY HEALTH, COUNCIL ON COMMUNITY PEDIATRICS. Runaway Youth: Caring for the Nation's Largest Segment of Missing Children. *Pediatrics.* 2020;145(2):e20193752

INTRODUCTION

The largest segment of missing children in the United States includes runaways, children who run away from home, and thrownaways, children who are told to leave or stay away from home by a household adult.[1,2] This report aims to provide clinical guidance for pediatricians regarding (1) the identification of adolescents who are at risk for running away or being thrown away and (2) the management of the unique medical, mental health, and social needs of these youth.

American Academy
of Pediatrics

DEDICATED TO THE HEALTH OF ALL CHILDREN™

This Clinical Report was reaffirmed October 2020.

Child Sex Trafficking and Commercial Sexual Exploitation: Health Care Needs of Victims

Jordan Greenbaum, MD, James E. Crawford-Jakubiak, MD, FAAP, COMMITTEE ON CHILD ABUSE AND NEGLECT

abstract

Child sex trafficking and commercial sexual exploitation of children (CSEC) are major public health problems in the United States and throughout the world. Despite large numbers of American and foreign youth affected and a plethora of serious physical and mental health problems associated with CSEC, there is limited information available to pediatricians regarding the nature and scope of human trafficking and how pediatricians and other health care providers may help protect children. Knowledge of risk factors, recruitment practices, possible indicators of CSEC, and common medical and behavioral health problems experienced by victims will help pediatricians recognize potential victims and respond appropriately. As health care providers, educators, and leaders in child advocacy, pediatricians play an essential role in addressing the public health issues faced by child victims of CSEC. Their roles can include working to increase recognition of CSEC, providing direct care and anticipatory guidance related to CSEC, engaging in collaborative efforts with medical and nonmedical colleagues to provide for the complex needs of youth, and educating child-serving professionals and the public.

www.pediatrics.org/cgi/doi/10.1542/peds.2014-4138

DOI: 10.1542/peds.2014-4138

PEDIATRICS (ISSN Numbers: Print, 0031-4005; Online, 1098-4275).

INTRODUCTION

Human trafficking is a major global health and human rights problem, with reported victims in at least 152 countries.[1] The total number of victims is unknown, although estimates range into the millions.[2] Women and children predominate: in 1 global study, up to 49% of the victims were women and 33% were children.[3] Violence and psychological manipulation are common, and victims are at increased risk of injury, sexual assault, infectious diseases, substance misuse, untreated chronic medical conditions, malnutrition, post-traumatic stress disorder (PTSD), major depression and other mental health disorders, homicide, and suicide.[4–9] Given the large number of children and youth involved and the numerous adverse effects on the victim's physical and mental health, medical providers are in a unique position to help potential victims.[10]

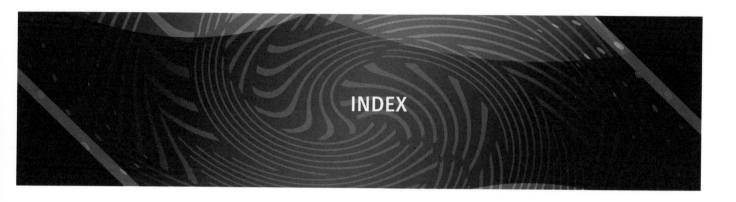

INDEX

Page numbers followed by *f* indicate a figure and by *t*, a table.

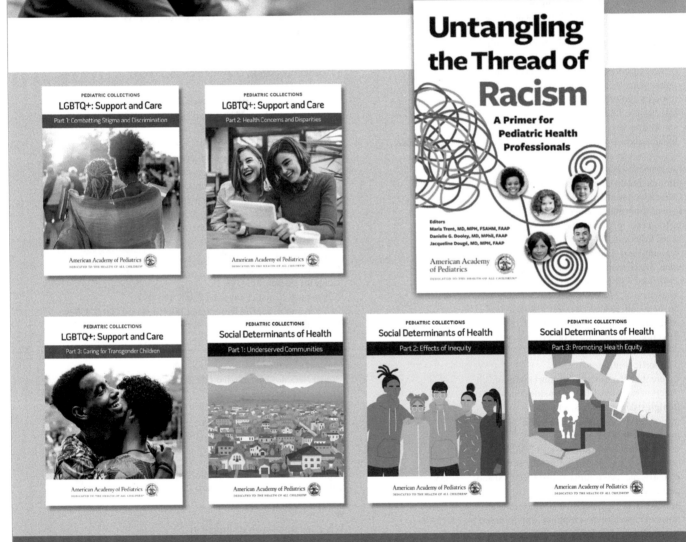
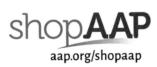